# Lecture Notes in Artificial Intelligence   8856

## Subseries of Lecture Notes in Computer Science

### LNAI Series Editors

Randy Goebel
  *University of Alberta, Edmonton, Canada*
Yuzuru Tanaka
  *Hokkaido University, Sapporo, Japan*
Wolfgang Wahlster
  *DFKI and Saarland University, Saarbrücken, Germany*

### LNAI Founding Series Editor

Joerg Siekmann
  *DFKI and Saarland University, Saarbrücken, Germany*

Alexander Gelbukh
Félix Castro Espinoza
Sofía N. Galicia-Haro (Eds.)

# Human-Inspired Computing and Its Applications

13th Mexican International Conference
on Artificial Intelligence, MICAI 2014
Tuxtla Gutiérrez, Mexico, November 16-22, 2014
Proceedings, Part I

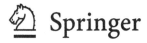 Springer

Volume Editors

Alexander Gelbukh
Centro de Investigación en Computación
Instituto Politécnico Nacional
Mexico City, Mexico
E-mail: gelbukh@gelbukh.com

Félix Castro Espinoza
Universidad Autónoma del Estado de Hidalgo
Área Académica de Computación y Electrónica
Hidalgo, Mexico
E-mail: fcastroe@gmail.com

Sofía N. Galicia-Haro
Universidad Autónoma Nacional de México
Facultad de Ciencias
Mexico City, Mexico
E-mail: sngh@fciencias.unam.mx

ISSN 0302-9743                           e-ISSN 1611-3349
ISBN 978-3-319-13646-2                   e-ISBN 978-3-319-13647-9
DOI 10.1007/978-3-319-13647-9
Springer Cham Heidelberg New York Dordrecht London

Library of Congress Control Number: 2014955199

LNCS Sublibrary: SL 7 – Artificial Intelligence

*Typesetting:* Camera-ready by author, data conversion by Scientific Publishing Services, Chennai, India

Printed on acid-free paper

Springer is part of Springer Science+Business Media (www.springer.com)

# Preface

The Mexican International Conference on Artificial Intelligence (MICAI) is a yearly international conference series organized by the Mexican Society of Artificial Intelligence (SMIA) since 2000. MICAI is a major international artificial intelligence forum and the main event in the academic life of the country's growing artificial intelligence community.

MICAI conferences publish high-quality papers in all areas of artificial intelligence and its applications. The proceedings of the previous MICAI events have been published by Springer in its *Lecture Notes in Artificial Intelligence* series, vols. 1793, 2313, 2972, 3789, 4293, 4827, 5317, 5845, 6437, 6438, 7094, 7095, 7629, 7630, 8265, and 8266. Since its foundation in 2000, the conference has been growing in popularity and improving in quality.

According to two main areas of artificial intelligence—modeling human mental abilities on the one hand and optimization and classification on the other hand—the proceedings of MICAI 2014 have been published in two volumes. The first volume, *Human-Inspired Computing and Its Applications*, contains 44 papers structured into seven sections:

- Natural Language Processing
- Natural Language Processing Applications
- Opinion Mining, Sentiment Analysis, and Social Network Applications
- Computer Vision
- Image Processing
- Logic, Reasoning, and Multi-agent Systems
- Intelligent Tutoring Systems

The second volume, *Nature-Inspired Computation and Machine Learning*, contains 44 papers structured into eight sections:

- Genetic and Evolutionary Algorithms
- Neural Networks
- Machine Learning
- Machine Learning Applications to Audio and Text
- Data Mining
- Fuzzy Logic
- Robotics, Planning, and Scheduling
- Biomedical Applications

This two-volume set will be of interest to researchers in all areas of artificial intelligence, students specializing in related topics, and to the general public interested in recent developments in artificial intelligence.

The conference received for evaluation 350 submissions by 823 authors from a record high number of 46 countries: Algeria, Argentina, Australia, Austria,

Brazil, Bulgaria, Canada, Chile, China, Colombia, Cuba, Czech Republic, Ecuador, Egypt, France, Germany, India, Iran, Ireland, Israel, Italy, Jordan, Kazakhstan, Lithuania, Malaysia, Mexico, Morocco, Nepal, Norway, Pakistan, Panama, Paraguay, Peru, Poland, Portugal, Russia, Singapore, Slovakia, South Africa, Spain, Sweden, Turkey, UK, Ukraine, USA, and Virgin Islands (USA); the distribution of papers by tracks is shown in Table 1. Of these submissions, 87 papers were selected for publication in these two volumes after a peer-reviewing process carried out by the international Program Committee. The acceptance rate was 24.8%.

In addition to regular papers, the second volume contains an invited paper by Oscar Castillo, Patricia Melin, and Fevrier Valdez: "Nature-Inspired Optimization of Type-2 Fuzzy Systems."

The international Program Committee consisted of 201 experts from 34 countries: Australia, Austria, Azerbaijan, Belgium, Brazil, Canada, China, Colombia, Czech Republic, Denmark, Finland, France, Germany, Greece, India, Israel, Italy, Japan, Mexico, The Netherlands, New Zealand, Norway, Poland, Portugal, Russia, Singapore, Slovenia, Spain, Sweden, Switzerland, Tunisia, Turkey, UK, and USA.

**Table 1.** Distribution of papers by tracks

| Track | Submissions | Accepted | Rate |
|---|---|---|---|
| Natural Language Processing | 59 | 19 | 32% |
| Machine Learning and Pattern Recognition | 42 | 12 | 29% |
| Logic, Knowledge-Based Systems, Multi-Agent Systems and Distributed AI | 40 | 8 | 20% |
| Computer Vision and Image Processing | 38 | 13 | 34% |
| Evolutionary and Nature-Inspired Metaheuristic Algorithms | 33 | 6 | 18% |
| Data Mining | 29 | 7 | 24% |
| Neural Networks and Hybrid Intelligent Systems | 28 | 7 | 25% |
| Robotics, Planning and Scheduling | 24 | 5 | 21% |
| Fuzzy Systems and Probabilistic Models in Decision Making | 23 | 4 | 17% |
| Bioinformatics and Medical Applications | 18 | 3 | 17% |
| Intelligent Tutoring Systems | 16 | 3 | 19% |

MICAI 2014 was honored by the presence of such renowned experts as Hojjat Adeli of The Ohio State University, USA, Oscar Castillo of Instituto Tecnológico de Tijuana, Mexico, Bonnie E. John of IBM T.J. Watson Research Center, USA, Bing Liu of the University of Illinois, USA, John Sowa of VivoMind Research, USA, and Vladimir Vapnik of the NEC Laboratories, USA, who gave excellent keynote lectures. The technical program of the conference also featured tutorials presented by Roman Bartak of Charles University, Czech Republic; Oscar Castillo of Tijuana Institute of Technology, Mexico; Héctor G. Ceballos of Clark & Parsia LLC, USA, and Héctor Pérez Urbina of Tecnológico de Monterrey, Mexico; Sanjoy Das of Kansas State University, USA; Alexander Gelbukh of

Instituto Politécnico Nacional, Mexico; Bonnie E. John of IBM T. J. Watson Research Center, USA; Bing Liu of University of Illinois, USA; Raúl Monroy of Tecnológico de Monterrey, Mexico; John Sowa of VivoMind Research, USA; and Luis Martín Torres Treviño of Universidad Autónoma de Nuevo León, Mexico, among others. Three workshops were held jointly with the conference: the 7th International Workshop on Hybrid Intelligent Systems, HIS 2014; the 7th International Workshop on Intelligent Learning Environments, WILE 2014, and the First International Workshop on Recognizing Textual Entailment and Question Answering, RTE-QA 2014.

The authors of the following papers received the Best Paper Award on the basis of the paper's overall quality, significance, and originality of the reported results:

1st place: "The Best Neural Network Architecture," by Angel Kuri-Morales (Mexico)

2nd place: "Multisensor-Based Obstacles Detection in Challenging Scenes," by Yong Fang, Cindy Cappelle, and Yassine Ruichek (France)

"Intelligent Control of Induction Motor-Based Comparative Study: Analysis of Two Topologies," by Moulay Rachid Douiri, El Batoul Mabrouki, Ouissam Belghazi, Mohamed Ferfra, and Mohamed Cherkaoui (Morocco)

3rd place: "A Fast Scheduling Algorithm for Detection and Localization of Hidden Objects Based on Data Gathering in Wireless Sensor Networks," by Eugene Levner, Boris Kriheli, Amir Elalouf, and Dmitry Tsadikovich (Israel)

The authors of the following papers selected among all papers of which the first author was a full-time student, excluding the papers listed above, received the Best Student Paper Award:

1st place: "Solving Binary Cutting Stock with Matheuristics," by Ivan Adrian Lopez Sanchez, Jaime Mora Vargas, Cipriano A. Santos, and Miguel Gonzalez Mendoza (Mexico)

"Novel Unsupervised Features for Czech Multi-label Document Classification," by Tomáš Brychcín and Pavel Král (Czech Republic)

We want to thank everyone involved in the organization of this conference. In the first place, these are the authors of the papers published in this book: It is their research work that gives value to the book and to the work of the organizers. We thank the track chairs for their hard work, the Program Committee members, and additional reviewers for their great effort spent on reviewing the submissions.

We are grateful to the Dean of the Instituto Tecnológico de Tuxtla Gutiérrez (ITTG), M.E.H. José Luis Méndez Navarro, the Dean of the Universidad Autónoma de Chiapas (UNACH), Professor Jaime Valls Esponda, and M.C. Francisco de Jesús Suárez Ruiz, Head of IT Department, for their instrumental support of MICAI and for providing the infrastructure for the keynote talks, tutorials, and workshops, and to all professors of the Engineering School of Computational Systems for their warm hospitality and hard work, as well as for their active participation in the organization of this conference. We greatly appreciate the generous sponsorship provided by the Government of Chiapas via the Conventions and Visitors Office (OCV).

We are deeply grateful to the conference staff and to all members of the Local Committee headed by Imelda Valles López. We gratefully acknowledge support received from the project WIQ-EI (Web Information Quality Evaluation Initiative, European project 269180). The entire submission, reviewing, and selection process, as well as preparation of the proceedings, was supported for free by the EasyChair system (www.easychair.org). Finally, yet importantly, we are very grateful to the staff at Springer for their patience and help in the preparation of this volume.

October 2014                                                        Alexander Gelbukh
Félix Castro Espinoza
Sofía N. Galicia-Haro

# Conference Organization

MICAI 2014 was organized by the Mexican Society of Artificial Intelligence (SMIA, Sociedad Mexicana de Inteligencia Artificial) in collaboration with the Instituto Tecnológico de Tuxtla Gutiérrez (ITTG), the Universidad Autónoma de Chiapas (UNACH), the Centro de Investigación en Computación del Instituto Politécnico Nacional (CIC-IPN), the Universidad Autónoma del Estado de Hidalgo (UAEH), and the Universidad Nacional Autónoma de México (UNAM).

The MICAI series website is www.MICAI.org. The website of the Mexican Society of Artificial Intelligence, SMIA, is www.SMIA.org.mx. Contact options and additional information can be found on these websites.

## Conference Committee

### General Chairs

| | |
|---|---|
| Alexander Gelbukh | Instituto Politécnico Nacional, Mexico |
| Grigori Sidorov | Instituto Politécnico Nacional, Mexico |

### Program Chairs

| | |
|---|---|
| Alexander Gelbukh | Instituto Politécnico Nacional, Mexico |
| Félix Castro Espinoza | Universidad Autónoma del Estado de Hidalgo, Mexico |
| Sofía N. Galicia Haro | Universidad Autónoma Nacional de México, Mexico |

### Workshop Chairs

| | |
|---|---|
| Obdulia Pichardo Lagunas | Instituto Politécnico Nacional, Mexico |
| Noé Alejandro Castro Sánchez | Centro Nacional de Investigación y Desarrollo Tecnológico, Mexico |

### Tutorials Chair

| | |
|---|---|
| Félix Castro Espinoza | Universidad Autónoma del Estado de Hidalgo, Mexico |

### Doctoral Consortium Chairs

| | |
|---|---|
| Miguel Gonzalez Mendoza | Tecnológico de Monterrey CEM, Mexico |
| Antonio Marín Hernandez | Universidad Veracruzana, Mexico |

### Keynote Talks Chair

| | |
|---|---|
| Sabino Miranda Jiménez | INFOTEC, Mexico |

**Publication Chair**

Miguel Gonzalez Mendoza    Tecnológico de Monterrey CEM, Mexico

**Financial Chair**

Ildar Batyrshin    Instituto Politécnico Nacional, Mexico

**Grant Chairs**

Grigori Sidorov    Instituto Politécnico Nacional, Mexico
Miguel Gonzalez Mendoza    Tecnológico de Monterrey CEM, Mexico

**Organizing Committee Chair**

Imelda Valles López    Instituto Tecnológico de Tuxtla Gutiérrez,
                       Mexico

## Track Chairs

**Natural Language Processing**

Grigori Sidorov    Instituto Politécnico Nacional, Mexico

**Machine Learning and Pattern Recognition**

Alexander Gelbukh    Instituto Politécnico Nacional, Mexico

**Data Mining**

Miguel Gonzalez-Mendoza    Tecnológico de Monterrey CEM, Mexico
Félix Castro Espinoza      Universidad Autónoma del Estado de Hidalgo,
                          Mexico

**Intelligent Tutoring Systems**

Alexander Gelbukh    Instituto Politécnico Nacional, Mexico

**Evolutionary and Nature-Inspired Metaheuristic Algorithms**

Oliver Schütze      CINVESTAV, Mexico
Jaime Mora Vargas   Tecnológico de Monterrey CEM, Mexico

**Computer Vision and Image Processing**

Oscar Herrera Alcántara    Universidad Autónoma Metropolitana
                          Azcapotzalco, Mexico

## Robotics, Planning and Scheduling

Fernando Martin
  Montes-Gonzalez                Universidad Veracruzana, Mexico

## Neural Networks and Hybrid Intelligent Systems

Sergio Ledesma-Orozco           Universidad de Guanajuato, Mexico

## Logic, Knowledge-Based Systems, Multi-Agent Systems and Distributed AI

Mauricio Osorio                 Universidad de las Américas, Mexico
Jose Raymundo                   Universidad Autónoma del Estado de México,
  Marcial Romero                Mexico

## Fuzzy Systems and Probabilistic Models in Decision Making

Ildar Batyrshin                 Instituto Politécnico Nacional, Mexico

## Bioinformatics and Medical Applications

Jesus A. Gonzalez               Instituto Nacional de Astrofísica, Óptica y
                                  Electrónica, Mexico
Felipe Orihuela-Espina          Instituto Nacional de Astrofísica, Óptica y
                                  Electrónica, Mexico

## Program Committee

Juan C. Acosta-Guadarrama       Universidad Autónoma del Estado de México,
                                  Mexico
Teresa Alarcón                  Universidad de Guadalajara, Mexico
Fernando Aldana                 Universidad Veracruzana, Mexico
Guillem Alenya                  IRI (CSIC-UPC), Spain
Adel Alimi                      University of Sfax, Tunisia
Jesus Angulo                    Ecole des Mines de Paris, France
Marianna Apidianaki             LIMSI-CNRS, France
Alfredo Arias-Montaño           Instituto Politécnico Nacional, Mexico
Jose Arrazola                   Universidad Autónoma de Puebla, Mexico
Gustavo Arroyo                  Instituto de Investigaciones Eléctricas, Mexico
Victor Ayala-Ramirez            Universidad de Guanajuato, Mexico
Alexandra Balahur               European Commission Joint Research Centre,
                                  Italy
Sivaji Bandyopadhyay            Jadavpur University, India
Maria Lucia Barrón-Estrada      Instituto Tecnológico de Culiacán, Mexico
Ildar Batyrshin                 Instituto Politécnico Nacional, Mexico
Anastasios Bezerianos           University of Patras, Greece

| | |
|---|---|
| Albert Bifet | University of Waikato, New Zealand |
| Eduardo Cabal-Yepez | Universidad de Guanajuato, Mexico |
| Felix Calderon | Universidad Michoacana de San Nicolás de Hidalgo, Mexico |
| Hiram Calvo | Instituto Politécnico Nacional, Mexico |
| Nicoletta Calzolari | Istituto di Linguistica Computazionale - CNR, Italy |
| Erik Cambria | Nanyang Technological University, Singapore |
| Jose Luis Carballido | Benemérita Universidad Autónoma de Puebla, Mexico |
| Michael Carl | Copenhagen Business School, Denmark |
| Heydy Castillejos | Universidad Autónoma del Estado de Hidalgo, Mexico |
| Oscar Castillo | Instituto Tecnológico de Tijuana, Mexico |
| Felix Castro Espinoza | Universidad Autónoma del Estado de Hidalgo, Mexico |
| Noé Alejandro Castro-Sánchez | Centro Nacional de Investigación y Desarrollo Tecnológico, Mexico |
| Gustavo Cerda-Villafana | Universidad de Guanajuato, Mexico |
| Stefano A. Cerri | University of Montpellier and CNRS, France |
| Niladri Chatterjee | Indian Institute of Technology Delhi, India |
| David Claudio Gonzalez | Universidad de Guanajuato, Mexico |
| Stefania Costantini | Università degli Studi dell'Aquila, Italy |
| Heriberto Cuayahuitl | Heriot-Watt University, UK |
| Erik Cuevas | Universidad de Guadalajara, Mexico |
| Iria Da Cunha | Universitat Pompeu Fabra, Spain |
| Oscar Dalmau | Centro de Investigación en Matemáticas, Mexico |
| Guillermo De Ita | Universidad Autónoma de Puebla, Mexico |
| Maria De Marsico | University of Rome La Sapienza, Italy |
| Vania Dimitrova | University of Leeds, UK |
| Asif Ekbal | Indian Institute of Technology Patna, India |
| Michael T.M. Emmerich | Leiden University, The Netherlands |
| Hugo Jair Escalante | Instituto Nacional de Astrofísica, Óptica y Electrónica, Mexico |
| Ponciano Jorge Escamilla-Ambrosio | Instituto Nacional de Astrofísica, Óptica y Electrónica, Mexico |
| Vlad Estivill-Castro | Griffith University, Australia |
| Gibran Etcheverry | Universidad de Sonora, Mexico |
| Denis Filatov | Instituto Politécnico Nacional, Mexico |
| Juan J. Flores | Universidad Michoacana de San Nicolás de Hidalgo, Mexico |
| Pedro Flores | Universidad de Sonora, Mexico |
| Andrea Formisano | Università di Perugia, Italy |

| | |
|---|---|
| Anilu Franco-Arcega | Instituto Nacional de Astrofísica, Óptica y Electrónica, Mexico |
| Claude Frasson | University of Montreal, Canada |
| Alfredo Gabaldon | Carnegie Mellon University, USA |
| Sofia N. Galicia-Haro | Universidad Nacional Autónoma de México, Mexico |
| Ana Gabriela Gallardo-Hernández | Universidad Nacional Autónoma de México, Mexico |
| Carlos Garcia-Capulin | Instituto Tecnológico Superior de Irapuato, Mexico |
| Ma. de Guadalupe Garcia-Hernandez | Universidad de Guanajuato, Mexico |
| Arturo Garcia-Perez | Universidad de Guanajuato, Mexico |
| Alexander Gelbukh | Instituto Politécnico Nacional, Mexico |
| Onofrio Gigliotta | University of Naples Federico II, Italy |
| Roxana Girju | University of Illinois at Urbana-Champaign, USA |
| Eduardo Gomez-Ramirez | Universidad La Salle, Mexico |
| Arturo Gonzalez | Universidad de Guanajuato, Mexico |
| Miguel Gonzalez-Mendoza | Tecnológico de Monterrey CEM, Mexico |
| Felix F. Gonzalez-Navarro | Universidad Autónoma de Baja California, Mexico |
| Efren Gorrostieta | Universidad Autónoma de Querétaro, Mexico |
| Carlos Arturo Gracios-Marin | CERN, Switzerland |
| Joaquin Gutierrez | Centro de Investigaciones Biológicas del Noroeste S.C., Mexico |
| Yasunari Harada | Waseda University, Japan |
| Mark Hasegawa-Johnson | University of Illinois at Urbana-Champaign, USA |
| Rogelio Hasimoto | Centro de Investigación en Matemáticas, Mexico |
| Antonio Hernandez | Instituto Politécnico Nacional, Mexico |
| Oscar Herrera | Universidad Autónoma Metropolitana Azcapotzalco, Mexico |
| Dieter Hutter | DFKI GmbH, Germany |
| Pablo H. Ibarguengoytia | Instituto de Investigaciones Eléctricas, Mexico |
| Rodolfo Ibarra | Tecnológico de Monterrey, Mexico |
| Oscar G. Ibarra-Manzano | Universidad de Guanajuato, Mexico |
| Diana Inkpen | University of Ottawa, Canada |
| Héctor Jiménez Salazar | Universidad Autónoma Metropolitana, Mexico |
| Laetitia Jourdan | Inria/LIFL/CNRS, France |
| Pinar Karagoz | Middle East Technical University, Turkey |
| Olga Kolesnikova | Instituto Politécnico Nacional, Mexico |
| Valia Kordoni | Humboldt University Berlin, Germany |

| | |
|---|---|
| Konstantinos Koutroumbas | National Observatory of Athens, Greece |
| Vladik Kreinovich | University of Texas at El Paso, USA |
| Angel Kuri-Morales | Instituto Tecnológico Autónomo de México, Mexico |
| Mathieu Lafourcade | Le Laboratoire d'Informatique, de Robotique et de Microélectronique de Montpellier (UM2/CNRS), France |
| Ricardo Landa | CINVESTAV Tamaulipas, Mexico |
| Dario Landa-Silva | University of Nottingham, UK |
| Bruno Lara | Universidad Autónoma del Estado de Morelos, Mexico |
| Yulia Ledeneva | Universidad Autónoma del Estado de México, Mexico |
| Sergio Ledesma | Universidad de Guanajuato, Mexico |
| Yoel Ledo Mezquita | Universidad de las Américas, Mexico |
| Eugene Levner | Ashkelon Academic College, Israel |
| Aristidis Likas | University of Ioannina, Greece |
| Rocio Lizarraga-Morales | Universidad de Guanajuato, Mexico |
| Aurelio Lopez | Instituto Nacional de Astrofísica, Óptica y Electrónica, Mexico |
| Virgilio Lopez-Morales | Universidad Autónoma del Estado de Hidalgo, Mexico |
| Omar López-Ortega | Universidad Autónoma del Estado de Hidalgo, Mexico |
| Tanja Magoc | University of Texas at El Paso, USA |
| Stephane Marchand-Maillet | University of Geneva, Switzerland |
| J. Raymundo Marcial-Romero | Universidad Autónoma del Estado de México, Mexico |
| Ricardo Martinez | Instituto Tecnológico de Tijuana, Mexico |
| Luis Martí | Pontifícia Universidade Católica do Rio de Janeiro, Brazil |
| Lourdes Martínez | Tecnológico de Monterrey CEM, Mexico |
| Francisco Martínez-Álvarez | Universidad Pablo de Olavide, Spain |
| María Auxilio Medina Nieto | Universidad Politécnica de Puebla, Mexico |
| R. Carolina Medina-Ramirez | Universidad Autónoma Metropolitana Iztapalapa, Mexico |
| Patricia Melin | Instituto Tecnológico de Tijuana, Mexico |
| Ivan Vladimir Meza Ruiz | Universidad Nacional Autónoma de México, Mexico |
| Efrén Mezura-Montes | Universidad Veracruzana, Mexico |
| Mikhail Mikhailov | University of Tampere, Finland |
| Sabino Miranda | INFOTEC, Mexico |
| Dieter Mitsche | Universitat Politècnica de Catalunya, Spain |

| | |
|---|---|
| Dunja Mladenic | Jozef Stefan Institute, Slovenia |
| Raul Monroy | Tecnologico de Monterrey CEM, Mexico |
| Manuel Montes-y-Gómez | Instituto Nacional de Astrofísica, Óptica y Electrónica, Mexico |
| Carlos Montoro | Universidad de Guanajuato, Mexico |
| Jaime Mora-Vargas | Tecnológico de Monterrey CEM, Mexico |
| Guillermo Morales-Luna | CINVESTAV, Mexico |
| Masaki Murata | Tottori University, Japan |
| Victor Muñiz | Centro de Investigación en Matemáticas, Mexico |
| Michele Nappi | Dipartimento di Matematica e Informatica, Italy |
| Jesús Emeterio Navarro-Barrientos | Society for the Promotion of Applied Computer Science (GFaI e.V.), Germany |
| Juan Carlos Nieves | Umeå University, Sweden |
| Roger Nkambou | Université du Québec à Montréal, Canada |
| Juan Arturo Nolazco Flores | Tecnológico de Monterrey CM, Mexico |
| Leszek Nowak | Jagiellonian University, Poland |
| C. Alberto Ochoa-Zezatti | Universidad Autónoma de Ciudad Juárez, Mexico |
| Ivan Olmos | Benemérita Universidad Autónoma de Puebla, Mexico |
| Sonia Ordoñez | Universidad Distrital Francisco Jose de Caldas, Colombia |
| Felipe Orihuela-Espina | Instituto Nacional de Astrofísica, Óptica y Electrónica, Mexico |
| Eber Enrique Orozco Guillén | Universidad Politécnica de Sinaloa, Mexico |
| Magdalena Ortiz | Vienna University of Technology, Austria |
| Mauricio Osorio | Universidad de Las Américas, Mexico |
| Ekaterina Ovchinnikova | Information Sciences Institute, University of Southern California, USA |
| Partha Pakray | Norwegian University of Science and Technology, Norway |
| Ivandre Paraboni | University of Sao Paulo, Brazil |
| Mario Pavone | University of Catania, Italy |
| Ted Pedersen | University of Minnesota Duluth, USA |
| Obdulia Pichardo | Instituto Politécnico Nacional, Mexico |
| David Pinto | Benemérita Universidad Autónoma de Puebla, Mexico |
| Volodymyr Ponomaryov | Instituto Politécnico Nacional, Mexico |
| Héctor Pérez-Urbina | Clark & Parsia, LLC, USA |
| Marta R. Costa-Jussà | Institute For Infocomm Research, Singapore |
| Risto Fermin Rangel Kuoppa | Universidad Autónoma Metropolitana Azcapotzalco, Mexico |

| | |
|---|---|
| Ivan Razo | Université libre de Bruxelles, Belgium |
| Alberto Reyes | Instituto de Investigaciones Eléctricas, Mexico |
| Orion Reyes | University of Alberta Edmonton AB, Canada |
| Bernardete Ribeiro | University of Coimbra, Portugal |
| Alessandro Ricci | University of Bologna, Italy |
| Erik Rodner | Friedrich Schiller University of Jena, Germany |
| Arles Rodriguez | Universidad Nacional de Colombia, Colombia |
| Eduardo Rodriguez-Tello | CINVESTAV Tamaulipas, Mexico |
| Alejandro Rosales | Instituto Nacional de Astrofísica, Óptica y Electrónica, Mexico |
| Paolo Rosso | Technical University of Valencia, Spain |
| Horacio Rostro Gonzalez | Universidad de Guanajuato, Mexico |
| Salvador Ruiz Correa | Centro de Investigación en Matemáticas, Mexico |
| Jose Ruiz-Pinales | Universidad de Guanajuato, Mexico |
| Klempous Ryszard | Wroclaw University of Technology, Poland |
| Chaman Sabharwal | Missouri University of Science and Technology, USA |
| Abraham Sánchez López | Benemérita Universidad Autónoma de Puebla, Mexico |
| Luciano Sanchez | Universidad de Oviedo, Spain |
| Guillermo Sanchez-Diaz | Universidad Autónoma de San Luis Potosí, Mexico |
| Jose Santos | University of A Coruña, Spain |
| Oliver Schuetze | CINVESTAV, Mexico |
| Friedhelm Schwenker | Ulm University, Germany |
| Shahnaz Shahbazova | Azerbaijan Technical University, Azerbaijan |
| Bernadette Sharp | Staffordshire University, UK |
| Oleksiy Shulika | Universidad de Guanajuato, Mexico |
| Patrick Siarry | Université de Paris 12, France |
| Grigori Sidorov | Instituto Politécnico Nacional, Mexico |
| Bogdan Smolka | Silesian University of Technology, Poland |
| Jorge Solis | Waseda University, Japan |
| Thamar Solorio | University of Alabama at Birmingham, USA |
| Juan Humberto Sossa Azuela | Instituto Politécnico Nacional, Mexico |
| Efstathios Stamatatos | University of the Aegean, Greece |
| Josef Steinberger | University of West Bohemia, Czech Republic |
| Vera Lúcia Strube de Lima | Pontifícia Universidade Católica do Rio Grande do Sul, Brazil |
| Luis Enrique Sucar | Instituto Nacional de Astrofísica, Óptica y Electrónica, Mexico |
| Shiliang Sun | East China Normal University, China |
| Johan Suykens | Katholieke Universiteit Leuven, Belgium |
| Antonio-José Sánchez-Salmerón | Universitat Politècnica de València, Spain |

Anastasios Tefas                          Aristotle University of Thessaloniki, Greece
Gregorio Toscano Pulido                   CINVESTAV Tamaulipas, Mexico
Kostas Triantafyllopoulos                 University of Sheffield, UK
Leonardo Trujillo                         Instituto Tecnológico de Tijuana, Mexico
Alexander Tulupyev                        St. Petersburg Institute for Informatics and
                                          Automation of Russian Academy of Sciences,
                                          Russia
Fevrier Valdez                            Instituto Tecnológico de Tijuana, Mexico
Edgar Vallejo                             Tecnológico de Monterrey CEM, Mexico
Manuel Vilares Ferro                      University of Vigo, Spain
Aline Villavicencio                       Universidade Federal do Rio Grande do Sul,
                                          Brazil
Francisco Viveros Jiménez                 Instituto Politécnico Nacional, Mexico
Panagiotis Vlamos                         Ionian University, Greece
Piotr W. Fuglewicz                        TiP Sp. z o. o., Poland
Fanhai Yang                               University of Massachusetts Lowell, USA
Nicolas Younan                            Mississippi State University, USA
Carlos Mario Zapata Jaramillo             Universidad Nacional de Colombia, Colombia
Ramon Zatarain                            Instituto Tecnológico de Culiacán, Mexico
Claudia Zepeda Cortes                     Benemérita Universidad Autónoma de Puebla,
                                          Mexico
Reyer Zwiggelaar                          Aberystwyth University, UK

## Additional Reviewers

Roberto Alonso                    Homero Miranda
Ricardo Alvarez Salas             Soujanya Poria
Igor Bolshakov                    Pedro Reta
Michael Emmerich                  Daniel Rivera
Victor Ferman                     Carlos Rodriguez-Donate
Esteban Guerrero                  Salvador Ruiz-Correa
Goffredo Haus                     Chrysostomos Stylios
Misael Lopez Ramirez              Yasushi Tsubota
José Lozano                       Dan-El Vila-Rosado
Ana Martinez

## Organizing Committee

### Local Chair
Imelda Valles López                       Instituto Tecnológico de Tuxtla Gutiérrez,
                                          Mexico

## Logistics Chairs

Delina Culebro Farrera              Instituto Tecnológico de Tuxtla Gutiérrez,
                                    Mexico

Adolfo Solís                        Universidad Autónoma de Chiapas, Mexico

## Marketing Chair

Aida Cossio Martínez                Instituto Tecnológico de Tuxtla Gutiérrez,
                                    Mexico

## Registration Chair

Héctor Guerra Crespo                Instituto Tecnológico de Tuxtla Gutiérrez,
                                    Mexico

## Workshop Chair

Octavio Guzmán Sánchez              Instituto Tecnológico de Tuxtla Gutiérrez,
                                    Mexico

## International Relations Chair

María Candelaria                    Instituto Tecnológico de Tuxtla Gutiérrez,
  Gutiérrez Gómez                   Mexico

## Finance Chair

Jacinta Luna Villalobos             Instituto Tecnológico de Tuxtla Gutiérrez,
                                    Mexico

## Student Chair

Sebastián Moreno Vázquez            Instituto Tecnológico de Tuxtla Gutiérrez,
                                    Mexico

# Table of Contents – Part I

## Natural Language Processing

## Natural Language Processing Applications

### Best Student Paper Award

## Opinion Mining, Sentiment Analysis, and Social Network Applications

# Computer Vision

## Best Paper Award, Second Place

# Image Processing

## Logic, Reasoning, and Multi-agent Systems

## Intelligent Tutoring Systems

# Table of Contents – Part II

## Genetic and Evolutionary Algorithms

## Neural Networks

### Best Paper Award, First Place

# Machine Learning

# Machine Learning Applications to Audio and Text

# Data Mining

### Best Student Paper Award

# Fuzzy Logic

## Invited Paper

# Robotics, Planning, and Scheduling

## Best Paper Award, Third Place

## Biomedical Applications

# Finding the Most Frequent Sense of a Word by the Length of Its Definition

Hiram Calvo and Alexander Gelbukh

Centro de Investigación en Computación, Instituto Politécnico Nacional,
Av. Juan de Dios Bátiz s/n, esq. Av. Mendizábal, D.F., 07738, Mexico
hcalvo@cic.ipn.mx,
www.gelbukh.com

**Abstract.** Most frequent sense (MFS) is a very powerful heuristic in word sense disambiguation, extremely difficult to outperform with sophisticated methods. We show that counting the number of words, characters, or relationships of a word's sense definitions allows guessing the most frequent sense of the word: the MFS usually has a longer gloss, more examples of usage, and more relationships with other words (synonyms, hyponyms, etc.). In addition, we show that this effect is resource-dependent, making some algorithms to perform differently with different dictionaries.

## 1 Introduction

Word sense disambiguation is required in several natural language applications such as text mining, information retrieval or question answering. For solving this task, several approaches have been proposed. Of course, many of them propose considering the context of a word in order to determine its sense (for example *bank* can be disambiguated if there is a word nearby such as *money* or *fishing*). However, an interesting baseline has been defined, which consists on selecting always the most frequent sense of a word. The Most Frequent Sense (MFS) of a word is calculated in different ways. WordNet itself includes a frequency count for each one of the senses of a word. As reported by Hawker and Honnibal (2006), the sense ranks in WordNet are derived from semantic concordance texts used in the construction of the database. Most senses have explicit counts listed in the database, although sometimes the counts will be reported as 0. In these cases, the senses are presumably ranked by the lexicographer's intuition.

Another important resource used for counting the frequency of senses are sense-tagged texts such as **SemCor** (SEMantic COncoRdance). The SemCor corpus (Miller *et al.*, 1994), contains approximately 700,000 English words. In SemCor, all words are grammatically tagged, and more than 200,000 are lemmatized and sense-tagged with the WordNet 1.6 senses inventory (and thus, a particular sense for a word). With this resource, it is also possible to calculate the MFS for many words. Usually the frequency counts of senses in WordNet are higher than the frequency of the sense in the SemCor sense-tagged corpus (Miller *et al.*, 1993), although not always.

A. Gelbukh et al. (Eds.): MICAI 2014, Part I, LNAI 8856, pp. 1–8, 2014.

On the side of non-manually tagged resources, an interesting way of calculating the MFS was reported by Dianna McCarthy *et al.* (2007). They propose a method for obtaining the predominant sense using raw text as source of information. Their method consists of two stages:

- First, a Lin Thesaurus (Lin, 1998) is queried to obtain a list of weighted terms related with the ambiguous word. This list is static; this means that it is always the same for each instance of the ambiguous word, no matter its context.

- Second, a maximization algorithm allows each one of the elements of the list to vote for a sense of the ambiguous word, so that the sense with the greatest number of votes is chosen as the most frequent sense.

In this work, we propose finding the most frequent sense by considering the amount of information available for each synset in WordNet, that is, its gloss, the number of words that conform it, the number of characters, the number of relationships, including all of them, or some of them, etc. Results of experimenting with different ways of choosing the MFS will be evaluated with several widely available tests, namely, the Senseval tests and the SemCor corpus, detailed in the following sections.

**Table 1.** Top-10 Systems of Senseval-2

| Rank | System | Type | Precision | Recall | Attempted |
|------|--------|------|-----------|--------|-----------|
| 1 | SMUaw | supervised | 0.690 | 0.690 | 100% |
| 2 | CNTS-Antwerp | supervised | 0.636 | 0.636 | 100% |
| 3 | Sinequa-LIA - HMM | supervised | 0.618 | 0.618 | 100% |
| – | **WordNet MFS (McCarthy *et al.*)** | **unsupervised** | **0.605** | **0.605** | **100%** |
| 4 | UNED - AW-U2 | unsupervised | 0.575 | 0.569 | 98.908% |
| 5 | UNED - AW-U | unsupervised | 0.556 | 0.550 | 98.908% |
| 6 | UCLA - gchao2 | supervised | 0.475 | 0.454 | 95.552% |
| 7 | UCLA - gchao3 | supervised | 0.474 | 0.453 | 95.552% |
| 8 | CL Research - DIMAP | unsupervised | 0.416 | 0.451 | 100% |
| 9 | CL Research - DIMAP (R) | unsupervised | 0.451 | 0.451 | 100% |
| 10 | UCLA - gchao | supervised | 0.500 | 0.449 | 89.729% |

## 2    The Senseval Tests

The purpose of the Senseval tests is to evaluate semantic analysis systems. Particularly, the Senseval-2 and Senseval-3 focus on two different tasks: *All words sense disambiguation*, and *Lexical Sample disambiguation*, where only one word per sentence has to be disambiguated.

Senseval-2 is a test based on the British National Corpus (BNC); the *English all words* dataset contains approximately 5,000 words of texts that have been extracted from *The Wall Street Journal* and an extract of *The Brown Corpus* (Snyder and Palmer, 2004) tagged according to the *Penn Treebank II* (Marcus *et al.*, 1993) using the version 1.7.1 of WordNet. The dataset for the task *English lexical sample* provides for training and test, around 60 nouns, adjectives and ambiguous verbs. The examples were extracted from the *British National Corpus*. The dictionary used for the senses inventory for nouns and adjectives was WordNet 1.7.1, and for verb senses, the dictionary *Wordsmyth* was used (Mihalcea *et al.*, 2004). Both Senseval-2 and Senseval-3 include tests for other languages as well.

McCarthy *et al.* (2007) determined automatically the most frequent sense in English all-words Senseval-2 (as raw text) based on the British National Corpus (BNC). For Word Sense Disambiguation—using always the most frequent sense identified by their method—they obtained 64% precision and 63% recall. This value is better than any other unsupervised method, as can be seen from Table 1. Note that this method does not consider the context of the ambiguous word. In addition, they compared the MFSs found by their method with the most frequent sense from tagged SemCor and Senseval-2. Choosing the most frequent sense from tagged SemCor gives a precision of 69% and 68% recall. By choosing the most frequent sense from Senseval-2 for WSD in Senseval-2 itself, they obtained a precision of 92% and a recall of 72%; this shows that the strategy of choosing the MFS for WSD is indeed a good solution.

## 3    The Longest Definition Algorithm

Our hypothesis is that the longest sense definition would correspond to the most frequent sense; it is based on the notion that it is possible to say more about a sense that is more frequent, compared with what it can be said about a less frequent sense, *i.e.*, the most frequent sense has more synonyms, more examples, a more detailed definition, etc. Let us consider the length of the gloss, and the number of relationships each synset has in WordNet 2.0. We assume that a long gloss has more probability of being the MFS for a word. In WordNet 2.0 there are 144,307 different words (many of them correspond to several synsets, and one synset can be tagged with different words). If we consider the MFS as the one with the longest gloss, we obtain that 127,935 (88.6%) correspond with the manually tagged MFS in WordNet. If we consider the MFS to be the one with the largest number of relations for each word, this number increases to 128,613 (89.1%) words that correspond with the "gold standard" provided by WordNet, including monosemous words in both cases.

We will see how this affects results in the Senseval tests. The Spanish Lexical Sample in the Senseval-3 test includes different words that have a different MFS distribution, so that WSD algorithms have a different performance for each word, see Màrquez *et al.* (2004). The Spanish Lexical Sample task in Senseval-3 is different from English in the fact that it provides a sense inventory called *Minidir* which includes *ex*amples, *syn*onyms and frequent *collo*cations; see Figure 1.

---

**banda.1**: Cinta que se coloca cruzada sobre el pecho y que es señal de un cargo o una distinción
*Ex*: ha conseguido unas cuantas bandas, incluyendo la novedosa de Miss Internet

**banda.2**: Tira de tela u otro material
*Ex*: unas bandas de lona, unas bandas de velcro
*Syn*: tira, cinta

**banda.3**: Conjunto de músicos que tocan juntos
*Ex*: banda de jazz, banda de cornetas y tambores
*Syn*: grupo
*Collo*: banda militar, banda de música, banda de rock, banda musical

**banda.4**: Grupo de personas que se une con fines comunes, especialmente delictivos
*Ex*: banda de atracadores, banda de traficantes
*Syn*: grupo
*Collo*: banda armada, banda callejera, banda de delincuentes, banda juvenil, banda militar, banda organizada, banda para-militar, banda terrorista, banda ultra

**banda.5**: Zona lateral de un objeto o lugar
*Ex*: recorrió toda la banda derecha con el balón cosido a sus botas
*Syn*: margen, lateral, lado, costado
*Collo*: banda derecha, banda izquierda, línea de banda, saque de banda

**banda.6**: Conjunto de animales que pertenecen a una misma especie y se desplazan en grupo
*Ex*: banda de gaviotas
*Syn*: bandada, manada

**banda.7**: Intervalo de frecuencias entre dos puntos que permite transmitir una señal por medio de ondas electromagnéticas
*Ex*: los radiofaros trabajan en la banda 280
*Syn*: frecuencia
*Collo*: banda de frecuencia

---

**Fig. 1.** Fragment of the Minidir sense inventory supplied in Senseval-3

We have chosen this sense inventory for a first test of our hypothesis, yielding the results for the Longest Definition Algorithm shown in Table 2. We can see from this table that, by choosing always the most frequent sense according to the Senseval-3 provided training corpus, independently from the context in which a word is used, we obtain a precision of 65.03%. If we count the number of words for each sense definition in Minidir, and select as the MFS the one that has the largest number of words per definition, we obtain 45% of precision. If we count the longest number of chars of this definition, we obtain a slightly higher score. If we filter out the non-content words, then we obtain 46.75% of precision, which is the highest value we obtained. As we are attempting all cases (our coverage is 100%), the recall figures, and the F-measures are the same as the precision values reported in Table 2.

**Table 2.** Results for the Longest Definition Algorithm (counting bags of words). (Coverage=100%). Spanish Lexical Sample, Senseval-3.

| Precision | Method |
|---|---|
| 65.03% | Most frequent sense from answers of Senseval-3 training corpus |
| 45.01% | MFS: largest number of words per definition in Minidir |
| 46.08% | MFS: largest number of chars per definition in Minidir |
| **46.75%** | MFS: largest number of content words per definition in Minidir |
| 45.31% | MFS: largest number of chars of content words per def. in Minidir |

In order to verify if this would replicate in English, we experimented with the Lexical Sample test for English, in Senseval-2. The results were around 20% (20.7% counting words and 20.5% counting chars). This was done considering words from the glosses. The next experiment was to consider also words from the glosses of related synsets (hypernyms, synonyms, antonyms, meronyms, etc.). This led to 29.17% when counting number of words, and 29.22% when counting number of chars. Note that using all words of Minidir would be similar to *counting words from glosses and related synsets*, because in Minidir the definitions already include relationships of each sense.

Additionally, we experimented with counting different words only once. Previous experiments counted every occurrence of every word ('life is life' are three words, *life* counts twice). Counting words only once did not improve results: the result was 28.75% accuracy. Finally, these results contrast with choosing the MFS in WordNet (using the first sense listed in WordNet): 36.11%. Results are summarized in Table 3.

**Table 3.** Results of our algorithm on the English Lexical Sample, Senseval-2

| Precision | Method |
|---|---|
| 18.78% | Selecting a random sense |
| 20.70% | Counting words from glosses |
| 20.50% | Counting chars from glosses |
| 29.17% | Counting words from glosses and related synsets |
| **29.22%** | Counting chars from glosses and related synsets |
| 28.75% | Counting words from glosses and related synsets only once per word |
| 36.11% | Choosing the first sense listed in WordNet |
| 28.67% | Counting number of relations |
| 47.94% | Using the most frequent sense in the Senseval-2 Lexical Sample test |

Apparently, from these results, the Longest Definition Algorithm works better for Spanish than for English, probably due to the construction of the sense inventory (Minidir) and the MFS distribution of the test set as well. Now we will attest results with another English resource, SemCor, in the following section.

## 4    Experiments with SemCor

The SemCor test corpus has 88,143 instances (tokens), from which 70,920 are polysemous nouns, and 17,223 are not polysemous. We will only work with the subset of 70,920 instances of polysemous nouns; that is, 5577 types of polysemous nouns. Results are shown in Table 4.

First, we calculated the most frequent sense from SemCor itself. This will be the upper bound, as we are trying to disambiguate the entire corpus by selecting always the same sense for each word. This yielded 74.14%.

If we always select the MFS provided by WordNet, we obtain a precision of 60.45%. In contrast, our lower baseline will be given by choosing a random sense (22.13%). The algorithm of McCarthy *et al.* (2007), consisting on automatically finding the MFSs given a fixed corpus from which a distributional thesaurus is built, yields 49% for the polysemous nouns in SemCor.

**Table 4.** Results of the Longest Definition Algorithm on SemCor. Methods are additive, *i.e.* adding related glosses + different chars + suppressing stop-words yields 40.59%.

| Method | | | Prec. (%) |
|---|---|---|---|
| MFS (SemCor) | | | 74.14 |
| WordNet first sense | | | 60.45 |
| Random sense | | | 22.13 |
| McCarthy *et. al.* (2007) | | | 49.20 |
| Longest definition measured by number of characters is MFS | | | |
| | no-preprocessing | | 25.72 |
| | adding related glosses | | **40.60** |
| | | different chars | **40.57** |
| | | suppressing stop-words | **40.59** |
| | removing non-alphabetic | | 25.78 |
| | suppressing stop-words | | 26.14 |
| | | multiplied by the number of relations | **39.68** |
| | | removing non-alphabetic | 26.01 |
| Longest definition counting by words is MFS | | | |
| | no-preprocessing | | 26.22 |
| | | different words (number of types) | 25.98 |
| | removing non-alphabetic | | 26.13 |
| | | different words (number of types) | 26.64 |
| | suppressing stop-words | | 27.48 |
| | | different words (number of types) | 28.14 |
| | | adding related glosses | **40.58** |
| | removing non-alphabetic and suppressing stop-words | | 27.60 |
| | | different words (number of types) | 27.89 |
| | | adding related glosses | **40.45** |
| Number of relationships | First order | | **42.48** |
| | Second order | | 30.27 |

Our longest definition algorithm was split in three main variants, one considering the longest definition by counting the number of characters; another by counting the number of words; and lastly, counting the number of relationships.

The first variant, **measuring by longest char definition**, yielded 25.72% precision with no pre-processing. When adding the strings of related glosses, the results increased above 40%. The *different chars* feature involved counting chars as types, that is, counting only the variety of characters present in the word, and its related chars itself. Finally, in addition to this, we experimented with removing stop-words from related glosses, and counting the different characters present in them.

Another option we tried with the first variant was to remove everything that was not an alphabetic character. We can see very little difference with previous results. We tried independently suppressing stop-words (without adding related glosses or counting chars as types), observing again that when we involved counting each word's relationships, results improved.

For the second variant, **counting by words**, we tried no-preprocessing, considering only different words, that is, different word types only; removing non-alphabetic characters and word types again, suppressing stop-words, with low results (26 to 28% approximately), except when adding words from related glosses (40.58%). The same happened when we tried different combinations, such as removing all non-alphabetic characters + suppressing stop-words (27.60%), the same + counting number of types, and finally, this latter + adding words from related glosses. Again, adding related glosses resulted in an increase of more than 12 percent.

Finally, for the third variant, **number of relationships**, we tried two methods. The first one consisted in counting the number of relationships a word has, and the second one consisted in counting the number of relationships plus the number of relationships of each word related to the original word; that is, *second order* relationship count. We obtained 42.48% and 30.97% for each one, respectively, concluding that adding second order relationships does not help finding the MFS.

## 5    Conclusions and Future Work

We have explored finding the Most Frequent Sense (MFS) of a word by counting the length of its definition in WordNet. We were motivated by the hypothesis that, the more frequent a sense is, the more examples is possible to find for this sense, as well as having a longer explanation, and a greater number of relationships. First we have measured the number of senses in WordNet that were manually labeled as the MFS compared with those selected as the MFS by our Longest Definition Algorithm. We found that nearly 90% of synsets selected by our algorithm are actually listed as the first sense for a word (near 44% if we remove the monosemous words). Then we tested several variations of our Longest Definition Algorithm in the Spanish Lexical Sample of Senseval-3 and obtained the best results by finding the largest number of content words per definition in Minidir (the sense inventory for this test). We tried similar variations with the English Lexical Sample of Senseval-2, and we obtained the best results by counting chars from glosses and *related synsets*. Finally, we tested our method with SemCor, and found the best results whenever we included the count of the different relations each synset had, with little effect from the length of the gloss definition. The best results were obtained by counting only the number of relationships without considering any word's gloss. This would mean that if we consider examples of usage, synonyms, and other related words as part of a word's definition, we are able to approximate the MFS.

We have found that relationship count of each synset provides indeed a good clue for selecting the MFS, giving another measure from WordNet apart from the listed MFS within the same resource. This could yield to other ways of calculating the MFS when a ranked sense inventory is not available. As future work, we plan to experiment with other gloss sources aside from WordNet, as well as a deeper analysis of the kind of relationships that help us the most to find the MFS from the WordNet structure.

**Acknowledgment.** The work was partially supported by the Mexican Government: SNI, SIP-IPN, COFAA-IPN, and SIP-IPN 20144534.

# References

1. Hawker, T., Honnibal, M.: Improved Default Sense Selection for Word Sense Disambiguation. In: Proceedings of the 2006 Australasian Language Technology Workshop (ALTW 2006), pp. 11–17 (2006)
2. Lesk, M.: Automatic sense disambiguation using machine readable dictionaries: how to tell a pine cone from an ice cream cone. In: Proceedings of the 5th Annual International Conference on Systems Documentation, pp. 24–26. ACM (1986)
3. Lin, D.: An information-theoretic definition of similarity. In: International Conference on Machine Learning, vol. 98, pp. 296–304 (1998)
4. Marcus, M.P., Marcinkiewicz, M.A., Santorini, B.: Building a large annotated corpus of English: The Penn Treebank. Computational linguistics 19(2), 313–330 (1993)
5. Màrquez, L., Taulé, M., Martí, M.A., García, M., Artigas, N., Real, F.J., Ferrés, D.: Senseval-3: The Spanish Lexical Sample Task. In: Senseval-3: Third International Workshop on the Evaluation of Systems for the Semantic Analysis of Text. Association for Computational Linguistics, Barcelona (2004)
6. McCarthy, D., Koeling, R., Weeds, R.J., Carroll, J.: Unsupervised acquisition of predominant word senses. Computational Linguistics 33(4), 553–590 (2007)
7. Mihalcea, R., Chklovski, T., Kilgarriff, A.: The Senseval-3 English lexical sample task. In: Senseval-3: Third International Workshop on the Evaluation of Systems for the Semantic Analysis of Text, pp. 25–28 (2004)
8. Miller, G., Leacock, C., Tengi, R., Bunker, R.T.: A Semantic Concordance. In: Proceedings of ARPA Workshop on Human Language Technology, pp. 303–308 (1993)
9. Miller, G.A., Chodorow, M., Landes, S., Leacock, C., Thomas, R.G.: Using a semantic concordance for sense identification. In: Proceedings of the ARPA Human Language Technology Workshop, pp. 240–243 (1994)
10. Snyder, B., Palmer, M.: The English all-words task. In: ACL 2004 Senseval-3 Workshop, Barcelona, Spain (2004)

# Complete Syntactic N-grams
# as Style Markers for Authorship Attribution

Juan-Pablo Posadas-Duran, Grigori Sidorov, and Ildar Batyrshin

Center for Computing Research (CIC),
Instituto Politécnico Nacional (IPN),
Mexico City, Mexico
http://www.cic.ipn.mx/~sidorov

**Abstract.** In this paper we present an authorship attribution method based on the use of complete (non-continuous, with bifurcations) syntactic n-grams as style markers. Syntactic n-grams are obtained by following paths in subtrees of a syntactic tree. We work with relatively short text fragments and build authors' profiles of various sizes using tf-idf scheme. We train SVM classifier to perform the task. We compare the method with the application of character n-grams and show that the accuracy increases when using complete syntactic n-grams.

**Keywords:** authorship attribution, style markers, syntactic markers, syntactic n-grams, syntactic paths, SVM.

## 1 Introduction

Various approaches were proposed for authorship attribution and hence many style markers were used in this task. The information used as the style markers includes most concepts of the natural language theory, from the explicit information contained in texts at the character level, word level or formatting to more complex levels like syntax or semantics.

For authorship attribution, character n-grams of sizes between 3 and 5 have shown to be very powerful style markers [13,1]. By using the frequency of character n-grams in the vector space representation, it is possible to identify the writing style of an author using supervised machine learning algorithms. In addition, the advantage of character n-grams is their simplicity, i.e., no special natural language processing tools are required and they can be applied to various languages without any special preprocessing.

Character n-grams focus on the occurrence of character patterns at the surface level of texts, preserving the natural order, in which the text was written. The information provided by character n-grams only reflects lexical and morphological features in texts, leaving aside important aspects related to the preferences of the author while using language, that are contained at the higher levels, such as syntax and semantics [8,13].

The main idea of our work is to show that complete syntactic n-grams (sn-gramas with bifurcations, non-continuous sn-grams) proposed in [10] can serve

A. Gelbukh et al. (Eds.): MICAI 2014, Part I, LNAI 8856, pp. 9–17, 2014.
© Springer International Publishing Switzerland 2014

as style markers for the problem of authorship attribution. We show that they overcome character n-grams. Although syntactic n-grams require a special tool for their obtaining (a parser), we consider that this is not a real limitation, because nowadays there are many such tools with good performance for many languages available on the *Web*.

In addition, our specific situation is that we work with relatively short texts, because we want to apply our results in future in the unsupervised task of plagiarism detection based on changes in writing style. In this work we are defining the relevant features for this future task. So, for our experiments, we used corpora of relatively short texts extracted from the corpora of novels of 7 authors used in [12]: we selected randomly only one chapter of each novel. The size of each corpus corresponds to the scenario with scarce number of examples. Note that this kind of texts does not have the problem of specific content (specific theme).

The rest of the paper is organized as follows: the problem of authorship attribution is briefly introduced in Section 2, the concept of complete syntactic n-grams is presented in Section 3, experimental results of the proposal are presented and compared with baseline in Section 4 and, finally, we draw conclusions in Section 5.

## 2   Authorship Attribution

The problem of authorship attribution can be defined as follows: identify, from a set of possible authors, the author or authors of a text, prior analysis of examples of their writing style. The authorship attribution can be applied in many areas, especially those related with the law issues, like copyright, plagiarism, identity theft, and many others.

The process of authorship attribution, in general, can be described by these steps [2]:

1. Select possible authors and gather some text examples of their authorship.
2. Model the style of writing of each author and the style of the unknown authorship text.
3. Associate the text of the unknown authorship with at least one of the known authors.

From the computational point of view, the authorship attribution can be stated as a multiclass classification problem of a text that is known to belong to one class only. The style of each of the possible authors represents one class and the main goal is to associate the style of the text of the unknown authorship with one of the known styles using machine learning algorithms.

Various strategies were proposed to solve the problem of authorship attribution. They vary in the features they use for modeling the style of authors and the machine learning algorithms they use as classifiers.

The features used to model the style of an author are known as *style markers*, which are the essence of the active area of research called *Stylometry*.

A style marker tries to identify how an author writes through the knowledge of the language. Therefore, the style markers can be classified by the level of the information they use, for example, character level, lexical level, syntactic level, and semantic level [13].

On the other hand, there are many algorithms of machine learning that can be applied to solve the problem of authorship attribution, one of the most popular is the Support Vector Machines (SVM) [12,4]. There are many other machine learning methods like decision trees [15], neural networks [14] and even genetic algorithms [7], to mention some of them.

## 3   Complete Syntactic N-grams

The concept of n-gram refers to a sequence of elements, when each sequence can be viewed as a helpful feature for modeling a phenomenon. This concept is widely used in Natural Language Processing field for representing text in terms of it's elements. It is commonly implemented by using an imaginary window that covers certain number of elements (the value of n), usually words or characters, and it slides with certain offset over the rest of the text.

A modern variant of n-grams approach proposed in [10,12,11] consists in obtaining the n-grams from dependency trees of sentences. In this way, the n-gram can represent the real preferences of an author when composing a text, overcoming the limitations of traditional n-grams based only on the surface information of the text. The elements that constitute syntactic n-grams can be of various types contained in the dependency relation tree, for example, lexical elements (words, lemmas, stems), POS tags, SR tags (tags of names of syntactic relations) [12,11]. There can be also mixed syntactic n-grams that contain elements of different types.

One kind of syntactic n-grams can be obtained from the dependency relation tree by following the paths in the branches of the tree without entering in bifurcations. These syntactic n-grams are called continuous [12,11]. A more general idea consists in extending the concept of syntactic n-grams so that it includes the bifurcations in the syntactic tree [10,11]. In this way, syntactic n-grams represent the complete set of relations contained in the syntactic tree. The complete syntactic n-grams (continuous sn-grams, sn-grams with bifurcations) are obtained from the syntactic tree as subtrees, when the size of the subtree corresponds to the length of the syntactic n-gram.

Let us consider an example sentence *John smoked with a little more dignity and surveyed them in silence.* Using the parser of Stanford University [9], the following information is obtained: part of speech tags (POS tags) of each word, lemmas of each word and syntactic relation tags (SR tags) that correspond to realtions between words. This information is shown in Table 1.

The information obtained from the parser is graphically represented as the dependency tree, where the nodes refer to words of the sentence and the arrows represent dependency relations between words. Figure 1 shows the dependency tree for the example sentence.

**Table 1.** Example of the results of the syntactic analysis

| Word Id | Word | Lemma | POS tag | SR tag | Dependent word |
|---------|------|-------|---------|--------|----------------|
| 1 | John | John | NNP | nsubj | 2 |
| 2 | smoked | smoke | VBD | root | 0 |
| 3 | with | with | IN | prep | 2 |
| 4 | a | a | DT | det | 7 |
| 5 | little | little | RB | advmod | 6 |
| 6 | more | more | JJR | amod | 7 |
| 7 | dignity | dignity | NN | pobj | 3 |
| 8 | and | and | CC | cc | 2 |
| 9 | surveyed | survey | VBD | conj | 2 |
| 10 | them | they | PRP | dobj | 9 |
| 11 | in | in | IN | prep | 9 |
| 12 | silence | silence | NN | pobj | 11 |

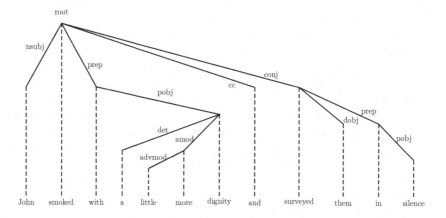

**Fig. 1.** Dependency tree for the example sentence

Complete syntactic n-grams are obtained by using a recursive algorithm that traverses the dependency tree[1]. It uses the metalanguage for represetnation of sn-grams proposed in [12]. In this software, the size of the n-grams is fixed to certain range (determined by user), so they capture the discriminative patterns. In Table 2 the n-grams of SR tags of size 3 are shown along with their frequencies for the example sentence.

The use of syntactic n-grams brings new information about the writing style of the authors that is contained in the syntactic rules that they tend to use unconsciously. This information is not available using traditional character or word n-grams. In case of continuous syntactic n-grams, as it was done in [12], the syntactic information is present but it reflects different syntactic properties.

---

[1] It is available at http://www.cic.ipn.mx/~sidorov/#Downloads

**Table 2.** N-grams of SR tags for the example sentence

| 3-gram | Frequency |
|---|---|
| VBD[IN[NN]] | 2 |
| VBD[NNP,IN] | 1 |
| NN[DT,JJR] | 1 |
| VBD[VBD[PRP]] | 1 |
| VBD[IN,CC] | 1 |
| VBD[VBD[IN]] | 1 |
| IN[NN[JJR]] | 1 |
| VBD[IN,VBD] | 1 |
| VBD[CC,VBD] | 1 |
| VBBD[NNP,VBD] | 1 |
| IN[NN[DT]] | 1 |
| VBD[PRP,IN] | 1 |
| NN[JJR[RB]] | 1 |

## 4    Proposed Method

In this article we propose a method that solves the traditional problem of authorship attribution using complete syntactic n-grams. The problem of the authorship attribution is formulated as follows: given a set of known authors and few examples of texts written by them, try to associate a text of the unknown authorship to one of them. The proposed method uses a machine learning technique because the problem of the authorship attribution is formulated as a multiclass classification problem and in our case is solved by using support vector machine algorithm.

The main contribution of the method lies in the application of the complete syntactic n-grams for modeling the writing style of an author. The method uses a vector space model, in which the writing style of each text is represented as a vector of features and their values. Each dimension in the vector space represents the frequency of a given syntactic n-gram in the text, each text is considered as an instance and the support vector machine algorithm is applied to the generated vector.

As a way to avoid less significant syntactic n-grams, the method reduces the space of features by implementing two strategies: on the one hand, it fixes the size of the syntactic n-grams to sizes from 3 to 7 in order to avoid either very common or unique syntactic n-grams: cases that are not representative for the style of an author. On the other hand, it uses tf-idf weighting scheme, very often used strategy in Information Retrieval that tends to assign high weights to those n-grams that are representative for each author and assigns low weights to the cases that appears too few or too often in the corpora.

The set of the representative syntactic n-grams is generated in a two steps process: (1) the method obtains a profile for each known author in terms of syntactic n-grams [6,5], i.e., gets the top frequent n-grams from all examples of each known author using the tf-idf weights as a selection parameter, (2) a common feature space is generated by intersecting the syntactic n-grams contained in the profiles.

Once the common feature space is formed, the vector representations of the training corpus are generated and provided to the support vector machine as the instance of an author (a class). For a text of the unknown authorship, the method obtains its representation as the vector using the common feature space mentioned before and associates it to the known author using the trained support vector machine.

The method was evaluated using a collection of novels of seven English writers that were obtained from the project Gutenberg repository[2]. We had a collection of 7 authors with 13 novels for each author, and we prepared a reduced collection selecting randomly chapters from each novel (from 1 to 2 chapters per novel) in order to work within a scenario for our task: relatively short texts. The details of the collection are shown in Table 3, the last column represents the range of texts sizes for each author.

**Table 3.** Details of the text collection used in our experiments

| Author | Number of samples | Size of the samples (KB) |
|---|---|---|
| Booth Tarkington | 13 | 9 - 33 |
| Charles Dickens | 13 | 10 - 33 |
| Frederick Marryat | 13 | 10 - 48 |
| George Donald | 13 | 7 - 29 |
| George Vaizey | 13 | 8 - 30 |
| Louis Tracy | 13 | 15 - 36 |
| Mark Twain | 13 | 8 - 17 |

In our work, we use three different types of elements of syntactic n-grams: SR tags, POS tags and lemmas. All of them are obtained from the dependency trees of the sentences using the Stanford parser [9]. As the baseline, we used character n-grams because it shows good performance as it is mentioned in [13].

For the implementation of the support vector machine, we used the SVMlib [3] library for training and testing focusing on the use of the RBF kernel because of its simplicity. The accuracy presented is the best obtained using the standard k-fold cross validation with 5 folds after implementing the grid search for the best values of the parameters $C$ and $\gamma$ of the RBF kernel using the tools provided by the SVMlib. The accuracy represents the percentage of instances which are correctly classified and is defined in terms of true positives (TP), false positives (FP), true negatives (TN) and false negatives (FN) as follows:

$$accuracy = \frac{TP + TN}{TP + TN + FP + FN} \qquad (1)$$

---

[2] See http://www.gutenberg.org/

In the experiments, different sizes for the set of features were tried. For certain sizes of the set we try to keep an equally distributed representation over all authors using in almost all cases the same number of the most representative n-grams from the profiles of the authors.

In Table 4 we present the accuracy for the sn-grams of SR tags with sizes of sets of features that have shown relevant variance and for the sizes of syntactic n-grams of our interest.

**Table 4.** Accuracy for sn-grams of SR tags

| Number of features (Profile size) | $n = 3$ | $n = 4$ | $n = 5$ | $n = 6$ | $n = 7$ |
|---|---|---|---|---|---|
| 100 | 66.07% | 78.57% | 57.14% | 39.28% | 32.14% |
| 500 | 78.57% | **96.42%** | 91.07% | 75.00% | 53.57% |
| 1000 | 89.27% | 87.50% | 91.07% | 69.64% | 64.28% |
| 2000 | 94.64% | 91.07% | 92.85% | 91.07% | 69.64% |
| 3000 | 94.64% | 91.07% | 92.85% | 96.42% | 76.78% |

In Table 5 and Table 6 we show the accuracy for the sn-grams of POS tag and lemmas respectively.

**Table 5.** Accuracy for sn-grams of POS tags

| Number of features (Profile size) | $n = 3$ | $n = 4$ | $n = 5$ | $n = 6$ | $n = 7$ |
|---|---|---|---|---|---|
| 100 | 78.57% | 67.85% | 60.71% | 37.50% | 25.00% |
| 500 | 82.14% | 92.85% | 83.92% | 66.07% | 46.42% |
| 1000 | 83.93% | 91.07% | 87.50% | 60.71% | 53.57% |
| 2000 | 92.85% | 89.28% | 92.85% | 83.92% | 58.92% |
| 3000 | 89.28% | 92.85% | **94.64%** | 87.50% | 60.71% |

**Table 6.** Accuracy for sn-grams of lemmas

| Number of features (Profile size) | $n = 3$ | $n = 4$ | $n = 5$ | $n = 6$ | $n = 7$ |
|---|---|---|---|---|---|
| 100 | 62.50% | 44.64% | 26.78% | 19.64% | 23.21% |
| 500 | 83.92% | 58.92% | 28.57% | 26.78% | 28.57% |
| 1000 | 87.50% | 66.07% | 35.71% | 28.57% | 26.78% |
| 2000 | 91.07% | 76.78% | 39.28% | 22.75% | 19.64% |
| 3000 | **94.64%** | 76.78% | 39.28% | 22.75% | 19.64% |

On the other hand, in Table 7 we present the accuracy of the application of character n-grams (baseline) for the same sizes of feature sets. It can be observed that the application of syntactic n-grams of various types works much better than the baseline method. Let us remind that in our specific problem we have the reduced size of the corpus.

**Table 7.** Accuracy for character n-grams (baseline)

| Number of features (Profile size) | $n = 3$ | $n = 4$ | $n = 5$ | $n = 6$ | $n = 7$ |
|---|---|---|---|---|---|
| 100 | 55.35% | 42.85% | 46.42% | 46.42% | 37.50% |
| 500 | 62.50% | 66.07% | 66.07% | 73.21% | 67.85% |
| 1000 | 71.42% | 73.21% | 67.85% | 75.00% | 76.78% |
| 2000 | 76.78% | 73.21% | 76.78% | 76.78% | 76.78% |
| 3000 | 80.35% | 76.78% | 76.78% | 80.35% | **85.71%** |

## 5   Conclusions

The complete syntactic n-grams allow obtaining full description of the information expressed in the syntactic trees that correspond to the sentences of texts. Its application allows better identification and comparison of syntactic centered features that can be useful in many tasks in the Natural Language Processing. Complete syntactic n-grams are suitable as style markers, because they explore directly the syntactic information.

We considered a task of the authorship attribution for relatively short texts. In the presented experiments, it is shown that complete syntactic n-grams are more efficient style markers than character n-grams, not only because they achieve more accurate results but also because they use smaller sets of features evaluated in a scenario with several authors and reduced samples for each author (at most 48 KB). The best results were obtained using syntactic n-grams of SR tags with sizes from 3 to 5.

## References

1. Argamon, S., Juola, P.: Overview of the international authorship identification competition at pan-2011. In: CLEF (Notebook Papers/Labs/Workshop) (2011)
2. Bozkurt, I.N., Baghoglu, O., Uyar, E.: Authorship attribution. In: 22nd International Symposium on Computer and information sciences, ISCIS 2007, pp. 1–5. IEEE (2007)
3. Chang, C.C., Lin, C.J.: Libsvm: a library for support vector machines. ACM Transactions on Intelligent Systems and Technology (TIST) 2(3), 27 (2011)
4. Diederich, J., Kindermann, J., Leopold, E., Paass, G.: Authorship attribution with support vector machines. Applied intelligence 19(1-2), 109–123 (2003)
5. Escalante, H.J., Solorio, T., Montes-y Gómez, M.: Local histograms of character n-grams for authorship attribution. In: Proceedings of the 49th Annual Meeting of the Association for Computational Linguistics: Human Language Technologies, vol. 1, pp. 288–298. Association for Computational Linguistics (2011)
6. Halteren, H.V.: Author verification by linguistic profiling: An exploration of the parameter space. ACM Transactions on Speech and Language Processing (TSLP) 4(1), 1 (2007)
7. Holmes, D.I., Forsyth, R.S.: The federalist revisited: New directions in authorship attribution. Literary and Linguistic Computing 10(2), 111–127 (1995)
8. Juola, P.: Future trends in authorship attribution. In: Advances in digital forensics III, pp. 119–132. Springer (2007)

9. Klein, D., Manning, C.D.: Accurate unlexicalized parsing. In: Proceedings of the 41st Annual Meeting on Association for Computational Linguistics, vol. 1, pp. 423–430. Association for Computational Linguistics (2003)

10. Sidorov, G.: Non-continuous syntactic n-grams. Polibits 48, 67–75 (2013)

11. Sidorov, G.: Syntactic dependency based n-grams in rule based automatic english as second language grammar correction. International Journal of Computational Linguistics and Applications 4(2), 169–188 (2013)

12. Sidorov, G., Velasquez, F., Stamatatos, E., Gelbukh, A., Chanona-Hernández, L.: Syntactic n-grams as machine learning features for natural language processing. Expert Systems with Applications 41(3), 853–860 (2014)

13. Stamatatos, E.: A survey of modern authorship attribution methods. Journal of the American Society for information Science and Technology 60(3), 538–556 (2009)

14. Tweedie, F.J., Singh, S., Holmes, D.I.: Neural network applications in stylometry: The federalist papers. Computers and the Humanities 30(1), 1–10 (1996)

15. Zhao, Y., Zobel, J., Vines, P.: Using relative entropy for authorship attribution. In: Information Retrieval Technology, pp. 92–105. Springer (2006)

# Extracting Frame-Like Structures
# from Google Books NGram Dataset

Vladimir Ivanov[1,2,3]

[1] Kazan Federal University
420008 Kazan, Kremlevskaya st., 18
http://www.kpfu.ru
[2] National University of Science and Technology "MISIS"
119049 Moscow, Leninskiy pr., 4
http://www.misis.ru
[3] Institute of Informatics, Tatarstan Academy of Sciences,
Levoboulachnaya St., 36a, Kazan, Russia

**Abstract.** We propose a method that facilitates a process of semi-automatic FrameNet construction. The method requires Google Books NGram dataset and WordNet or another thesaurus for a particular language. We evaluated the method for Russian ngrams. Due to a huge amount of available data the method does not require sophisticated natural language processing techniques (e.g. for word sense disambiguation), and it shows a promising result.

**Keywords:** natural language processing, framenet, information extraction, subordination models, ngrams.

## 1 Introduction

FrameNet and similar resources (PropBank[7] and VerbNet[9]) are important from both theoretical and practical points of view. The most developed resource, English FrameNet [1], is used in semantic role labeling of unstructured text. Frames, Frame Elements (FEs), Lexical Units (LU) and Valences, that expose a frame structure in example sentences, are core elements of the FrameNet. Manual construction of a FrameNet-like resource is a time-consuming task, that is based on parsing and semantic annotation of text corpora. In the paper we propose a method that helps semi-automatic FrameNet construction. The method requires Google Books N-gram dataset (or similar huge ngram statistics) and a thesaurus for a particular language. Essentially, the following linguistic resources are needed to run the method:

- a thesaurus (Wordnet or a similar resource);
- a subordination dictionary;
- a dependency parser and a large corpus.

The result is a set of FEs for a particular language. Each FE describes some subordination model enriched with semantic types from the thesaurus. The next

A. Gelbukh et al. (Eds.): MICAI 2014, Part I, LNAI 8856, pp. 18–27, 2014.

step in developing a FrameNet, to organize some FEs into a frame structure, is out of scope in this paper. In section 2 we describe linguistic resources that are necessary in semi-automatic construction of FrameNet. Section 3 presents the method for frame element extraction. Section 4 provides few samples from the resulting dataset.

## 2   Related Work

### 2.1   FrameNets

There are FrameNets for Bulgarian[3] and other languages (German, Danish, Japanese to name a few). These resources share many mutual features, as all of them are based on the Frame Semantics theory. Manual construction of a FrameNet-like resource is a time-consuming task, that is based on parsing and semantic annotation of text corpora. Development of FrameNet for Russian described in [6]. This resource has a specific structure and contains about 1300 verbs, and it is still far from full coverage of more than 20,000 Russian verbs. Tonelli et al. [12] tried to build FrameNet for Italian semi-automatically. Authors populated Italian frames exploiting existing resources: Wikipedia, Wordnet and English FrameNet. They provide algorithms for translating English FrameNet into Italian as well as annotated corpora (about 50,000 sentences in total).

### 2.2   Russian Wordnet and RuThes-Lite

Despite few attempts of developing Russian WordNet, there is still no such resource available. However, there is a large thesaurus, RuThes-lite, developed in Moscow State University[1]. The thesaurus has a hierarchical structure similar to Wordnet's structure, but the two resources also have significant differences. We will not describe all features of the thesaurus here and recommend an interested reader to refer to the recent work [5]. One important feature of the RuThes-lite is that it covers top-level concepts, like Physical Object or Abstract Entity.

### 2.3   A Subordination Dictionary for Russian

Another type of resource important in FrameNet development is a subordination dictionary (a dictionary that describes valences of verbs). An attempt to generate such a dictionary has been carried out in [8].

A number of research has been carried out so far in the area of generating subordination models for Russian verbs. Most work use large corpora such as Russian National Corpora[2]. Klyshinsky et al. [8] use web corpus. They developed a method for automatic generation of dictionary of subordination models for verbs and prepositions. The system deals only with lexical information,

---

[1] The resource is available at http://www.labinform.ru/pub/ruthes/index.htm

[2] http://ruscorpora.ru

i.e. information about case of nouns that controlled by verb through specified preposition.

Authors review previous works and their limitations like insufficient dictionary size that prevents to use such dictionaries in a computer system. Existing treebanks of Russian language also have insufficient corpus size for automatic generation of a complete verbal subordination dictionary.

There is a difference with previous woks that ambiguous part of text is not processed at all. Authors note that ambiguity in Russian language has a big difference from ambiguity in English. The extraction of verb(-preposition)-noun dependencies is done with six simple finite automaton. Parsing was not used in corpus processing. Result dataset is filtered to exclude grammatical ambiguity, rare word combinations and combinations that are not allowed in Russian grammar. Unfortunately, the dictionary is not available. In this paper we present an alternative method for generating a subordination dictionary using Google Books Ngram Corpus (GBNC).

### 2.4   Google Books Ngram Corpus

This Corpus describes how often words and phrases were used over a period of five centuries, in eight languages; it reflects about 6% of all books ever published. Russian subset of GBNC contains 67,137,666,353 tokens extracted from 591,310 volumes [4] mostly from past three centuries. Each book was scanned with custom equipment and the text was digitized by means of OCR. Only those n-grams that appear over 40 times, are included into the dataset.

The original the GBNC data set contains statistics on occurrences of n-grams (n=1 ... 5) as well as frequencies of binary dependencies between words[3]. These binary dependencies represent syntactic links between words from Google Books texts. The GBNC stores all statistics on a year-by-year basis, each datafile contain tab-separated data in the following format[4]:

```
n-gram, year, match_count, volume_count
```

Latest version of GBNC introduced syntactic annotations: words were tagged with their part-of-speech, and head-modifier relationships were recorded. An accuracy of unlabeled attachment for Russian dependency parser reported in [4] is 86.2% . Syntactic ngrams have been studied by Sidorov et al. in [11], [10] Here, we use these ngrams for generating of new dictionaries.

## 3   A Method for Frame-Like Elements Extraction

We propose a method for extraction basic FrameNet structures from the Google Books N-gram dataset: Frame Elements (FE), Lexical Units (LU) . For each LU, the method provides possible frame candidates and a list of frame elements with

---

[3] http://books.google.com/ngrams/
[4] http://storage.googleapis.com/books/ngrams/books/datasetsv2.html

optional semantic types as well as syntactic realization of the FE. The method
has two main steps. First, the method extracts subordination models for a verb,
and then associates each model with a FE. We describe both steps in a separate
subsections. Due to both steps use a preprocessed GBNC dataset, we describe
the preprocessing step in the first place.

### 3.1 Google Books Dataset Preprocessing

The main preprocessing step that allows using the GBNC is enrichment of the
corpus with morphological information. We have preprocessed the original data
set in a special way. First, for each dependency 2-gram (the same step for each
3-gram), we have collected all its occurrences on the whole data set and added
up all "match_count" values since 1900. Aggregated data set consists of pairs
(n-gram, count), n=2, 3. This step also lowered case of letters in each n-grams
in order to decrease variability.

In the next step we assigned each word in a 1-gram data set a PoS-tag and
morphological features. For this purpose we used an OpenCorpora morphological
dictionary. This resulted in a dataset, that has the following format:

```
n1, match_count, pos, lemma, gram.
```

For ambiguous words we will obtain several records.

```
n1, match_count, pos, lemma, gramA;
n1, match_count, pos, lemma, gramB;
. . .
```

In all such cases, we omitted rows with alternative grammatical interpretations from the dataset, because taking these records into account adds a lot of
noise. This step omit all homonyms from the dataset, but remaining words are
still enough for further steps. We denote a morphologically enriched dataset as
m-GBNC.

### 3.2 A Subordination Dictionary of Russian verbs

When constructing the dictionary of subordination models, we focus on subordination models for Russian verbs. Let us briefly describe a technique we use
to generate a dictionary of subordination models. First, we capture all pairs
(head, dependent) with PoS-tag of the "head" part equals to 'VERB' and with
a certain grammatical case of the "dependent" part, say, 'gent' for the Genitive.
Finally, we group all these pairs by "lemma" (different forms of the verb share
the same "lemma") and count the number of records in each group and add
up match_count values. Basically, we run the following SQL-query against the
m-GBNC dataset ("dep_bigrams" is a name of the table with enriched dependencies data):

```
SELECT dep_bigrams.lemma_id,
    SUM(CASE
      WHEN dep_bigrams.gram LIKE '%nomn%'
      THEN dep_bigrams.count
      ELSE 0 END) AS nomn,
  ...
    SUM(CASE
      WHEN dep_bigrams.gram LIKE '%loct%'
      THEN dep_bigrams.count
      ELSE 0 END) AS loct,
    FROM dep_bigrams
    WHERE dep_bigrams.pos='VERB'
    GROUP BY dep_bigrams.lemma_id;
```

In this example we have six aggregation (sum) functions (one for each grammatical case, e.g. 'loct' for the Locative, 'nomn' for the Nominative). Each aggregation function in the query calculates total amount of dependency links between verbs given a lemma_id and arbitrary word forms in a certain grammatical case. We apply the same technique when generating a model for subordination of a preposition in the 3-gram dataset. These two types of queries differ only in the WHEN-conditions and the GROUP-BY operator that includes additional restriction on the second word (that has to be a preposition) in a 3-gram.

The result of this step is a set of merged records. Each record descries a basic part of subordination model for some verb and has the following format:

```
VERB,
  Nominative_COUNT,
  Genitive_COUNT,
  Dative_COUNT,
  Accusative_COUNT,
  Instrumental_COUNT.
```

We eliminated the Locative case, because in Russian it requires a preposition. This dataset contains about 24 thousand rows (one row per verb). If the verb subordinates a preposition then record has different format:

```
VERB, PREP,
  Nominative_COUNT,
  Genitive_COUNT,
  Dative_COUNT,
  Accusative_COUNT,
  Instrumental_COUNT,
  Locative_COUNT.
```

This dataset contains about 51.5 thousand rows (a verb + preposition per row). Then, we have carried out an additional postprocessing step of the GBNC, a conceptual indexing step. In this step if the second word in 2-gram (or the third word in the 3-gram) have the "NOUN" PoS-tag, then the word is a matter for looking up the RuThes-lite thesaurus for a corresponding concepts. In the case of multiple matches (e. g. multiple word senses), we exclude the corresponding n-gram from the resulting dataset. This preprocessing step resulted in a conceptually enriched dataset (we will refer to it as c-GBNC), that contains the following information for each n-gram:

1) an unambiguous part-of-speech tag and lemma for each word in the n-gram;
2) an unambiguous set of grammatical features (e.g. case, gender, number) for each word in the n-gram;
3) an unambiguous RuThes-lite concept for the last word in the n-gram.

Thus, after this step the dataset is enriched with grammatical and semantic information.

### 3.3   A Dictionary of Semantic Types and Frame Elements Extraction

Frame elements can be discovered from the c-GBNC dataset using valences of a given verb. But, FEs form different frames may share the same verb and its subordination model. In this case, FEs can be discovered using differences in senses of a subordinate noun. Thus, the next step is building a dictionary of semantic types and attaching a subordination model of a given verb to one or more semantic types from the dictionary.

We use top level concepts of the RuThes-lite as a dictionary of basic semantic types. As the RuThes-lite has too few concepts (such as "Persistent Entity", "Occurrent Entity", "Role, Place", etc.) at the top level, we consider such distinctions as insufficient. We extended the dictionary with immediate descendants of the top concepts and obtained about 150 concepts (further we call them "semantic types"). Using a hierarchy of the RuThes-lite, each concept can be mapped to a certain semantic type from the dictionary.

The main idea behind creating the dictionary of semantic types is discovering of frame elements. We claim that a FE may be defined by a unique combination of a verb sense, a case of a subordinated noun (or noun phrase), and the semantic type of the noun. Distinct semantic types will describe differences between FEs sharing the same verb and noun case. Of course, the unique combination should include prepositions if it is the case in a subordinate model of the given verb. This is illustrated in the following examples: ходить в одиночестве (to walk alone), ходить в шортах (to walk in shorts), ходить в городе (to walk in the city). All three phrases have the same syntactic realization, but have different semantic types of subordinate nouns. We discovered FEs for about 10,000 Russian verbs.

## 4   Experiments and Discussion

We have run few experiments for the proposed methods, i.e. extraction of subordination models and discovering FEs. We also evaluated FE discovery algorithm on English GBNC dataset, using English FrameNet and Wordnet. We observed a possibility for extension of the English FrameNet using our FE discovery method.

## 4.1  Extraction of Subordination Models

In order to extract subordination models, we have run two types of SQL-queries, described in the previous section, against the m-GBNC dataset. We have got about 24 thousand rows (one row per verb) from the dependency pair dataset and about 51.5 thousand rows from the 3-gram dataset (a verb + preposition per row). Samples from the resulted subordination models dictionary are provided in Table 1 and Table 2. The normalized weights (representing fraction of corresponding grammatical case) can further be used in modeling a probability for a given verb to superordinate a word in particular case.

The interesting result is that many verbs can superordinate nouns (as direct object) in almost any grammatical form. However, in most rows there is a singe dominating grammatical case (or two). Subordination of preposition is different.

**Table 1.** Generated subordination models of direct object for frequent Russian verbs

| Major case | Genitive | Dative | Accusative | Instrum. | Infinitive form |
|---|---|---|---|---|---|
| Dative | 0.024 | 0.905 | 0.002 | 0.060 | помочь - to help |
| Dative | 0.067 | 0.679 | 0.174 | 0.060 | передать - to transmit |
| Dative | 0.183 | 0.573 | 0.057 | 0.133 | сказать - to say |
| Dative | 0.194 | 0.511 | 0.252 | 0.025 | дать - to give |
| Dative | 0.171 | 0.504 | 0.005 | 0.296 | ответить - to answer |
| Dative | 0.192 | 0.434 | 0.070 | 0.166 | говорить - to talk |
| Dative | 0.163 | 0.433 | 0.191 | 0.041 | строить - to build |
| Dative | 0.185 | 0.433 | 0.170 | 0.178 | показать - to show |
| Dative | 0.207 | 0.389 | 0.174 | 0.123 | писать - to write |
| Dative | 0.299 | 0.380 | 0.252 | 0.046 | давать - to give |
| Dative | 0.216 | 0.377 | 0.338 | 0.056 | указать - to point |
| Dative | 0.109 | 0.371 | 0.323 | 0.188 | доказать - to prove |
| Dative | 0.239 | 0.366 | 0.046 | 0.228 | судить - to judge |
| Genitive | 0.409 | 0.359 | 0.127 | 0.080 | делать - to do |
| Accusative | 0.131 | 0.338 | 0.352 | 0.115 | изменить - to change |
| Instrum. | 0.093 | 0.292 | 0.113 | 0.489 | объяснить - to explain |
| Instrum. | 0.149 | 0.280 | 0.006 | 0.498 | действовать - to act |
| Accusative | 0.148 | 0.271 | 0.454 | 0.075 | написать - to write |
| Instrum. | 0.147 | 0.264 | 0.083 | 0.462 | смотреть - to look |
| Accusative | 0.157 | 0.264 | 0.377 | 0.176 | представить - to represent |
| Accusative | 0.203 | 0.227 | 0.397 | 0.063 | оставить - to leave |
| Instrum. | 0.050 | 0.209 | 0.008 | 0.724 | служить - to serve |
| Accusative | 0.196 | 0.198 | 0.449 | 0.102 | читать - to read |
| Instrum. | 0.171 | 0.190 | 0.015 | 0.530 | жить - to live |
| Genitive | 0.377 | 0.188 | 0.087 | 0.210 | есть - to be |

**Table 2.** Generated subordination models of prepositions for verb "купить" (to buy)

| Preposition | Major case | Genitive | Dative | Accusative | Instrum. | Locative |
|---|---|---|---|---|---|---|
| для (for) | Genitive | 1.0 | 0.0 | 0.0 | 0.0 | 0.0 |
| из (from) | Genitive | 1.0 | 0.0 | 0.0 | 0.0 | 0.0 |
| без (without) | Genitive | 1.0 | 0.0 | 0.0 | 0.0 | 0.0 |
| до (before) | Genitive | 1.0 | 0.0 | 0.0 | 0.0 | 0.0 |
| с (with) | Genitive | 0.595 | 0.0 | 0.0 | 0.405 | 0.0 |
| в (in) | Locative | 0.0 | 0.011 | 0.068 | 0.0 | 0.921 |
| к (to) | Dative | 0.0 | 1.0 | 0.0 | 0.0 | 0.0 |
| на (on) | Locative | 0.0 | 0.049 | 0.138 | 0.005 | 0.808 |
| по (for) | Dative | 0.0 | 1.000 | 0.0 | 0.0 | 0.0 |
| под (under) | Instrum. | 0.0 | 0.0 | 0.0 | 1.0 | 0.0 |

**Table 3.** Frame elements extracted from GBNC for verb "купить" (to buy)

| Case | Preposition | Nouns | RuThes Concepts | Semantic Types | Count of Concepts |
|---|---|---|---|---|---|
| Locative | в - in | Лондоне (London), *среднем (average)*, магазинах (shops), ... | ЛОНДОН (London), *СРЕДНИЙ (average)* , МАГАЗИН (shop), ... | ФИЗИЧЕСКАЯ СУЩНОСТЬ (PHYSICAL ENTITY), *АБСТРАКТНАЯ СУЩНОСТЬ (ABSTRACT ENTITY)* ФИЗИЧЕСКАЯ СУЩНОСТЬ (PHYSICAL ENTITY) | 15 |
| Locative | на - at | базаре (Bazaar), рынке (Market), *аукционе (Auction)* ... | РЫНОК (MARKET), БАЗАР (BAZAAR), *РЫНОЧНАЯ ЭКОНОМИКА (MARKET ECONOMY)*, *АУКЦИОН (AUCTION)* ... | ФИЗИЧЕСКАЯ СУЩНОСТЬ (PHYSICAL ENTITY), *ЗАНЯТИЕ (ACTIVITY)*, *ДЕЯТЕЛЬНОСТЬ (ACTIVITY)* ... | 5 |
| Genitive | для - for | колхоза (farm), жены (wife) | КОЛХОЗ (FARM), ЖЕНА (WIFE) | СУБЪЕКТ ДЕЯТЕЛЬНОСТИ (ACTOR), ФИЗИЧЕСКАЯ СУЩНОСТЬ (PHYSICAL ENTITY) | 2 |
| Dative | – | сыну (son), мальчику (boy), правительству (government), крестьянам (peasants), ... | СЫН (SON), МАЛЬЧИК (BOY), ПРАВИТЕЛЬСТВО (GOVERNMENT), КРЕСТЬЯНИН (PEASANT), ... | ФИЗИЧЕСКАЯ СУЩНОСТЬ (PHYSICAL ENTITY), СОВОКУПНОСТЬ ЛЮДЕЙ (GROUP OF PEOPLE), ... | 23 |

## 4.2   Frame Elements Extraction

In the second experiment we discovered frame elements. The total amount of discovered FEs cover about 10,000 verbs, due to elimination of nouns with multiple senses. Table 3 shows a sample of the result dataset for verb купить (to buy). The sample illustrates both situations when splitting of FE (Locative-rows) and merging of FE (Genitive- and Dative-rows) are needed. The result dataset of extracted FEs is available on-line[5].

In the Table 3 we labeled few rows with bold. These rows include concepts with significantly different meanings. This heterogeneity in a set of frame elements indicates that corresponding combination of verb, preposition and case covers more than one semantic role, and possibly needs splitting into two or more roles.

In a separate experiment we evaluated our method on English GBNC dataset. For English both GBNC data and WordNet are available, so we used Wordnet instead of the RuThes-lite. We run FE extraction algorithm on the English GBNC dataset and compared results to the English FrameNet. We examined all extracted FEs for the a single verb "to buy". Each FE that appears in English FrameNet (as of version 1.5) also appears in the set of extracted FEs. Additionally, our method extracted several FEs that were not described in the FrameNet. For example, the following FE:

"to buy *into* the house, firm, business, company, etc."

This FEs should not be confused with another one "to buy into the idea". The latter was extracted too, but it has different meaning and should be considered as a part of another frame.

## 5   Conclusion

In this article we propose a method that facilitates a process of semi-automatic FrameNet construction. The method extracts a subordination dictionary from n-gram dataset. The resulting dictionary for Russian contains more than 75 thousand units: both pairs (verb + case of subordinated word) and triples (verb + preposition + case of subordinated word). The dictionary is bigger than others and includes frequency information about a syntactic construction. Using this dictionary and RuThes-lite thesaurus we conducted a set of semantic frame elements for more than 10 thousand of Russian verbs. The resulting dataset forms a basis for semi-automatic construction of a FrameNet for Russian.

In our future work we plan to evaluate the quality of method by running the FE extraction algorithm on datasets for other languages (German and Spanish). For those languages both GBNC data and thesauri as well as parsers are available. We plan to compare results to existing approaches (e.g. to the method proposed in [2]). Another direction is to develop a Russian FrameNet by aggregating similar senses of verbs together.

---

[5] http://framenet.s3-website-us-east-1.amazonaws.com/

**Acknowledgments.** This work was funded by the subsidy allocated to Kazan Federal University for the state assignment in the sphere of scientific activities. This research was partially supported by Russian Foundation for Basic Research (grant 13-07-00773).

# References

1. Baker, C.F., Fillmore, C.J., Cronin, B.: The structure of the framenet database. International Journal of Lexicography 16(3), 281–296 (2003)
2. Castro-Sánchez, N.A., Sidorov, G.: Analysis of definitions of verbs in an explanatory dictionary for automatic extraction of actants based on detection of patterns. In: Hopfe, C.J., Rezgui, Y., Métais, E., Preece, A., Li, H. (eds.) NLDB 2010. LNCS, vol. 6177, pp. 233–239. Springer, Heidelberg (2010)
3. Koeva, S.: Lexicon and grammar in bulgarian framenet. In: LREC (2010)
4. Lin, Y., Michel, J.-B., Aiden, E.L., Orwant, J., Brockman, W., Petrov, S.: Syntactic annotations for the google books ngram corpus. In: Proceedings of the ACL 2012 System Demonstrations, pp. 169–174. Association for Computational Linguistics (2012)
5. Loukachevitch, N., Dobrov, B.: Ruthes linguistic ontology vs. russian wordnets. In: Proceedings of Global WordNet Conference GWC-2014, Tartu (2014)
6. Lyashevskaya, O.: Dictionary of valencies meets corpus annotation: A case of russian framebank. Proceedings of EURALEX 15 (2012)
7. Palmer, M., Gildea, D., Kingsbury, P.: The proposition bank: An annotated corpus of semantic roles. Computational linguistics 31(1), 71–106 (2005)
8. Kochetkova, N.A., Klyshinsky, E.S.: A method of automatic generating of russian verb subordination models. In: Proceedings of the In XII National Conference of Artificial Intelligence (2013)
9. Schuler, K.K.: Verbnet: A broad-coverage, comprehensive verb lexicon (2005)
10. Sidorov, G.: Syntactic dependency based n-grams in rule based automatic english as second language grammar correction. International Journal of Computational Linguistics and Applications 4(2), 169–188 (2013)
11. Sidorov, G., Velasquez, F., Stamatatos, E., Gelbukh, A., Chanona-Hernández, L.: Syntactic n-grams as machine learning features for natural language processing. Expert Systems with Applications 41(3), 853–860 (2014)
12. Tonelli, S., Pianta, E.: Frame information transfer from english to italian. In: LREC (2008)

# Modeling Natural Language Metaphors
# with an Answer Set Programming Framework

Juan Carlos Acosta-Guadarrama[1], Rogelio Dávila-Pérez[2], Mauricio Osorio[3],
and Victor Hugo Zaldivar[4],*

[1] Universidad Autónoma del Estado de México,
Toluca, Estado de México, México
jguadarrama@gmail.com

[2] División de Posgrado, Universidad Autónoma de Guadalajara,
Zapopan, Jal., México
rdav90@gmail.com

[3] Universidad de las Américas, Puebla,
Cholula, Puebla, México
osoriomauri@gmail.com

[4] Departamento de Electrónica, Sistemas e Informática,
Instituto Tecnológico y de Estudios Superiores de Occidente,
Tlaquepaque, Jal., México
victorhugo@iteso.mx

**Abstract.** Metaphors are natural language constructions that play an
important role in the way human beings communicate knowledge and understand
the world. Some formal philosophers such as Searle and Lakoff
claim that the semantic analysis of expressions that involve fictional stories
and metaphors are examples of the inadequacy of using predicate
logic for the analysis of the meaning of language. D'Hanis proposes that
using predicate logic in combination of non-monotonic reasoning is possible
to interpret metaphorical expressions. In this paper, we introduce
an approach for modelling metaphorical thinking using a particular form
of logic programming called *answer set programming* (ASP). ASP essentially
enhances the logical apparatus of predicate calculus by introducing
mechanisms such as *negation as a failure* that enable the system to
accomplish *non-monotonic reasoning*. We show that using ASP is possible
to model the meaning of some expressions involving metaphorical
constructions and the implementation of metaphorical reasoning mechanisms
that could be a great addition to any knowledge-based application.

**Keywords:** metaphors, metaphorical thinking, philosophical logic, non-monotonic
reasoning, answer-set programming.

## 1 Introduction

Metaphors are not just a linguistic phenomenon or an atypical use of language.
Either from a philosophical point of view, such as Wittgenstein's family resem-

---

* Authors are listed in alphabetical order, their position does not represent their contribution
to the present document.

A. Gelbukh et al. (Eds.): MICAI 2014, Part I, LNAI 8856, pp. 28–36, 2014.

blance [1] or from a more empirical point of view such as Searle [2] and Lakoff [3, 4] , one can say that metaphors play a central role in human cognition, a role that has not been properly addressed in knowledge representation or natural language processing systems.

What is a metaphor and why is it so important? According to Indurkhya [5], in a metaphor we must have a source and a target. A metaphor consists in describing the target, an object or an event, in terms of concepts that belongs to the source. A metaphor is made meaningful by interpreting the source unconventionally in the target. Metaphor interpretation is subjective, in part because the conventional meaning of words and phrases are also subjective. Moreover, metaphors are asymmetric.[1]

Thus, the metaphorical content of a description is a notion of degree. There are statements that are clearly metaphorical such as: "The sky is crying". While for some others it is not clear, such as: "The chairman of the meeting plowed through the agenda". Some authors [6] consider that the metaphorical content dissolves as the phrases are used in daily basis. This issue is an open discussion and is beyond the scope of this paper.

As we can see, metaphors play a central role in the way people *see* the world. That is, in the way that people organize and interact with their knowledge of the world. That means that any knowledge system aiming at understanding and using metaphors must consider not only assigning a meaning to a metaphorical description, but also some metaphorical mechanisms used in building categories and reasoning with them. These metaphorical reasoning mechanisms will be a great addition to any knowledge-based application, especially those aiming at dealing with ontologies.

In the following section, we introduce briefly Answer-Set Programming[2]. In section 3, a formal framework is build to accomplish the analysis of metaphorical expressions. In section 4, we undertake the modeling of metaphorical expressions. In section 5, we draw some conclusions pointing out the simplicity in which this reasoning mechanism could be integrated in a knowledge-based system.

## 2    Preliminaries

Finally, in this paper we assume that the reader is familiar with basic notions of logic programming [6] and in particular with Answer-Sets Programming, ASP.

*Answer-Set Programming*, also known as A-Prolog [7], represents a relatively new paradigm for *logic programming*. ASP is a declarative knowledge representation that is implemented as a logic programming language. ASP allows solving problems with default knowledge and produce *non-monotonic reasoning* using the notion of *negation as a failure*. ASP in contrast with Prolog, covers the whole

---

[1] That is, when the source and target of a metaphor are reversed, the meaning can change and the description may even cease to be a metaphor. Consider for instance "Computers are brains" vs. "Brains are Computers".

[2] In this paper we assume that the reader is familiar with basic notions of logic programming [16] and in particular with ASP.

language of predicate logic, introducing the classical negation (represented by the symbol "−" in the formulae), which is different from the symbol for negation as a failure: *not*.

There are several popular software implementations to compute *answer sets*. In this work, we verified our experiments with an open source solver called **dlv**.[3] The efficiency of such solvers has increased the practical list of applications in the areas of planning, intelligent agents and artificial intelligence.

We represent knowledge by means of Answer Set Programming (ASP), as it is one of the most studied and successful semantics to reason about incomplete (unknown) information; in this section, we provide a very-short description of ASP, which is identified with other names like *Stable Semantics for Logic Programming* or *Stable Model Semantics* [8] and **A-Prolog**. Its formal language and some more notation are introduced in our context as follows:

**Definition 1 (ASP Language of logic programs, $\mathcal{L}_{ASP}$).** *In the following $\mathcal{L}_{ASP}$ is a language of propositional logic with symbols: $a_0, a_1, \ldots$; connectives: "," (conjunction) and meta-connective ";"; disjunction $\vee$, also denoted as $|$; $\leftarrow$ (also denoted as $\rightarrow$); $\neg$ (negation as failure or weak negation, also denoted with the word* not*); "$\sim$" (strong negation, equally denoted as "−"). The propositional symbols, $\Sigma$, are also called atoms or atomic propositions. A literal is an atom or a strong-negated atom. A rule $\rho$ is an ordered pair $h(\rho) \leftarrow b(\rho)$, where $h(\rho)$ is a possibly-empty set of literals, and $b(\rho)$ is a possibly-empty set of literals or $\neg$-negated literals.*

For convenience, we shall constrain to a finite set of literals. With the notation just introduced in Definition 1, one may construct program clauses of several forms that are well known in the literature, such as Extended Logic Program (ELP), Extended Disjunctive Logic Program (EDLP), etc. In particular we shall use **EDLP**, as in Definition 1.

We can also have a shorthand notation when using *variables* in a rule, which we call a schema for the set of its *ground instantiations*. Finally, a *logic program* (or just program) is a possibly empty finite set of such rules.

Informally, the semantics of such programs consists in reducing the general rules to rules without negation-as-failture "$\neg$", because the latter are universally well understood. For page limitation, we just skip the formal definition of such reduct, which can be easily found in the literature [8].

## 3 Metaphors in ASP

The modelling of metaphorical reasoning in a non-monotonic framework is proposed by D'Hanis[9]. In her paper, she models the meaning of metaphorical expressions in a formal system that she calls *adaptive logic*. Adaptive logic is structured in three layers: an Upper Limit Logic (ULL), a Lower Limit Logic (LLL) and an *adaptive strategy* . The adaptive strategy is what makes the system

---

[3] **DLV** solver, could be downloaded from: http://www.dbai.tuwien.ac.at/proj/dlv

non-monotonic, the logic layers are standard first order logic. Different expressions are stated at both levels and represent the before/after states of the system. Expressions are first modelled in ULL, then the adaptive strategy makes a revision of which formulae hold and which do not hold anymore leaving in LLL just the consistent formulae. Even thought the idea is quite interesting we have no evidence of any system in which this approach could be implemented for automatic reasoning. In this document we show how metaphorical expressions can be modelled in first order logic and implemented in an appealing form of *logic programming* called *Answer Set Programming*. As far as we know this is the first attempt to analyse metaphorical expressions using ASP.

## 3.1   Metaphors

Inspired iin [10, 11], we can summarize some general characteristics of a metaphor interpretation as follows:

**mechanism:** Metaphor is a mechanism through which we learn abstract concepts and conclude abstractions.
**context:** Most of our conceptual system is not metaphorical.
**grounding:** Metaphors are grounded in non-metaphorical knowledge.
**concretion:** Metaphors allow us to understand them in terms of a more concrete ground.
**mapping:** Metaphors are asymmetrical partial ontological relations across conceptual domains.
**projection:** Metaphors can project source inference patterns onto target ones.
**invariance:** This principle states that mappings from the metaphor domain structure shall be consistent with the target structure.

Although very general, these characteristics should be some how featured in our following framework.

## 3.2   The Logical Framework

In this section we define a program transformation to ensure which features one wishes to keep from a given ontology, not to rise empty models.

We call *ontological rule* $\rho$ an ASP rule, $h(\rho) \leftarrow b(\rho)$, where cardinalities $|h(\rho)| = |b(\rho)| = 1$ and $h(\rho)$ is called a *property* of $b(\rho)$. An *ontology* $\mathcal{T}$ is a collection of ontological rules. Finally, a *rhetoric theory* is an EDLP, $\mathcal{P}$, where $\mathcal{T}_1 \subset \mathcal{P}$ is an ontology.

Formally, given an ontological rule $\rho$ over $\mathcal{L}_{\mathsf{ASP}}$, its *metaphorical form* corresponds to rule $h(\rho) \leftarrow b(\rho) \cup \{\neg \widetilde{h(\rho)}\}$, where $\widetilde{\alpha} = \sim\alpha$ and $\widetilde{\sim\alpha} = \alpha$, for all $\mathcal{L}_{\mathsf{ASP}}$-atom $\alpha$.

In addition, a *metaphorical ontology* is a collection of *metaphorical propositions*. We can define another program transformation out of an original rhetoric theory as follows:

**Definition 2 (Metaphoric Program).** *Given a rhetoric theory* $\mathcal{P}$ *over a set of atoms* $\Sigma$ *and its corresponding ontology* $\mathcal{T} \subseteq \mathcal{P}$*, its corresponding* metaphoric program *is* $(\mathcal{P} \setminus \mathcal{T}) \cup \mathcal{T}'$*, where* $\mathcal{T}'$ *is the metaphorical ontology of* $\mathcal{T}$*.*

The model of a metaphoric program corresponds to the minimal set inclusion from the answer sets of the former.

**Definition 3 (Metaphoric Model).** *Given a rhetoric theory* $\mathcal{P}$ *over a set of atoms* $\Sigma$*, the set* $\mathcal{M} \subseteq \Sigma$ *is a* metaphoric model *of* $\mathcal{P}$ *if and only if* $\mathcal{M}$ *is minimal with respect to set inclusion from the answer sets of the resulting metaphoric program out of* $\mathcal{P}$

### 3.3    Reasoning with Ontological Theories in **ASP**

Language is mainly devised for communication, that is, the aim of language is to allow for transference of ideas from one individual to others. Metaphors are powerful language constructions that communicate ideas. With the background introduced in previous section and inspired with the works from [9], we can model the following story.

*Example 1.* Consider the following scenario:

1. Mary and Paul and John work at Isaac Newton College.
2. Mary and Paul are teachers.

We are interested in analysing the meaning of the two metaphoric expressions:

1. *"John is a donkey"*.
2. *"Paul is a donkey"*.

In order to formalize the original scenario, we assume that we have a finite language including among other, *john, mary*, etc., and we have a metaphoric program, $\mathcal{P}$ over the language. We need to introduce some dot-separated facts, like membership $M^2$ to Isaac Newton College—*inc*:

$$M(mary, inc).$$
$$M(john, inc).$$
$$M(paul, inc).$$

We keep this list open as we do not know if there are more employees that work for the same school, who can be *updated* at a later state. Then we proceed to add a list of teachers, $T$:

$$T(mary).$$
$$T(paul).$$

In this case, we add a *closed-word assumption* saying that any human $x$ is not teacher when we have no evidence of it:

$$\sim T(x) \leftarrow H(x), \neg T(x).$$

Then we include the fact that "*a teacher $x$ can not be a stupid $x \notin D_s$*":

$$\sim D_s(x) \leftarrow T(x).$$

Then we add some facts about gender, where $G_m$ stands for man and $G_w$ woman:

$$G_w(mary).$$
$$G_m(paul).$$
$$G_m(john).$$

Now, some well-known facts about humans and donkeys are needed:

1. *Every man and all womans are humans $H$, all donkeys and every human are mammals $M_m$, every mammal is an animal $A$, and every animal is something that is alive $L$.* We can express these facts in predicate logic using properties, and in ASP introducing rules into our ontology $\mathcal{T}$ as:

$$H(x) \leftarrow G_m(x). \ \ H(x) \leftarrow G_w(x).$$
$$M_m(x) \leftarrow D(x). \ \ M_m(x) \leftarrow H(x).$$
$$A(x) \leftarrow M_m(x). \ \ L(x) \leftarrow A(x).$$

2. We also have some constraints: "*men are not donkeys*", or in other words: "*no individual can be both a donkey and a human being*". This constrain is introduced as a rule with empty head:

$$\emptyset \leftarrow H(x), D(x) \tag{1}$$

which means that being a donkey and a human is a contradiction (i.e. has no model). In other words,

$$\bot \leftarrow H(x), D(x)$$

where $\bot$ is our logical constant for *false*.

But it will be worth for this proposition being stated in a more general way by considering that for any animal $x$ for which we do not have evidence that is a donkey, we can assume that it is not a donkey:

$$\sim D(x) \leftarrow A(x), \neg D(x).$$

Now, when we model the meaning of the metaphoric expression "*John is a donkey*":

$$\mathcal{P} \cup \{D(john)\}.$$

By adding this fact to the original theory, we can make some inferences in $\mathcal{L}_{\mathsf{ASP}}$:

$$G_m(john),$$
$$H(john),$$
$$D(john)$$

which leads up to a contradiction, just because of the constraint we introduced in (1): Equivalently, $\sim D(john) \leftarrow H(john)$, which makes us conclude that both $\sim D(john)$ and $D(john)$!

The source of the problem is that the sentence "*John is a donkey*" is a *metaphoric expression*, which means it should not be taken literally. The general idea is as follows:

There is a knowledge base $\mathcal{P}$, and a new formula $\alpha \notin \mathcal{P}$, that you want to add up to $\mathcal{P}$. Then, if the result of introducing $\alpha$ into $\mathcal{P}$, introduces a contradiction, i.e. $\mathcal{P} \cup \{\alpha\}$ has no model.

Then, before discarding $\alpha$, we must consider the possibility that it is not a typical expression but might be a metaphoric expression.

## 4   Modeling Metaphorical Expressions

We have a knowledge base $\mathcal{P}$ called rhetoric, than contains different forms of knowledge. We have to introduce a subset of $\mathcal{P}$, which contains general knowledge related to the predicate donkey. By following our framework, let us call this set ontology, $\mathcal{T} \subset \mathcal{P}$. It contains well-known properties of a donkey that includes:

1. Donkeys have long ears, $D_e(x) \leftarrow D(x)$.
2. Donkeys are stupid, $D_s(x) \leftarrow D(x)$.
3. Donkeys are stubborn, $D_m(x) \leftarrow D(x)$.
4. Donkeys bray, $D_b(x) \leftarrow D(x)$.

These facts can be introduced as rules in ASP.

Now, to analyse the metaphorical expression, "*John is a donkey*", we must introduce the notion of metaphorical donkey, that is, a donkey that has certain properties that can be inherited by a human being.

The metaphorical program in our approach corresponds to $(\mathcal{P} \setminus \mathcal{T}) \cup \mathcal{T}'$, where $\mathcal{P}$ corresponds the rhetoric theory out of the ontology $\mathcal{T}$ and the original set of rules.

The proposition that asserts that "*John is a metaphorical donkey*" is: $D(john)$. We call this formula a *metaphorical proposition*. To interpret a rhetoric theory in our approach, we shall transform it into a *metaphoric program* in which we will include some properties about metaphorical donkeys $\mathcal{T}'$—these properties are metaphoric forms of the donkey properties. Take for example:

1. Metaphorical donkeys are normally stupid.

$$D_s(x) \leftarrow D(x), \neg \sim D_s(x).$$

This clause should be read as: If $x$ is a metaphorical donkey, and there is no evidence that it is not a stupid, then we conclude that it is a stupid.
2. Similarly, metaphorical donkeys are normally stubborn:

$$D_m(x) \leftarrow D(x), \neg \sim D_m(x).$$

With this example we can analyse the reasoning process: Since John is a metaphorical donkey and there is no evidence that John is not stupid and there is no evidence as well that John is not stubborn, then the extended metaphoric program in ASP concludes that John is stupid and stubborn:

$$D_s(john).D_m(john).$$

Now, to understand how the non-monotonic reasoning framework works, when adding to the metaphoric program the fact that *"Paul is a donkey"*: $\mathcal{P}' \cup \{D(paul)\}$, it concludes that he is stubborn:

$$D_m(paul).$$

But, why did the system not conclude that *"Paul is a stupid"* as it happened with John? The reason is that *"Paul is a teacher"* and the metaphoric program knows that *"a teacher can not be a stupid"*.

## 5   Experimental Results

By interpreting the principles in Section 3.1, we can introduce a generalised metaphor interpretation, $\mu$, and encode them in a few properties as follows, which are met and can be easily verified.

Given a *rhetoric theory* $\mathcal{T}$, a possibly-empty metaphorical ontology $\mathcal{T}_m \subset \mathcal{T}$, any proposition $\psi \in \mathcal{T}$ and $\psi \notin \mathcal{T}_m$,

*Closure*: $\mu(\mathcal{T}) = \mathsf{Cn}(\mu(\mathcal{T}))$ is a rhetoric theory.
*Success*: $\mathcal{T}_m \subseteq \mathcal{T}$.
*Inclusion*: $\mu(\mathcal{T}_m) \subseteq \mathsf{Cn}(\mathcal{T})$.

which correspond to the three properties listed in th previous section.

## 6   Conclusions and Further Work

We have introduced some metaphorical expressions and shown possible problems with attempting an interpretation of them. Then we incorporated a new kind of *entity* called *metaphorical entity* [9], and an extension for the knowledge base that incorporates knowledge that can be applied to the target of the metaphorical expression. Then we showed how clear and easily we could formalize a system based in ASP for interpreting some metaphoric constructions with great possibilities of being part of an automatic reasoning system.

The approach proposed in this document is just a first glance of what could be achieved if we combine first order predicate logic in a framework of Answer Set Programming. As far as we know this is the first attempt to analyse metaphorical expressions using ASP.

# References

[1] Wittgenstein, L.: Philosophical Investigations. Macmillan (1953)
[2] Searle, J.R.: Speech Acts. Cambridge University Press, Cambridge (1969)
[3] Lakoff, G., Johnson, M.: Metaphors we live by. University of Chicago Press (1980)
[4] Lakoff, G.: Women, Fire and Dangerous Things. University of Chicago Press, Chicago (1987)
[5] Indurkhya, B.: Metaphor and Cognition. Kluwer Academic Publishers, Dordrecht (1992)
[6] Lloyd, J.W.: Foundations of Logic Programming, 2nd edn. Springer, Berlin (1987)
[7] Gelfond, M., Kahl, Y.: Knowledge Representation, Reasoning, and de Design of Intelligent Agents: The Answer-Set Programming Approach. Cambridge University Press, Cambridge (2014)
[8] Gelfond, M., Lifschitz, V.: The stable model semantics for logic programming. In: Kowalski, R.A., Bowen, K.A. (eds.) Proceedings of the Fifth International Conference and Symposium ICLP/SLP, pp. 1070–1080. MIT Press, Seattle (1988)
[9] D'Hanis, I.: A logical approach to the analysis of metaphors. In: Logic and Computational Aspects of Model–Based Reasoning, San Jose, CA. Applied Logic Series, vol. 25, pp. 21–37 (2002)
[10] Ortony, A.: Metaphor and though. Cambridge University Press, Cambridge (1993)
[11] Gibbs, R.W.: The Cambridge handbook of metaphor and thought. Cambridge University Press, Cambridge (2008)

# Whole-Part Relations Rule-Based Automatic Identification: Issues from Fine-Grained Error Analysis

Ilia Markov[1], Nuno Mamede[2,3], and Jorge Baptista[3,4]

[1] Centro de Investigación en Computación (CIC),
Instituto Politécnico Nacional (IPN)
México D.F., Mexico
`markovilya@yahoo.com`
[2] Universidade do Algarve/FCHS and CECL
Faro, Portugal
`jbaptis@ualg.pt`
[3] INESC-ID Lisboa/L2F – Spoken Language Lab
Lisboa, Portugal
`{Nuno.Mamede,jbaptis}l2f.inesc-id.pt`
[4] Universidade de Lisboa/IST
Lisboa, Portugal
`Nuno.Mamede@ist.utl.pt`

**Abstract.** In this paper, we focus on the most frequent errors that occurred during the implementation of a rule-based module for semantic relations extraction, which has been integrated in STRING, a hybrid statistical and rule-based Natural Language Processing chain for Portuguese. We focus on *whole-part* relations (*meronymy*), that is, a semantic relation between an entity that is perceived as a constituent part of another entity, or a member of a set. In this case, we target the type of meronymy involving human entities and *body-part nouns*. We describe with some detail the decisions that were made in order to overcome the errors produced by the system and the solutions adopted to improve its performance.

**Keywords:** whole-part relation, meronymy, body-part noun, Portuguese, error analysis.

## 1 Introduction

Automatic identification of semantic relations contributes to cohesion and coherence of a text and can be useful in several other Natural Language Processing (NLP) tasks such as opinion mining, question answering, text summarization, machine translation, information extraction, information retrieval, and others [10].

The goal of this work is to improve the extraction of semantic relations between textual elements in STRING, a hybrid statistical and rule-based NLP

A. Gelbukh et al. (Eds.): MICAI 2014, Part I, LNAI 8856, pp. 37–50, 2014.

chain for Portuguese[1] [17], by targeting the most frequent errors that occured during the implementation of the whole-part relations extraction module. Whole-part relations (*meronymy*) is a semantic relation between an entity that is perceived as a constituent part of another entity, or a member of a set. In this case, we focus on the type of meronymy involving human entities and *body-part nouns* (henceforward, *Nbp*) when they co-occur in texts.

This paper is structured as follows: Section 2 briefly describes related work on whole-part dependencies extraction, while Section 3 explains how this task was implemented in STRING; Section 4 presents the evaluation procedure; Section 5 describes with some detail how the error analysis was carried out; Section 6 illustrates the results of the performance of the system after the error analysis; and Section 7 draws the conclusions.

## 2   Related Work

Meronymy is a complex relation that "should be treated as a collection of relations, not as a single relation" [15]. In NLP, various information extraction techniques have been developed in order to capture whole-part relations from texts.

Hearst [13] tried to find lexical correlates to the *hyponymic* relations (type-of relations) by searching in unrestricted, domain-independent text for cases where known hyponyms appear in proximity. The author proposed six lexico-syntactic patterns; he then tested the patterns for validity and used them to extract relations from a corpus. To validate his acquisition method, the author compared the results of the algorithm with information found in WordNet [4]. The author reports that when the set of 152 relations that fit the restrictions of the experiment (both the hyponyms and the hypernyms are unmodified) was looked up in WordNet: "180 out of the 226 unique words involved in the relations actually existed in the hierarchy, and 61 out of the 106 feasible relations (*i.e.*, relations in which both terms were already registered in WordNet) were found." [13, p. 544]. The author claims that he tried applying the same technique to meronymy, but without great success.

Girju *et al.* [10,11] present a supervised, domain independent approach for the automatic detection of whole-part relations in text. The algorithm identifies lexico-syntactic patterns that encode whole-part relations. The authors report an overall average precision of 80.95% and recall of 75.91%. The authors also state that they came across a large number of difficulties due to the highly ambiguous nature of syntactic constructions.

Van Hage *et al.* [12] developed a method for learning whole-part relations from vocabularies and text sources. The authors reported that they were able to acquire 503 whole-part pairs from the AGROVOC Thesaurus[2] to learn 91 reliable whole-part patterns. They changed the patterns' part arguments with known entities to

---

[1] https://string.l2f.inesc-id.pt/ [last access: 22/09/2014].

[2] http://www.fao.org/agrovoc [last access: 12.08.2014].

introduce web-search queries. Corresponding whole entities were then extracted from documents in the query results, with a precision of 74%.

The Espresso algorithm [24] was developed in order to harvest semantic relations in a text. The algorithm extracts surface patterns by connecting the seeds (tuples) in a given corpus. The algorithm obtains a precision of 80% in learning whole-part relations from the Acquaint (TREC-9) newswire text collection, with almost 6 million words.

Some work has already been done on building *knowledge bases* for Portuguese, most of which include the concept of whole-part relations. These knowledge bases are often referred to as *lexical ontologies*, because they have properties of a lexicon as well as properties of an ontology [14,26]. Well-known, existing lexical ontologies for Portuguese are Portuguese WordNet.PT [19,20], later extended to WordNet.PT Global (Rede Léxico-Conceptual das Variedades do Português) [21]; MWN.PT-MultiWordNet of Portuguese [25]; PAPEL (Palavras Associadas Porto Editora Linguateca) [23]; and Onto.PT [22]. Some of these ontologies are not freely available for the general public, while others just provide the definitions associated to each lexical entry without the information on whole-part relations. Furthermore, the type of whole-part relation targeted in this work, involving any human entity and its related *Nbp*, can not be adequately captured using those resources (or, at least, only those resources)[3].

Attention was also paid to two well-known parsers of Portuguese, in order to discern how do they handle the whole-part relations extraction: the PALAVRAS parser [2], consulted using the Visual Interactive Syntax Learning (*VISL*) environment, and LX Semantic Role Labeller [3]. Judging from the available online versions/demos of these systems, apparently, none of these parsers extracts whole-part relations, at least explicitly.

## 3 Whole-Part Dependency Extraction Module in STRING

### 3.1 STRING Overview

STRING is a fully-fledged NLP chain that performs all the basic steps of natural language processing (tokenization, sentence splitting, POS-tagging, POS-disambiguation and parsing) for Portuguese texts. The architecture of STRING is given in Fig. 1.

STRING has a modular, pipe-line structure, where: (i) the preprocessing stage (tokenization, sentence splitting, text normalization) and lexical analysis are performed by LexMan; (ii) followed by RuDriCo, which applies disambiguation rules, handles contractions and several special types of compound words; (iii) the MARv module then performs POS-disambiguation, using HMM and the Viterbi

---

[3] At the later stages of our research (May, 2014), we came to know the work of Cláudia Freitas [7]; however, since all the lexicon, grammar rules and evaluation procedures had been already accomplished by then, we decided not to take it into consideration at this moment but to use it in future work.

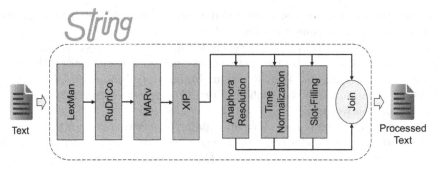

**Fig. 1.** STRING Architecture

algorithm; and, finally, (iv) the XIP parser (Xerox Incremental Parser) [1] segments sentences into chunks (or elementary sentence constituents: NP, PP, etc.) and extracts dependency relations among chunks' heads (SUBJect, MODifier, etc.). XIP also performs named entities recognition (NER). A set of post-parser modules have also been developed to handle certain NLP tasks such as anaphora resolution, temporal expressions' normalization and slot-filling. As part of the parsing process, XIP executes *dependency rules*. Dependency rules extract different types of dependencies between nodes of the sentence chunking tree, namely, the chunks' heads. Dependencies can thus be viewed as equivalent to (or representing) the syntactic relations holding between different elements in a sentence. Some of the dependencies extracted by XIP represent rather complex relations, such as the notion of *subject* (SUBJ) or *direct object* (CDIR), which imply a higher level of analysis of a given sentence. Other dependencies are much simpler and sometimes quite straightforward, like the determinative dependency DETD, holding between an article and the noun it determines, *e.g.*, *o livro* 'the book' – DETD(livro,o). Some dependencies can also be seen as auxiliary dependencies, and are required to build the more complex ones.

## 3.2   A Whole-Part Extraction Module in STRING

Next, we describe the way a whole-part dependency involving *Nbp* is extracted in the Portuguese grammar for XIP. To this end, a new module of the rule-based grammar was built, which contains most of the rules required for this work. Example (1) is a simple case where there is a determinative PP, complement *de* 'of' N of the *Nbp*, so that the meronymy is overtly expressed in the text:

(1)  *O Pedro partiu o braço do João* 'Pedro broke the arm of João'

The next rule captures the meronymy relation between *João* and *braço* 'arm':

```
IF( MOD[POST](#2[UMB-Anatomical-human],#1[human]) & PREPD(#1,?[lemma:de]) &
    CDIR[POST](#3,#2) & ~WHOLE-PART(#1,#2) )
    WHOLE-PART(#1,#2)
```

This rule is built using the XIP dependency rules' syntax, and it reads as follows: first, the parser determines the existence of a [MOD]ifier dependency, already calculated, between an *Nbp* (variable #2) and a human noun (variable #1); notice that, according to XIP conventions, the governor of the dependency is its first argument, hence *João* is said to be a modifier of *braço* 'arm'; this modifier must also be introduced by preposition *de* 'of', which is expressed by the dependency PREPD; then, a constraint is defined that the *Nbp* must be a direct object (CDIR) of a given verb (variable #3); and, finally, that there is still no previously calculated WHOLE-PART dependency between the *Nbp* and the human noun (variable #1); this last constraint is meant to ensure that there is only one meronymy relation between each *Nbp* and a given noun; if all these conditions are met, then, the parser builds the WHOLE-PART relation between the human determinative complement and the *Nbp*.

The meronymy extraction module contains 29 general rules addressing the most relevant syntactic constructions triggering this type of meronymic relations, and a set of 87 rules for the 29 *disease nouns* (*Nsick*), in order to capture the underlying *Nbp* (*e.g.*, *gastrite-estômago* 'gastritis-stomach'). A set of around 400 rules has also been devised to prevent the whole-part relations being extracted in the case the *Nbp* are elements of idiomatic expressions (*e.g.*, *O Pedro partiu o coração à Ana* 'Pedro broke the heart to Ana'). This work also addresses the cases where a whole-part relation holds between two *Nbp* in the same sentence (*e.g.*, *A Ana pinta as unhas dos pés* (lit: Ana paints the nails of the feet) 'Ana paints her toes' nails') and the case of determinative nouns that designate parts of an *Nbp*, though they are not themselves *Nbp* (*e.g.*, *O Pedro encostou a ponta da língua ao gelado da Ana* 'Pedro touched with the tip of the tongue the ice cream of Ana'). Each one of these cases triggers different sets of dependencies. 54 rules were built to associate the *Nbp* with their respective parts, to handle the cases where there is an *Nbp* and a noun that designates a part of that same *Nbp*.

# 4   Evaluation

For the evaluation of the work the first fragment of the CETEMPúblico corpus [27] (14,7 million tokens and 6,25 million words) was used in order to extract sentences that involve *Nbp* and *Nsick*. Using the *Nbp* (151 lemmas) and the *Nsick* (29 lemmas) dictionaries, specifically built for STRING lexicon, 16,746 *Nbp* and 79 *Nsick* instances were extracted from the corpus. In order to produce a golden standard for the evaluation, a random stratified sample of 1,000 sentences was selected, keeping the proportion of the total frequency of *Nbp* in the source corpus. This sample also includes a small number of *Nsick* (6 lemmas, 17 sentences). The 1,000 output sentences were divided into 4 subsets of 225 sentences each. Each subset was then given to a different annotator (native Portuguese speaker), and a common set of 100 sentences was added to each subset in order to assess inter-annotator agreement. The annotators were asked to append the whole-part dependency, as it was previously defined in a set of guidelines, using the XIP format. To assess inter-annotator agreement we used ReCal3: Reliability Calculator [6], for 3 or more annotators. The results showed that the Average Pairwise Percent Agreement equals 0.85, the Fleiss' Kappa inter-annotator agreement is 0.62, and the Average Pairwise Cohen's Kappa 0.63. According to Landis and Koch [16] these figures correspond to the lower bound of the "substantial" agreement; however, according to Fleiss [5], these results correspond to an inter-annotator agreement halfway between "fair" and "good". In view of these results, we assumed that the remaining, independent and non-overlapping annotation of the corpus by the four annotators is sufficiently consistent, and can be used as a golden standard for the evaluation of the system output.

The results of the system performance are showed in Table 1, where TP=*true-positives*; TN=*true-negatives*; FP=*false positives*; FN=*false negatives*; and the first line correspond to the 100 sentences that were subject to multiple annotators' classification, while the 900 sentences are the remainder instances of the sample taken form the corpus. The number of instances is higher than the number of sentences, as one sentence may involve several instances, and we count 5 partial TP as 0.5. The relative percentages of the TP, TN, FP and FN instances are similar between the 100 and the 900 set of sentences. This explains the similarity of the evaluation results and seems to confirm our decision to use the remaining 900 sentences' set as a golden standard for the evaluation of the system's output with enough confidence.

**Table 1.** System's performance for *Nbp*

| Number of sentences | TP | TN | FP | FN | Precision | Recall | F-measure | Accuracy |
|---|---|---|---|---|---|---|---|---|
| 100 | 8 | 73 | 7 | 14 | 0.53 | 0.36 | 0.43 | 0.79 |
| 900 | 73.5 | 673 | 55 | 118 | 0.57 | 0.38 | 0.46 | 0.81 |
| Total: | 81.5 | 746 | 62 | 132 | 0.57 | 0.38 | 0.46 | 0.81 |

## 5    Error Analysis

The results of the evaluation of the task showed that there were 62 false positive cases and 132 false negatives. We begin this section by the analysis of some false positives cases and then move on to the false negatives.

### 5.1    False Positives

**Disambiguation of *Nbp* in Context.** To begin with, we tackled a number of cases with the ambiguous noun *língua* 'tongue/language'. In order to preclude the building of whole-part relation in cases such as *língua portuguesa* 'Portuguese language', *a língua de Camões* 'the language of Camões', *professor de língua* (lit: teacher of language) 'language teacher', etc., where the noun *língua* 'language' is not used in the meanining of an anatomical part, we adopted one of the following strategies: we removed the *Nbp* (sem-anmov) feature from the nouns lexical set of features. This is carried out by the following rules, which are applied before the chunking stage:

— in the case of gentilic adjectives, one rule had to be done for each one of this type of adjectives:

```
2> noun[lemma:língua,sem-anmov=~], adj[gentcontinent=+].
2> noun[lemma:língua,sem-anmov=~], adj[gentregion=+].
2> noun[lemma:língua,sem-anmov=~], adj[gentcountry=+].
2> noun[lemma:língua,sem-anmov=~], adj[gentcity=+].
```

— in the case of combinations of *língua* 'tongue/language' with renowned authors of a given language, a PP structure has to be spelled out; so far, we built rules for over a dozen authors, epitomes of their national languages, which occurred with some frequency in the CETEMPúblico corpus:

```
2> noun[lemma:língua,sem-anmov=~], prep[lemma:de], noun[lemma:Camões].
2> noun[lemma:língua,sem-anmov=~], prep[lemma:de], noun[lemma:Shakespeare].
```

— a similar rule is necessary for PP complements with country names (*a língua de Portugal* 'Portugal's language'):

```
2> noun[lemma:língua,sem-anmov=~], prep[lemma:de], noun[country=+].
```

Besides, there could also be a determiner for examples such as *a língua do Brasil é o Português* 'the language of the Brazil is the Portuguese' Thus, a second rule is necessary:

```
2> noun[lemma:língua,sem-anmov=~], prep[lemma:de], art[lemma:o], noun[country=+].
```

This second rule is required because some country names are obligatorily preceded by a definite article (*o Brasil* 'the Brazil', *os Estados Unidos* 'the United States', *etc.*)

**Difficult Cases.** A certain number of cases were found where the use of the *Nbp* is clearly figurative, but it is not neither an idiom nor a compound word, so we were unable to devise any strategy to avoid capturing the whole-part relation:

(2) *À farta ementa associou-se um acontecimento a que certamente não foi alheio o **dedo** organizativo de José Perdigão, que no filho encontrou precioso instrumento...*

'To the abundant menu, an event was associated, which was certainly not unconnected with the organizational finger of José Perdigão, who found in [his] son a [precious=] most valuable tool...'

WHOLE-PART(José Perdigão,dedo) 'WHOLE-PART(José Perdigão,finger)'
In this case, the whole-part relation is correctly extracted, but the *Nbp dedo* 'finger' is not to be interpreted literally, but figuratively, and can be connoted with several idiomatic expressions such as *meter o dedo/a mão em* 'sb. put [one's] finger/hand in sth.' 'to have a role in / to interfere with'.

## 5.2 False Negatives

**Noun or NP Modifiers (not involving verbs).** The rules that have been developed only involve verb arguments (subject or complements) and did not consider the situations where an *Nbp* is a modifier of a noun or an adjective. Therefore, in several situations, the whole-part relations have not been captured. For example:

(3) *Um mágico de carapuço na cabeça*
'A magician with a hood over the head'

In this case, there is only a complex NP, with all the PP depending on the head noun *mágico* 'magician'. It is also possible to consider that in these cases an adjective or a verb past participle has been zeroed (*e.g.*, *Um mágico de carapuço enfiado/posto/colocado na cabeça* 'A magician with a hood stucked/placed over the head'). The meronymy module did not contemplate these complex NPs, including those with a zeroed adjective/past-participle, as most of the rules always involved a verb argument. This will have to be taken into consideration in future work.

**Missing Features.** One of the main reasons why the whole-part relation has not been captured derived from the fact that many human nouns are still unmarked with the human feature (or any of its subsumed features). For example, in the sentence:

(4) *Numa espécie de altar, um transexual padece com uma coroa de agulhas espetadas na cabeça, apoiado a umas muletas, provavelmente a sua cruz, nesta paródia à crucificação*
'In a kind of altar, a transsexual suffers with a crown of needles stuck in his head, supported by crutches, probably his cross, in this parody of the crucifixion'

In this case, the whole-part relation between the subject of *padecer* 'suffer' and the body-part *cabeça* 'head' was not captured just because the noun *transexual* (*id.*) had not been attributed the feature human.

In some cases, the rules were not triggered because the human entity is expressed by a personal pronoun and this category is not marked with the human feature. In the next sentence, the system failed to establish the whole-part relation because it can not ascribe the human feature to the relative pronoun *que* 'who' that is the subject of the relative clause.

(5) *Segundo o responsável do hospital, o doente – **que** também sofreu graves ferimentos na cabeça – poderia ser ainda sujeito a uma segunda intervenção cirúrgica*
'According to the head of the hospital, the patient - **who** also suffered serious head injuries - could still be subjected to a second surgical intervention'

However, the antecedent of the pronoun has been correctly extracted:
ANTECEDENT_RELAT(doente,que) 'ANTECEDENT_RELAT(patient,who)'

According to [18], relative pronouns are among the most successful cases of anaphora resolution in STRING. Therefore, it is possible that after this module comes into play, the features of the antecedent are inherited by the pronoun and the whole-part module be allowed to process the sentence again.

An opposite situation occurs when some features associated to the *Nbp* preclude the correct extraction of the whole-part dependency. The noun *corpo* 'body' is one of that cases and a very complex one. It is an element of several compound nouns, which are identified during lexical analysis and do not interfere in the dependency extraction step. Furthermore, it can be considered as an *Nbp* (*e.g.*, *o corpo da vítima* 'the body of the victim') and also a collective noun, functioning as a type of determiner, as in

(6) *O corpo (=conjunto) dos docentes da faculdade*
'The staff of the (= set) of the teachers of the faculty'

Because of this a QUANTD (quantifying) dependency is extracted between *corpo* 'body' and the immediately following PP, which prevents the extraction of whole-part relation; therefore, rules were build to partially disambiguate this particular noun by removing the features associated to its collective noun interpretation.

```
3> noun[lemma:corpo,sem-anmov=+,sem-sign=~,sem-cc=~, sem-ac=~,sem-hh=~,sem-group-of-things=~],
prep[lemma:de], (art[lemma:o]), noun[lastname=+].
3> noun[lemma:corpo,sem-anmov=+,sem-sign=~,sem-cc=~, sem-ac=~,sem-hh=~,sem-group-of-things=~],
prep[lemma:de], (art[lemma:o]), noun[firstname=+].
```

These rules read as follows: if the noun *corpo* 'body' is followed by preposition *de* 'of' and a first or a last proper name, then we remove all the other features of *corpo* 'body' except the one that marks it as an *Nbp*.

They do not solve all the cases, naturally, since the distinction between the determiner and the *Nbp* can not yet be done, as it would require a previous word sense disambiguation module.

**Ambiguous FIXED Expressions, Incorrectly Captured.** In some cases, the FIXED expressions have been incorrectly captured instead of the whole-part relations, because they are ambiguous and have been used in the literal sense. For example:

(7) *Ele arrancava-me os cabelos todos* 'He pulled out all my hair'

FIXED(arrancava,cabelos) 'FIXED(pulled out,hair)'

In the idiom *arrancar os cabelos* 'to despair', there is obligatory correference between the subject and the *Nbp*, so there is no way the sentence could be interpreted figuratively. The problem, thus, relies in the incorrect representation of the constraints of the idiom, not of the grammar.

In this case, the correct relation should be:
WHOLE-PART(me,cabelos) 'WHOLE-PART(my,hair)'

**No Syntactic Relation Between *Whole* and *Part*.** In some cases, the *whole* and the *part* are not syntactically related (and can be far away from each other in a sentence):

(8) *O facto do corpo ter sido encontrado na cozinha, leva os bombeiros a suspeitar que a vítima, com graves problemas de saúde, tenha desmaiado e caído à lareira, o que poderá ter estado na origem do incêndio*
'The fact that the body was found in the kitchen, makes the firefighters to suspect that the victim, with serious health problems, had fainted and fallen into the hearth, which may have been the origin of the fire'

In this example, the *part corpo* 'body' is the subject of the *ter sido encontrado* 'have been found', while the *whole vítima* 'victim' is the subject of *tenha desmaiado* 'had fainted'; each noun is in a different subclause, and there is no syntactic dependency between the two nouns. However, the annotator was able to identify this meronymic relation `WHOLE-PART(vítima,corpo)` `'WHOLE-PART(victim,body)'`, which is beyond the scope of our current parser. Eventually, a bag-of-words machine learning approach could overcome this difficulty, which can not be done by this rule-based approach.

**Difficult Cases.** In spite of our best efforts, some *Nbp* were still missing from the lexicon, as in the case of *defesas imunitárias* 'immune defenses':

(9) *O que se pensa que acontece na artrite reumatóide é que a cartilagem é atacada pelas defesas imunitárias do doente, como se ela fosse um autêntico "corpo estranho"*
'What we think happens in rheumatoid arthritis is that the cartilage is attacked by the immune defenses of the patient as if it was an authentic "foreign body"'

In such cases, we have completed the dictionary, naturally.

In the next example, there is also a problem with the compound noun *cabelo(s) branco(s)* 'white hair(s)':

(10) *Um deles, de óculos e cabelo branco, olha para o relógio e depois perscruta com alguma inquietação as bancadas a meia nau*
'One of them, wearing glasses and with white hair, looks at his watch and then peers restlessly to the seats at midship'

For the moment, even though *cabelo(s) branco(s)* 'white hair(s)' is already tokenized as a compound noun, it has not been given the *Nbp* feature; therefore, the system did not capture any meronymic relation for this element. Even so, the problem is in the missed apposition relation of the two PPs with the subject complex NP, whose head is a pronoun (namely, *um deles* 'one of them'). Since no dependency exists between the subject (*um* ''one') and the apposition and also because the subject is a pronoun, no feature is there to trigger the meronymy rules.

## 6    Evaluation after Error Analysis

Ones all the corrections were taken into consideration, we ran the system again in order to carry out a second evaluation of the system's performance. The results are shown in Table 2 (the abbreviations and the legend are explained in Table 1).

**Table 2.** Post-error analysis system's performance for *Nbp*

| Number of sentences | TP | TN | FP | FN | Precision | Recall | F-measure | Accuracy |
|---|---|---|---|---|---|---|---|---|
| 100 | 10 | 75 | 4 | 12 | 0.71 | 0.45 | 0.56 | 0.84 |
| 900 | 90 | 688 | 39 | 91 | 0.70 | 0.50 | 0.58 | 0.86 |
| Total: | 100 | 763 | 43 | 103 | 0.70 | 0.49 | 0.58 | 0.85 |

The precision improved by 0.13 (from 0.57 to 0.70), the recall by 0.11 (from 0.38 to 0.49), the F-measure by 0.12 (from 0.46 to 0.58), and the accuracy by 0.04 (from 0.81 to 0.85). Since only some of the errors detected, particularly the most frequent, were we able to correct at this stage, and some can still be improved by extending the current work to so far unaddressed situations (dependencies on nouns, anaphora resolution, to name a few) it is expectable that higher levels of performance will be achieved in future work.

## 7    Conclusions

In this paper, we present the most frequent errors in a rule-based module for whole-part relations extraction involving human entities and body-part nouns (*Nbp*) in Portuguese, which has been implemented and integrated in the STRING NLP system. Around 17 thousand sentences with *Nbp* and disease nouns were extracted from a corpus. 4 Portuguese native speakers annotated a stratified random sample of 1,000 sentences and produced a golden standard, which was confronted against the system's output. The results show 0.57 precision, 0.38 recall, 0.46 F-measure, and 0.81 accuracy. The recall is relatively small (0.38), which can be explained by the fact that in many sentences, the *whole* and the *part* are not syntactically related and are quite far away from each other; naturally, human annotators were able to overcome these difficulties. In some cases, the rules were not triggered because some human nouns and personal pronouns are unmarked with the human feature. Besides, as we focused on verb complements alone, the situations where an *Nbp* is a modifier of a noun or an adjective (and not a verb) have not been contemplated in this work, which produced a significant number of *false negatives*. Other, quantitatively less relevant, cases were also presented in the detailed error analysis made after the systems' first evaluation. The problem derived from pronouns (especially relative pronouns) not having the human feature raises the issue of the adequate placing of the meronymy module in the STRING pipeline architecture: if some part of this task could also be performed *after* anaphora resolution, it is likely that better results would be produced. The precision of the task is somewhat better (0.57). The accuracy is relatively high (0.81) since there is a large number of *true-negative* cases. A detailed error analysis was performed to determine the most relevant cases for these results, which led to some situations being implemented. A second evaluation of the system's performance was carried out, with the same golden standard, and the results showed that the precision improved by 0.13 (from 0.57 to 0.70), the recall by 0.11 (from 0.38 to 0.49), the F-measure by 0.12 (from 0.46 to 0.58), and the accuracy by 0.04 (from 0.81 to 0.85).

From the observations above, it is clear that most of the phenomena here described are not exclusive of the Portuguese language, for example, the *Nbp*-disease noun relations, though there may be language-specific lexical gaps. It is also obvious that the structural descriptions involved in the transformational processes (sentence alternations) here analyzed depend on the particulars of every language syntax (and morphology), which should be modeled independently from the meronymy extraction task. In this respect, this paper may hint both on similar and on different linguistic aspects of the meronymy here tackled, and the observations here made might be useful for other approaches to meronymy extraction, in other languages.

In future work, the extraction of other types of whole-part relations will be addressed such as component-integral object (*pedal - bicycle*), member-collection (*player - team*), place-area (*grove - forest*), and others [30]. We intend to target the extraction of these types of whole-part relations using *syntactic dependency-based n-grams* (the concept is introduced in detail in [28,29]) and other syntactic information, such as subcategorization frames [8,9] in a machine learning approach. Another line of future work will be to use the lists of *Nbp* and several *Nbp*-related words provided by Cláudia Freitas [7] in order to complete the existing *Nbp* lexicon in STRING and to improve the recall by focusing on the *false negative* cases already found, which have shown that several syntactic patterns have not been paid enough attention yet.

**Acknowledgments.**   This work was supported by national funds through FCT – Fundação para a Ciência e a Tecnologia, under project PEst-OE/EEI/LA0021/2013; Erasmus Mundus Action 2 2011-2574 Triple I - Integration, Interaction and Institutions; and the Mexican Government (scholarship CONACYT).

# References

1. Ait-Mokhtar, S., Chanod, J., Roux, C.: Robustness beyond shallowness: incremental dependency parsing. Natural Language Engineering 8(2/3), 121–144 (2002)
2. Bick, E.: The Parsing System "Palavras": Automatic Grammatical Analysis of Portuguese in a Constraint Grammar Framework. Ph.D. thesis, Aarhus Univ. Aarhus, Denmark: Aarhus Univ. Press (2000)

3. Costa, F., Branco, A.: LXGram: A Deep Linguistic Processing Grammar for Portuguese. In: Pardo, T.A.S., Branco, A., Klautau, A., Vieira, R., de Lima, V.L.S. (eds.) PROPOR 2010. LNCS, vol. 6001, pp. 86–89. Springer, Heidelberg (2010)

4. Fellbaum, C.: WordNet: An Electronic Lexical Database. MIT Press, Cambridge (1998)

5. Fleiss, J.L.: Statistical methods for rates and proportions, 2nd edn., pp. 38–46. John Wiley, New York (1981)

6. Freelon, D.: ReCal: Intercoder Reliability Calculation as a Web Service. Intl. J. of Internet Science 5(1), 20–33 (2010)

7. Freitas, C.: ESQUELETO - Anotaçã das palavras do corpo humano. Tech. Rep. Versão 5 (May 20, 2014), http://www.linguateca.pt/acesso/Esqueleto.pdf

8. Gelbukh, A.: Syntactic disambiguation with weighted extended subcategorization frames. In: Proceedings of PACLING-99, Pacific Association for Computational Linguistics, pp. 244–249. University of Waterloo, Canada (1999)

9. Gelbukh, A.: Unsupervised Learning for Syntactic Disambiguation. Computación y Sistemas 18(2), 329–344 (2014)

10. Girju, R., Badulescu, A., Moldovan, D.: Learning Semantic Constraints for the Automatic Discovery of Part-Whole Relations. In: Proceedings of HLT-NAACL, vol. 3, pp. 80–87 (2003)

11. Girju, R., Badulescu, A., Moldovan, D.: Automatic discovery of part-whole relations. Computational Linguistics 21(1), 83–135 (2006)

12. van Hage, W.R., Kolb, H., Schreiber, G.: A method for learning part-whole relations. In: Cruz, I., Decker, S., Allemang, D., Preist, C., Schwabe, D., Mika, P., Uschold, M., Aroyo, L.M. (eds.) ISWC 2006. LNCS, vol. 4273, pp. 723–735. Springer, Heidelberg (2006)

13. Hearst, M.: Automatic acquisition of hyponyms from large text corpora. In: Proceedings of the 14th Conf. on Computational Linguistics, COLING 1992, vol. 2, pp. 539–545. ACL Morristown, NJ (1992)

14. Hirst, G.: Ontology and the lexicon. In: Staab, S., Studer, R. (eds.) Handbook on Ontologies, pp. 209–230. Springer (2004)

15. Iris, M., Litowitz, B., Evens, M.: Problems of the Part-Whole Relation. In: Evens, M. (ed.) Relational Models of the Lexicon: Representing Knowledge in Semantic Networks, pp. 261–288. Cambridge Univ. Press (1988)

16. Landis, J., Koch, G.: The measurement of observer agreement for categorical data. Biometrics 33(1), 159–174 (1977)

17. Mamede, N., Baptista, J., Diniz, C., Cabarrão, V.: STRING: An Hybrid Statistical and Rule-Based Natural Language Processing Chain for Portuguese. In: Computational Processing of Portuguese, PROPOR 2012, vol. Demo Session (2012), http://www.propor2012.org/demos/DemoSTRING.pdf

18. Marques, J.: Anaphora Resolution. Master's thesis, Univ. of Lisbon/IST and INESC-ID Lisboa/L2F (2013)

19. Marrafa, P.: WordNet do Português: uma base de dados de conhecimento linguístico. Instituto Camões (2001)

20. Marrafa, P.: Portuguese WordNet: general architecture and internal semantic relations. DELTA 18, 131–146 (2002)

21. Marrafa, P., Amaro, R., Mendes, S.: WordNet.PT Global – extending WordNet.PT to Portuguese varieties. In: Proceedings of the 1st Workshop on Algorithms and Resources for Modelling of Dialects and Language Varieties, pp. 70–74. ACL Press, Edinburgh (2011)

22. Oliveira, H.: Onto.PT: Towards the Automatic Construction of a Lexical Ontology for Portuguese. Ph.D. thesis, Univ. of Coimbra/Faculty of Science and Technology (2012)

23. Oliveira, H.G., Santos, D., Gomes, P., Seco, N.: PAPEL: A Dictionary-Based Lexical Ontology for Portuguese. In: Teixeira, A., de Lima, V.L.S., de Oliveira, L.C., Quaresma, P. (eds.) PROPOR 2008. LNCS (LNAI), vol. 5190, pp. 31–40. Springer, Heidelberg (2008)

24. Pantel, P., Pennacchiotti, M.: Espresso: Leveraging generic patterns for automatically harvesting semantic relations. In: Proceedings of Conf. on Computational Linguistics/ACL, COLING/ACL 2006, pp. 113–120. Sydney, Australia (2006)

25. Pianta, E., Bentivogli, L., Girardi, C.: MultiWordNet: developing an aligned multilingual database. In: 1st Intl. Conf. on Global WordNet, Mysore, India, pp. 293–302 (2002)

26. Prévot, L., Huang, C., Calzolari, N., Gangemi, A., Lenci, A., Oltramari, A.: Ontology and the lexicon: a multi-disciplinary perspective (introduction). In: Huang, C., Calzolari, N., Gangemi, A., Lenci, A., Oltramari, A., Prévot, L. (eds.) Ontology and the Lexicon: A Natural Language Processing Perspective. Studies in Natural Language Processing, ch. 1, pp. 3–24. Cambridge Univ. Press (2010)

27. Rocha, P., Santos, D.: CETEMPúblico: Um corpus de grandes dimensões de linguagem jornalística portuguesa. In: Nunes, M. (ed.) V Encontro para o processamento computacional da língua portuguesa escrita e falada (PROPOR 2000), pp. 131–140. São Paulo, ICMC/USP (2000)

28. Sidorov, G.: Non-continuous Syntactic N-grams. Polibits 48, 67–75 (2013)

29. Sidorov, G., Velasquez, F., Stamatatos, E., Gelbukh, A., Chanona-Hernandez, L.: Syntactic N-grams as Machine Learning Features for Natural Language Processing. Expert Systems with Applications 41(3), 853–860 (2013)

30. Winston, M., Chaffin, R., Herrmann, D.: A Taxonomy of Part-Whole Relations. Cognitive Science 11, 417–444 (1987)

# Statistical Recognition of References in Czech Court Decisions

Vincent Kríž[1], Barbora Hladká[1], Jan Dědek[2], and Martin Nečaský[2]

[1] Institute of Formal and Applied Linguistics
[2] Department of Software Engineering
Faculty of Mathematics and Physics, Charles University in Prague
Malostranské nám. 25, 118 00 Praha 1, Czech Republic

**Abstract.** We address the task of detection and classification of references in Czech court decisions, mainly we focus on references to other court decisions and acts. In addition, we are interested in detection of institutions that issued documents under consideration. We handle these references like entities in the task of Named Entity Recognition. We approach the task using machine learning methods, namely HMM and Perceptron algorithm and we report F-measure over 90% averaged over all entities. The results significantly outperform the systems published previously.

## 1 Introduction

Information extraction from unstructured documents is an important and still open issue. Its relevance is increasing with the exponential growth of digital data. Every day new documents are made available[1] and there is a need to identify and extract relevant information automatically from them. Although this is a general domain issue, it has a special relevance in the legal domain.

Our main goal is to increase one's comfort when searching for a particular legal data. Detecting references in court decisions presents a specific task of this general goal. We approach it as the task of Named Entity Recognition (NER) handling references like named entities. A NER system detects named entities in a text and classifies their semantic type (e.g., names of people, places, organizations, products, dates). Various NER systems were designed and implemented employing both linguistic grammar-based techniques and statistical models [2], some of them focus on legal texts [3]. We can see reference recognition as a medium of document interlinking.

The paper is organized as follows: we report previous related works in Section 2. A detailed description of court decisions, their characteristics and annotation are provided in Section 3. We present experiments with machine learning methods, detailed evaluation and error analysis in Section 4. We briefly describe the application of our system in Section 5. Section 6 presents some conclusions and points out possible future work.

---

[1] According to International Data Corporation[1], 90% of all available digital data is unstructured and its amount currently grows twice as fast as structured data.

A. Gelbukh et al. (Eds.): MICAI 2014, Part I, LNAI 8856, pp. 51–61, 2014.

## 2   Related Works

In the past decade, several approaches to entity recognition in legal texts were reported. [4] summarizes three methodologically different approaches, namely *lookup*, *rule-based*, and *statistical models*.

The *lookup method* creates a list of entities and then simply tags entity mentions in texts. [4] addresses named entity recognition and resolution in US legal documents classifying entities into five classes, namely judges, attorneys, companies, jurisdictions, and courts. Their test set consists of 600 documents randomly selected from a large collection of legal documents. They report 84.76% F-measure averaged over all entities. [5] developed and empirically tested parser effectiveness on reference detection in Dutch laws. Their evaluation is provided on randomly selected six documents. As they report, "the references follow a very strict structure, which can easily be represented using a regular expression or context free grammar". However, law names (or names of any other regulation) do not follow a unique pattern. They can even contain commas and other names, which make the entity detection task more difficult. Therefore, they decided not to recognize names by matching them with regular expressions. Instead they compare texts with a list of law names. They report accuracy higher than 95%. The lookup method may generate many false positives if a list of entities contains many ambiguous words. Applying this method on flective languages requires manipulating several word forms per lemma and lemmatization makes this method language dependent. Another drawback of this approach is that if a name is not in the list, it will not be recognized. In addition, within a document, new law names may be defined (typically abbreviations and acronyms). These names will be missed unless they are added to the list.

By looking at development data, one can define a *rule-based* system with a set of rules that recognize the majority of entities in texts and do not produce many false positives. [6] worked out a set of regular expressions to recognize references to legal documents. They reported F-Measure of 85% evaluated on a database of IT legislation. [7] presented an approach to populate a legal ontology from legal texts through NER automatically. Their NER module identifies Law, Act and Rule entities and classifies them. The system uses NLP tools for sentence splitting, tokenization and POS tagging to identify syntactic and positional patterns. The evaluation was carried out on a corpus of 25 texts and approximately 200,000 words composed by different types of documents from legislation. They report F-Measure of 33.49%. [8] proposed identifying document references using syntactic information generated by an automatic parser. They report precision around 35%. The high error rate value is explained by a complex syntactic structure of references. [9] presented a procedure detecting legal references in Italian court decisions. The parser implements four finite state automata, based on regular expressions. In the preliminary experiments the parser showed high reliability for detecting case citations, however no exact evaluation is reported. Development of rule-based systems requires manually annotated development data and a large amount of effort from experienced rule writers. Even more, maintenance of such rule sets can be tricky because rules often intricate interdependencies that are easy to forget and make modification risky.

*Statistical models* offer an alternative to contextual rules for encoding contextual cues. One way of thinking about such statistical models is as a set of cues that receive weights and these weights are combined based on probability and statistical concepts. A knowledge engineer must develop features that correspond to cues, pick an appropriate statistical model, and train the model using training data. Development of statistical models requires manually annotated training data and a large amount of effort from an experienced machine learning expert. Adding new development data is definitely more straightforward than editing contextual rules.

**Table 1.** An overview of systems for reference detection in legal texts. Their evaluation was performed on different data sets, we provide reported accuracy (Acc.), precision (Prec.) and F-measure (F-1).

| System | Lang. | Tools | Technique | Acc. | Prec. | F-1 |
|--------|-------|-------|-----------|------|-------|-----|
| [4] | ENG | Lists | Hybrid | | | 85 % |
| [7] | ENG | POS tagger | Rule-based | | | 34 % |
| [8] | ENG | Parser | Rule-based | 35 % | | |
| [9] | ITA | Regexps | Rule-based | | | |
| [6] | ITA | Regexps | Rule-based | | | 85 % |
| [10] | DUT | Regexps, Lists | Rule-based | 95 % | | |

Table 1 presents the systems for detecting references in legal English, Italian and Dutch texts developed recently. The systems apply different detecting techniques, like lists, POS tagger, parser, regular expressions and they belong to either hybrid or rule-based strategies. Their evaluation was performed on different data sets, we provide reported accuracy (Acc.), precision (Prec.) and F-measure (F-1).

At least to our knowledge, no research applying pure statistical models to reference detection in legal texts has been done yet. It is rather surprising, because the state of the art NER systems exploit almost exclusively statistical approaches. The systems that showed high scores on the CoNLL-2003 task [11] include [12], [13] and [2]. To our knowledge, the best currently known results on this dataset were published in 2009 by [2] and reached 90.80% F-measure on the test portion of the data. For Czech language, [14] presents a system based on Maximum Entropy Markov Model. The system achieves F-measure of 82.82% and it significantly outperforms the existing system designed by [15] that achieves 72.94% F-measure.

## 3   Building an Annotated Corpus of Czech Court Decisions

The most successful system for detecting references in law texts is reported in [16]. However, the nature of case law references in decisions is quite different from references contained in law texts in general. The text of decisions is typically more verbose, less formally structured and the details of a reference are often mixed with a sparse text or expressions leaving important details as implicit, causing ambiguity not easy to solve.

The Czech Republic has a system of courts of *general* jurisdiction (Supreme Court, High, Regional and District courts), *administrative* jurisdiction (Supreme Administrative Court) and *constitutional* jurisdiction (Constitutional Court). Decisions of the

Constitutional and the Supreme Court are available on-line.[2] None of them has a unified style of citations. Even more, there are different opinions what to cite. Some judges cite other court decisions only, some of them cite various types of literature as well, some of them cite *everything* (blogs, internet sources, Bible, novels, etc.). In our system, we distinguish references to court decisions and acts.

*References to Court Decisions.* They have several formats (e.g., *III. US 321/03, 0 P 58/2008-135*). Identification numbers of court decisions are not unique and two courts may publish decisions with the same identification number. For a unique identification of the document, it is essential to know which court published a given decision.

*References to Acts.* We adopt the reference terminology used in [16] to describe a structure of references to acts in Czech decisions:

- **simple references** to acts are represented in three ways: (1) name (e.g., *Act on Customs Administration in the Czech Republic*), (2) label and number (e.g, *§12, Head 1*), (3) anaphors, indirect references and acronyms (e.g., *Charter* standing for *Charter of Fundamental Rights and Freedoms*).
  There can appear a reference to a particular version of some act as well. This version corresponds to a version valid since a specific time, called *applicability* (effectiveness), e.g., *Act on Customs Administrations, valid from 1.1.1997.*
- **complex references** can be (1) multi-valued and (2) multi-layered.
  Multi-valued references consist of a label-numbers pair. Numbers can be represented as a list (e.g., *§2, 3 and 14*), as a range (e.g., *Section 13-18*) and as a combination of lists and ranges (e.g., *§2, 3-6 and 14*).
  A multi-layered reference is a reference that consists of several simple references, which navigate through a structure of a target document. Multi-layered references can be ordered in one of three ways: (1) zooming in, when the reference starts with the broadest part and ends with the narrowest part (e.g., *Accounting Act, §2, section 1, letter a*); (2) zooming out, when the reference starts with the narrowest part and ends with the broadest part (e.g., *section 1, §2, of the Charter*); and (3) zooming in, then zooming out (e.g., *§2, section 1 of the Accounting Act*). In Czech court decisions, we observe zooming in references only.

### 3.1   Czech Court Decisions Annotation

*Data Set.* We work with a sample of 300 court decisions published on-line by The Supreme Court (SC) and The Constitutional Court (CC). The sample from SC consists of documents published in 2012 and we selected them with respect to their distribution over senates. The sample from CC consists of the decisions published from 2004 to 2012 dealing with lease agreement issues.[3]

---

[2] http://usoud.cz, http://nsoud.cz/

[3] We selected a sample from CC with respect to the goals formulated in the INTLIB project (http://ufal.mff.cuni.cz/intlib).

*Annotation.* To obtain the training and test set for our experiments, we manually annotated the sample documents. We distinguish four types of entities: (1) reference to a court decision (D); (2) reference to an act (Ac); (3) applicability of an act (Ap), and (4) an institution (I). In addition, we define relation between D and I if a given institution issued a given decision.

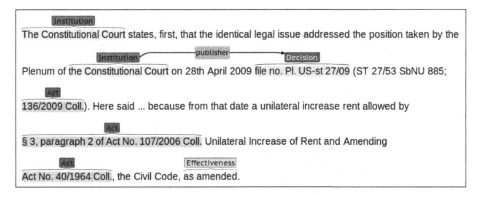

**Fig. 1.** Annotation of court decisions

We used a web-based annotation tool *Brat* [17].[4] Annotators marked entity occurrences and label them with an appropriate tag. Then they marked relations between D and I if they appear in a text. It can happen that a (multi-word) token can be annotated with more than one tag, e.g., a document reference contains an institution reference – *The Constitutional Court Act* contains *The Constitutional Court*. An annotator marks and tags an institution first and an act afterwards. See Figure 1 for illustration. We run experiments based on the cross-validation strategy. Therefore, Table 2 presents statistics on the 300 annotated documents averaged over 10 cross-validation folds.

We did a single annotation of 300 court decisions. However, to assess task difficulty, we selected 15 documents from the sample and annotated them by three independent annotators. In average, the annotators marked 551 institutions, 258 references to court decisions, 402 references to acts and 42 applicabilities. We used the Fleiss' kappa [18] to calculate the inter-annotator agreement. We interpret $\kappa = 0.85$ as almost perfect agreement. Therefore, we consider the task of reference detection quite easy for human annotators.

## 4   Experiments

We compare performance of two machine learning approaches, namely Perceptron Algorithm with Uneven Margins (PAUM) and Hidden Markov model algorithm (HMM).

---

[4] http://brat.nlplab.org/

**Table 2.** Entity and token distribution in the training and test data averaged over 10 cross-validation folds

| | | | Ac | D | Ap | I | Total |
|---|---|---|---|---|---|---|---|
| SC | # of Tokens | Training | 43,117 | 11,074 | 1,262 | 12,425 | 332,535 |
| | | Test | 5,348 | 1,855 | 265 | 1,450 | 36,999 |
| | # of Entities | Training | 3,949 | 1,304 | 222 | 2,485 | 7,487 |
| | | Test | 439 | 145 | 25 | 276 | 943 |
| CC | # of Tokens | Training | 19,675 | 12,780 | 843 | 14,767 | 312,191 |
| | | Test | 2,707 | 2,127 | 102 | 1,743 | 34,701 |
| | # of Entities | Training | 2,338 | 1,481 | 210 | 3,206 | 7,910 |
| | | Test | 260 | 165 | 23 | 356 | 879 |

### 4.1 Systems

*PAUM.* The PAUM algorithm [20] is one of the machine learning alternatives provided by the GATE framework [21].[5] The algorithm represents a slight modification of the classical Perceptron algorithm [22] used in neural networks and extended by SVM [23]. It provides comparable performance to SVM, with much reduced training times.

PAUM was already applied to the NER task by [24]. Authors compare their modification of SVM, standard SVM and PAUM. They use CoNLL-2003 [11] data set for the experiments. PAUM system (F-measure of $84.36\%$) performed worse than the SVM system. On the other hand, training time of PAUM is only 1% of that for the SVM and the PAUM implementation is much simpler than that of SVM.

In our experiments, PAUM was used in the chunk learning mode with the features listed in Table 3 and we proposed four models: the `PM small` and `PM` models use word forms only and the `PM pos` and `PM pos ext` models use lemmatization and POS tagging.

**Table 3.** Features used by PAUM

| PAUM model | Features |
|---|---|
| PM small | trigrams of word forms: $(w_{i-2}, w_{i-1}, w_i)$ |
| PM | 5-grams of word forms: $(w_{i-2}, w_{i-1}, w_i, w_{i+1}, w_{i+2})$ |
| PM pos | 5-grams of lemmas and part of speech tags: $(l_{i-2}, l_{i-1}, l_i, l_{i+1}, l_{i+2}), (t_{i-2}, t_{i-1}, t_i, t_{i+1}, t_{i+2})$ |
| PM pos ext | It extends PM pos with an orthography feature and it distinguishes first and last tokens in a sentence. The following orthographic categories are used: *upper initial* (e.g. Czech), *lowercase* (e.g. language), *all caps* (e.g. PAUM) and *mixedCaps* (e.g. JTagger). |

*HMM.* Hidden Markov Models present historically a very first statistical model applied in the field of natural language processing [25]. The natural language processing community has effectively employed HMM models for many kinds of efforts starting with POS tagging, NER including. HMM based IdentiFinder [26] have achieved remarkably good performance.

---

[5] http://gate.ac.uk

In our task, the output alphabet consists of all possible words occurring in the training data and the states contain reference tags that we assign to the words. The goal is to compute the most likely sequence of tags that has generated the input text. While PAUM models identify the beginning and end tokens for each entity, HMM annotates each token.

## 4.2   Experiment Evaluation

We evaluated performance of individual approaches using standard evaluation measures, namely Precision, Recall and F-measure.

Strict $F_1$ on entities

|  | Entity | HMM | PM pos ext | PM pos | PM | PM small |
|---|---|---|---|---|---|---|
| SC | Act | 0.75±0.02 | 0.91±0.02 ○ | 0.91±0.03 ○ | 0.89±0.03 ○ | 0.88±0.03 ○ |
| | Decision | 0.82±0.08 | 0.97±0.02 ○ | 0.96±0.02 ○ | 0.95±0.03 ○ | 0.94±0.02 ○ |
| | Effectiveness | 0.89±0.04 | 0.90±0.05 | 0.89±0.05 | 0.88±0.08 | 0.82±0.10 |
| | Institution | 0.92±0.03 | 0.96±0.02 ○ | 0.96±0.02 ○ | 0.95±0.02 ○ | 0.96±0.02 ○ |
| CC | Act | 0.63±0.05 | 0.87±0.02 ○ | 0.86±0.02 ○ | 0.84±0.03 ○ | 0.78±0.03 ○ |
| | Decision | 0.83±0.05 | 0.95±0.03 ○ | 0.95±0.03 ○ | 0.93±0.03 ○ | 0.92±0.03 ○ |
| | Effectiveness | 0.96±0.03 | 0.96±0.03 | 0.96±0.03 | 0.96±0.03 | 0.96±0.03 |
| | Institution | 0.91±0.02 | 0.93±0.02 ○ | 0.93±0.02 ○ | 0.92±0.01 ○ | 0.92±0.01 ○ |

Lenient $F_1$ on entities

|  | Entity | HMM | PM pos ext | PM pos | PM | PM small |
|---|---|---|---|---|---|---|
| SC | Act | 0.93±0.02 | 0.96±0.01 ○ | 0.96±0.01 ○ | 0.95±0.01 ○ | 0.95±0.02 ○ |
| | Decision | 0.91±0.03 | 0.98±0.01 ○ | 0.97±0.02 ○ | 0.96±0.02 ○ | 0.95±0.02 ○ |
| | Effectiveness | 0.94±0.04 | 0.91±0.05 | 0.90±0.05 ● | 0.90±0.06 ● | 0.83±0.10 ● |
| | Institution | 0.97±0.01 | 0.98±0.00 ○ | 0.98±0.01 ○ | 0.97±0.01 | 0.97±0.01 |
| CC | Act | 0.89±0.02 | 0.94±0.01 ○ | 0.94±0.01 ○ | 0.94±0.01 ○ | 0.93±0.02 ○ |
| | Decision | 0.93±0.03 | 0.97±0.02 ○ | 0.97±0.02 ○ | 0.96±0.02 ○ | 0.95±0.03 |
| | Effectiveness | 0.96±0.03 | 0.96±0.03 | 0.96±0.03 | 0.96±0.03 | 0.96±0.03 |
| | Institution | 0.97±0.01 | 0.98±0.01 ○ | 0.98±0.01 ○ | 0.97±0.01 | 0.97±0.01 |

$F_1$ on tokens

|  | Entity | HMM | PM pos ext | PM pos | PM | PM small |
|---|---|---|---|---|---|---|
| SC | Act | 0.96±0.01 | 0.96±0.01 | 0.96±0.01 | 0.96±0.02 | 0.95±0.02 |
| | Decision | 0.95±0.02 | 0.98±0.01 ○ | 0.98±0.02 ○ | 0.97±0.02 ○ | 0.96±0.02 |
| | Effectiveness | 0.94±0.03 | 0.89±0.06 ● | 0.88±0.06 ● | 0.88±0.06 ● | 0.79±0.12 ● |
| | Institution | 0.96±0.01 | 0.97±0.01 ○ | 0.97±0.01 ○ | 0.97±0.01 | 0.96±0.02 |
| CC | Act | 0.94±0.01 | 0.94±0.01 | 0.93±0.01 | 0.93±0.02 | 0.89±0.02 ● |
| | Decision | 0.95±0.02 | 0.96±0.02 ○ | 0.96±0.01 | 0.96±0.02 | 0.94±0.02 |
| | Effectiveness | 0.96±0.03 | 0.96±0.04 | 0.96±0.04 | 0.96±0.04 | 0.96±0.04 |
| | Institution | 0.95±0.01 | 0.95±0.01 | 0.95±0.02 | 0.95±0.01 | 0.94±0.01 |

○, ● statistically significant improvement or degradation w.r.t. HMM

**Table 4.** Cross-validation results – entities and tokens

When evaluation is being done on potentially multi-token entities, partially correct (or overlapping) matches can occur. The evaluation can be calculated in two ways, depending on what units are compared. We can use either individual (potentially multi-token) entities or tokens from which the entities are composed of. Evaluation using tokens is easier to calculate since there is no need to construct any pairing between discovered and gold-standard entities as in the other case. It also reflects the proportion of partially correct matches, but it does not reflect situations when e.g., two directly following entities are mistaken for one long entity and we also do not know how many entities are entirely correct and how many only overlap. The entity evaluation is computed analogically to the token evaluation, except the number of true negatives can not be taken into account because it does not make sense in this case, therefore also accuracy can not be used in this case.

*Strict* and *Lenient* variants of performance measures allow dealing with partially correct matches in different ways: Strict measures consider all partially correct matches as incorrect (spurious, false positive), while Lenient measures consider all partially correct matches as correct (true positive).[6]

We performed an experiment using 10-fold cross-validation. Statistical significance was computed using the corrected resampled (two tailed) t-Test [27], which is suitable for cross validation based experiments. Test significance was 0.05.

Table 4 shows the results of cross-validation, both token- and entity- based F-measure for CC and SC decisions separately. The results are presented in a form of confidence intervals. The first column is always the baseline and remaining columns are evaluated against it; statistically significant increase/decrease is indicated by ∘/•, resp.

We can formulate a preliminary conclusion that PAUM shows better performance than HMM (especially, `PM small` works with the same features as HMM and its results are better).

### 4.3  Error Analysis

We manually checked the output of both HMM and PAUM algorithms and we identified the following rather frequent errors:

– References labeled with two separate tags instead of one tag. For example, in the reference *file no. 7 To 346/2011*, token *To* is not recognized as a part of document reference.
– An institution's name ends with a number, like *Disctrict Court for Prague 4*, and the last token *4* is not recognized as a part of the reference entity.
– Names of foreign courts, e.g. *Land Court in Norimberg, Germany*.

## 5  JTagger

We present the system *JTagger* for reference recognition in Czech court decisions. Demo, data and source codes are available at `http://kpmd.eu/jtagger`. JTagger is the first component in a pipeline processing Czech court decisions. JTagger built

---

[6] See also the GATE documentation chapter about performance evaluation – `http://gate.ac.uk/userguide/chap:eval`

upon the HMM model is used in the ODCleanStore system.[7] This system publishes court decisions according to the principles of Linked Data [28]. Every day, new decisions published by SC and CC are automaticaly processed by JTagger and converted to the Resource Description Framework (RDF, [29]) in the Linked Open Data Cloud.[8]

# 6   Conclusion

In our paper, we presented the statistical-based systems of reference detection in Czech court decisions. At least to our knowledge, there exists no other system for reference detection in legal texts employing statistical models. We achieved performance that outperforms the results published in literature so far. The given system, *JTagger*, has been published online.

Having recognized references in court decisions, we will compose a so-called *case story* that will track a storyline of a given case since its beginning to its end. Formally, the story will be represented as an oriented graph with decisions being nodes and relations between decisions being oriented edges. Both nodes and edges will be built upon the output of reference recognition.

**Acknowledgements.** The authors would like to thank annotators for their work. We gratefully acknowledge support from the Technology Agency of the Czech Republic (grant no. TA02010182). This work has been using language resources developed and/or stored and/or distributed by the LINDAT/CLARIN project.

# References

1. Gantz, J., Reinsel, D.: The digital universe decade – are you ready (2010), `http://goo.gl/ZaO0PR`
2. Ratinov, L., Roth, D.: Design challenges and misconceptions in named entity recognition. In: Proceedings of the Thirteenth Conference on Computational Natural Language Learning, pp. 147–155. Association for Computational Linguistics (2009)
3. Quaresma, P., Gonçalves, T.: Using linguistic information and machine learning techniques to identify entities from juridical documents. In: Francesconi, E., Montemagni, S., Peters, W., Tiscornia, D. (eds.) Semantic Processing of Legal Texts. LNCS, vol. 6036, pp. 44–59. Springer, Heidelberg (2010)
4. Dozier, C., Kondadadi, R., Light, M., Vachher, A., Veeramachaneni, S., Wudali, R.: Named entity recognition and resolution in legal text. In: Francesconi, E., Montemagni, S., Peters, W., Tiscornia, D. (eds.) Semantic Processing of Legal Texts. LNCS, vol. 6036, pp. 27–43. Springer, Heidelberg (2010)
5. de Maat, E., Winkels, R., van Engers, T.M.: Automated detection of reference structures in law. In: van Engers, T.M. (ed.) JURIX. Frontiers in Artificial Intelligence and Applications, vol. 152, pp. 41–50. IOS Press (2006)
6. Palmirani, M., Brighi, R., Massini, M.: Automated extraction of normative references in legal texts. In: Proceedings of the 9th International Conference on Artificial Intelligence and Law, pp. 105–106. ACM (2003)

---

[7] `http://sourceforge.net/projects/odcleanstore/`
[8] `http://datahub.io/group/lodcloud`

7. Bruckschen, M., Northfleet, C., Silva, D., Bridi, P., Granada, R., Vieira, R., Rao, P., Sander, T.: Named entity recognition in the legal domain for ontology population. In: Workshop Programme, p. 16 (2010)

8. Quaresma, P., Gonçalves, T.: Using linguistic information and machine learning techniques to identify entities from juridical documents. In: Francesconi, E., Montemagni, S., Peters, W., Tiscornia, D. (eds.) Semantic Processing of Legal Texts. LNCS, vol. 6036, pp. 44–59. Springer, Heidelberg (2010)

9. Bacci, L., Francesconi, E., Sagri, M.: A rule-based parsing approach for detecting case law references in italian court decisions. In: Semantic Processing of Legal Texts (SPLeT-2012) Workshop Programme, p. 27 (2012)

10. De, E., Winkels, R., van Engers, T.: Automated detection of reference structures in law. In: Frontiers in Artificial Intelligence and Applications, p. 41 (2006)

11. Tjong Kim Sang, E.F., De Meulder, F.: Introduction to the CoNLL-2003 shared task: Language-independent named entity recognition. In: Proceedings of the Seventh Conference on Natural Language Learning at HLT-NAACL 2003, vol. 4, pp. 142–147. Association for Computational Linguistics (2003)

12. Suzuki, J., Isozaki, H.: Semi-supervised sequential labeling and segmentation using giga-word scale unlabeled data. In: ACL, pp. 665–673. Citeseer (2008)

13. Ando, R.K., Zhang, T.: A high-performance semi-supervised learning method for text chunking. In: Proceedings of the 43rd Annual Meeting on Association for Computational Linguistics, pp. 1–9. Association for Computational Linguistics (2005)

14. Straková, J., Straka, M., Hajič, J.: A new state-of-the-art czech named entity recognizer. In: Habernal, I., Matousek, V. (eds.) TSD 2013. LNCS, vol. 8082, pp. 68–75. Springer, Heidelberg (2013)

15. Konkol, M., Konopík, M.: Maximum entropy named entity recognition for czech language. In: Habernal, I., Matoušek, V. (eds.) TSD 2011. LNCS, vol. 6836, pp. 203–210. Springer, Heidelberg (2011)

16. de Maat, E., Krabben, K., Winkels, R.: Machine Learning versus Knowledge Based Classification of Legal Texts. In: Proceedings of the 2010 Conference on Legal Knowledge and Information Systems: JURIX 2010: The Twenty-Third Annual Conference, pp. 87–96. IOS Press, Amsterdam (2010)

17. Stenetorp, P., Pyysalo, S., Topić, G., Ohta, T., Ananiadou, S., Tsujii, J.: brat: a web-based tool for nlp-assisted text annotation. In: Proceedings of the Demonstrations at the 13th Conference of the European Chapter of the Association for Computational Linguistics, pp. 102–107. Association for Computational Linguistics (2012)

18. Fleiss, J.L.: Measuring nominal scale agreement among many raters. Psychological Bulletin 76, 378 (1971)

19. Carletta, J.: Assessing agreement on classification tasks: the kappa statistic. Computational linguistics 22, 249–254 (1996)

20. Li, Y., Zaragoza, H., Herbrich, R., Shawe-Taylor, J., Kandola, J.S.: The perceptron algorithm with uneven margins. In: Proceedings of the Nineteenth International Conference on Machine Learning, ICML 2002, pp. 379–386. Morgan Kaufmann Publishers Inc., San Francisco (2002)

21. Cunningham, H., Maynard, D., Bontcheva, K., Tablan, V.: GATE: A Framework and Graphical Development Environment for Robust NLP Tools and Applications. In: Proceedings of the 40th Anniversary Meeting of the Association for Computational Linguistics, ACL 2002 (2002)

22. Kim, K.-B., Kim, S., Joo, Y., Oh, A.-S.: Enhanced fuzzy single layer perceptron. In: Wang, J., Liao, X.-F., Yi, Z. (eds.) ISNN 2005. LNCS, vol. 3496, pp. 603–608. Springer, Heidelberg (2005)

23. Cortes, C., Vapnik, V.: Support-vector networks. Mach. Learn. 20, 273–297 (1995)
24. Li, Y., Bontcheva, K., Cunningham, H.: Using uneven margins svm and perceptron for information extraction. In: Proceedings of the Ninth Conference on Computational Natural Language Learning, pp. 72–79. Association for Computational Linguistics (2005)
25. Merialdo, B.: Tagging english text with a probabilistic model. Comput. Linguist. 20, 155–171 (1994)
26. Bikel, D.M., Miller, S., Schwartz, R., Weischedel, R.: Nymble: a high-performance learning name-finder. In: Proceedings of the Fifth Conference on Applied Natural Language Processing, pp. 194–201. Association for Computational Linguistics (1997)
27. Nadeau, C., Bengio, Y.: Inference for the generalization error. Machine Learning 52, 239–281 (2003)
28. Berners-Lee, T.: Linked data - design issues. W3C (2006)
29. Lassila, O., Swick, R.R.: Resource description framework (RDF) model and syntax specification. Technical report (1999), `http://www.w3.org/TR/1999/REC-rdf-syntax-19990222/`

# LSA Based Approach to Domain Detection

Diego Uribe

Instituto Tecnológico de la Laguna
División de Estudios de Posgrado e Investigación
Revolución y Cuauhtémoc, Torreón, Coah., MX
diego@itlalaguna.edu.mx

**Abstract.** In this paper we consider the key role of corpus homogeneity in the problem of domain adaptation. Domain adaptation is an interesting research topic concerned with the capability of portability that a linguistic tool is able to display. Since a linguistic tool is commonly developed for a specific domain, to make use of the tool with a different domain decrease its performance. In this way, determining the homogeneity of the implicated corpora is crucial for the purpose of minimising the portability cost. We examine the semantic relatedness between domains by analysing the co-occurrence of the terms. By mapping the texts and corresponding terms into the latent semantic space we identify the underlying semantic similarity between different domains. We evaluate a collection of reviews corresponding to four different domains and the results obtained so far have shown how our method is a plausible alternative in measuring the homogeneity of the collection.

## 1 Introduction

Domain adaptation is an interesting research subject concerned with the capability of portability that a linguistic tool is able to display. For example, information extraction is a linguistic task that takes unseen texts as input and produces structured-unambiguous data as output. However, it is a domain dependent task since when we need to extract information from a new domain, a new ad-hoc system is demanded. For this reason, building an information extraction system is difficult and time consuming [1], [2]. Similar challenges are also addressed by an open domain question answering system, a system to obtain concise answers to questions stated in natural language, that needs to be adaptable to play a crucial role in business intelligence applications [3].

Corpora homogeneity plays a crucial role in domain adaptation since there is an intuitive assumption that high similarity between corpora contribute to reduce the portability cost. In this way, it is paramount to determine how different is a new domain from the one used to develop a linguistic tool. In fact, Oakes mentions how important is to characterise corpora in order to minimise the impact on the replicability of the results [4]; furthermore, the necessity of characterisation of the corpora as a guide for developing NLP systems and for estimation of transferability is also emphasised by Bank et al. [5].

A. Gelbukh et al. (Eds.): MICAI 2014, Part I, LNAI 8856, pp. 62–69, 2014.

In this paper, we make use of *text categorisation* (TC) as the framework for identification of similar domains. A common application of TC occurs when a user manifests his interest in a particular type of news: a TC system classifies the topic of new stories to show the user the preferred stories only. How do we contemplate corpus homogeneity from a TC perspective? In our case, instead of being interested in a particular type of news, we are interested in a particular type of domain: a TC system classifies the domain of new information to show the user the most similar of the pre-defined domains. Once the most similar domain is identified, the user is more confident about selecting an appropriated linguistic tool.

In this way, we identify the underlying semantic similarity between different domains by mapping the texts and corresponding terms into the latent semantic space. We evaluate a collection of reviews corresponding to four different domains and the results obtained so far have shown how our method is a plausible alternative to measure the homogeneity of the collection.

The description of our work is organised as follows. The next section 2 makes a brief description of related work on corpus homogeneity. Section 3 describes in detail the semantic similarity approach used in our analysis. Section 4 defines the dataset used in our experimentation as well as the pre-processing task for the extraction of the linguistic terms to which we submitted our data collection. Then, the results of the experimentation are exhibited and discussed. Finally, conclusions and future work are given in section 5.

## 2   Related Work

In this section, we briefly describe some of the substantial works dealing with the problems of corpus homogeneity and domain adaptation. First, we make reference to the classic work on corpus homogeneity developed by Kilgarriff [6]. In this work, Kilgarriff claims that similarity can only be interpreted in the light of corpus homogeneity. Since small (or large) within-corpus distance denotes homogeneity (or heterogeneity), it is interesting to observe some of the multiple combinations when working on comparison of corpora. For example, when comparing corpus A and corpus B, where each one exhibits homogeneity (small within-corpus distance), a large distance between them suggests A and B represent different language varieties or domains. It is also interesting the way in which Kilgarriff prepares the corpora for assessing similarity measures such as Spearman, $\chi^2$ and cross-entropy. The composition is based on the combination of different percentages from two different corpora (*Known-Similarity Corpora*), but not so different since they share some varieties.

Oakes also presented another interesting work concerned with the impact of corpus characteristics in the development of a linguistic tool [4]. He analyses differences between corpora by using multiple measures that allow not only to determine similarity between corpora but also to identify individual features.

In fact, he emphasises the exploration of features, such as the frequencies of phrase structures rather than individual words, for the characterisation of corpora as a useful guide to minimise the portability cost. The chi-squared measure, information radius and factor analysis were some of the statistical measures implemented in this work.

Finally, a different but also interesting work focused on measuring the semantic similarity of short texts was developed by Mihalcea [7]. Multiple similarity measures implemented in this work are grouped into two categories: corpus-based and knowledge-based measures in order to derive a text-to-text similarity metric. The experimentation is conducted on a paraphrase data set and the achieved results show how the similarity metric proposed outperforms the vector-based similarity approach.

## 3    Approach

We describe in detail in this section our semantic similarity approach. Basically, we look into the semantic relatedness between domains by analysing the co-occurrence of the terms. Since *Latent Semantic Analysis* (LSA) is a technique based on the co-occurrence of the terms (the coincidence of the terms) rather than the occurrence of the terms only, the use of LSA as semantic similarity measure represents a plausible alternative to determine the homogeneity of corpora. The first step in LSA is to create the term-by-document matrix where each cell denotes the weight of the term [8]. In this work, the weight of the term has been determined by using *Term Frequency* ($tf_{ij}$) and *Document Frequency* ($df_i$). Whereas Term Frequency is an indicator of how important is a term for a document, Document Frequency is an indicator of how specific (or general) a term is across the documents.

Once we have built our matrix, the next step is the application of the mathematical technique *Singular Value Decomposition* (SVD) to factorise our matrix into three matrices. In addition to being useful as a method of co-occurrence analysis, SVD can also be useful as a method for dimensionality reduction. This is the reason why we factorise our term-by-document model: to find a reduced dimensional representation that lead us to the reconstruction of the matrix with the least possible information.

A formal description of the decomposition technique is as follows. Let $A_{td}$ denotes the term-by-document matrix. The factorisation of $A_{td}$ is represented by:

$$A_{td} = T_{tn}S_{nn}(D_{dn})^T \tag{1}$$

where $n = min(t, d)$ and the matrices T and D represent terms and documents in this new space. The S matrix is the diagonal matrix containing the singular values of $A_{td}$ [9]. Once a new space has been modelled, not only can similarity assessment be carried out with standard similarity measures, but also can visualise such similarity assessment.

# 4    Experimental Evaluation

In this section the corpora used in our experimentation is described. Because we intend to identify the semantic similarity between different domains, different language varieties are being considering in this work.

## 4.1    Data and Pre-processing

Our experimentation is based on corpora that consist in a collection of Epinions reviews developed by Taboada et al. [10]. Such dataset consists of eight different categories: books, cars computers, cookware, hotels, movies, music and phones. There are 50 opinions per category, giving a total of 400 reviews in the collection, which contains a grand total of 279,761 words. Also, each category contains 25 reviews per polarity that denote balance within each domain.

From the whole collection, we consider those domains with at least 4,000 terms. Thus, we discarded two domains: Cookware and Phones. These domains have been discarded because we can consider them as *outliers*: their number of terms is clearly separated from the rest of the domains. Then, from the remaining six, four domains were selected: Books, Computers, Movies and Music.

The set of sentences corresponding to each review in the collection was submitted to a tagger based on a broad use of lexical features: The Stanford Tagger with a remarkable degree of accuracy [11]. We model each review as a set of terms where the linguistic granularity of each term consists of unigrams; these are defined for our particular purpose as a word and its corresponding part of speech (e.g. *touched/Verb*). To optimise the set of terms to be analysed, the collection was also submitted to the lemmatisation process provided by the rich functionality of the Stanford Tagger. In this way, the term *touch/Verb* is different from the term *touch/Noun*.

Besides obtaining the unigrams corresponding to each review, two kind of linguistic terms are removed: *functions words* and *proper nouns*. Whereas the former are very common and not very useful for distinction purposes, the latter are very specific to a particular domain. In other words, we discard terms that occur practically in any domain and we discard terms that occur just about in one domain.

This pre-processing task leads to the definition of the term-by-document matrix. We first use *Document Frequency* $(df_i)$ to remove peculiar terms (terms that dont exhibit co-occurrence) and then, the value of each cell (i.e. the weight of the term) is determined by using *Term Frequency* $(tf_{ij})$.

## 4.2    Results and Analysis

Figure 1 gives evidence on how different language varieties are being considering in this work. Taking advantage of the new space created by LSA: a new reduced dimensional model, the D matrix allows us to obtain the coordinates of each domain. We observe for example how each domain can be clearly noticed as each one keeps enough distance from the rest; thus, the set of reviews corresponding to each domain keeps small within-domain distance across them. Also, we see in Figure 1 how a small distance between Movies and Music may indicate some degree of similarity. In addition to visual evidence, Table 1 shows the distance across domains by using Euclidean measure.

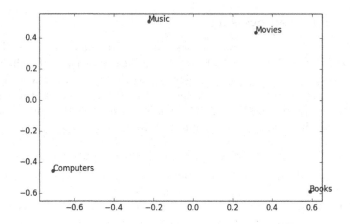

**Fig. 1.** Geometric representation of domains diversity

**Table 1.** Euclidean distance across domains

|        | Books  | Compu  | Movies | Music  |
|--------|--------|--------|--------|--------|
| **Books**  |        | 1.3054 | 1.0598 | 1.3640 |
| **Compu**  | 1.3054 |        | 1.3578 | 1.0774 |
| **Movies** | 1.0598 | 1.3578 |        | 0.5442 |
| **Music**  | 1.3640 | 1.0774 | 0.5442 |        |

Now, we make use of Text Categorisation (TC) as the framework for the evaluation of the homogeneity of the collection. For identification of similar domains, we adopt the approach suggested for the optimisation of the Information Retrieval (IR) task: "to avoid every query to be compared with every document in the collection, to define a set of clusters in such a way that queries can be first compared with each cluster" [12]. However, considering that we apply TC as our similarity context, we adapt such approach: the set of clusters correspond to the set of different domains and the queries correspond to new reviews.

The method to evaluate the performance is based on the *train and test* method so we randomly split the reviews corresponding to each domain in proportion 80:20. Table 2 shows the similarity results across domains by using Euclidean distance and Figure 2 shows the particular results for the similarity evaluation of new Books reviews. Two points are worth to notice. First, the new Books reviews are clearly categorised as Books reviews. Second, the closest similar domain after Books is Movies, denoting consistency with the results (illustrated by Table 1 and Table 2) that show the diversity of the corpora. In fact, as Table 1 shows how

Movies is the closest domain to Books, Table 2 also does. So we can suggest that the cost of portability of a linguistic tool developed for Movies is less than the cost of adaptability of a tool designed for Music. In this way, adapting a linguistic tool to a new domain such as Books, a tool based on Movies is recommended for its customisation.

**Table 2.** Euclidean distance between domains and new reviews

|        | Books  | Compu  | Movies | Music  |
|--------|--------|--------|--------|--------|
| **Books**  | 0.3603 | 0.9173 | 0.8421 | 1.0370 |
| **Compu**  | 1.0213 | 0.3733 | 0.9360 | 1.2477 |
| **Movies** | 0.8906 | 0.9414 | 0.5150 | 0.7888 |
| **Music**  | 1.1179 | 1.2553 | 0.9991 | 0.1312 |

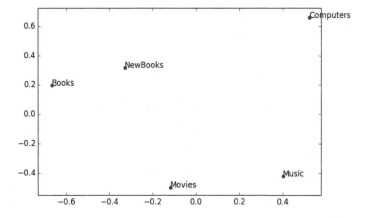

**Fig. 2.** Geometric representation of domains and NewBooks as query

In addition to Books, the results for Movies and Music also denote consistency with the results that show the diversity of the collection. Table 1 and Table 2 show how Music is the closest domain to Movies and vice versa. However, this consistency is not observed on Computers. We attribute this variation to the identification of high semantic similarity between Movies and Music (Figure 1 and Table 1), suggesting that for the adaptation of a linguistic tool to a new domain such as Computers, a tool based on Movies or Music is recommended for its customisation.

We can also visualise the obtained results with colours. However, to make use of colours, we use the values of the D matrix from a different perspective. We select two different colours: one for negatives values and the other one for positives. For the sake of illustration, we also choose four different-colour intensities for the singular values. Figure 3 shows the colour bar corresponding to the results for new Books reviews. Similar colours in both bars denoting more semantic similarity, we can see how Movies is the closest domain to Books.

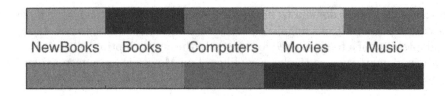

**Fig. 3.** Similarity results for NewBooks reviews based on colours

A note of caution: the semantic similarity of the method does not entail that a linguistic tool for a particular task and domain exhibits almost the same performance for a similar foreign domain. For example, in opinion mining, the adaptability of a linguistic tool such as a sentiment classifier is different from a tool for the extraction of comparative relations. The analysis of a polarity-feature distribution is crucial for a classifier [13], whereas the analysis of a comparative-feature distribution is essential for a relations-extractor [14].

## 5    Conclusions and Future Work

In this paper, we focus our attention in the key role of corpus homogeneity in the problem of domain adaptation. As initial step to cope with domain adaptation, to determine the homogeneity of the implicated corpora is crucial. By mapping the texts and corresponding terms into the latent semantic space we identify the semantic relatedness between domains. The evaluation conducted with four different domains shows how the use of text categorisation, as the frame for detection of semantic similarity, is a plausible method to measure the homogeneity of the collection.

As part of our future work, we intend to extend our investigation on the cost of adaptability of two different linguistic tools. For example, according to our results, a linguistic tool based on Movies is recommended for the customisation to Books. To investigate the difference in the cost of customisation between a classifier and a relations-extractor sounds interesting.

Also, we are interested in the implications of the analysis of more datasets collections. For example, the dataset collected by Blitzer et al. [15] is an interesting collection of product reviews corresponding to four domains: books, DVDs, electronics, and kitchen appliances. We think this collection is worth our attention to improve and optimise our analysis.

## References

1. Glickman, O., Jones, R.: Examining machine learning for adaptable end-to-end information extraction systems (1999)
2. Cardie, C.: Empirical methods in information extraction. AI Magazine 39(1), 65–79 (1997)

3. Vila, K., Ferrández, A.: Model-driven restricted-domain adaptation of question answering systems for business intelligence. In: Proceedings of the 2nd International Workshop on Business Intelligence and the WEB, pp. 36–43 (2011)
4. Oakes, M.P.: Statistical measures for corpus profiling. In: BCS Offices, London (eds.) Proceedings of the Open University Workshop on Corpus Profiling (2008)
5. Bank, M., Remus, R., Schierle, M.: Textual characteristics for language engineering (2012)
6. Kilgarriff, A.: Comparig corpora. International Journal of Corpus Linguistics 6(1), 97–133 (2001)
7. Mihalcea, R., Corley, C., Strapparava, C.: Corpus-based and knowledge-based measures of text semantic similarity. In: Proceedings of the 21st National Conference on Artificial Intelligence, vol. 1, pp. 775–780 (2006)
8. Landauer, T.K., Foltz, P., Laham, D.: Introduction to latent semantic analysis. Discourse Processes 25 (1998)
9. Manning, C., Schutze, H.: Foundations of Statistical Natural Language Processing. MIT Press (1999)
10. Taboada, M., Anthony, C., Voll, K.: Creating semantic orientation dictionaries, pp. 427–432 (2006)
11. Toutanova, K., Klein, D., Manning, C., Singer, Y.: Feature-rich part-of-speech tagging with a cyclic dependency network, pp. 252–259 (2003)
12. Jurafsky, D., Martin, J.H.: Speech and Language Processing. 2nd edn. Prentice Hall (2008)
13. Aue, A., Gamon, M.: Customizing sentiment classifiers to new domains: A case study (2005)
14. Jindal, N., Liu, B.: Mining comparative sentences and relations (2006)
15. Blitzer, J., Dredze, M., Pereira, F.: Biographies, bollywood, boom-boxes and blenders: Domain adaptation for sentiment classification (2007)

# Novel Unsupervised Features for Czech Multi-label Document Classification

Tomáš Brychcín[1,2] and Pavel Král[1,2]

[1] Dept. of Computer Science & Engineering,
Faculty of Applied Sciences,
University of West Bohemia,
Plzeň, Czech Republic
[2] NTIS - New Technologies for the Information Society,
Faculty of Applied Sciences,
University of West Bohemia,
Plzeň, Czech Republic
{brychcin,pkral}@kiv.zcu.cz

**Abstract.** This paper deals with automatic multi-label document classification in the context of a real application for the Czech News Agency. The main goal of this work consists in proposing novel fully unsupervised features based on an unsupervised stemmer, Latent Dirichlet Allocation and semantic spaces (HAL and COALS). The proposed features are integrated into the document classification task. Another interesting contribution is that these two semantic spaces have never been used in the context of document classification before. The proposed approaches are evaluated on a Czech newspaper corpus. We experimentally show that almost all proposed features significantly improve the document classification score. The corpus is freely available for research purposes.

**Keywords:** Multi-label Document Classification, LDA, Semantic spaces, HAL, COALS, HPS, Stemming, Czech, Czech News Agency, Maximum Entropy.

## 1 Introduction

Nowadays, the amount of electronic text documents and the size of the World Wide Web increase extremely rapidly. Therefore, automatic document classification (or categorization) becomes very important for information retrieval.

In this work, we focus on the *multi-label* document classification[1] in the context of a real application for the Czech News Agency (ČTK)[2]. ČTK produces daily about one thousand of text documents. These documents belong to different categories such as politics, sport, culture, business, etc. In the current application, documents are manually annotated. Unfortunately, the manual labeling represents a very time consuming and

---

[1] *Multi-label* document classification: one document is usually labeled with more than one label from a predefined set of labels vs. *Single-label* document classification: one document is assigned exactly to one label.
[2] http://www.ctk.eu

A. Gelbukh et al. (Eds.): MICAI 2014, Part I, LNAI 8856, pp. 70–79, 2014.

expensive task. It is thus beneficial to propose and implement an automatic document classification system.

One important issue in the document classification field is the high dimensionality and insufficient precision of the feature vector. Several feature selection methods and sophisticated language specific features have been proposed. The main drawback of these methods is that they need a significant amount of the annotated data. Furthermore, a complete re-annotation is necessary when the target language is modified.

In this work, we address these issues by proposing novel fully unsupervised features based on an unsupervised stemmer, Latent Dirichlet Allocation (LDA) and semantic spaces (HAL and COALS). We further integrate these features into the document classification task.

The next scientific contribution is evaluating a new simple LDA model, called S-LDA, which integrates stem features into the topic modeling. Another interesting contribution is the use of semantic space models (i.e. HAL and COALS), because they have not been used for the document classification yet. The last contribution consists in the evaluation of the proposed approaches on Czech, as a representative of morphologically rich language.

The paper structure is as follows. Section 2 introduces the document classification approaches with a particular focus on the document representation. Section 3 describes our proposed features and their integration into the document classification task. Section 4 deals with the experiments on the ČTK corpus. In the last section, we discuss the research results and we propose some future research directions.

## 2    Related Work

The today's document classification relies usually on supervised machine learning methods that exploit a manually annotated training corpus to train a classifier, which in turn identifies the class of new unlabeled documents. Most approaches are based on the Vector Space Models (VSMs), which mostly represent each document as a vector of all occurring words usually weighted by their Term Frequency-Inverse Document Frequency (TF-IDF).

Several classification algorithms have been successfully applied [3,7], e.g. Bayesian classifiers, decision trees, k-Nearest Neighbor (kNN), rule learning algorithms, neural networks, fuzzy logic based algorithms, Maximum Entropy (ME) and Support Vector Machines (SVMs). However, one important issue of this task is that the feature space in VSM has a high dimension which negatively affects the performance of the classifiers.

Numerous feature selection/reduction approaches have been proposed in order to solve this problem. The successfully used feature selection methods include Document Frequency (DF), Mutual Information (MI), Information Gain (IG), Chi-square test or Gallavotti, Sebastiani & Simi metric [8,9].

In the last years, multi-label document classification becomes a popular research field, because it corresponds usually better to the needs of the real applications than the single-label document classification. One popular approach presented in [27] uses $n$ binary *class/no class* classifiers. A final classification is then given by an union of these partial results. Another approach presented by the authors of [27] simplifies the multi-label document classification task by replacing *each different* set of labels by a new *single label.* Then, a single-label document classifier is created on such data. Note that this approach suffers by the data sparsity problem. Zhu et al. propose in [30] another multi-label document classification approach. The same classifier as in the single-label document classification task is created. The document is associated with a set of labels based on an acceptance *threshold.* The other methods are presented for instance in survey [26].

Furthermore, a better document representation may lead to decreasing the feature vector dimension, e.g. using lexical and syntactic features as shown in [18]. Chandrasekar et al. further show in [6] that it is beneficial to use POS-tag filtration in order to represent a document more accurate. The authors of [21] and [28] use a set of linguistic features. Unfortunately, they do not show any impact to the document classification task. However, they conclude that more complex linguistic features may improve the classification score.

More recently, an advanced technique based on Labeled Latent Dirichlet Allocation (L-LDA) [24] has been introduced. Unlike our approach, L-LDA incorporates supervision by constraining the topic model to use only those topics that correspond to document labels. Principal Component Analysis (PCA) [10] incorporating semantic concepts [29] has been also successfully proposed for the document classification. Semi-supervised approaches, which augment labeled training corpus with unlabeled data [22] were also used.

The most of the proposed approaches is focused on English. Unfortunately, only little work about the document classification in other non-mainstream languages, particularly in Czech, exits. Hrala et al. [14] use lemmatization and POS-tag filtering for a precise representation of the Czech documents. The authors further show the performance of three multi-label classification approaches [13].

## 3    Document Classification

In the following sections we describe the proposed unsupervised features and classification approaches.

### 3.1    Unsupervised Stemming

Stemming is a task to replace a particular (inflected) word form by its "stem" (an unique label for all morphological forms of a word). It is used in many Natural Language Processing (NLP) fields (e.g. information retrieval) to reduce the number of parameters with a positive impact to the classification accuracy. Therefore, we assume that stems should improve the results of the document classification.

We propose two approaches to integrate the stem features into the document classification. In the first approach, the stem occurrences are used directly as the features, while in the second one, we use stems as a preprocessing step for LDA. We use an unsupervised stemming algorithm called HPS [5] This stemmer have been already proved to be very efficient in the NLP, see for example [12].

Note that this task is very similar to lemmatization. However, the main advantage of our stemming approach is that it is fully unsupervised and thus it does not need any annotated data (only plain text).

## 3.2    Latent Dirichlet Allocation

Latent Dirichlet Allocation (LDA) [2] is a popular topic model that assigns a topic to each word in the document collection. In our first approach, we use a standard LDA model as follows. We calculate the topic probabilities for each document. The probability of each topic $t$ is given by the number of times the topic $t$ occurs in a document divided by the document size. These probabilities are used directly as new features for a classifier.

In our second approach, we use stems instead of words. This concept is motivated by the following assumptions. LDA is a bag-of-word model, thus the word role in a sentence is inhibited. We assume that the morphosyntactic information in a document is useless for inferring topics. Moreover, the word normalization (i.e. stemming in our case) can reduce the data sparsity problem, which is particularly significant in the processing of morphologically rich languages (e.g. Czech). The parameters of such model should be better estimated than the parameters of the standard LDA. The features for the classifier are calculated in the same way as for the word-based LDA. This model will be hereafter called the *S-LDA* (Stem-based LDA).

## 3.3    Semantic Spaces

Semantic spaces represent words as high dimensional vectors. Semantically close words should be represented by similar vectors and the vector space gives an opportunity to use a clustering method to create word clusters.

The authors of [4] have proved that word clusters created by the semantic spaces improve significantly language modeling. We assume that these models can play an important role for document classification. We use two semantic space models, namely: HAL (Hyperspace Analogue to Language) [19] and COALS (Correlated Occurrence Analogue to Lexical Semantic) [25]. The word clusters are created using Repeated bisection algorithm. The document is then represented as a bag of clusters and we use a tf-idf weighting scheme for each cluster to create the features.

We assume that these models should reduce (analogically as in the previous case) the data sparsity problem. It is worth of mentioning that these two semantic space models have never been used in the context of document classification before.

## 3.4    Document Classification

For multi-label classification, we use (as presented in [27]) $n$ binary classifiers $C_{i=1}^{n}$ : $d \rightarrow l, \neg l$ (i.e. each binary classifier assigns the document $d$ to the label $l$ iff the label is included in the document, $\neg l$ otherwise). The classification result is given by the following equation:

$$C(d) = \cup_{i=1}^{n} : C_i(d) \qquad (1)$$

The Maximum Entropy (ME) [1] classifier is used. As a baseline, we use the tf-idf weighting of the word features. Then, this set is progressively extended by the novel unsupervised features. In order to facilitate the reading of the paper, all features are summarized next.

- **Words (baseline)** – Occurrence of a word in a document. Tf-idf weighting is used.
- **Stems** – Occurrence of a stem in a document. Tf-idf weighting is used.
- **LDA** – LDA topic probabilities for a document.
- **S-LDA** – S-LDA topic probabilities for a document.
- **HAL** – Occurrence of a HAL cluster in a document. Tf-idf weighting is used.
- **COALS** – Occurrence of a COALS cluster in a document. Tf-idf weighting is used.

## 4   Experiments

In our experiments we use LDA implementation from the MALLET [20] tool-kit. For each experiment, we train LDA with 1,000 iterations of the Gibbs sampling. The hyperparameters of the Dirichlet distributions were (as proposed in [11]) initially set to $\alpha = 50/K$, where $K$ is the number of topics and $\beta = 0.1$.

The S-Space package [15] is used for implementation of the HAL and COALS algorithms. For each semantic space, we use a four-word context window (in both directions). HAL uses a matrix consisting of 50,000 columns. COALS uses a matrix with 14,000 columns (as suggested by the authors of the algorithm). SVD (Singular Value Decomposition) was not used in our experiments.

We created the word clusters in the similar way as described in [4], i.e. by using Repeated Bisection algorithm and cosine similarity metric. For clustering, we use an implementation from the CLUTO software package [16]. For both semantic spaces, the word vectors are clustered into four depths: 100, 500, 1,000, and 5,000 clusters.

For multi-label classification we use Brainy [17] implementation of Maximum Entropy classifier.

### 4.1   Corpus

As mentioned previously, the results of this work will be used by the ČTK. Therefore, we use Czech document collection provided by the ČTK for the training of our models (i.e. LDA, S-LDA, semantic spaces and multi-label classifier).

This corpus contains 2,974,040 words belonging to 11,955 documents annotated from a set of 37 categories. Figure 1 illustrates the distribution of the documents depending on the number of labels. This corpus is freely available for research purposes at http://home.zcu.cz/~pkral/sw/.

In all experiments, we use the five-fold cross-validation procedure, where 20% of the corpus is reserved for the test. For evaluation of the document classification accuracy, we use the standard Precision $(P)$, Recall $(R)$ and F-measure $(F_m)$ metrics [23]. The confidence interval of the experimental results is 0.6% at a confidence level of 0.95.

No feature selection has been done in our experiments to clearly show the impact of the proposed features. In the following tables, the term *words* denotes the word features and *stems* denotes the stem features.

### 4.2   Classification Results of the LDA and S-LDA Models

In this experiment, we would like to compare the classification results of the stand-alone LDA and S-LDA model (see Table 1). This table shows that the larger number of

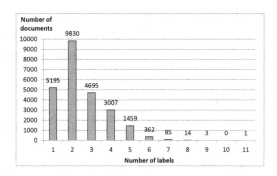

**Fig. 1.** Distribution of the documents depending on the number of labels

**Table 1.** Results of stand-alone LDA and S-LDA models

| topics | LDA | | | S-LDA | | |
|---|---|---|---|---|---|---|
| | $P[\%]$ | $R[\%]$ | $F_m[\%]$ | $P[\%]$ | $R[\%]$ | $F_m[\%]$ |
| 100 | 82.9 | 65.9 | 73.4 | 83.1 | 66.0 | 73.6 |
| 200 | 83.4 | 69.1 | 75.6 | 83.7 | 70.3 | 76.4 |
| 300 | 84.0 | 71.1 | 77.0 | 85.3 | 72.6 | 78.4 |
| 400 | 83.3 | 70.7 | 77.5 | 85.5 | 73.2 | 78.8 |
| 500 | 84.7 | 72.6 | 78.2 | 85.9 | 74.0 | 79.5 |

the topics is better for document classification. Moreover, the proposed S-LDA slightly outperforms the stand-alone LDA model for all topic numbers.

### 4.3 Classification Results of the LDA and S-LDA Models with Baseline Word Features

This experiment compares the classification results of the stand-alone LDA and S-LDA models when the baseline word features are also used (see Table 2). Unlike the previous experiment, the recognition score remains almost constant for every topic number and both LDA models. The topic number and LDA type thus no longer play any role for document classification.

**Table 2.** Results of LDA models with baseline word features

| topics | Words+LDA | | | Words+S-LDA | | |
|---|---|---|---|---|---|---|
| | $P[\%]$ | $R[\%]$ | $F_m[\%]$ | $P[\%]$ | $R[\%]$ | $F_m[\%]$ |
| 100 | 89.0 | 74.0 | 80.8 | 88.9 | 74.0 | 80.8 |
| 200 | 88.9 | 73.8 | 80.7 | 88.9 | 73.6 | 80.5 |
| 300 | 88.9 | 73.6 | 80.6 | 89.0 | 73.6 | 80.6 |
| 400 | 88.8 | 73.7 | 80.5 | 88.8 | 73.7 | 80.5 |
| 500 | 88.8 | 73.7 | 80.5 | 88.8 | 73.5 | 80.4 |

### 4.4 Classification Results of the Semantic Space Models

This experiment compares the classification results of the HAL and COALS models (see Table 3). The table shows that with rising number of clusters the classification score increases. At the level of 5,000 clusters the score is almost the same as for the baseline. However, the number of the parameters in the classifier is significantly reduced.

In the case of COALS and 5,000 clusters the F-measure is slightly better than the baseline. However, we believe this deviation is caused by a chance. In all these experiments COALS outperforms the HAL model.

**Table 3.** Results of semantic space models

| clusters | HAL | | | COALS | | |
|---|---|---|---|---|---|---|
| | $P[\%]$ | $R[\%]$ | $F_m[\%]$ | $P[\%]$ | $R[\%]$ | $F_m[\%]$ |
| 100 | 58.5 | 14.7 | 23.6 | 66.9 | 25.2 | 36.6 |
| 500 | 76.1 | 51.3 | 61.3 | 79.6 | 59.3 | 68.0 |
| 1000 | 80.2 | 62.0 | 70.0 | 81.6 | 64.8 | 72.2 |
| 5000 | 87.9 | 72.1 | 79.2 | 88.5 | 73.5 | 80.3 |

### 4.5 Classification Results of the Semantic Space Models with Baseline Word Features

This experiment compares the classification results of the HAL and COALS models when the baseline word features are also used. The results are reported in Table 4. Unlike the previous experiment, the recognition score remains almost constant for all clusters and for both semantic space models.

We can explain this behavior by the fact that the clusters from semantic spaces do not bring any useful additional information compared to the baseline.

**Table 4.** Results of semantic space models with baseline word features

| clusters | Words+HAL | | | Words+COALS | | |
|---|---|---|---|---|---|---|
| | $P[\%]$ | $R[\%]$ | $F_m[\%]$ | $P[\%]$ | $R[\%]$ | $F_m[\%]$ |
| 100 | 88.2 | 72.6 | 79.7 | 88.2 | 72.8 | 79.7 |
| 500 | 88.2 | 72.7 | 79.7 | 88.2 | 72.7 | 79.7 |
| 1000 | 88.3 | 72.8 | 79.8 | 88.2 | 72.7 | 79.7 |
| 5000 | 88.3 | 72.8 | 79.8 | 88.3 | 72.7 | 79.7 |

### 4.6 Classification Results of the Different Model Combinations

In this section we evaluate and compare several combinations of our models (see Table 5). The best model configurations from the previous experiments are used. These configurations are compared over the baseline "word" approach (first line in the table). This experiment clearly shows that almost all proposed features significantly improve the document classification accuracy. The F-measure improvement is 2.1% in the absolute value when all proposed features are used. Only the semantic space models do not have any significant impact to improve the classification score. Note that this behavior has been already justified in the previous section.

**Table 5.** Results of different model combinations. The term COALS denotes the combination of all four COALS models (i.e. 100, 500, 1000, and 5000 clusters). The term HAL denotes the combination of all HAL models. The term S-LDA means the combination of the S-LDA models with 100 and 400 topics.

| model | $P[\%]$ | $R[\%]$ | $F_m[\%]$ | impr. $F_m[\%]$ |
|---|---|---|---|---|
| words | 88.1 | 72.7 | 79.7 | |
| stems | 86.4 | 75.0 | 80.3 | +0.7 |
| words+stems | 88.3 | 74.8 | 81.0 | +1.3 |
| words+HAL | 88.4 | 72.8 | 79.9 | +0.2 |
| words+COALS | 88.5 | 72.8 | 79.9 | +0.2 |
| words+S-LDA | 89.2 | 74.6 | 81.2 | +1.6 |
| words+stems+S-LDA | 88.8 | 75.5 | 81.6 | +1.9 |
| words+stems+S-LDA+COALS | 89.0 | 75.6 | 81.7 | +2.1 |

## 5 Conclusions and Future Work

In this work, we have proposed novel fully unsupervised features based on an unsupervised stemmer HPS, Latent Dirichlet Allocation and semantic spaces (HAL and COALS). These features were further integrated into the multi-label document classification task.

We have evaluated the proposed approaches on the ČTK corpus in Czech that is a representative of morphologically rich languages.

We have experimentally shown that almost all proposed unsupervised features significantly improve the document classification score. The F-measure improvement over the baseline is 2.1% absolute, when all proposed features are used.

We plan to extend our work by experiments with different languages and language families. Due to the unsupervised character of the proposed methods, no additional annotations are required.

**Acknowledgements.** This work has been partly supported by the UWB grant SGS-2013-029 Advanced Computer and Information Systems and by the European Regional Development Fund (ERDF), project "NTIS - New Technologies for Information Society", European Centre of Excellence, CZ.1.05/1.1.00/02.0090. We also would like to thank Czech New Agency (ČTK) for support and for providing the data.

## References

1. Berger, A.L., Pietra, V.J.D., Pietra, S.A.D.: A maximum entropy approach to natural language processing. Computational linguistics 22(1), 39–71 (1996)
2. Blei, D.M., Ng, A.Y., Jordan, M.I., Lafferty, J.: Latent dirichlet allocation. Journal of Machine Learning Research 3, 2003 (2003)
3. Bratko, A., Filipič, B.: Exploiting structural information for semi-structured document categorization. In: Information Processing and Management, pp. 679–694 (2004)
4. Brychcín, T., Konopík, M.: Semantic spaces for improving language modeling. Computer Speech & Language 28(1), 192 (2014)

5. Brychcín, T., Konopík, M.: Hps: High precision stemmer. Information Processing & Management 51(1), 68–91 (2015), `http://www.sciencedirect.com/science/article/pii/S0306457314000843`

6. Chandrasekar, R., Srinivas, B.: Using syntactic information in document filtering: A comparative study of part-of-speech tagging and supertagging (1996)

7. Della Pietra, S., Della Pietra, V., Lafferty, J.: Inducing features of random fields. IEEE Transactions on Pattern Analysis and Machine Intelligence 19(4), 380–393 (1997), `http://ieeexplore.ieee.org/lpdocs/epic03/wrapper.htm?arnumber=588021`

8. Forman, G.: An extensive empirical study of feature selection metrics for text classification. The Journal of Machine Learning Research 3, 1289–1305 (2003)

9. Galavotti, L., Sebastiani, F., Simi, M.: Experiments on the use of feature selection and negative evidence in automated text categorization. In: Borbinha, J.L., Baker, T. (eds.) ECDL 2000. LNCS, vol. 1923, pp. 59–68. Springer, Heidelberg (2000), `http://dl.acm.org/citation.cfm?id=646633.699638`

10. Gomez, J.C., Moens, M.-F.: Pca document reconstruction for email classification. Computer Statistics and Data Analysis 56(3), 741–751 (2012)

11. Griffiths, T.L., Steyvers, M.: Finding scientific topics. Proceedings of the National Academy of Sciences of the United States of America 101(Suppl. 1), 5228–5235 (2004)

12. Habernal, I., Ptáček, T., Steinberger, J.: Sentiment analysis in czech social media using supervised machine learning. In: Proceedings of the 4th Workshop on Computational Approaches to Subjectivity, Sentiment and Social Media Analysis, pp. 65–74. Association for Computational Linguistics, Atlanta (2013)

13. Hrala, M., Král, P.: Multi-label document classification in czech. In: Habernal, I., Matousek, V. (eds.) TSD 2013. LNCS, vol. 8082, pp. 343–351. Springer, Heidelberg (2013)

14. Hrala, M., Král, P.: Evaluation of the document classification approaches. In: Burduk, R., Jackowski, K., Kurzynski, M., Wozniak, M., Zolnierek, A. (eds.) CORES 2013. Advances in Intelligent Systems and Computing, vol. 226, pp. 875–884. Springer, Heidelberg (2013)

15. Jurgens, D., Stevens, K.: The s-space package: An open source package for word space models. System Papers of the Association of Computational Linguistics (2010)

16. Karypis, G.: Cluto - a clustering toolkit (2003), `www.cs.umn.edu/~karypis/cluto`

17. Konkol, M.: Brainy: A machine learning library. In: Rutkowski, L., Korytkowski, M., Scherer, R., Tadeusiewicz, R., Zadeh, L.A., Zurada, J.M. (eds.) ICAISC 2014, Part II. LNCS, vol. 8468, pp. 490–499. Springer, Heidelberg (2014)

18. Lim, C.S., Lee, K.J., Kim, G.C.: Multiple sets of features for automatic genre classification of web documents. Information Processing and Management 41(5), 1263–1276 (2005), `http://www.sciencedirect.com/science/article/pii/S0306457304000676`

19. Lund, K., Burgess, C.: Producing high-dimensional semantic spaces from lexical co-occurrence. Behavior Research Methods Instruments and Computers 28(2), 203–208 (1996)

20. McCallum, A.K.: Mallet: A machine learning for language toolkit (2002), `http://mallet.cs.umass.edu`

21. Moschitti, A., Basili, R.: Complex linguistic features for text classification: A comprehensive study. In: McDonald, S., Tait, J.I. (eds.) ECIR 2004. LNCS, vol. 2997, pp. 181–196. Springer, Heidelberg (2004), `http://dx.doi.org/10.1007/978-3-540-24752-4_14`

22. Nigam, K., McCallum, A.K., Thrun, S., Mitchell, T.: Text Classification from Labeled and Unlabeled Documents Using EM. Mach. Learn. 39(2-3), 103–134 (2000), `http://dx.doi.org/10.1023/A:1007692713085`

23. Powers, D.: From precision, recall and f-measure to roc., informedness, markedness & correlation. Journal of Machine Learning Technologies 2(1), 37–63 (2011)

24. Ramage, D., Hall, D., Nallapati, R., Manning, C.D.: Labeled lda: A supervised topic model for credit attribution in multi-labeled corpora. In: Proceedings of the 2009 Conference on Empirical Methods in Natural Language Processing, EMNLP 2009, vol. 1, pp. 248–256. Association for Computational Linguistics, Stroudsburg (2009), `http://dl.acm.org/citation.cfm?id=1699510.1699543`
25. Rohde, D.L.T., Gonnerman, L.M., Plaut, D.C.: An improved method for deriving word meaning from lexical co-occurrence. Cognitive Psychology 7, 573–605 (2004)
26. Sebastiani, F.: Machine learning in automated text categorization. ACM computing surveys (CSUR) 34(1), 1–47 (2002)
27. Tsoumakas, G., Katakis, I.: Multi-label classification: An overview. International Journal of Data Warehousing and Mining (IJDWM) 3(3), 1–13 (2007)
28. Wong, A.K., Lee, J.W., Yeung, D.S.: Using complex linguistic features in context-sensitive text classification techniques. In: Proceedings of 2005 International Conference on Machine Learning and Cybernetics, vol. 5, pp. 3183–3188. IEEE (2005)
29. Yun, J., Jing, L., Yu, J., Huang, H.: A multi-layer text classification framework based on two-level representation model. Expert Systems with Applications 39(2), 2035–2046 (2012)
30. Zhu, S., Ji, X., Xu, W., Gong, Y.: Multi-labelled classification using maximum entropy method. In: Proceedings of the 28th Annual International ACM SIGIR Conference on Research and Development in Information Retrieval, pp. 274–281. ACM (2005)

# Feature Selection Based on Sampling and C4.5 Algorithm to Improve the Quality of Text Classification Using Naïve Bayes

Viviana Molano[1], Carlos Cobos[1], Martha Mendoza[1], Enrique Herrera-Viedma[2,3], and Milos Manic[4]

[1] Computer Science Department, University of Cauca, Colombia
{jvmolano,ccobos,mmendoza}@unicauca.edu.co
[2] Department of Computer Science and Artificial Intelligence, University of Granada, Spain
viedma@decsai.ugr.es
[3] Department of Electrical and Computer Engineering, Faculty of Engineering,
King Abdulaziz University, Jeddah 21589, Saudi Arabia
[4] School of Engineering East Hall, Virginia Commonwealth University, Virginia, U.S.A.
misko@ieee.org

**Abstract.** Automatic text classification into predefined categories is an increasingly important task given the vast number of electronic documents available on the Internet and enterprise servers. Successful text classification relies heavily on the vital task of dimensionality reduction, which aims to improve classification accuracy, give greater expression to the classification process, and improve classification computational efficiency. In this paper, two algorithms for feature selection are presented, based on sampling and weighted sampling that build on the C4.5 algorithm. The results demonstrate considerable improvements with regard to classification accuracy - up to 10% - compared to traditional algorithms such as C4.5, Naïve Bayes and Support Vector Machines. The classification process is performed using the Naïve Bayes model in the space of reduced dimensionality. Experiments were carried out using data sets based on the Reuters-21578 collection.

## 1 Introduction

Thanks to the continued growth of digital information and the increasing accessibility, the classification of text documents has become a task of great interest to the world. The classification task supports key tasks related to electronic trading, search engines, antivirus, email, etc. A great deal of research has been devoted to the subject, and a variety of solutions proposed that apply or adapt such algorithms as Naïve Bayes [1-3], K Nearest Neighbors (KNN) [4-7], Support Vector Machines (SVM) [8, 9] and Neural Networks [10].

The text classification process begins by characterizing the documents. This leads to a structured representation that encapsulates the information in them. A reliable representation of a document is the result of the extraction and selection of its most representative characteristics and its encoding and organization in order to be processed by a classification algorithm. Feature extraction is the process of segmentation

A. Gelbukh et al. (Eds.): MICAI 2014, Part I, LNAI 8856, pp. 80–91, 2014.

and analysis of the text, from which it is possible to differentiate components such as paragraphs, sentences, words, relationships of frequencies, among others, that define the document's content or structure. These components represent the characteristics and work at a syntactic or semantic level. The syntactic characteristics (features) refer to statistical data on occurrences of segmented components (words or phrases), while the semantic features are linked with the sense that they are given and relationships that may exist between them. When features have been extracted, it is crucial to measure their amount of representativeness (importance), i.e. measure of the degree of differentiation that these features provide between the two documents. With this in mind, it is determined whether or not features need to be taken into account during the classification process. This is the task of feature selection, which predominantly seeks to reduce dimensionality, improving the accuracy of the classification process. This reduction can also be done by finding nontrivial relationships between features.

With the feature set defined, each document is differentiated according to its content and represented so that it can be processed by a classification algorithm. This algorithm is responsible for categorizing the content, by using a classifier model that is obtained in a training phase with labeled data (with a defined class), or by comparing its similarity to other documents that have a class assigned.

During the process previously explained, the principal points comprise: 1) managing of the high dimensionality of the feature sets obtained in the text collections, and 2) increasing the expressivity of the classification models generated. In seeking to alleviate the previously stated problems, this paper presents a review of the state of the art and proposes two algorithms that apply C4.5 under the concept of sampling and weighted sampling to reduce dimensionality, and build upon Naïve Bayes algorithm for executing the classification process on the reduced feature space. The novel method exhibits better results in classification accuracy and generates models that are easier to understand by users than the methods typically used.

The rest of the paper goes as follows. Section 2 presents recent research work related to text classification. Section 3 describes the proposed algorithm and its variations. Section 4 describes the data set for evaluation and the comparative analysis against C4.5, Naïve Bayes and Support Vector Machines techniques. Finally, the conclusions and future work the authors plan to pursue are presented in Section 5.

## 2    Related Works

A very widely based state of the art already exists with regard to automatic text classification. As a result, there may be a number solutions designed to meet the varied challenges this field offers. The following takes a brief look at some established methods, first related to document representation (extraction and feature selection) and then focused on the task of classification.

### 2.1    Document Representation: Extraction and Feature Selection

Many researchers have focused their attention on finding the best representation mechanism, knowing that this task is critical to the success of the classification.

Vector Space Model (VSM) based on the model Bag Of Words (BOW), represents a document as a vector of words or phrases associated with their frequency of occurrence, which is commonly calculated using TF-IDF [6, 11, 12]. VSM is the most used method, for its simple implementation, easy interpretation and because it achieves highly significant condensed document content information [11-13]. However, the information it provides is only syntactic in nature and does not take into account the meaning and distribution of terms or structure of the document, in addition to the vectors being high-dimensional [1, 14, 15]. Another widely used model is Latent Semantic Indexing (LSI), which analyzes co-occurrence of high order to find latent semantic relationships between terms. This model finds synonymy and polysemy relationships [11, 15, 16] but has a high computational cost [11].

As a result of the shortcomings of these methods, there are new proposals which explore other data structures and semantic relationships. In [17] a two-level representation is proposed: building a VSM using TF-IDF terms (syntax), and generating concepts, associating each term, depending on the context, with a corresponding definition in Wikipedia (semantic). In [14], graphs to represent both content and structure are used, supported by WordNet. In [16], the authors also use graphs to represent patterns of association between terms. These patterns are roads that are given by the co-occurrence of terms in documents belonging to the same class. In [18] BOW is extended by analyzing grammatical relations between terms to determine patterns of lexical dependency. In [15] a document is represented by a vector that includes concepts, which are combinations of semantically related terms (according to predefined syntactic features). The work done [19] in presents a model for feature extraction composite (c-features) based on the co-occurrence of pairs of terms for each category, regardless of position, order or distance. In [20] the document title importance is highlighted and even though its terms may not be high frequency, they propose to assign greater weight in the feature matrix (TF-IDF), to the terms that it contains. Similarly to [21] except that it analyzes semantically the title to extract concepts before to the weighting.

Other works done in this area apply the concept of clustering. In [9] clusters of words closely related at semantic level (based on co-occurrences of terms across categories) are created and each is treated as a new feature. Some studies have also been done in relation to selection measures: the study in [22] concludes that the best performance is obtained when signed X2 and signed information gain are combined. In [23] it is determined that the measures in which Naïve Bayes achieves the greatest accuracy in the selection task are Multi-class Odds Ratio (MOR) and Class Discriminating Measure (CDM), CDM being the highest simplicity.

All the above mentioned proposals seek to enrich the semantic representation of a document and emphasize the importance of selecting the really significant features prior to classification. However, it is important to note that none of these proposals is clear as to whether all selected features are contributing to the classification process, which indicates that the level of reduction could be carried out further. In most of the work reviewed so far, the selection process and reduction are developed based on the analysis of certain metrics such as Information Gain (IG), Mutual Information (MI), or generally posting frequency. However, what is not taken into account is the inclusion of a classifier, which could contribute to refine the set of features needed to improve the classification task. In many cases a threshold is required, which is difficult to optimally define. In [24], an objective function of feature selection based on probability is presented, which defines a Bayesian adaptive model selection. However, this approach is computationally very expensive.

## 2.2   Classification

In classification there are also many research papers and hence many proposals developed that revolve around improving the accuracy of the results and reduce computing costs. In [25], the ISOBagC4.5 algorithm is proposed, which implements Isomap for feature reduction and Bagging with C4.5 algorithm for classification. Their results are better than Bagging C4.5 but the optimum values are not defined for the parameters and the complexity of the algorithm Isomap is very high.

In [26] and [27] methods for generating clusters are proposed based on similarity of features using K-means (or an extension thereof). Each cluster is trained to generate a specific classification. These approaches based on clustering have an expensive training phase, especially when large and unbalanced data sets are involved. Furthermore, in [10], it is shown how to generate clusters using a neural network using frequency matrix of terms by document. The results improve as the size of the training set increases.

There are other proposals that have sought to extend and enhance traditional classification algorithms, e.g. [28] proposes the use of KNN with the Mahalanobis distance. [29] authors improve K-NN to reduce the search space of the immediate neighbors. In [13], the importance of data distribution is highlighted. They use a measure of density to increase or decrease the distance between a sample to be classified and its K nearest neighbors. In this work, the increase in accuracy is more visible as the training set grows. [12] describes an algorithm based on KNN classifier with feature selection after taking into account the frequency, distribution and concentration of the data. In [4], an improved KNN is put forward where the parameter K is optimized based on the features selected by cross validation, and that uses IG as a metric for comparison. The accuracy of the results is much higher than conventional KNN, but not very significant compared with SVM. The work proposed in [30] is based on a graph representation where the weights are calculated using KNN (cosine measure) from TF-IDF matrix. On average, the results are more accurate than the comparison algorithms (including SVM, TSVM, and LP), but in the comparison of accuracy by category it is not always better.

The idea presented in [8] is based on combining SVM and KNN by classification in two stages. The first stage uses VPRSVM (SVM based on Variable Precision Rough sets - VPRS) to filter noise and partition the feature space by category (according to the level of confidence in the assignment of the class). The second stage focuses on RKNN (Restrictive K Nearest Neighbor) to reduce class candidates from partitions generated. In [31], the authors propose to construct a combined classifier from SVM, Naïve Bayes and Rocchio that trains with positive data and is capable of generating negative from unlabeled data.

In [1], a Naïve Bayes Multinomial extension (MNB) is shown, which presents a semi-supervised algorithm for learning parameters: Semi-Supervised Frequency Estimate (SFE). Precision results obtained do not exceed MNB for all sets of test data. In [16], the Higher Order Naïve Bayes (HONB) algorithm is put forward; this algorithm takes advantage of the connectivity of the search terms by chains that co-occur among the documents of the same category. This proposal has a search phase connectivity that greatly increases the complexity of Naïve Bayes.

In [32], the authors present the High Relevance Keyword Extraction (HRKE) method to achieve text pre-processing and feature selection. In [33], a modeling language based on n-grams applied to the classification is used. In [34], the learning process is performed based on two types of related documents. A set of pre-labeled documents and other unlabeled documents set. The method performs automatic classification of the second data set through knowledge extracted from the features it shares with the first.

Some researchers elaborated more on the metrics used to compare two documents. For example, in [35], a generalization of the cosine measure using the Mahalanobis distance was proposed. This measure considers the correlation between terms. In [36], some measures for the KNN classification according to the results are explored. In this document, the authors argue that the choice of metric is dependent on the application domain. Other research has been directed toward specific applications of text classification. For example, in [2], Naïve Bayes Shrinkage for analysis based on medical diagnoses is presented, while in [3] web classification by Naïve Bayes algorithm that handles HTML tags and hyperlinks is presented. In [37], an extension of TF-IDF for unbalanced data representation given its distribution for the discovery of behavioral patterns between proteins from published literature is presented.

## 3    The Proposed Method

The method of feature selection (dimensionality reduction) presented in this paper has four stages: preprocessing, model generation, feature selection and classification. In the following, a detailed description of these stages is presented.

The method is based on the Terms by Documents Matrix (TDM) commonly used in Information Retrieval (IR). This matrix is built in the preprocessing stage. This stage use Lucene [38] and includes: terms tokenizer, lower case filter, stop word removal, Porter's stemming algorithm [39] and the building of the TDM matrix. TDM is based on the vector space model [39]. In this model, the documents are designed as bags of words, the document collection is represented by a matrix of D-terms by N-documents, each document is represented by a vector of normalized frequency term ($tf_i$) by the inverse document frequency for that term, in what is known as TF-IDF value (see Eq. (1)).

$$w_{i,j} = \frac{freq_{i,j}}{\max(freq_i)} \times \log\left(\frac{N}{n_j}\right)$$

$$(1)$$

Where $freq_{i,j}$ relates the number of occurrences of the term j-th in the document i-th, $max(freq_i)$ is the maximum frequency found in the document i-th, $N$ is the total number of documents in the collection and $n_j$ is the number of documents containing the j-th term.

The proposed method, called 10-WS-C4.5-TDM-NB-TDMR, uses ten (10) samples obtained with weighting techniques (WS). The document representation model is the TDM matrix. Each sample is used to create a specific decision tree based on C4.5 algorithm. Next, all different attributes in the 10 decision trees are used in order to build a reduced TDM matrix of documents (TDMR), and finally, the Naïve Bayes (NB) algorithm is used to classify new documents. **Fig. 1** shows the general pseudo-code of this method, including the model generation stage. An alternative method, called 10-S-C4.5-TDM-NB-TDMR, uses sampling with replacement (S in the name of this method instead of WS in previous one) instead of sampling with weighting, as is shown in **Fig. 2**. The final product of this stage is a list of terms that appears in all C4.5 decision trees. This list of terms is a subset of the D-terms in TDM matrix.

```
Preprocessing
Read text collection.
Create a TDM matrix including: Tokenize, lower case filter, stop word re-
moval, and stemming process.

Model generation
Assign equal weight to each training instance.
Initialize list of terms (L).
For each of I iterations:
   Apply C4.5 to weighted dataset.
   Extract terms (t) from C4.5 tree and include in list (L ← L U t).
   Compute error e of model on weighted dataset and store error.
   If e equal to zero:
    Terminate model generation.
   For each instance in dataset:
    If instance is not classified correctly by model:
        Multiply weight of instance by e / (1 - e).
   End For
   Normalize weight of all instances.
End For

Feature Selection
TDMR ← Reduce TDM matrix to selected terms in List L.
Build a Naïve Bayes model on TDMR and stored.

Classification
Predict class of new instances using Naïve Bayes model on TDMR representa-
tion.
```

**Fig. 1.** Pseudo-code for 10-WS-C4.5-TDM-NB-TDMR method

The next stage, called Feature Selection, focuses on the reduction of the TDM matrix. This new TDM matrix is called TDM Reduced (TDMR) and includes only the set of terms stored in the previous built list. Then, a Naïve Bayes (NB) model is applied to this new matrix (TDMR). Finally, the classification stage occurs when users need to classify a new instance (document). The document is represented in the reduced space (same terms on TDMR) and classified based on the Naïve Bayes model previously built and stored. It should be noted that just one model is needed in the classification stage.

```
Model generation
Let n be the number of instances in the training data.
Initialize list of terms (L)
For each of I iterations:
  Sample n instances with replacement from training data.
  Apply C4.5 to the sample.
  Extract terms (t) from C4.5 tree and include in list (L ← L U t).
End For
```

**Fig. 2.** Model generation stage in 10-S-C4.5-TDM-NB-TDMR method

The proposed method has an estimated time complexity of $O(m \times n)$ in the preprocessing stage, $O(I \times m \times n^2)$ in the model generation stage (based on complexity of C4.5 algorithm), $O(m \times n)$ in the feature selection stage, and $O(c \times r)$ in the classification stage, where I is the number of iterations (C4.5 models), m is the size of the training data, n is the number of attributes of the training data, c is the number of classes, and r is the number of attributes of the reduced training data ($r \ll n$). In general, the training phase (preprocessing, model generation, and features selection stages) is $O(m \times n^2)$, and will therefore have linear complexity with regard to the size of the training dataset and have a quadratic complexity with regard to the number of attributes in the training dataset. The testing (classification) phase is very fast (linear complexity with regard to the number of classes and the number of reduced attributes).

## 4     Experimentation

**Datasets for assessment:** The Reuters-21578 collection is commonly used as a neutral third party classifier, using human editors to classify manually and store thousands of news items. In this research a total of one hundred datasets were randomly built from this collection (these datasets are called Reuters-100; for details see www.unicauca. edu.co/~ccobos/wdc/reuters-100.htm). On average, datasets have 81.2 documents, 4.9 topics and 1,945 terms. **Table 1** shows detailed information from each dataset.

**Measures:** There are many different methods proposed for measuring the quality of classification. Three of the best known are precision, recall and F-measure, commonly used in IR [39]. In this research, the measures of weighted Precision, weighted Recall and weighted F-measure (the harmonic means of precision and recall) are used to evaluate the quality of solution. The True Positive Rate, the False Positive Rate, the True Negative Rate, and the False Negative Rate were also used to compare method results.

**Results with datasets:** The proposed algorithms were compared with C4.5, Naïve Bayes, and Support Vector Machines algorithms (all of them available in Weka). **Table 1** shows detailed results of Precision, Recall, and F-measure for each dataset. **Table 2** shows general results (mean, standard deviation, minimum value, and maximum value) of Precision, Recall and F-measure over all datasets. **Table 3** shows results of other important indexes, namely: True Positive Rate (TPR), True Negative Rate (TNR), False Positive Rate (FPR), False Negative Rate (FNR), and Receiver Operating Characteristic (ROC). Tests were carried out using cross validation with 10-folds.

**Table 1.** Description of Datasets (#Docs for number of documents, #Class for number of classes, #Attr for number of attributes, P for Precision, R for Recall and F for F-Measure)

| * Best results in bold | | | | C4.5 | | | NB | | | SVM | | | 10-S-C4.5-TDM-NB- TDMR | | | 10-WS-C4.5-TDM-NB-TDMR | | |
|---|---|---|---|---|---|---|---|---|---|---|---|---|---|---|---|---|---|---|
| Id | #Docs | #Class | #Attr | P | R | F | P | R | F | P | R | F | P | R | F | P | R | F |
| 0 | 49 | 2 | 1427 | 0.96 | 0.96 | 0.96 | 0.94 | 0.94 | 0.93 | 0.93 | 0.92 | 0.91 | 0.98 | 0.98 | 0.98 | **1.00** | **1.00** | **1.00** |
| 1 | 103 | 8 | 2601 | 0.83 | 0.83 | 0.82 | 0.78 | 0.75 | 0.75 | 0.87 | 0.86 | 0.86 | **0.94** | **0.92** | **0.93** | 0.82 | 0.83 | 0.82 |
| 2 | 77 | 4 | 1824 | 0.90 | 0.90 | 0.90 | 0.91 | 0.90 | 0.89 | 0.91 | 0.91 | 0.91 | 0.84 | 0.82 | 0.82 | **0.94** | **0.94** | **0.94** |
| 3 | 93 | 4 | 2100 | 0.91 | 0.90 | 0.90 | 0.94 | 0.94 | 0.94 | **0.97** | **0.97** | **0.97** | 0.92 | 0.90 | 0.90 | **0.97** | **0.97** | **0.97** |
| 4 | 78 | 3 | 1957 | 0.92 | 0.92 | 0.92 | 0.91 | 0.91 | 0.91 | 0.87 | 0.87 | 0.87 | **1.00** | **1.00** | **1.00** | 0.97 | 0.97 | 0.97 |
| 5 | 74 | 7 | 1989 | 0.97 | 0.97 | 0.97 | 0.74 | 0.73 | 0.73 | 0.84 | 0.81 | 0.81 | **0.99** | **0.99** | **0.99** | **0.99** | **0.99** | **0.99** |
| 6 | 81 | 4 | 1899 | 0.90 | 0.91 | 0.91 | 0.89 | 0.89 | 0.89 | 0.92 | 0.93 | 0.92 | 0.94 | 0.95 | 0.94 | **0.96** | **0.98** | **0.97** |
| 7 | 91 | 4 | 2254 | **0.95** | **0.95** | **0.95** | 0.82 | 0.81 | 0.81 | 0.86 | 0.85 | 0.84 | 0.84 | 0.81 | 0.82 | 0.92 | 0.90 | 0.90 |
| 8 | 78 | 6 | 1993 | 0.77 | 0.76 | 0.76 | 0.75 | 0.71 | 0.71 | **0.89** | **0.88** | **0.89** | 0.85 | 0.82 | 0.82 | 0.84 | 0.83 | 0.83 |
| 9 | 60 | 2 | 1578 | 0.94 | 0.93 | 0.93 | 0.93 | 0.92 | 0.91 | **0.98** | **0.98** | **0.98** | **0.98** | **0.98** | **0.98** | **0.98** | **0.98** | **0.98** |
| 10 | 75 | 7 | 2156 | 0.90 | 0.89 | 0.89 | 0.69 | 0.65 | 0.64 | 0.81 | 0.73 | 0.71 | 0.90 | 0.89 | 0.89 | **0.96** | **0.96** | **0.96** |
| 11 | 76 | 8 | 1891 | 0.81 | 0.80 | 0.80 | 0.86 | 0.84 | 0.83 | 0.86 | 0.82 | 0.81 | 0.83 | 0.82 | 0.82 | **0.92** | **0.91** | **0.91** |
| 12 | 102 | 3 | 2394 | 0.95 | 0.94 | 0.94 | 0.92 | 0.92 | 0.92 | 0.96 | 0.96 | 0.96 | 0.96 | 0.95 | 0.95 | **0.98** | **0.98** | **0.98** |
| 13 | 32 | 2 | 838 | 0.97 | 0.97 | 0.97 | 0.97 | 0.97 | 0.97 | 0.97 | 0.97 | 0.97 | 0.97 | 0.97 | 0.97 | **1.00** | **1.00** | **1.00** |
| 14 | 71 | 3 | 1774 | 0.96 | 0.96 | 0.96 | 0.93 | 0.92 | 0.91 | 0.92 | 0.92 | 0.90 | **0.97** | **0.97** | **0.97** | **0.97** | **0.97** | **0.97** |
| 15 | 91 | 3 | 1968 | 0.88 | 0.88 | 0.88 | 0.93 | 0.92 | 0.92 | 0.93 | 0.93 | 0.93 | 0.94 | 0.93 | 0.94 | **0.96** | **0.96** | **0.96** |
| 16 | 68 | 2 | 1729 | **1.00** | **1.00** | **1.00** | 0.96 | 0.96 | 0.96 | 0.99 | 0.99 | 0.99 | **1.00** | **1.00** | **1.00** | **1.00** | **1.00** | **1.00** |
| 17 | 96 | 6 | 2381 | **0.88** | **0.88** | **0.88** | 0.61 | 0.60 | 0.60 | 0.73 | 0.69 | 0.70 | 0.79 | 0.79 | 0.79 | 0.81 | 0.80 | 0.80 |
| 18 | 52 | 3 | 1458 | 0.97 | 0.96 | 0.96 | 0.89 | 0.87 | 0.85 | 0.88 | 0.85 | 0.83 | 0.97 | 0.96 | 0.96 | **1.00** | **1.00** | **1.00** |
| 19 | 78 | 6 | 1898 | 0.65 | 0.67 | 0.65 | 0.68 | 0.64 | 0.62 | 0.68 | 0.73 | 0.69 | **0.85** | **0.81** | **0.81** | 0.82 | 0.78 | 0.77 |
| 20 | 72 | 5 | 1885 | 0.86 | 0.88 | 0.87 | 0.76 | 0.76 | 0.76 | 0.85 | 0.85 | 0.83 | **0.94** | **0.94** | **0.94** | 0.92 | 0.93 | 0.92 |
| 21 | 28 | 3 | 838 | 0.89 | 0.93 | 0.91 | 0.94 | 0.96 | 0.95 | 0.73 | 0.86 | 0.79 | 0.93 | 0.96 | 0.95 | 0.93 | 0.96 | 0.95 |
| 22 | 63 | 2 | 1519 | 0.96 | 0.95 | 0.95 | **1.00** | **1.00** | **1.00** | 0.98 | 0.98 | 0.98 | 0.95 | 0.95 | 0.95 | 0.97 | 0.97 | 0.97 |
| 23 | 83 | 6 | 2264 | 0.72 | 0.73 | 0.72 | 0.77 | 0.71 | 0.71 | **0.91** | **0.90** | **0.90** | 0.84 | 0.83 | 0.83 | 0.81 | 0.81 | 0.81 |
| 24 | 104 | 5 | 2565 | 0.94 | 0.93 | 0.93 | 0.83 | 0.76 | 0.76 | 0.91 | 0.91 | 0.91 | 0.94 | 0.93 | 0.93 | **0.95** | **0.95** | **0.95** |
| 25 | 62 | 4 | 1372 | **1.00** | **1.00** | **1.00** | 0.90 | 0.87 | 0.86 | 0.92 | 0.90 | 0.90 | **1.00** | **1.00** | **1.00** | **1.00** | **1.00** | **1.00** |
| 26 | 91 | 3 | 2189 | 0.87 | 0.87 | 0.87 | 0.91 | 0.91 | 0.91 | 0.93 | 0.93 | 0.93 | 0.94 | 0.93 | 0.93 | **0.99** | **0.99** | **0.99** |
| 27 | 69 | 5 | 1871 | **0.88** | **0.87** | **0.87** | 0.77 | 0.74 | 0.74 | 0.79 | 0.78 | 0.78 | 0.85 | 0.84 | 0.84 | 0.85 | 0.86 | 0.85 |
| 28 | 41 | 3 | 1293 | 0.94 | 0.93 | 0.93 | **0.98** | **0.98** | **0.97** | 0.88 | 0.85 | 0.84 | 0.98 | 0.98 | 0.97 | **0.98** | **0.98** | **0.97** |
| 29 | 81 | 5 | 2028 | 0.90 | 0.90 | 0.90 | 0.78 | 0.75 | 0.76 | 0.87 | 0.84 | 0.83 | 0.82 | 0.81 | 0.81 | **0.96** | **0.95** | **0.95** |
| 30 | 46 | 3 | 1061 | **0.96** | **0.98** | **0.97** | 0.90 | 0.91 | 0.90 | 0.88 | 0.89 | 0.87 | **0.96** | **0.98** | **0.97** | 0.94 | 0.96 | 0.95 |
| 31 | 73 | 6 | 1696 | 0.81 | 0.82 | 0.82 | 0.78 | 0.75 | 0.75 | 0.84 | 0.82 | 0.82 | 0.90 | 0.89 | 0.89 | **0.90** | **0.90** | **0.90** |
| 32 | 85 | 5 | 2008 | 0.84 | 0.85 | 0.84 | 0.85 | 0.85 | 0.84 | **0.92** | **0.93** | **0.92** | 0.91 | 0.91 | 0.91 | 0.91 | **0.92** | 0.91 |
| 33 | 44 | 3 | 1716 | **1.00** | **1.00** | **1.00** | 0.94 | 0.93 | 0.93 | 0.94 | 0.93 | 0.93 | 0.98 | 0.98 | 0.98 | 0.98 | 0.98 | 0.98 |
| 34 | 103 | 9 | 2445 | 0.94 | 0.93 | 0.93 | 0.70 | 0.70 | 0.69 | 0.82 | 0.81 | 0.81 | **0.97** | **0.98** | **0.98** | 0.94 | 0.94 | 0.94 |
| 35 | 84 | 7 | 2045 | 0.67 | 0.68 | 0.66 | 0.79 | 0.76 | 0.76 | 0.73 | 0.79 | 0.76 | **0.84** | **0.83** | **0.84** | 0.84 | 0.83 | 0.83 |
| 36 | 33 | 3 | 945 | **1.00** | **1.00** | **1.00** | 0.86 | 0.82 | 0.80 | 0.88 | 0.85 | 0.84 | **1.00** | **1.00** | **1.00** | **1.00** | **1.00** | **1.00** |
| 37 | 110 | 8 | 2317 | 0.85 | 0.85 | 0.84 | 0.75 | 0.71 | 0.71 | 0.83 | 0.82 | 0.81 | **0.93** | **0.93** | **0.93** | 0.92 | 0.92 | 0.92 |
| 38 | 99 | 6 | 2290 | 0.93 | 0.91 | 0.91 | 0.75 | 0.71 | 0.71 | 0.83 | 0.79 | 0.78 | 0.88 | 0.87 | 0.87 | **0.94** | **0.94** | **0.94** |
| 39 | 103 | 5 | 2584 | 0.88 | 0.87 | 0.87 | 0.84 | 0.82 | 0.82 | 0.87 | 0.85 | 0.85 | 0.93 | 0.92 | 0.92 | **0.94** | **0.94** | **0.94** |
| 40 | 103 | 6 | 2261 | 0.82 | 0.79 | 0.79 | 0.73 | 0.72 | 0.72 | 0.88 | 0.84 | 0.85 | 0.80 | 0.80 | 0.79 | **0.87** | **0.85** | **0.86** |
| 41 | 72 | 4 | 1651 | 0.93 | 0.92 | 0.91 | 0.89 | 0.88 | 0.88 | 0.90 | 0.88 | 0.87 | 0.97 | 0.97 | 0.97 | **0.99** | **0.99** | **0.99** |
| 42 | 32 | 4 | 981 | **0.94** | **0.97** | **0.95** | 0.83 | 0.84 | 0.83 | 0.89 | 0.91 | 0.89 | 0.91 | 0.94 | 0.92 | 0.89 | 0.91 | 0.89 |
| 43 | 65 | 6 | 1949 | 0.87 | 0.83 | 0.82 | 0.70 | 0.65 | 0.66 | 0.73 | 0.66 | 0.61 | **0.94** | **0.94** | **0.93** | 0.91 | 0.91 | 0.91 |
| 44 | 92 | 8 | 2209 | 0.85 | 0.86 | 0.85 | 0.75 | 0.72 | 0.72 | 0.88 | 0.89 | 0.89 | **0.92** | **0.90** | **0.90** | 0.89 | 0.89 | 0.89 |
| 45 | 51 | 2 | 1146 | **1.00** | **1.00** | **1.00** | 0.96 | 0.96 | 0.96 | 0.96 | 0.96 | 0.96 | **1.00** | **1.00** | **1.00** | **1.00** | **1.00** | **1.00** |
| 46 | 55 | 2 | 1476 | 0.90 | 0.89 | 0.89 | 0.97 | 0.96 | 0.96 | **0.98** | **0.98** | **0.98** | 0.98 | **0.98** | 0.98 | 0.93 | 0.93 | 0.93 |
| 47 | 75 | 4 | 1620 | **0.97** | **0.97** | **0.97** | 0.81 | 0.80 | 0.80 | 0.90 | 0.89 | 0.89 | 0.95 | 0.95 | 0.95 | 0.96 | 0.96 | 0.96 |
| 48 | 82 | 4 | 1824 | **0.97** | **0.96** | **0.96** | 0.91 | 0.90 | 0.90 | 0.96 | 0.95 | 0.95 | 0.96 | 0.95 | 0.95 | 0.95 | 0.95 | 0.95 |
| 49 | 77 | 6 | 1796 | 0.87 | 0.87 | 0.87 | 0.78 | 0.74 | 0.75 | 0.80 | 0.78 | 0.78 | 0.90 | 0.88 | 0.88 | **0.94** | **0.92** | **0.92** |
| 50 | 80 | 2 | 1971 | 0.99 | 0.99 | 0.99 | 0.95 | 0.95 | 0.95 | 0.98 | 0.98 | 0.98 | 0.99 | 0.99 | 0.99 | **1.00** | **1.00** | **1.00** |
| 51 | 61 | 4 | 1665 | 0.80 | 0.84 | 0.81 | 0.83 | 0.82 | 0.81 | 0.82 | 0.84 | 0.81 | 0.87 | 0.87 | 0.87 | **0.89** | **0.90** | **0.90** |
| 52 | 71 | 3 | 1781 | **0.99** | **0.99** | **0.99** | 0.96 | 0.96 | 0.96 | 0.94 | 0.93 | 0.93 | **0.99** | **0.99** | **0.99** | **0.99** | **0.99** | **0.99** |
| 53 | 104 | 9 | 2422 | 0.81 | 0.81 | 0.80 | 0.82 | 0.81 | 0.79 | 0.87 | 0.87 | 0.86 | 0.86 | 0.86 | 0.85 | **0.91** | **0.90** | **0.90** |
| 54 | 105 | 7 | 2036 | 0.84 | 0.84 | 0.84 | 0.82 | 0.81 | 0.81 | **0.89** | **0.88** | **0.88** | **0.89** | **0.89** | **0.89** | 0.85 | 0.83 | 0.83 |
| 55 | 96 | 7 | 2238 | 0.88 | 0.88 | 0.87 | 0.80 | 0.75 | 0.76 | 0.93 | 0.92 | 0.92 | 0.85 | 0.84 | 0.84 | **0.91** | **0.90** | **0.90** |
| 56 | 105 | 7 | 2105 | 0.84 | 0.83 | 0.83 | 0.68 | 0.66 | 0.67 | 0.78 | 0.74 | 0.74 | 0.90 | **0.89** | 0.89 | 0.82 | 0.80 | 0.80 |
| 57 | 86 | 6 | 2217 | 0.86 | 0.84 | 0.83 | 0.86 | 0.80 | 0.80 | 0.90 | 0.88 | 0.87 | 0.89 | 0.88 | 0.88 | **0.95** | **0.94** | **0.94** |
| 58 | 115 | 6 | 2605 | 0.87 | 0.87 | 0.87 | 0.77 | 0.73 | 0.73 | 0.90 | 0.89 | 0.88 | **0.93** | **0.92** | **0.92** | 0.90 | 0.89 | 0.89 |
| 59 | 89 | 7 | 2115 | 0.72 | 0.71 | 0.71 | 0.73 | 0.73 | 0.72 | 0.79 | 0.78 | 0.74 | 0.89 | **0.90** | 0.90 | 0.90 | 0.89 | 0.89 |
| 60 | 95 | 6 | 2256 | 0.78 | 0.77 | 0.77 | 0.75 | 0.72 | 0.72 | 0.80 | 0.76 | 0.75 | **0.94** | **0.94** | **0.94** | 0.91 | 0.91 | 0.91 |
| 61 | 102 | 5 | 2410 | **0.94** | **0.93** | **0.93** | 0.82 | 0.76 | 0.76 | 0.86 | 0.84 | 0.83 | 0.92 | 0.92 | 0.92 | 0.93 | 0.92 | 0.92 |
| 62 | 56 | 4 | 1445 | 0.95 | 0.96 | 0.96 | 0.91 | 0.93 | 0.92 | 0.89 | 0.89 | 0.88 | **0.98** | **0.98** | **0.98** | 0.96 | **0.98** | 0.97 |
| 63 | 100 | 6 | 2128 | 0.87 | 0.85 | 0.85 | 0.76 | 0.77 | 0.76 | 0.87 | 0.87 | 0.86 | **0.89** | **0.88** | **0.88** | 0.80 | 0.81 | 0.80 |
| 64 | 76 | 4 | 1963 | 0.88 | 0.88 | 0.88 | 0.87 | 0.87 | 0.87 | **0.92** | 0.91 | 0.90 | 0.92 | 0.92 | 0.92 | 0.92 | 0.92 | 0.92 |
| 65 | 120 | 3 | 2744 | **0.98** | **0.98** | **0.97** | 0.91 | 0.89 | 0.89 | 0.98 | 0.98 | 0.98 | 0.98 | 0.98 | 0.98 | 0.98 | 0.98 | 0.98 |
| 66 | 68 | 3 | 1968 | 0.94 | 0.94 | 0.94 | 0.83 | 0.81 | 0.81 | 0.95 | 0.94 | 0.94 | **0.96** | **0.96** | **0.96** | 0.96 | 0.96 | 0.95 |
| 67 | 78 | 6 | 1936 | 0.87 | 0.86 | 0.86 | 0.72 | 0.71 | 0.71 | 0.84 | 0.82 | 0.82 | **0.94** | **0.94** | **0.94** | 0.90 | 0.90 | 0.89 |
| 68 | 69 | 6 | 1508 | **0.91** | **0.86** | **0.86** | 0.80 | 0.78 | 0.78 | 0.83 | 0.83 | 0.82 | 0.90 | 0.88 | 0.88 | 0.89 | 0.87 | 0.87 |
| 69 | 65 | 2 | 1799 | **1.00** | **1.00** | **1.00** | 0.93 | 0.92 | 0.92 | 0.99 | 0.98 | 0.98 | **1.00** | **1.00** | **1.00** | **1.00** | **1.00** | **1.00** |
| 70 | 94 | 8 | 2249 | 0.75 | 0.76 | 0.75 | 0.65 | 0.63 | 0.62 | 0.80 | **0.83** | 0.81 | 0.79 | 0.79 | 0.78 | **0.81** | 0.82 | **0.81** |
| 71 | 76 | 4 | 2000 | 0.84 | 0.83 | 0.83 | 0.86 | 0.86 | 0.86 | 0.91 | 0.91 | 0.91 | 0.92 | 0.92 | 0.92 | **0.97** | **0.97** | **0.97** |
| 72 | 60 | 2 | 1231 | 0.97 | 0.97 | 0.97 | **1.00** | **1.00** | **1.00** | 0.95 | 0.95 | 0.95 | 0.97 | 0.97 | 0.97 | 0.98 | 0.98 | 0.98 |
| 73 | 119 | 7 | 2757 | 0.83 | 0.82 | 0.81 | 0.84 | 0.82 | 0.82 | **0.93** | **0.92** | **0.92** | 0.91 | 0.90 | 0.90 | 0.91 | 0.90 | 0.90 |
| 74 | 86 | 6 | 2033 | 0.79 | 0.77 | **0.77** | 0.67 | 0.65 | 0.65 | 0.74 | 0.72 | 0.72 | **0.83** | **0.78** | **0.77** | 0.79 | 0.78 | 0.78 |
| 75 | 76 | 3 | 1645 | 0.86 | 0.86 | 0.85 | 0.96 | 0.96 | 0.96 | 0.92 | 0.96 | 0.94 | 0.98 | 0.97 | 0.97 | **0.99** | **0.99** | **0.99** |
| 76 | 89 | 7 | 2161 | 0.77 | 0.74 | 0.75 | 0.72 | 0.66 | 0.67 | 0.78 | 0.76 | 0.77 | 0.87 | 0.87 | 0.86 | **0.89** | **0.89** | **0.89** |
| 77 | 77 | 5 | 1833 | 0.97 | 0.97 | 0.97 | 0.90 | 0.88 | 0.88 | 0.93 | 0.92 | 0.92 | **1.00** | **1.00** | **1.00** | 0.99 | 0.99 | 0.99 |

| | | | | P | R | F | P | R | F | P | R | F | P | R | F | P | R | F |
|---|---|---|---|---|---|---|---|---|---|---|---|---|---|---|---|---|---|---|
| 78 | 91 | 7 | 2300 | 0.85 | 0.86 | 0.85 | 0.78 | 0.78 | 0.78 | 0.90 | 0.87 | 0.87 | **0.91** | **0.91** | **0.91** | 0.82 | 0.82 | 0.82 |
| 79 | 73 | 8 | 1759 | 0.80 | 0.78 | 0.78 | 0.75 | 0.70 | 0.70 | 0.68 | 0.70 | 0.68 | **0.87** | **0.86** | **0.86** | 0.86 | 0.85 | 0.84 |
| 80 | 91 | 7 | 2245 | 0.92 | 0.91 | 0.91 | 0.78 | 0.76 | 0.76 | 0.87 | 0.88 | 0.87 | **0.95** | **0.96** | **0.95** | **0.95** | **0.96** | **0.95** |
| 81 | 120 | 4 | 2582 | 0.95 | 0.95 | 0.95 | 0.89 | 0.84 | 0.85 | 0.95 | 0.95 | 0.95 | **0.98** | **0.98** | **0.97** | 0.96 | 0.96 | 0.96 |
| 82 | 86 | 3 | 1532 | 0.88 | 0.88 | 0.88 | 0.97 | 0.97 | 0.96 | 0.95 | 0.95 | 0.95 | 0.94 | 0.93 | 0.93 | **0.98** | **0.98** | **0.98** |
| 83 | 87 | 9 | 2057 | 0.77 | 0.74 | 0.72 | 0.65 | 0.68 | 0.66 | 0.73 | 0.77 | 0.74 | **0.78** | **0.76** | **0.76** | 0.71 | 0.74 | 0.72 |
| 84 | 80 | 4 | 2055 | 0.84 | 0.84 | 0.84 | 0.90 | 0.90 | 0.90 | 0.92 | 0.91 | 0.91 | 0.95 | 0.95 | 0.95 | **0.96** | **0.96** | **0.96** |
| 85 | 104 | 6 | 1890 | 0.77 | 0.77 | 0.77 | 0.88 | 0.87 | 0.86 | 0.94 | 0.94 | 0.94 | **0.96** | **0.96** | **0.96** | 0.93 | 0.92 | 0.92 |
| 86 | 107 | 5 | 2486 | 0.88 | 0.88 | 0.88 | **0.91** | 0.90 | **0.90** | **0.91** | **0.91** | **0.90** | 0.86 | 0.86 | 0.86 | **0.91** | 0.90 | **0.90** |
| 87 | 83 | 7 | 1642 | 0.82 | 0.83 | 0.82 | 0.82 | 0.82 | 0.81 | 0.83 | 0.82 | 0.82 | **0.93** | **0.94** | **0.93** | 0.90 | 0.90 | 0.90 |
| 88 | 63 | 4 | 1904 | 0.91 | 0.90 | 0.90 | 0.85 | 0.79 | 0.78 | 0.80 | 0.76 | 0.73 | 0.93 | 0.92 | 0.92 | **0.97** | **0.97** | **0.97** |
| 89 | 105 | 5 | 2599 | 0.93 | 0.92 | 0.92 | 0.84 | 0.81 | 0.81 | 0.92 | 0.91 | 0.91 | **0.93** | **0.92** | **0.92** | 0.92 | 0.91 | 0.92 |
| 90 | 53 | 4 | 1465 | 0.95 | 0.96 | 0.95 | 0.87 | 0.89 | 0.88 | 0.88 | 0.89 | 0.88 | **1.00** | **1.00** | **1.00** | 0.96 | 0.98 | 0.97 |
| 91 | 120 | 4 | 2149 | 0.90 | 0.90 | 0.90 | 0.93 | 0.93 | 0.93 | 0.96 | 0.96 | 0.96 | 0.97 | 0.97 | 0.97 | **0.98** | **0.98** | **0.98** |
| 92 | 100 | 3 | 2166 | **1.00** | **1.00** | **1.00** | 0.94 | 0.94 | 0.94 | 0.95 | 0.95 | 0.95 | **1.00** | **1.00** | **1.00** | **1.00** | **1.00** | **1.00** |
| 93 | 68 | 3 | 1371 | 0.97 | 0.97 | 0.97 | 0.96 | 0.96 | 0.96 | 0.96 | 0.96 | 0.96 | **0.99** | **0.99** | **0.99** | **0.99** | **0.99** | **0.99** |
| 94 | 120 | 4 | 2284 | 0.96 | 0.96 | 0.96 | 0.93 | 0.93 | 0.93 | **0.98** | **0.98** | 0.97 | 0.93 | 0.93 | 0.93 | **0.98** | **0.98** | **0.98** |
| 95 | 83 | 4 | 2211 | 0.91 | **0.90** | **0.90** | 0.81 | 0.78 | 0.78 | 0.88 | 0.87 | 0.86 | 0.89 | 0.89 | 0.89 | **0.92** | **0.90** | **0.90** |
| 96 | 91 | 7 | 2188 | 0.78 | 0.76 | 0.75 | 0.87 | 0.87 | 0.86 | 0.87 | 0.85 | 0.85 | 0.91 | 0.91 | 0.91 | **0.92** | **0.92** | **0.92** |
| 97 | 101 | 9 | 2187 | 0.67 | 0.65 | 0.65 | 0.71 | 0.67 | 0.68 | 0.75 | 0.76 | 0.73 | **0.80** | **0.78** | **0.78** | 0.79 | **0.78** | **0.78** |
| 98 | 80 | 3 | 2027 | **0.99** | **0.99** | **0.99** | 0.89 | 0.89 | 0.89 | 0.96 | 0.95 | 0.95 | 0.98 | 0.98 | 0.97 | 0.95 | 0.95 | 0.95 |
| 99 | 95 | 4 | 2226 | 0.86 | 0.85 | 0.85 | 0.85 | 0.83 | 0.83 | 0.94 | 0.94 | 0.94 | **0.98** | **0.98** | **0.98** | 0.97 | 0.97 | 0.97 |

**Table 2.** General Results Part I: Number of documents (#Docs), number of classes (#Class), number of attributes (#Attr), Precision (P), Recall (R), and F-Measure (F)

| | C4.5 | | | NB | | | SVM | | | 10-S-C4.5-TDM-NB- TDMR | | | 10-WS-C4.5-TDM-NB-TDMR | | |
|---|---|---|---|---|---|---|---|---|---|---|---|---|---|---|---|
| | P | R | F | P | R | F | P | R | F | P | R | F | P | R | F |
| **Mean** | 0.89 | 0.88 | 0.88 | 0.84 | 0.82 | 0.82 | 0.88 | 0.88 | 0.87 | 0.92 | 0.92 | **0.92** | **0.93** | **0.93** | 0.92 |
| Std.Dev. | 0.08 | 0.08 | 0.08 | 0.09 | 0.10 | 0.10 | 0.07 | 0.08 | 0.08 | **0.06** | **0.06** | **0.06** | **0.06** | **0.06** | **0.06** |
| Min | 0.65 | 0.65 | 0.65 | 0.61 | 0.60 | 0.60 | 0.68 | 0.66 | 0.61 | **0.78** | **0.76** | **0.76** | 0.71 | 0.74 | 0.72 |
| Max | **1.00** | **1.00** | **1.00** | **1.00** | **1.00** | **1.00** | 0.99 | 0.99 | 0.99 | **1.00** | **1.00** | **1.00** | **1.00** | **1.00** | **1.00** |

**Table 3.** General Results Part II

| * Best results in bold | TPR | TNR | FPR | FNR | ROC |
|---|---|---|---|---|---|
| C4.5 | 0.884 | 0.962 | 0.038 | 0.116 | 0.926 |
| NB | 0.824 | 0.932 | 0.068 | 0.176 | 0.904 |
| SVM | 0.876 | 0.934 | 0.066 | 0.124 | 0.927 |
| 10-S-C4.5-TDM-NB- TDMR | **0.920** | **0.975** | **0.025** | **0.080** | **0.981** |
| 10-WS-C4.5-TDM-NB-TDMR | **0.927** | **0.977** | **0.023** | **0.073** | **0.985** |

On average, the results on all 100 datasets show that 10-WS-C4.5-TDM-NB-TDMR and 10-S-C4.5-TDM-NB-TDMR are better (based on all index: precision, recall, f-measure, true positive rate, true negative rate, false positive rate, false negative rate, and receiver operating characteristics) than other methods; therefore, the general performance of the proposed methods are better in Reuters-100 collection. Improvements in precision, recall, F-measure, TPR, and FNR are between 4% and 10%. Improvements in TNR and FPR are between 1.5% and 4.5%. Improvements in ROC are between 6% and 8%.

The feature selection process allows a more understandable model to be obtained. The models are more compact and clear to users. They are also very light and computationally very cheap (in classification stage). With 10-S-C4.5-TDM-NB-TDMR the average feature reduction is 99.06%. For example, the data set 92 with 2166 attributes is reduced to 3 attributes and the data set 35 with 2045 attributes is reduced to 47 attributes.

Some specific datasets do not follow the general tendency, for example, dataset number 1 shows better results for 10-S-C4.5-TDM-NB-TDMR and then for SVM. Therefore, it is necessary to review the pruned process on C4.5 trees and some tuning parameters (for example the number of iterations or models). Also, it is necessary to use concepts instead of terms in the Term by Document Matrix (TDM) e.g. using tools based on science mapping to identify the concepts [40].

## 5    Conclusions and Future Work

Two novel methods for feature selection and text classification, called 10-S-C4.5-TDM-NB-TDMR and 10-WS-C4.5-TDM-NB-TDMR, were presented in this paper. These approaches are aimed at applications such as spam filtering, where additional clarity, efficiency, and ease of use is needed for human operators to be effective. The methods presented were tested on publicly available datasets (Reuters-100). Comparisons with C4.5, Naïve Bayes, and Support Vector Machine techniques demonstrated consistent improvements of up to 10% in precision, recall and F-measure. TPR (true positive rates), FNR (false negative rates), and ROC (receiver operating characteristic), demonstrated similar improvements.

As future work, the authors are planning on including ontologies and parts of speech detection techniques in the preprocessing stage. Also, a detailed study will be conducted to define the best value for the number of iterations (the number of models) it is required to use in the model generation stage. It is necessary to evaluate the proposed model over different test sets, such as LingSpam, and evaluate other combinations of models, e.g. C4.5 with Neural Networks or CART with Naïve Bayes. Finally, tuning some parameters of C4.5 and Naïve Bayes algorithms in order to increase the accuracy of the entire method will be considered.

**Acknowledgments.** This paper has been developed with the Federal financing of Projects FuzzyLIng-II TIN2010-17876, Andalucian Excellence Projects TIC5299 and TIC-5991, and the Vicerrectoría de Investigaciones of the Universidad del Cauca. We are especially grateful to Colin McLachlan for suggestions relating to English text.

## References

1. Su, J., Sayyad-Shirab, J., Stan, M.: Large Scale Text Classification using Semi-supervised Multinomial Naive Bayes. In: Proceedings of the 28th International Conference on Machine Learning (ICML 2011), pp. 97–104 (2011)
2. Laur, E.J.M., March, A.D.: Combining Bayesian Text Classification and Shrinkage to Automate Healthcare Coding: A Data Quality Analysis. J. Data and Information Quality 2(3), 1–22 (2011)
3. He, Y., Xie, J., Xu, C.: An improved Naive Bayesian algorithm for Web page text classification. In: 2011 Eighth International Conference on Fuzzy Systems and Knowledge Discovery, FSKD (2011)
4. Ambert, K.H., Cohen, A.M.: k-Information Gain Scaled Nearest Neighbors: A Novel Approach to Classifying Protein-Protein Interaction-Related Documents. IEEE/ACM Transactions on Computational Biology and Bioinformatics 9(1), 305–310 (2012)

5. Wajeed, M.A., Adilakshmi, T.: Semi-supervised text classification using enhanced KNN algorithm. In: 2011 World Congress on Information and Communication Technologies, WICT (2011)
6. Trstenjak, B., Mikac, S., Donko, D.: KNN with TF-IDF based Framework for Text Categorization. Procedia Engineering 69, 1356–1364 (2014)
7. Bhadri Raju, M.S.V.S., Vishnu Vardhan, B., Sowmya, V.: Variant Nearest Neighbor Classification Algorithm for Text Document. In: Satapathy, S.C., et al. (eds.) ICT and Critical Infrastructure: Proceedings of the 48th Annual Convention of Computer Society of India-Vol II, pp. 243–251. Springer International Publishing (2014)
8. Li, W., Miao, D., Wang, W.: Two-level hierarchical combination method for text classification. Expert Systems with Applications 38(3), 2030–2039 (2011)
9. Jung-Yi, J., Ren-Jia, L., Shie-Jue, L.: A Fuzzy Self-Constructing Feature Clustering Algorithm for Text Classification. IEEE Transactions on Knowledge and Data Engineering 23(3), 335–349 (2011)
10. Saha, D.: Web Text Classification Using a Neural Network. In: 2011 Second International Conference on Emerging Applications of Information Technology, EAIT (2011)
11. Zhang, W., Yoshida, T., Tang, X.: A comparative study of TF-IDF, LSI and multi-words for text classification. Expert Systems with Applications 38(3), 2758–2765 (2011)
12. Shi, K., et al.: Efficient text classification method based on improved term reduction and term weighting. The Journal of China Universities of Posts and Telecommunications 18(Suppl.1), 131–135 (2011)
13. Shi, K., Li, L., He, J., Liu, H., Zhang, N., Song, W.: An improved KNN text classification algorithm based on density. In: 2011 IEEE International Conference on Cloud Computing and Intelligence Systems (CCIS), pp. 113–117 (2011)
14. Jiang, C., et al.: Text classification using graph mining-based feature extraction. Knowledge-Based Systems 23(4), 302–308 (2010)
15. Sun, Y., Liu, X., Cui, X.: The Mining of Term Semantic Relationships and its Application in Text Classification. In: 2012 Fifth International Conference on Intelligent Computation Technology and Automation, ICICTA (2012)
16. Ganiz, M.C., George, C., Pottenger, W.M.: Higher Order Naïve Bayes: A Novel Non-IID Approach to Text Classification. IEEE Transactions on Knowledge and Data Engineering 23(7), 1022–1034 (2011)
17. Yun, J., et al.: A multi-layer text classification framework based on two-level representation model. Expert Systems with Applications 39(2), 2035–2046 (2012)
18. Özgür, L., Güngör, T.: Text classification with the support of pruned dependency patterns. Pattern Recognition Letters 31(12), 1598–1607 (2010)
19. Figueiredo, F., et al.: Word co-occurrence features for text classification. Information Systems 36(5), 843–858 (2011)
20. Xia, T., Du Improve, Y.: VSM text classification by title vector based document representation method. In: 2011 6th International Conference on Computer Science & Education (ICCSE), pp. 210–213 (2011)
21. Zhang, P.Y.: The Application of Semantic Similarity in Text Classification. Modern Development in Materials, Machinery and Automation 346, 141–144 (2013)
22. Hiroshi Ogura, H.A., Kondo, M.: Comparison of metrics for feature selection in imbalanced text classification. Expert Systems with Applications 38(5), 4978–4989 (2011)
23. Chen, J., et al.: Feature selection for text classification with Naïve Bayes. Expert Systems with Applications 36(3, pt. 1), 5432–5435 (2009)
24. Guozhong Feng, J.G., Jing, B.-Y., Hao, L.: A Bayesian feature selection paradigm for text classification. Information Processing & Management 48(2), 283–302 (2012)

25. Li, F.G., Fan, J.L., Wang, L., Zhang, H.L., Duan, R.: A method based on manifold learning and Bagging for text classification. In: 2011 2nd International Conference on Artificial Intelligence, Management Science and Electronic Commerce (AIMSEC), pp. 2713–2716 (2011)

26. Li, Y., Hung, E., Chung, K.: A subspace decision cluster classifier for text classification. Expert Systems with Applications 38(10), 12475–12482 (2011)

27. Nizamani, S., Memon, N., Wiil, U.K., Karampelas, P.: CCM: A Text Classification Model by Clustering. In: 2011 International Conference on Advances in Social Networks Analysis and Mining (ASONAM), pp. 461–467 (2011)

28. Suli, Z., Xin, P.: A novel text classification based on Mahalanobis distance. In: 2011 3rd International Conference on Computer Research and Development, ICCRD (2011)

29. Nedungadi, P., Harikumar, H., Ramesh, M.: A high performance hybrid algorithm for text classification. In: 2014 Fifth International Conference on the Applications of Digital Information and Web Technologies, ICADIWT (2014)

30. Subramanya, A., Bilmes, J.: Soft-supervised learning for text classification. In: Proceedings of the Conference on Empirical Methods in Natural Language Processing 2008, pp. 1090–1099. Association for Computational Linguistics, Honolulu (2008)

31. Shi, L., et al.: Rough set and ensemble learning based semi-supervised algorithm for text classification. Expert Systems with Applications 38(5), 6300–6306 (2011)

32. Lee, L.H., et al.: High Relevance Keyword Extraction facility for Bayesian text classification on different domains of varying characteristic. Expert Systems with Applications: An International Journal 39(1), 1147–1155 (2012)

33. Farhoodi, M., Yari, A., Sayah, A.: N-gram based text classification for Persian newspaper corpus. In: 2011 7th International Conference on Digital Content, Multimedia Technology and its Applications, IDCTA (2011)

34. Meng, J., Lin, H., Li, Y.: Knowledge transfer based on feature representation mapping for text classification. Expert Systems with Applications: An International Journal, 2011 38(8), 10562–10567 (2011)

35. Mikawa, K.I.T., Goto, M.: A proposal of extended cosine measure for distance metric learning in text classification. In: 2011 IEEE International Conference on Systems, Man, and Cybernetics (SMC), pp. 1741–1746 (2011)

36. Wajeed, M.A., Adilakshmi, T.: Different similarity measures for text classification using KNN. In: 2011 2nd International Conference on Computer and Communication Technology (ICCCT), pp. 41–45 (2011)

37. Xu, G., et al.: Improved TFIDF weighting for imbalanced biomedical text classification, pp. 2360–2367. Elsevier Science Energy Procedia (2011)

38. Gospodnetic, O., E. Hatcher, and D. Cutting.: Lucene in action, Mannaging (2005)

39. Manning, C., Raghavan, P., Schütze, H.: Introduction to Information Retrieval. Cambridge University Press, Cambridge (2008)

40. Cobo, M.J., et al.: Science Mapping Software Tools: Review, Analysis and Cooperative Study among Tools. Journal of the American Society for Information Science and Technology 62(7), 1382–1402 (2011)

# Detailed Description of the Development of a MOOC in the Topic of Statistical Machine Translation

Marta R. Costa-jussà, Lluís Formiga, Jordi Petit*, and José A.R. Fonollosa

Departament de Teoria de Senyal i Comunicacions
*Departament de Ciències de la Computació
Universitat Politècnica de Catalunya, 08034 Barcelona
{marta.ruiz,lluis.formiga,jose.fonollosa}@upc.edu,
jpetit@cs.upc.edu

**Abstract.** This paper describes the design, development and execution of a MOOC entitled "Approaches to Machine Translation: rule-based, statistical and hybrid". The course is launched from the Canvas platform used by recognized European universities. The course contains video-lecture, quizzes and laboratory assignments. Evaluation is done using a virtual learning environment for computer programming and peer-to-peer strategies. This MOOC allows to introduce people from various areas to the Machine Translation theory and practice. It also allows to internationalize different tools developed at the Universitat Politècnica de Catalunya.

## 1 Introduction

The Massive Open On-line Courses (MOOCs) have received large acceptance among the academics to develop their courses. Among the different advantages, MOOCs require low resources in comparison to the international impact that they potentially have.

In the context of Natural Language Processing (NLP), there is the discipline of Machine Translation (MT) that puts together different communities from linguists to engineers. From the Universitat Politècnica de Catalunya, with more than 12 years of experience in the topic, we have launched a MOOC that overviews the basis behind the most popular MT systems. The main motivations to develop this course are listed as follows:

1. To improve the contents and digital resources of MT.
2. To adapt an MT course to an international public.
3. To propose the course in complete platform that is used by large European universities.
4. To use and publisize the open-source NLP tools developed at the UPC that are useful in the MT community.

This rest of this decriptive paper is organized as follows. Section 2 presents the course topic and contents. Next section details the activities proposed to the students. Section 4 describes the procedure to record the videolectures and the promotional video and section 5 explains which are the functionalities of the Canvas platform. Finally, section 7 concludes the paper with final remarks.

---

* Corresponding author.

A. Gelbukh et al. (Eds.): MICAI 2014, Part I, LNAI 8856, pp. 92–98, 2014.

## 2   Course Topic and Contents

The course aims at giving a broad view of MT. Given that MT is a multidisciplinary field involving linguists, computer scientists, engineers and informatics, this course is targeted for all these profiles.

The course will review the most important paradigms of MT including statistical, rule-based and hybrid translation, focusing on giving an overview of the state-of-the-art techniques and algorithms and outline the most challenging problems in the field. In addition, an overview of several evaluation approaches will be presented: automatic measures, human perception evaluation, and human linguistic evaluation, putting, emphasis on the advantages and disadvantages of each method. The course will underline how statistics and linguistics are combined in both development and evaluation.

From the theoretical point of view, at the end of the course the student will understand the theory behind rulebased, statistical and hybrid MT systems. The student will have to pass several theoretical tests to show his skills. From the practical point of view, at the end of the course the student will be able to build a rule and a statistical-based MT system. The student will be asked to build parts of the systems along the course.

References that are pillars of the course include the Statistical Machine Translation book [1] and the survey of Linguistics applied to Statistical Machine Translation [2]. Other references have been the slides from Adam Lopez[1] and the corresponding activities [3].

## 3   Activities

Activities constitute the main differential linchpin of MOOC and its main identity. In addition they represent a breeding ground in order to obtain qualitative and quantitative metrics to further understand the MOOC phenomena.

However, when facing the design of activities, we have to consider that not all MOOC contents are inclusive to all participants. Especially people coming from areas such as linguistics, humanities, fine-arts or translation and interpretation do not have a solid mathematical basis. Thus two non exclusionary are profiles are set to achieve the syllabus certificate of accomplishment. One, i.e. *mt-developer*, with a complex and strong mathematical background and one i.e., *mt-manager*, based on a linguistic basis and the understanding of various concepts along with their interaction.

From the first day, teaching assistants will try to identify the roles of leader and follower from within the participants based on different parameters such as participation in the forums, test grading, behavioral pattern both on slide consultation and viewing the video lectures. Leaders will be publicly reputed gaining some extra-motivation with techniques based on authority, popularity and typical metrics from social networks (like, dislike, mention, badges...).

Even so, we set the focus of collective work beyond forum or feedback activities. Therefore, the activities are not only limited to Programming Assignments, Weekly Quizzes but they also try to go deeper on other skills of the student in order to gain joint responsibility of the knowledge path alongside their peers making the learning

---

[1] http://mt-class.org

process more a journey together better than an individual landmark. In that sense, for instance, scientific assignment seek the complicity of students to cooperate to solve several challenges they may encounter during the course by mutually correcting scientific-paper reviews or make a competition of brainstorming ideas to guide the MT research community.

In addition, we are also centered in deploying a methodology under Problem Based Learning perspective. Thus, programming assignment pretend not only to fulfill the *mt-advanced* profile while programming critical lines of source code concerning alignment, scoring, decoding or evaluation but also we want the *mt-manager* profile to be able to build a bash script to train a complete ad-hoc MT-system based on freely available tools.

Programming assignments will be automatically evaluated using the Jutge.org platform [4]. Jutge.org is an open access educational online programming judge where students can try to solve a broad range of programming problems using several programming languages. The verdict of their solutions is computed using exhaustive test sets run under time, memory and security restrictions.

As a whole, the detailed structure of the activities is as follows:

**Weekly Quizes:** Try-and-error tests with random questions and answers to measure the student's level of acquisition of the syllabus contents.

**Elementary Programming Assignments:** They are based on bash scripting evaluating the appropriate calls to freely available toolkits such as SRILM, Moses or Asiya [5] in terms of argument passing and coherence. In that sense, the tools are neither downloaded nor on-line executed as we just do a script-checking and provide previously generated files to the student.

**Avanced Programming Assignments:** An automatic software evaluator based on DreaMT [3] problems and the "jutge.org". Grades will also be set depending on the efficiency and precision/recall scores of students code.

**Scientific assignment:** The students will have the duty to review a state-of-the-art MT paper and provide some dissemination alongside future research ideas. They will be evaluated by other peers.

**Competition on fresh ideas:** The ideas on research from the students will be put in a public voting competition where the students with better ideas will get better social reputation.

**Final Exam:** The final exam will give a global perspective to the student. However, it will only have a marginal weight on the final grading.

At last we have to mention that most part of the success is due to the flexibility and re-usability of the Canvas platform.

## 4    Recording Set

The video recording sessions of the MOOC pose different challenges to be solved. The most important issue is to get the student's attention in order to transfer the course knowledge efficiently. A MOOC presents certain traits that differ from a real class based lecture. For example, it is mandatory to avoid long sessions with a high mathematical or conceptual development. In that sense, communication is more direct and therefore requires of delivery structured in pills where each one of the pills is responsible of transmitting very few concepts but so well prepared.

In this sense aesthetics or means of obtaining audio and video are key compared to the means in which a master class takes place at the faculty. It is important to consider that the main quality of the video session is evaluated as much as it is able to transmit a specific knowledge in an affordable way, as well as it is able to unlock the student from jamming situation, which it can be caused by a misunderstanding of the slides or the fact that they are not self-explanatory enough.

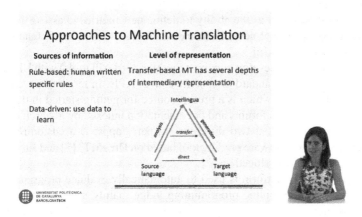

**Fig. 1.** Screen composed of recorded teacher and the slides of the presentation

In this section we detail the design decisions MOOC video recordings in order to increase the course success. First a maximum duration of the videos is set lasting between 10 and 15 minutes. Moreover sound quality is prioritized using a directional lapel microphone: it is the main means of communication between teacher and student. As for aesthetics, the sessions are held on a set with a minimalist environment: a flat white background and a close-up of the teacher sitting waist up towards capturing her facial expressions or communicative gestures. Moreover the main display to the student will consist of the presentation slides, occupying most of the area of the screen, leaving the teacher in a discreet corner with a corporate background (see Figure 1).

On the recording set, the teacher can view the presentation in two places, first in a touch device on the table such as a Wacom table or iPad[2] that allows to delete, write, annotate, or make clarifications of any kind to the student's screen to focus to specific aspects. Moreover, the presentation will also be on teleprompter off camera allowing the teacher to focus its eyes on the target and not thus not giving the student the feeling that the teacher is only interested on the table device. Therefore, we minimize the possibility that the student gets distracted.

Finally, the practical sessions will be developed through screen-casting technology. More precisely, the teacher's computer screen is captured and the student can see all

---

[2] Using an application as *ExplainEverything*.

the actions made by the teacher while she simultaneously records her voice to give explanations for everything that occurs. For this kind of session is also essential to use a good microphone to ensure students understanding.

## 5  Platform

The course will be deployed on the CANVAS[3,4] platform.

Canvas is a new, open-source Learning Management System (LMS) that has several interesting properties aligned with our interests. First it is fully open-source and downloadable making it suitable for being installed on the faculty servers to have full control on the course activity as well as the ability to define new metrics to assess the course. In addition, has a strong social-network focus as it borrows a number of features from Facebook, Twitter, Youtube...[6]

Furthermore, it allows to develop your own modules (3rd API tools) with LTI (Learning Tools Interoperability) standard or specific canvas APIs. In terms of development, it has a "dev & friends" site which is a great resource for getting started in developing on canvas itself as it contains forums and documentation indexed by a search engine.

In that sense we implement two different 3rd-party apps: *i)* a customized video streaming server and a *ii)* software grading tool based on DreaMT[5] [3] and Jutge.org [4] in a similar way that was developed on [7]

As said, the Jutge.org platform is used to automatically evaluate programming assignments. Jutge.org is an online programming judge mainly used at UPC to assist students and instructors in massive regular courses in the Computer Science and Mathematics schools. It currently offers more than 1500 problems and has corrected more than one million submissions so far. Its average response time is six seconds for submission.

The architecture of Jutge.org offers a web front-end that exposes all its capacities for its users, and a back-end that handles the submissions of its clients. As this MOOC uses the Canvas platform in order to provide its contents and administrate its courses, only the back-end of Jutge.org is used. In our case, the integration between this back-end and Canvas is solved by LTI[6].

Internally, Jutge.org's back-end is designed as a distributed master-slave system, with a master server that offers a queue in which clients post submissions and retrieve corrections, and several slave servers that host the different virtual machines that perform the actual correction tasks under a secure environment [4]. In order to correct a submission, a virtual machine receives the problem description (including the solution written by the problem setler), the candidate solution and a driver module, which guides the compilation, execution and checking process to produce a correction.

Note that executing arbitrary code submitted by arbitrary users is an important security concern. In order to isolate possible threads (see [8] for a nice summary), the correction

---

[3] http://www.instructure.com

[4] https://github.com/instructure/canvas-lms/wiki

[5] http://alopez.github.io/dreamt/

[6] http://www.imsglobal.org/toolsinteroperability2.cfm

system of Jutge.org uses virtual machines with immutable drives that continually reboot and are placed behind a network firewall.

Thanks to the modular architecture and the secure environment that Jutge.org offers, handling problems for the area of this MOOC has been an easy task: It was only needed to create a new driver to guide the correction of problems on Machine Translation. Since this driver shares many similar capacities to the already existing ones in Jutge.org, developing it just took a couple of days.

## 6    Promotion

This MOOC has been promoted in under a low-resource strategy. Before any promotion took place, we started with a web page[7] which exposes the promotional video. This video shows basically a dialog between the MOOC professors and a selection of images presenting the university and the contents of the course that pretend to motivate the students to enroll. The dialog of the professors was recorded under the same conditions than the videolectures. In addition to the promotional video, the web page presents the structure of the course and some previous experiences of students that did the course before the launching. With the web page as reference, promotion was done via distribution lists. There was also an internal promotion in the Spanish University system.

## 7    Final Remark

This paper shows our experience in the development of a MOOC in the topic of MT under the Canvas platform. Details about students are not available yet since the course is launched early October 2014.

**Acknowledgments.** This work has been partially supported by the AGAUR under the MOOCs 2013 contract; by the Spanish Ministerio de Economía y Competitividad, contract TEC2012-38939-C03-02 as well as from the European Regional Development Fund (ERDF/FEDER) and the Seventh Framework Program of the European Commission through the International Outgoing Fellowship Marie Curie Action (IMTraP-2011-29951).

## References

1. Koehn, P.: Statistical Machine Translation. Cambridge University Press (2010)
2. Costa-jussà, M.R., Farrús, M.: Statistical machine translation enhancements through linguistic levels: A survey. ACM Computing Surveys (2014)
3. Lopez, A., Post, M., Callison-Burch, C., Weese, J., Ganitkevitch, J., Ahmidi, N., Buzek, O., Hanson, L., Jamil, B., Lee, M., Lin, Y.T., Pao, H., Rivera, F., Shahriyari, L., Sinha, D., Teichert, A.R., Wampler, S., Weinberger, M., Xu, D., Yang, L., Zhao, S.: Learning to translate with products of novices: a suite of open-ended challenge problems for teaching mt. TACL 1, 165–178 (2013)

---

[7] Please, visit http://www.mt-mooc.upc.edu

4. Petit, J., Giménez, O., Roura, S.: Jutge.org: An educational programming judge. In: Proc. of the 43rd ACM Technical Symposium on Computer Science Education (SIGCSE-2012), pp. 445–450. Association for Computing Machinery (2012)
5. Giménez, J., Màrquez, L.: Asiya: An Open Toolkit for Automatic Machine Translation (Meta) Evaluation. The Prague Bulletin of Mathematical Linguistics, 77–86 (2010)
6. Godwin-Jones, R.: Emerging technologies challenging hegemonies in online learning. Language Learning & Technology 16(2), 4–13 (2012)
7. Staubitz, T., Renz, J., Willems, C., Jasper, J., Meinel, C.: Lightweight ad hoc assessment of practical programming skills at scale. In: 2014 IEEE Global Engineering Education Conference (EDUCON), pp. 475–483 (2014)
8. Forišek, M.: Security of Programming Contest Systems. In: Dagiene, V., Mittermeir, R. (eds.) Information Technologies at School, pp. 553–563 (2006)

# NEBEL: Never-Ending Bilingual Equivalent Learner

Thiago Lima Vieira and Helena de Medeiros Caseli

Federal University of São Carlos,
São Carlos, São Paulo, Brazil
{thiago.lima.vieira,helenacaseli}@dc.ufscar.br
http://www.lalic.dc.ufscar.br

**Abstract.** In this paper, we present NEBEL: an automatic system able to learn bilingual equivalents (translations) using the never-ending machine learning (NEML) strategy. Motivated by the way humans learn, the NEML is a continuous learning strategy which uses the knowledge already acquired to learn new information and, therefore, to improve its performance. The NEML was chosen to be applied in our context because it has two desirable features to deal with our intended problem: (i) it uses the Internet as knowledge source and (ii) it combines different extractions methods to improve the final result. In the experiments presented in this paper, NEBEL reached 65% accuracy in the English-Portuguese pair of languages.

**Keywords:** bilingual lexicon, never-ending machine learning, natural language processing.

## 1 Introduction

In the context of this paper, a Bilingual Lexicon can be a set of lexical items (single words or multiword units) from a source language accompanied by their equivalents (translation) in the target language. For example, sample entries of an English-Portuguese bilingual lexicon could be the pairs "bread" (in English) and "pão" (in Portuguese), or "throw away" (in English) and "jogar fora" (in Portuguese). In the automatically extracted lexicons, generally to each entry is assigned the probability or frequency of the pair in the corpus to indicate the pair confidence.

A bilingual lexicon is an important resource for multilingual applications, mainly Machine Translation (MT). In the statistical MT, for example, bilingual lexicon entries can be used to improve the language and translation models augmenting the lexical coverage and, consequently, improving the MT final result. According to studies carried out by [3] and [4], the highest percentage of errors found in the English-Portuguese MT was due to lexical errors. Thus the bilingual lexicon never-ending learning is an alternative to improve the outcome of the MT and other multilingual applications.

A bilingual lexicon can be manually or automatically built. The manually built lexicon is more accurate but demands time and skilled labor. Instead, the bilingual

A. Gelbukh et al. (Eds.): MICAI 2014, Part I, LNAI 8856, pp. 99–103, 2014.

equivalent pairs which constitute the lexicon can be automatically learned using parallel *corpus*[1]. In this context, the Never-Ending Machine Learning (NEML) strategy is an alternative way for automatically building bilingual lexicons.

The NEML is a semi-supervised machine learning strategy that tries to reproduce the human way of learning: first the simpler facts are learned and these facts are used to learn new and more complex facts in the future [5]. NEML systems run constantly and use the Internet as source of knowledge (training data), mainly, due to the constant growing of available knowledge [1].

The NEML was chosen for the development of NEBEL, the never-ending bilingual equivalent learner, due to thee main aspects. First, the resulting bilingual lexicon, extracted from a dynamic source of knowledge (the Internet), will have a bigger coverage. Second, the linguistic variations can be identified by the constant execution, even though they are not frequent enough to be considered by the traditional lexicon extraction methods. Finally, using NEML, the bilingual lexicon is built almost at the same speed of the linguistic variations emergence.

This paper is organized as follows: the next section presents a overview of the architecture and operation of NEBEL; then, we describe a first experiment carried out with NEBEL and some preliminary results; finally, we finish this paper drawing some conclusions and presenting our future work.

## 2    Never-Ending Bilingual Equivalent Learner

The never-ending bilingual equivalent learner, NEBEL, is based on the Never-Ending Language Learner (NELL)[2], the first NEML system developed in the context of the Read The Web project [5].

Although an inspiration for NEBEL, NELL differs from NEBEL in many aspects. While NELL reads the Internet to extract categories (facts) and relations between categories in English, NEBEL has only one relationship (is_translation) and the categories learned are the lexical equivalents in two different natural languages (English and Portuguese in our first experiments). So, while NELL learns relations such as is_a(shakespeare, writer) or writer_wrote_book(shakespeare, hamlet), NEBEL learns pairs of bilingual equivalents, for instance, is_translation ("love", "amor") and is_translation("let it go", "deixe para lá"). Thus, the training input data, the extraction methods and the resulting knowledge are different.

Regarding the training input data, the NEBEL's current lexicon automatic induction strategy involves parallel corpus. Possible sources of parallel knowledge on the Internet are the lyrics[3] and the movies or series subtitles[4]. Parallel texts are collected from the Internet by one of the four modules of NEBEL, illustrated in Figura 1.

---

[1] Parallel *corpus* is a set of text pairs where the source language text is accompanied by its translation in the target language.

[2] NELL: http://rtw.ml.cmu.edu/rtw/

[3] Such as: http://www.lyrics.com.br/

[4] Such as: http://www.opensubtitles.org

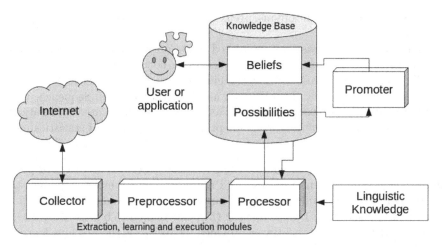

**Fig. 1.** Basic NEBEL architecture

The Collector module is the first of the four NEBEL's modules. It is responsible for retrieving the parallel versions of lyrics and subtitles available in online repositories.

Lyrics and subtitles are very different in structure and content, so, to deal adequately with each one, some preprocessing steps are performed to prepare them to the learning phase. These preprocessing steps are performed by the Preprocessor module and involve cleaning the text, tokenization, part-of-speech tagging[5], automatic sentence[6] and word[7] alignment.

After preprocessing, the Processor module uses the existing knowledge (beliefs), stored in the knowledge base, to extract possibilities (candidates to bilingual entries). In each iteration, the Processor has as input a pair of automatically aligned and tagged parallel sentences. Since it is possible that any adjacent tokens in the source sentence be the translation of any adjacent tokens in the target sentence, all possibilities are generated, and similarity measures are applied to measure how likely the possibilities are.

The NEBEL currently implements 23 similarities measures grouped into four groups:

1. **Simple Measures** calculated based on easy observation and fulfillment features regarding lexical items. Examples of simple measures are: the frequency, size (in tokens and in characters) and position of a lexical item, the source-target pair co-occurrence, among others.
2. **Linguistic Measures** calculated based in some deeper language observation taking into account the relation between languages or their features that may indicate a translation relationship. Examples of linguistic measures are those

---

[5] NEBEL uses the part-of-speech tagger of Apertium: http://www.apertium.org/
[6] NEBEL used the TCAlign [2] sentence aligner.
[7] NEBEL uses the GIZA++ [6] lexical aligner.

based on: synonyms, antonyms, prefix and suffix patterns, and part-of-speech tags.

3. **Edit Distance Measures** calculated based on similarities between words expressed by common character sequences in both languages. Examples of edit distance measures are: Levenshtein distance, Damerau Levenshtein distance, Dice coefficient, Jaro Winkler and Longest Common Sequence.

4. **Statistics Measures** calculated based on more sophisticated calculations, which involves the entire corpus for predicting. Examples of statistics measures are: Likelihood, Mutual Information and Inverse Document Frequency.

After calculating those measures, the Processor generates a cluster of possibilities which are then analyzed by the Promoter. The Promoter combines the results of all measures using a machine learning algorithm and classifies the possibilities as translation or not, promoting the positive ones to beliefs. The current version of NEBEL uses Naive Bayes provided by Weka[8] as the machine learning algorithm to train the Promoter.

To promote the first candidates to beliefs (S1), the classifier was trained with a seed bilingual lexicon (S0). The new beliefs learned in the first iteration and the seeds $(S1 + S0)$ are used to retrain the classifier and promote the candidates in the second iteration (S2). The retraining of the classifier is performed successively $(S_n + ... + S2 + S1 + S0)$ to improve its learning ability. However, it is already known that this approach can lead to errors accumulation, concepts 'drifts' and overfitting, therefore human supervision is necessary from time to time.

## 3  Experiment and Results

It is important to say that NEBEL is still under development, so, the experiment and results presented in this paper are preliminary and there is plenty of room for improvement. In a preliminary experiment, NEBEL processed 5989 pairs of parallel texts, which were automatically extracted from the subtitles and lyrics repositories. From this initial set, 1682 pairs of lexical equivalents were extracted.

Table 1 shows a sample of 10 lexical equivalents extracted in this experiment. All of these 10 examples are possible translations in English-Portuguese language pair.

With respect to accuracy, 1000 entries of the lexicon were manually evaluated[9] resulting in a accuracy of 65%. It is not feasible calculate the resulting lexicon coverage in this context, since it is not possible to know the total amount of lexical equivalents which could be extracted from the input corpus (the Internet).

## 4  Final Remarks

Until now, the NEBEL has demonstrated satisfactory results even with the requirement of high throughput computational demand.

---

[8] Weka: http://www.cs.waikato.ac.nz/ml/weka/

[9] It is worth to say that the evaluator had a good knowledge of both languages and could see the context in which the pairs were extracted.

**Table 1.** Ten lexical equivalents pairs extracted by NEBEL

| English | Portuguese |
|---|---|
| "hallelujah" | "aleluia" |
| "i feel" | "me sinto" |
| "right_now" | "agora" |
| "i don't wanna" | "eu não quero" |
| "i don't know" | "eu não sei" |
| "man" | "cara" |
| "'s" | "isso" |
| "you" | "lhe" |
| "cuz" | "porque" |
| "whatcha whatcha" | "o que" |

One of the most remarkable features of NEBEL is that it is language independent, so, with the right resources (seed bilingual lexicon, lists of synonyms and antonyms, etc.) and tools (tagger, aligners, etc.) it is possible to apply it to any pair of languages.

The authors believe that the NEML is a powerful alternative to automatically build resources for Natural Language Processing, not only bilingual resources but also monolingual ones such as lists of paraphrases, multiword expressions and semantic relations. All of these are already been investigated in parallel projects.

**Aknowledgments.** This work is part of grants #2013/11811-0 and #2013/50757-0 (AIM-WEST project), São Paulo Research Foundation (FAPESP) and it was partially funded by CAPES/CNPq.

# References

1. Carlson, A., Betteridge, J., Kisiel, B., Settles, B., Hruschka Jr, E.R., Mitchell, T.M.: Toward an architecture for never-ending language learning. In: Proceedings of the Twenty-Fourth Conference on Artificial Intelligence, AAAI 2010 (2010)
2. de Medeiros Caseli, H., da Paz Silva, A.M., das Graças Volpe Nunes, M.: Evaluation of methods for sentence and lexical alignment of brazilian portuguese and english parallel texts. In: Bazzan, A.L.C., Labidi, S. (eds.) SBIA 2004. LNCS (LNAI), vol. 3171, pp. 184–193. Springer, Heidelberg (2004)
3. Caseli, H.M., Nunes, M.G.V., Forcada, M.L.: Automatic induction of bilingual resources from aligned parallel corpora: application to shallow-transfer machine translation. Machine Translation 20(4), 227–245 (2006)
4. Martins, D.B.d.J.: Pós-edição automática de textos traduzidos automaticamente de inglês para português do Brasil. Master's thesis, Centro de Ciências Exatas e de Tecnologia – Programa de Pós-graduao em Ciência da Computação, Universidade de São Carlos (2014)
5. Mitchell, T.M., Betteridge, J., Carlson, A., Hong, S.A., Hruscka, E.A.L.M.E., Wang, S.: Never-ending language learning: The Readtheweb Manifesto (May 2008)
6. Och, F.J., Ney, H.: A systematic comparison of various statistical alignment models, vol. 29, pp. 19–51. Association for Computational Linguistics (2003)

# RI for IR: Capturing Term Contexts Using Random Indexing for Comprehensive Information Retrieval

Rajendra Prasath[1,2], Sudeshna Sarkar[1], and Philip O'Reilly[2]

[1] Department of Computer Science and Engineering
Indian Institute of Technology, Kharagpur - 721 302, India
{drrprasath,shudeshna}@gmail.com
[2] Department of Business Information Systems
University College Cork, Cork, Ireland
Philip.OReilly@ucc.ie

**Abstract.** In this paper, we present an approach, based on random indexing, to identify semantically related information that effectively disambiguate the user query and improves the retrieval efficiency of news documents. User query terms are expanded based on the terms with similar word senses that are discovered by implicitly considering the "associatedness" of the document context with that of the given query. This type of associatedness is guided by word space models, as described by Kanerva *et* al.(2000). The word-space model computes the meaning of the terms by implicitly utilizing the distributional patterns (contexts) of words collected over large text data. The distributional patterns represent semantic similarity between words in terms of their spatial proximity in the context space. In this space, words are represented by context vectors whose relative directions are assumed to indicate semantic similarity. Motivated by this distributional hypothesis, words with similar meanings are assumed to have similar contexts. For example, if we observe two words that constantly occur with the same context, we are justified in assuming that they mean similar things. Hence the word space methodology makes semantics computable and the underlying models do not require any linguistic or semantic expertise. Experimental results done on FIRE news collection show that the proposed approach effectively captures the term contexts using higher order term associations across the collection of news documents and use such information to assist the retrieval of documents.

**Keywords:** Random Indexing, Implicit Semantic Analysis, Topic Dynamics, Retrieval Effectiveness, Cross-Lingual Information Retrieval.

## 1 Introduction

In domain independent IR systems, the collection of documents is of a diversified nature and therefore we cannot use specific ontologies for such a collection. In this case, we propose to disambiguate the user query using semantically related terms

A. Gelbukh et al. (Eds.): MICAI 2014, Part I, LNAI 8856, pp. 104–112, 2014.

that are identified by higher order term co-occurrences. Identifying semantically related terms would assist the document retrieval by implicitly considering the "associatedness" of the document context with respect to the query. This type of associatedness can be explored with word space models that focus on semantic indexing of the text documents, as motivated by [1].

The word-space model, as described by [2,3], is a computational model of word meaning that utilizes the distributional patterns of words collected over large text data. These distributional patterns represent semantic similarity between words in terms of their spatial proximity in the context space. In this space, words are represented by context vectors whose relative directions are assumed to indicate semantic similarity. Motivated by this distributional hypothesis, words with similar meanings are assumed to have similar contexts. For example, if we observe two words that constantly occur in the same context, we are justified in assuming that they mean similar things. Hence the word space methodology makes semantics computable and allows to define semantic similarity in mathematical terms. Word space models constitute a purely descriptive approach to semantic modelling and does not require any linguistic or semantic knowledge.

## 2   Background on Random Indexing

Kanerva *et* al. [4] proposed a method namely Random Indexing (RI) - an approximate technique based on the word space model. The main intuition behind Random Indexing is derived as a result of Johnson-Lindenstrauss Lemma[1]. It suggests the fact that whenever a set of points in a higher dimensional space can be mapped into a reduced dimensional space, then the distance between any pair of points does not vary significantly[1]. Based on this intuition, the computational procedure behind Random Indexing, as suggested by Sahlgren [2] consists of two phases: allocation of elemental vectors and training. Random Indexing has been extensively used for many problems: synonym extraction [5], automatic bilingual lexicon acquisition  [6], nearest neighbor classification in combination with Reflective Random Indexing (RRI) - another scalable random indexing based method of distributional semantics [7], indirect inference in biomedical literature - finding meaningful connections between terms that are related but do not occur together in any document in a collection  [8], Cross-Lingual Query Expansion [9].

**Term Index Vectors:** RI projects term vectors into a low dimensional space (relative to the corpus size). Each term is assigned a unique and randomly generated representation of fixed size vectors. Index vectors are sparse, high-dimensional, and ternary and their dimensionality ($n$) is in the order of thousands. Also they consist of a small number of randomly distributed +1 and -1 values (referred to as seeds), with the rest of the elements of the vectors set to 0.

**Term Context Vectors:** Each context vector is produced by scanning through index vectors of the term present in the given text fragment. Whenever a term occurs in the context within a sliding context window of fixed size, then the context vector of that term is updated by adding its $n-$dimensional index vector multiplied with real coefficient which is based on the position of the occurrence of the term. Terms are thus represented by $n-$dimensional context vectors that collectively represent the sum of the terms' contexts. For each occurrence of a given term, a fixed window of size $(2k)+1$ centered at the given term (suggested window size is 5 (terms $+$ / $-$ $k$ terms; here $k = 2$)) is considered. Then the term context vector for $term_i$ is computed using the following equation:

$$C_{term_t} := C_{term_t} + \sum_{j=-k;j\neq0}^{+k} I_{term_j \times \frac{1}{d|j|}} \tag{1}$$

where $\frac{1}{d|j|}$ is the weight proportion relative to the size j of window ($d = 2$). Superposition is used to add two context vectors during the training. At the end of training process, the term context vectors are obtained one for each term. From these term context vectors, the document context vector (DCV) is computed for each document $d$ having $m$ terms by the following equation:

$$DCV(d) := \sum_m TF(t_i) \times C_{t_i} \tag{2}$$

where $TF(t_i)$ denotes the term frequency of the $term_i$ in document $d$.

Since RI reduces the dimensionality implicitly, it is a good alternative to Latent Semantic Indexing [10]. Kanerva et al. [4] used Random Indexing with document-based co-occurrence statistics to solve the synonym-finding part of the TOEFL, in which the synonym of the given word is to be found among four alternatives. Later Sahlgren and Cöster [11], used Random Indexing to improve the performance of text categorization. The idea was to produce concept-based text representations based on Random Indexing, and to use those representations as input to a support vector machine classifier. Then Sahlgren and Karlgren [12] demonstrated that Random Indexing can be applied to multilingual, parallel data to extract bilingual lexicon. In this approach, one random index vector is assigned to each aligned pair of text segments in the source and target languages. Then the context vectors are produced for the terms in both languages by adding an aligned segment's index vector to the context vector for a given term, every time the term occurs in the aligned segment. Then the cosine of the angles between the context vectors was used to estimate similar terms across languages.

Sahlgren et al. [13] used random indexing methodology for finding similar terms for query expansion. In this work, 1,800 dimensional random index vectors were used and context vector for each word was accumulated by adding the index vectors of $n$ ( here $n = 3$ ) surrounding words to it. Then using these vectors with the accumulated contexts, Sahlgren expanded the given query with its semantically similar terms. This was achieved by summing the context vectors of the words in the query, and then calculating the similarity between the query vector and the context vectors of the words in the vocabulary. Since Random Indexing has been applied to find semantically similar terms, it looks promising to try RI for IR tasks.

## 3    RI Applied to IR

User queries are short and ambiguous and users may not have used the appropriate query terms to express their retrieval context. So the query terms need to be expanded with more informative or semantically similar terms which could possibly help to disambiguate the retrieval context of users. Since Random indexing has the potential to explore the given terms with its semantically similar terms, we propose to adopt a random indexing methodology for document retrieval in IR systems.

The overview of our proposed approach can be explained in 3 steps:

(i) **Extract contextual information of terms**: The contextual information of terms may be extracted by detecting higher order term correlations in given text content

(ii) **Generate context vectors**: For each term in the given text content (query / document), generate context information in the form of feature vectors of fixed length.

(iii) **Computing similarity**: Compute the similarity between the query and the documents by their constituent term context vectors and then get the ranked list of documents sorted by their similarity score in decreasing order.

We adopted term vector weighting schemes, similar to [14], for computing the similarity between the query and the document:

Document terms weighting($W_{d_i}$):

$$\frac{w_{d_i}}{\sqrt{\sum_{i=1}^{m} w_{d_i}^2}} \tag{3}$$

where $w_{d_i}$ is the superposition of the term context vectors, each multiplied with its frequency, in the document $c_i$.

Query terms weighting($W_{q_i}$):

$$\frac{w_{q_i}}{\sqrt{\sum_{i=1}^{m} w_{q_i}^2}} \tag{4}$$

where $w_{q_i}$ is superposition of term context vectors, each multiplied with its frequency, in the query $q_i$.

Similarity between the query and the document in the corpora is computed using:

$$sim(q_i, d_i) = \sum_{matching\ terms} W_{q_i} \times W_{d_i} \tag{5}$$

During the training of the term context vectors, the values of the vector increase with the number of occurrences of the term in the documents collection. In such situations, we could apply progressive vector length normalization adopted from [14].

---

**Algorithm 1.** Creating Term Index and Context Vectors

---

**Input:** A collection of documents;

$w$ - the size of the text window;

**Description:**

1. **for** each document $d_i$ in the collection **do**
2.    Read the text content from the document $d_i$ and tokenize the content into individual terms
3.    **for** each of term $t_i$ in the document $d$ **do**
4.        create a unique index vector of dimension $k$ with distributed +1 and -1 at random positions
5.        Find the window of text having $\pm w$ terms from $t_i$
6.        Produce the context vector for $t_i$ by summing up the index vectors of the terms in the text window using the Equation 1
7.    **end for**
8.    store and update the term context information;
9. **end for**

**Output:** term context vectors

---

The description of the proposed algorithm is given in Algorithm 1 and 2:

We have performed the evaluation of the proposed domain independent document retrieval method. The experimental details and results are given in the following section.

# 4    Experimental Results

We have presented the results of our experiments with domain Independent IR. We have used the common evaluation infrastructure initiated by the Forum

---

**Algorithm 2.** Proposed Document Retrieval

---

**Input:** Given a user query having $k$ terms: $Q = \{t_1, t_2, t_3, \cdots, t_k\}$, $k > 0$ and the term context vectors;

**Description:**

1. For the given query, obtain the context vectors for the terms in the query by applying Algorithm. 1
2. Compute the query context vector of the given query (QCV) using Equation 2
3. Compute the document context vectors (DCV) for the documents using Equation 2

4. Compute the similarity between the QCV and each of the DCV in the context space using the cosine similarity
5. return top $k$ matching documents based on their decreasing similarity scores.

**Output:** The ranked list of retrieved documents

---

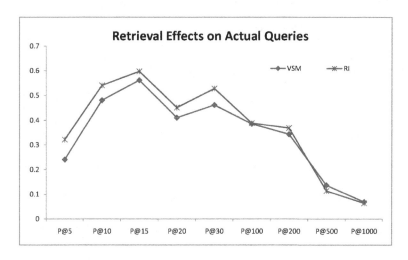

**Fig. 1.** VSM vs Random Indexing on Actual Queries

for Information Retrieval Evaluation (FIRE)[1] for comparing the performance of IR techniques applied by different IR systems [15,16]. FIRE releases data sets in Indian Languages including Hindi, Bengali, Tamil, Telugu, Malayalam, Marathi, Punjabi and also in English. At present, we have taken a subset of English corpora along with English queries for our experiments and evaluated the proposed method using the evaluation similar to TREC (Text REtrieval Conference) evaluation.

### 4.1 Corpora and Queries

We have selected 14,418 news articles from adhoc news collection of Forum for Information Retrieval Evaluation (FIRE) 2010 corpora in English. The collection contains documents that are of mixed types(news, sports, tourism, health and so on). We have selected 10 queries from the FIRE 2010 query set and the relevant judgments for evaluating our retrieved results. FIRE queries are in the standard TREC format with three fields: TITLE, DESC[2] and NARR[3]. Among these fields, we have used TITLE (the actual query) and DESC (the expanded query) fields for document retrieval. While retrieving the documents, the query words are connected by an OR operator so as to increase the number of search results, but compromises on the grounds of relevance.

We have done two experiments for domain independent information retrieval: one with the actual query and another one with the expanded query. Here we

---

[1] http://www.isical.ac.in/~fire/

[2] DESC stands for *description* tag in FIRE queries

[3] NARR stands for *narration* tag in FIRE queries

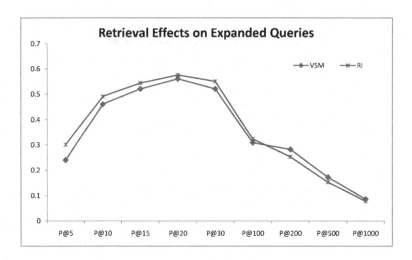

**Fig. 2.** VSM vs Random Indexing on Expanded Queries

compute the results of the cosine similarity against Random indexing. For each term, we obtained the term context vector as described in section 2. From these term context vectors, we compute document context vectors. Then using the term vector weighting schemes, similar to [14], we compute similarity between query and documents.

We have used actual and expanded queries for retrieving the documents. From the list of retrieved documents, the precision @ top $d$ documents ($p@d$ - $d = 5, 10, 15, 20, 30, 100, 200, 500, 1000$) were computed. In the first experiment, actual queries were used to retrieve the documents. Figure. 1 shows the comparison among retrieval accuracies obtained with Vector Space Model(VSM) and random indexing. Next we used DESC part of the queries (expanded queries) for the retrieval task. The performance of retrieval through the retrieval accuracies with VSM and random indexing is plotted in Figure. 2. From these results, RI is found to perform better in retrieving up to top 20 documents. Later on the performance of the proposed method degrades with respect to the cosine similarity method.

## 5   Conclusion

In this paper, we presented an random indexing based approach, to identify semantically related information that effectively disambiguate the user query and improves the retrieval efficiency of news documents. The proposed method captures the context of a term occurring in a specific context and also accumulates different contexts of the term across the collection of news documents. In this preliminary work, we have experimented the proposed approach with a fixed size window of texts and used these contexts for better retrieval of news documents. Also we have compared the proposed method with the standard vector space model. Experimental results done on FIRE news collection show that the proposed random indexing approach appears to be promising to effectively capture the term contexts using higher order term associations across the collection of news documents and use such information to assist the retrieval of documents. Subsequently, we plan to apply this proposed approach for the cross lingual retrieval of news documents.

**Acknowledgment.** This work has been supported by the BMIDEA project (UCC) and the School of Graduate Studies, Business and Law, UCC.

# References

1. Johnson, W., Lindenstrauss, L.: Extensions of lipschitz maps into a hilbert space. Contemporary Mathematics 26, 189–206 (1984)
2. Sahlgren, M.: An introduction to random indexing. In: Methods and Applications of Semantic Indexing Workshop at 7th Int. Conf. on Terminology and Knowledge Eng., TKE 2005 (2005)
3. Sahlgren, M.: The Word-Space Model: using distributional analysis to represent syntagmatic and paradigmatic relations between words in high-dimensional vector spaces. PhD thesis, Stockholm University (2006)
4. Kanerva, P., Kristoferson, J., Holst, A.: Random indexing of text samples for latent semantic analysis. In: Proceedings of the 22nd Annual Conference of the Cognitive Science Society, pp. 103–106. Erlbaum (2000)
5. Henriksson, A., Moen, H., Skeppstedt, M., Daudaravicius, V., Duneld, M.: Synonym extraction and abbreviation expansion with ensembles of semantic spaces. J. Biomedical Semantics 5, 6 (2014)
6. Sahlgren, M., Karlgren, J.: Automatic bilingual lexicon acquisition using random indexing of parallel corpora. Natural Language Engineering 11(3), 327–341 (2005)
7. Vasuki, V., Cohen, T.: Reflective random indexing for semi-automatic indexing of the biomedical literature. J. of Biomedical Informatics 43(5), 694–700 (2010)
8. Vasuki, V., Cohen, T.: Reflective random indexing for semi-automatic indexing of the biomedical literature. Journal of Biomedical Informatics 43(5), 694–700 (2010)
9. Sahlgren, M., Karlgren, J.: Vector-based semantic analysis using random indexing for cross-lingual query expansion. In: Peters, C., Braschler, M., Gonzalo, J., Kluck, M. (eds.) CLEF 2001. LNCS, vol. 2406, pp. 169–176. Springer, Heidelberg (2002)
10. Deerwester, S.C., Dumais, S.T., Landauer, T.K., Furnas, G.W., Harshman, R.A.: Indexing by Latent Semantic Analysis. Journal of the American Society of Information Science 41(6), 391–407 (1990)
11. Sahlgren, M., Cöster, R.: Using bag-of-concepts to improve the performance of support vector machines in text categorization. In: Proceedings of the 20th International Conference on Computational Linguistics. COLING 2004. Association for Computational Linguistics, Stroudsburg (2004)
12. Sahlgren, M., Karlgren, J.: Automatic bilingual lexicon acquisition using random indexing of parallel corpora. Nat. Lang. Eng. 11, 327–341 (2005)
13. Sahlgren, M., Karlgren, J., Cöster, R., Järvinen, T.: Sics at clef 2002: Automatic query expansion using random indexing. In: Peters, C., Braschler, M., Gonzalo, J. (eds.) CLEF 2002. LNCS, vol. 2785, pp. 311–320. Springer, Heidelberg (2003)

14. Singhal, A., Salton, G., Mitra, M., Buckley, C.: Document length normalization. Inf. Process. Manage. 32(5), 619–633 (1996)
15. Majumder. P., M.M., Dataa, K.: Multilingual information access: an indian language perspective. In: Proc. ACM SIGIR Workshop on New Directions in Multilingual Information Access, Seattle, pp. 22–27 (2006)
16. Majumder, P., Mitra, M., Pal, D., Bandyopadhyay, A., Maiti, S., Pal, S., Modak, D., Sanyal, S.: The fire 2008 evaluation exercise. ACM Transactions on Asian Language Information Processing (TALIP) 9, 10:1–10:24 (2010)

# Data Extraction Using NLP Techniques and Its Transformation to Linked Data

Vincent Kríž[1], Barbora Hladká[1], Martin Nečaský[2], and Tomáš Knap[2]

[1] Institute of Formal and Applied Linguistics
[2] Department of Software Engineering
Faculty of Mathematics and Physics, Charles University in Prague
Malostranské nám. 25, 118 00 Praha 1, Czech Republic

**Abstract.** We present a system that extracts a knowledge base from raw unstructured texts that is designed as a set of entities and their relations and represented in an ontological framework. The extraction pipeline processes input texts by linguistically-aware tools and extracts entities and relations from their syntactic representation. Consequently, the extracted data is represented according to the Linked Data principles. The system is designed both domain and language independent and provides users with data for more intelligent search than full-text search. We present our first case study on processing Czech legal texts.

## 1 Introduction

According to the statistics provided by International Data Corporation [1], 90% of all available digital data is unstructured and its amount currently grows twice as fast as structured data. In many domains, large collections of unstructured documents form main sources of information. Their efficient browsing and querying present key aspects in many areas of human activities. Typical approaches of searching large collections are *full-text search* and *metadata search*. In general, both approaches do not work with the semantic interpretation of documents.

We depict the relationship between the fields of Information Extraction (IE) and Semantic Web (SW) in the scheme displayed in Figure 1 where the components of Gathering data and Linguistic analysis belong to IE and while the components of Data representation and Data linking belong to SW. The components are characterized by general features that are typically domain and language independent. However, their design in an extraction pipeline must take into account specifications related to a domain under consideration.

In our work, we focus on the components of Linguistic analysis and Data representation. We deal with the semantics through a *knowledge base* composed of entities and their relations. The knowledge base is built from raw texts by extraction of entities and relations referring to real-world objects. Namely, we exploit dependency trees where both entities and relations are recognized. The outputs are presented according to the Linked Data Principles[1] in the Resource Description Framework (RDF, [2]) that is, in connection

---

[1] http://www.w3.org/wiki/LinkedData

A. Gelbukh et al. (Eds.): MICAI 2014, Part I, LNAI 8856, pp. 113–124, 2014.

with the SPARQL query language,[2] highly suitable not only as a database and querying tool, but for interpretation of the document semantics as well.

[3] proposed the ontology for representing the structure of Czech legal documents. Our motivation is to enrich this ontology with semantic information to provide users with more intelligent search in documents. We specify the semantic information through exploiting syntactic structures in documents. First, we detect entities in the documents, i.e., in syntactic structures of the sentences present in the document and then we link each entity occurrence with its ontological concept. Second, we detect relations in syntactic structures and we enrich the ontological concepts with formal definitions of entities, rights of entities, and obligations declared in documents. Such information can be useful for various users, e.g., an accountant can easily find the definition of a given accounting term and each occurrence of this term in documents; a patient can browse the insurance act to find his rights; an employer can obtain a list of his obligations to his employees.

We demonstrate the system for the legislative domain, namely we concentrate on acts, decrees and regulations published in the Collection of Laws of the Czech Republic. Although there are several systems where users can browse Czech legal texts (e.g. ASPI[3] or ZákonyProLidi.cz[4]), the systems do not offer any additional information, for example hyperlinks to refered documents.

Our paper is organized as follows: in Section 2, we provide an overview of works related to our topic. The RExtractor system is a complex system that (i) processes input documents by natural language processing (NLP) tools and (ii) queries linguistic structures to extract entities and their relations. Its architecture and components are described in Section 3. In general, the RExtractor system is designed to be domain independent but some modifications must be done when using it for a specific domain. In Section 4 we present the steps that we undertook during the processing of Czech legal texts. We also include the evaluation of this case study. Once the data from the legal texts is extracted, its representation according to a chosen data model follows. Details on this step are described in Section 5. In Section 6 we provide an outline of our future work that covers both improving syntactic parsing and linking ontological concepts.

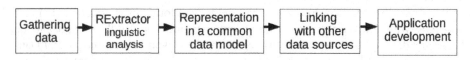

**Fig. 1.** A scheme of data extraction, its representation and exploitation

## 2   Related Work

Works on *relation extraction*: The extraction of relational facts from raw texts has been of interest in information extraction for last decade. With the emergence of the Semantic Web [4] and ontologies [5], data integration has become an additional challenge.

---

[2] http://www.w3.org/TR/rdf-sparql-query/

[3] http://systemaspi.cz

[4] http://zakonyprolidi.cz

There has been a considerable amount of research on applying semi-supervised methods for data integration [6,7,8]. Unsupervised approaches have contributed further improvements by not requiring hand-labeled data [9,10]. [11] presents SOFIE, a system for automated ontology extension. The system performance was evaluated on the corpus of 150 newspapers articles and the authors report 91.30% precision and 31.08% recall. [12] presents the platform MeTAE. It allows extraction and annotation of medical entities and relationships from medical texts and their representation in the RDF format. They evaluateed the extraction of treatment relations between a treatment (e.g., medication) and an illness (e.g., disease): they obtained 75.72% precision and 60.46% recall.[13] employs a combination of NLP tools, including semantic parsing, coreference resolution, and named entity linking. They proposed an end-to-end system, that extracts entity relations from plain text and attempted to map entities onto the DBpedia namespace. They reported precision of 74.3% and recall of 59.9%. [14] proposes a complex pipeline of NLP tools for Czech performing extraction of basic facts presented in a text. An automatic syntactic analysis is used for extracting phrases that are later classified using Czech WordNet into several semantic categories, such as *Location* or *Time*. They present the results of manual evaluation on 50 randomly selected sentences from internet news groups. They reported accuracy of 69.9%.

At least to our best knowledge, [15] presents the very first results on the legislative domain. The authors implemented two modules to qualify fragments of normative texts in terms of provision types and to extract their arguments. The evaluation set for their extractor consists of 473 law paragraphs. They report accuracy of 82%.

Works on *linked data*: In the proceedings [16], recent relevant developments are documented, mainly language archives for language documentation, typological databases, lexical-semantic resources in NLP, multi-layer annotations and semantic annotation of corpora.

Works on *NLP and the legislative domain*: An elaborated overview of current efforts in legal text processing is given by [17]. The main issues include information extraction, construction of knowledge resources, automatic summarization and translation. [18] showes that the state-of-the-art statistical parser can handle even complex syntactic constructions of an appellate court judge.A few attempts have been carried out to check the performance of parsers on legal texts. One of the main reasons lies in the absence of syntactically annotated gold corpora of legal texts. The first competition on dependency parsing of legal texts took place in 2012. The SPLet 2012 – First Shared Task on Dependency Parsing of Legal Texts [19] looked at different parsing systems which have been tested against Italian and English legal data sets. All submitted systems concentrated on tuning parameters of machine learning methods they applied.

The processing of Czech legal texts has been overviewed during the work on the Dictionary of law terms [20]. The authors used partial parsing to extract noun groups as the main candidates for legal terms and they explored the valency frames of verbs to link together the established law terms [21]. Processing of non-Czech legal texts is established as well, see e.g. [17] for a review of current efforts.

## 3   RExtractor Architecture

We have proposed a general, domain and language independent architecture called *RExtractor*. The RExtractor system is displayed in Figure 2 and it consists of four components:

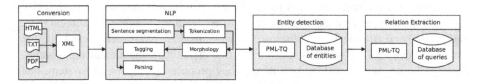

**Fig. 2.** RExtractor architecture

**Conversion** – a largely technical component converting various input formats into internal representation.

**Natural Language Processing** – a linguistic component providing various analyses of input texts, namely sentence segmentation, tokenization, morphological analysis, part-of-speech tagging, and syntactic parsing. Currently employed procedures fit the framework originally formulated in the Prague Dependency Treebank (PDT) [22,23].[5] The dependency approach to syntactic parsing with the main role of verb is applied and it results in a dependency tree where each token in the sentence has one corresponding node and dependencies are assigned with the syntactic dependency relation, as illustrated in Figure 4. The procedures are available in the Treex framework [24].

**Entity Detection** – an extraction component querying dependency trees to detect entities stored in Database of Entities (DBE, see Figure 2) in texts and it exploits the PML-TQ tool [25].[6] DBE is built by domain experts. We prefer querying dependency trees to matching texts with regular expressions because it allows us to detect entities with more complex structures, like coordination. Figure 3 displays the dependency tree of coordination *current tangible and intangible assets*. Using the PML-TQ query displayed in Figure 3, we detect the entity *current tangible assets* in the tree. Because of 1:1 correspondence between tokens in the sentence and nodes in its dependency tree, we can directly mark entities in the original input text.

**Relation Extraction** – an extraction component querying dependency trees with high-lighted entities to detect relations between them. It exploits the PML-TQ tool as well and poses queries stored in Database of Queries (DBQ, see Figure 2). DBS is built by both domain and PML-TQ experts.

For illustration, we assume the sentence *(3) Accounting units, which keep books in simplified extent, create fixed items and reserves according to special legal regulations*, its dependency tree and the query displayed in Figure 4. The query is designed to extract responsibilities of accounting units. Table 1 lists data extracted from the given tree by the given query.

---

[5] http://ufal.mff.cuni.cz/pdt3.0/
[6] http://ufal.mff.cuni.cz/pmltq/

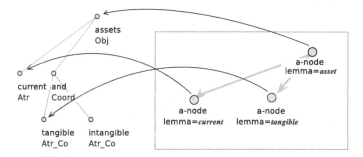

**Fig. 3.** Dependency tree of coordination *current tangible and intangible assets* and tree query for detection of the entity *current tangible assets*

**Table 1.** Data extracted by the query from the tree in Figure 4

| Subject | Predicate | Object |
|---------|-----------|--------|
| *Entity* | *hasToCreate* | *Something* |
| id:1 <br> Accounting units <br> Účetní jednotky | id:6 <br> create <br> tvoří | id:3 <br> fixed items <br> opravné položky |
| id:1 <br> Accounting units <br> Účetní jednotky | id:6 <br> create <br> tvoří | id:4 <br> reserves <br> rezervy |

# 4   RExtractor on Czech Legal Texts

In the pilot study, we used RExtractor for processing acts, decrees, and regulations published in the Collection of Laws of the Czech Republic. We list specifics related to the legislative domain for each RExtractor component.

**Conversion.** Although legal texts under consideration have strictly hierarchical structure, there is no official machine readable source of them. Therefore, we converted the input texts according to the RExtractor XML Schema.

**Natural Language Processing.** Legal texts are specialized texts operating in legal settings. In view of the fact that they should transmit legal norms to their recipients, they need to be clear, explicit and precise. Simple sentences in legal texts are very rare, with exception of headings, references and similar rather technical sections or their parts. Typically, the sentences are long and very complex, therefore, in order to ensure comprehensibility of the whole text they have to be clearly separated and hierarchized. Long sentences do not necessarily obstruct the understandability of texts. Moreover, the special structure is emphasized by a significant use of punctuation, such as semicolons and parentheses. However, the style of legal texts is "generally considered very difficult to read and understand". [26]

We can see the syntactic parsing as a key procedure employed in RExtractor. However, NLP procedures we have at our disposal for Czech are trained on newspaper texts.[7]

---

[7] http://ufal.mff.cuni.cz/pdt2.0/doc/pdt-guide/en/html/ch03.html

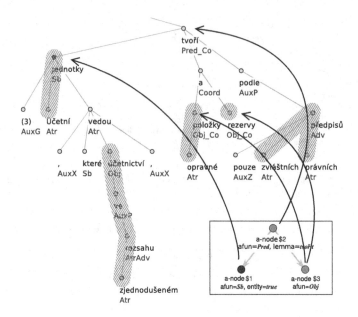

**Fig. 4.** Query matching in a dependency tree

Since legal texts and newspaper texts essentially differ in syntactic features, special attention must be payed to the verification whether we can use the parser trained on newspaper texts or some modifications are needed. To address this issue, we use the manually annotated Corpus of Czech legal texts (CCLT, [27]) consisting of two legal documents from the Collection of Laws of the Czech Republic.[8] The corpus contains 1,133 manually annotated dependency trees with 35,085 nodes in total. The document selection was motivated in the wider context of the INTLIB project.[9]

We have already implemented two preprocessing steps which potentially could improve parser performance, namely sentence splitting and re-tokenization. Both manual and automatic parsing become more difficult with the higher number of words in a sentence. Thus we split long sentences occurring in lists into several shorter sentences, see Table 2. In addition, we adopt the idea of re-tokenization [27] – joining several tokens into one token – that implies reduction of nodes in a tree.

**Entity Detection.** Entities in the decree from CCLT were manually recognized by accounting experts and automatically parsed to import their dependency trees into DBE. Consequently, the queries for entity detection were automatically generated from these trees.

Since CCLT is manually syntactically annotated, we evaluated the process of entity detection against it. We automatically parsed the decree, queryied its manual and automatic trees and compare the extracted entities. Table 3 presents the results. One can observe relatively low precision which is caused by the high number of false positives.

---

[8] The Accounting Act (563/1991 Coll.) and Decree on Double-entry Accounting for undertakers (500/2002 Coll.).

[9] http://ufal.mff.cuni.cz/intlib

**Table 2.** Long lists and enumerations replaced with several shorter sentences

| Input sentence | Output sentences |
|---|---|
| (1) The General Directorate of Customs | |
| a) is an administrative ... | The General Directorate of Customs is an administrative ... |
| b) administers the customs ... | The General Directorate of Customs administers the customs ... |
| c) functions as a ... | The General Directorate of Customs functions as ... |

It means that RExtractor detected entities which were not annotated manually in gold-standard data. We investigated, that almost in most of such cases, the goldstandard annotation is missing. The human annotators were not consistent and they did not annotate each occurrence of a given entity. Other conclusion from the experiment is positive and it says that the parser has very low influence on the performance of entity detection.

**Relation Extraction** We focus on three different types of relations: *definitions* (D) – sentences where entities are explained or defined; *Obligations* (O) – sentences bearing the information *Entity* is obligated to do *Something*; *Rights* (R) – sentences bearing the information *Entity* has a right to do *Something*. Tree queries for detecting these relations are designed manually by both domain and PML-TQ experts and should respect the strategy to cover the maximum number of relations with the minimum number of queries.

In the pilot study, we used the act from CCLT for the query development. Finally, we obtained 5 queries for Definitions, 4 queries for Rights and 2 queries for Obligations. A sample of the queries is presented in Table 7. We carried out the evaluation on the decree from CCLT where we manually detected relations. The decree consists of 762 sentences, 21,967 tokens and 467 relations. We compared them to the queries output and we obtained the results presented in Table 4: the row *Goldstandard* lists the number of manually detected relations. The next rows present the RExtractor output. We determined three types of errors for incorrectly detected relation, see false negatives and false positives in Table 4): (i) incorrect dependency tree, (ii) missing or incorrect query, (iii) missing or incorrect entity. The results are summarized in Table 6.

We collected a set of 28 laws on accounting and taxes provisions consisting of 27,808 sentences and 745,137 tokens. We run RExtractor on this collection and we obtained 2,645 relations in total, details are listed in Table 5.

**Table 3.** Evaluation of Entity Detection Component

| Entity Parsing | Extracted | True positives | False positives | False negatives | Precision | Recall |
|---|---|---|---|---|---|---|
| Manual | 16, 428 | 9, 549 | 6, 879 | 628 | 58.1% | 93.8% |
| Automatic | 16, 160 | 9, 278 | 6, 882 | 838 | 57.4% | 91.7% |

**Table 4.** Evaluation of Relation Extraction Component

|  | D | O | R | Total |
|---|---|---|---|---|
| # of queries | 5 | 4 | 2 | 11 |
| Goldstandard | 97 | 308 | 62 | 467 |
| Extracted | 70 | 255 | 41 | 366 |
| True positive | 53 | 206 | 36 | 295 |
| False negative | 44 | 102 | 26 | 172 |
| False positive | 17 | 49 | 5 | 71 |
| Precision (%) | 75.7 | 80.8 | 87.8 | 80.6 |
| Recall (%) | 54.6 | 66.9 | 58.1 | 63.2 |

**Table 5.** Number of relations extracted by tree queries from the collection of 28 laws

| D |  | R |  | O |  |
|---|---|---|---|---|---|
| $D_1$ | 36 | $R_1$ | 240 | $O_1$ | 183 |
| $D_2$ | 287 | $R_2$ | 470 | $O_2$ | 37 |
| $D_3$ | 35 | $R_3$ | 127 |  |  |
| $D_4$ | 466 | $R_4$ | 6 |  |  |
| $D_5$ | 46 |  |  |  |  |
| Total | 1580 | Total | 843 | Total | 220 |

**Table 6.** Error analysis of incorrectly detected relations

| Error | # of errors | Ratio |
|---|---|---|
| Parser | 145 | 59.7 % |
| Query | 93 | 38.3 % |
| Entity | 5 | 2.1 % |

**Table 7.** Simplyfied versions of the most successfull queries. In a PML-TQ query, both subject and object depend on predicate

| Query | Subject | Predicate | Object |
|---|---|---|---|
| $D_4$ | CASE = 7 | LEMMA = rozumět_se | POS = noun, CASE = 1 |
| $R_2$ | AFUN = Sb | LEMMA = odpovídat | LEMMA = za |
| $O_1$ | ENTITY = true | LEMMA = moci | AFUN = Obj, POS = verb |

## 5  RDF Representation of the Data from RExtractor

In our previous work [3], we presented the ontology for representing acts and consolidated expressions in RDF. The ontology represents each act and its consolidated expressions as an RDF resource which can be linked from other data sources according to the Linked Data principles. The ontology also considers representation of act sections and their consolidated expressions. Therefore, each section of each act is also an RDF resource. We considered only the structure of acts, i.e. their sections and links to those sections. However, we did not consider the semantics of acts, i.e. entities and relations between them defined in acts. Now, since we work with RExtractor, we extend our previously published ontology with new components to represent data extracted by RExtractor in RDF.

The extension has two parts. We describe each as a separate ontology. The first one is called *Legal Concepts Ontology*. Its URI is http://purl.org/lex/ontology/concepts# and we use a prefix lexc: to refer to it in this paper. The ontology enables to represent the extracted entities and relationships between them independently of the original text of the ontology. The classes and predicates introduced by the ontology are depicted in Figure 5.

The core class of the ontology is the class Concept whose instances represent the entities extracted by RExtractor. We call those instances *concepts*. A concept defined by an act exists independently of particular versions (consolidated expressions) of the act. However, because the act exists in one or more versions, there are also respective

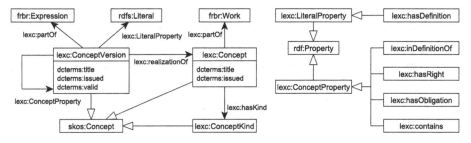

**Fig. 5.** Legal Concepts Ontology

versions of concepts defined by the act. There is a version in which the act defines a concept for the first time. The concept then exists in the following versions of the act until it is cancelled. For each following version, there is a respective version of the concept. Therefore, for each version of the act which speaks about the concept, we also create an instance of the class `ConceptVersion`. This instance represents a particular version of the concept defined by the respective version of the act. Each concept is linked to the act and its sections. This enables us to show users the list of concepts which appear in a chosen act or in any of its sections.

The extracted relations between concepts and their literal properties are represented with sub-properties of the abstract `ConceptProperty` and `LiteralProperty` properties, respectively. However, because each relationship and literal property is extracted from a particular version of an act, the domain of those properties is not the class `Concept` but the class `ConceptVersion`. As Figure 5 shows, there are various sub-properties of the abstract properties and it is easy to add new properties. Currently, there is a literal property `hasDefinition`, which enables to link a concept to its literal definition, and concept properties `hasRight`, `hasObligation`, `inDefinitionOf`, and `contains`, which enable to link a concept to another concept which is the right or obligation of the concept, or is contained in the definition of the concept, or is a part of that concept, respectively.

The `lexc:` ontology enables us to search for literal or concept properties. However, it is not possible to show users the original text of the consolidated act from which a property was extracted by RExtractor. This is very important for users because even precision and recall of RExtractor are relatively high, they are not perfect. Showing the extracted information out of the original textual context could be, therefore, insufficient. Thus, we provide the second extension that we call *Lingvistic Ontology*. Its URI is http://purl.org/lingv/ontology# and we use a prefix `lingv:` to refer to it in this paper. The classes and predicates defined by the ontology are depicted in Figure 6.

The core class of the ontology is the class `TextChunk`. It represents a part of the original text (called text chunk) which is the occurrence of some entity (see the sub-class `NamedEntityOccurrence`) or the occurrence of a relationship specification (see the sub-class `RelationOccurrence`). Each text chunk is annotated by its meaning which is a version of some concept (an instance of the class `ConceptVersion` from `lexc:` ontology), relationship between two concepts (a sub-property of `ConceptProperty` from `lexc:` ontology), or literal property (a sub-property of

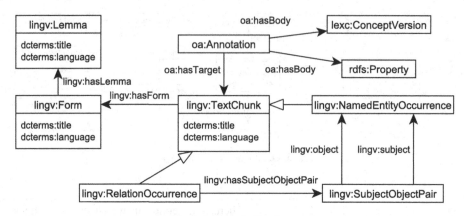

**Fig. 6.** Lingvistic Ontology

LiteralProperty from lexc: ontology). For representing annotations in RDF we use the Open Annotation Ontology (we use prefix oa:).[10]

The lingv: ontology enables us to display users text chunks from which RExtractor extracted particular concepts and relations between them. Because a text chunk is also a part of the original text, we are able to show users each text chunk in the context of original documents.

In our experiment we converted the results of RExtractor presented in Table 5 to RDF. The numbers of instances of the main classes from lexc: and lingv: ontologies are displayed in Table 8.

**Table 8.** The numbers of instances of the main classes from lexc: and lingv: ontologies

| Class or property | Number of instances |
|---|---|
| lexc:ConceptVersion | 3504 |
| lexc:hasDefinition | 727 |
| lexc:hasObligation | 546 |
| lexc:hasRight | 160 |
| lingv:TextChunk | 33086 |
| lingv:NamedEntityOccurrence | 23674 |
| lingv:RelationOccurrence | 1605 |
| oa:Annotation | 30800 |

## 6    Conclusion and Future Work

In this paper, we presented a general pipeline of tools for extraction and representation of data that is presented in raw texts. The extraction pipeline processes input texts by linguistically-aware tools and extracts entities and relations from their syntactic representation. Consequently, the extracted data is represented according to the Linked

---

[10] http://www.openannotation.org/spec/core/

Data principles. We applied the tools on texts from the legislative domain. Based on the experience that we acquired in the pilot study, we formulate topics to address in the future:

- improve RExtractor, in particular syntactic parsing and relation query development.
- improve linking of concepts of particular sections of acts to other data sources (e.g., life situations, agendas of public bodies, fines imposed by public bodies, etc.).
- develop web applications which enable users to work with the extracted concepts and relationships and to explore links between extracted concepts and other data sources.

In addition, we will place the emphasis on the evaluation considering a number of aspects, mainly gold standard data vs. practical use cases, developers' experience vs. users' expectations, scientific contribution vs. 'making life easier'.

**Acknowledgements.** We gratefully acknowledge support from the Technology Agency of the Czech Republic (grant no. TA02010182). This work has been using language resources developed and/or stored and/or distributed by the LINDAT/CLARIN project.

# References

1. Gantz, J., Reinsel, D.: The digital universe decade - are you ready? (2010), `http://goo.gl/ZaOOPR`
2. Lassila, O., Swick, R.R.: Resource description framework (RDF) model and syntax specification. Technical report (1999), `http://www.w3.org/TR/1999/REC-rdf-syntax-19990222/`
3. Nečaský, M., Knap, T., Klímek, J., Holubová, I., Vidová-Hladká, B.: Linked open data for legislative domain - ontology and experimental data. In: Abramowicz, W. (ed.) BIS Workshops 2013. LNBIP, vol. 160, pp. 172–183. Springer, Heidelberg (2013)
4. Berners-Lee, T., Hendler, J., Lassila, O., et al.: The semantic web. Scientific American 284, 28–37 (2001)
5. Biemann, C.: Ontology learning from text: A survey of methods. In: LDV forum, vol. 20, pp. 75–93 (2005)
6. Agichtein, E., Gravano, L.: Snowball: Extracting relations from large plain-text collections. In: Proceedings of the Fifth ACM Conference on Digital Libraries, DL 2000, pp. 85–94. ACM, New York (2000)
7. Etzioni, O., Cafarella, M., Downey, D., Kok, S., Popescu, A.M., Shaked, T., Soderland, S., Weld, D.S., Yates, A.: Web-scale information extraction in Knowitall (preliminary results). In: Proceedings of the 13th International Conference on World Wide Web, WWW 2004, pp. 100–110. ACM, New York (2004)
8. Carlson, A., Betteridge, J., Kisiel, B., Settles, B., Hruschka Jr, E.R., Mitchell, T.M.: Toward an architecture for never-ending language learning. In: AAAI (2010)
9. Banko, M., Etzioni, O.: Strategies for lifelong knowledge extraction from the web. In: Proceedings of the 4th International Conference on Knowledge Capture, K-CAP 2007, pp. 95–102. ACM, New York (2007)
10. Fader, A., Soderland, S., Etzioni, O.: Identifying relations for open information extraction. In: Proceedings of the Conference on Empirical Methods in Natural Language Processing, pp. 1535–1545. Association for Computational Linguistics (2011)

11. Suchanek, F.M., Sozio, M., Weikum, G.: Sofie: a self-organizing framework for information extraction. In: Proceedings of the 18th International Conference on World Wide Web, pp. 631–640. ACM (2009)

12. Abacha, A.B., Zweigenbaum, P.: Automatic extraction of semantic relations between medical entities: a rule based approach. J. Biomedical Semantics 2, S4 (2011)

13. Exner, P., Nugues, P.: Entity extraction: From unstructured text to dbpedia rdf triples. In: The Web of Linked Entities Workshop, WoLE 2012 (2012)

14. Baisa, V., Kovář, V.: Information extraction for czech based on syntactic analysis. In: Vetulani, Z. (ed.) Proceedings of 5th Language and Technology Conference on Human Language Technologies as a Challenge for Computer Science and Linguistics, Pozna, Funcacja Universytetu im. A. Mickiewicza, pp. 466–470 (2011)

15. Biagioli, C., Francesconi, E., Passerini, A., Montemagni, S., Soria, C.: Automatic semantics extraction in law documents. In: Proceedings of the 10th International Conference on Artificial Intelligence and Law, pp. 133–140. ACM (2005)

16. Chiarcos, C., Hellmann, S., Nordhoff, S.: Introduction and overview. In: Chiarcos, C., Nordhoff, S., Hellmann, S. (eds.) Linked Data in Linguistics, pp. 1–12. Springer, Heidelberg (2012)

17. Francesconi, E., Montemagni, S., Peters, W., Tiscornia, D. (eds.): Semantic Processing of Legal Texts. LNCS, vol. 6036. Springer, Heidelberg (2010)

18. McCarty, L.T.: Deep semantic interpretations of legal texts. In: Proceedings of the 11th International Conference on Artificial Intelligence and Law, ICAIL 2007, pp. 217–224. ACM, New York (2007)

19. Dell'Orletta, F., Marchi, S., Montemagni, S., Plank, B., Venturi, G.: The splet–2012 shared task on dependency parsing of legal texts. In: Proceedings of the 4th Workshop on Semantic Processing of Legal Texts 2012, Istanbul, Turkey (2012)

20. Pala, K., Rychlý, P., Šmerk, P.: Automatic identification of legal terms in czech law texts. In: Semantic Processing of Legal Texts, pp. 83–94. Springer, Berlin (2010)

21. Pala, K., Mráková, E.: Legal terms and word sketches: a case study. In: Sojka, P., Horák, A. (eds.) Proceedings of Fourth Workshop on Recent Advances in Slavonic Natural Languages Processing, RASLAN 2010, Brno, Tribun s.r.o, pp. 31–39 (2010)

22. Hajič, J., Panevová, J., Hajičová, E., Sgall, P., Pajas, P., Štěpánek, J., Havelka, J., Mikulová, M., Žabokrtský, Z., Ševčíková-Razímová, M.: Prague dependency treebank 2.0 (2006)

23. Bejček, E., Hajičová, E., Hajič, J., Jínová, P., Kettnerová, V., Kolářová, V., Mikulová, M., Mírovský, J., Nedoluzhko, A., Panevová, J., Poláková, L., Ševčíková, M., Štěpánek, J., Zikánová, Š.: Prague dependency treebank 3.0. (2013), http://ufal.mff.cuni.cz/pdt3.0

24. Popel, M., Žabokrtský, Z.: TectoMT: Modular NLP framework. In: Loftsson, H., Rögnvaldsson, E., Helgadóttir, S. (eds.) IceTAL 2010. LNCS, vol. 6233, pp. 293–304. Springer, Heidelberg (2010)

25. Pajas, P., Štěpánek, J.: System for querying syntactically annotated corpora. In: Lee, G., Im Walde, S.S. (eds.) Proceedings of the ACL-IJCNLP 2009 Software Demonstrations, pp. 33–36. Association for Computational Linguistics, Suntec (2009)

26. Tiersma, P.: The Creation, Structure, and Interpretation of the Legal Text (2010), http://www.languageandlaw.org/LEGALTEXT.HTM

27. Kříž, V.: Detecting semantic relations in texts and their integration with external data resources. In: WDS 2013 Proceedings of Contributed Papers, Praha, Czechia, pp. 18–23. Matematicko-fyzikální fakulta Univerzity Karlovy, Matfyzpress (2013)

# A New Memetic Algorithm
# for Multi-document Summarization Based on CHC
# Algorithm and Greedy Search

Martha Mendoza[1], Carlos Cobos[1], Elizabeth León[2], Manuel Lozano[3],
Francisco Rodríguez[3], and Enrique Herrera-Viedma[3]

[1] Universidad del Cauca, Popayán, Colombia
{mmendoza,ccobos}@unicauca.edu.co
[2] Universidad Nacional de Colombia, Bogotá D.C., Colombia
eleonguz@unal.edu.co
[3] Universidad de Granada, Granada, España
{lozano,fjrodriguez,viedma}@decsai.ugr.es

**Abstract.** Multi-document summarization has been used for extracting the most relevant sentences from a set of documents, allowing the user to more quickly address the content thereof. This paper addresses the generation of extractive summaries from multiple documents as a binary optimization problem and proposes a method, based on CHC evolutionary algorithm and greedy search, called MA-MultiSumm, in which objective function optimizes the lineal combination of coverage and redundancy factors. MA-MultiSumm was compared with other state-of-the-art methods using ROUGE measures. The results showed that MA-MultiSumm outperforms all methods on the DUC2005 dataset; and on DUC2006 the results are very close to the best method. Furthermore in a unified ranking MA-MultiSumm only was improved on by the DESAMC+DocSum method, which requires as many iterations of the evolutionary process as MA-MultiSumm. The experimental results show that the optimization-based approach for multiple document summarization is truly a promising research direction.

**Keywords:** Multi-document summarization, Memetic algorithms, CHC algorithm, Greedy search.

# 1    Introduction

Currently vast quantities of information are found in digital text documents on the internet and within organizations. When a user is interested in exploring a specific topic in depth, the information required may be contained in a large number of related texts that can be read in their entirety by the user only with great difficulty, the user having to invest much time and effort to find what they are looking for; it is therefore important to be able to rely on a summary in order to identify the main topics contained in the documents available. For many years, the automatic generation of summaries has been attempting to create summaries that closely approximate those generated by humans

A. Gelbukh et al. (Eds.): MICAI 2014, Part I, LNAI 8856, pp. 125–138, 2014.
© Springer International Publishing Switzerland 2014

[1, 2], enabling the user to engage the documents that satisfy their requirements in less time. Some of the application areas of the generation of extractive summaries from multiple documents are the summaries of news, web Summarization and email thread summarization [2].

Different taxonomies for summaries exist [1, 2], based on the way the summary is generated, the target audience of the summary, the number of documents to be summarized, and so on. According to the way in which the summary is generated, it can be either extractive or abstractive [1, 2]. Extractive summaries are formed from the reuse of portions of the original text. Abstractive summaries [3], on the other hand, are rather more complex, requiring linguistic analysis tools to construct new sentences from those previously extracted. Taking account of the target audience, summaries may be [1, 2]: generic, query-based, user-focused or topic-focused. Generic summaries do not depend on the audience for whom the summary is intended. Query-based summaries respond to a query made by the user. User-focused ones generate summaries to tailor the interests of a particular user, while topic-focused summaries emphasize those summaries on specific topics of documents. Depending to the number of documents that are processed, summaries [1, 2] can be either single document or multiple document. With regard the language of the document, they may be monolingual or multilingual, and regarding document genre may be scientific article, news, blogs, and so on.

The summarization algorithm (method) proposed in this paper is extractive; generic and multiple documents, allowing the summary is generated on any group of documents; and for any type of document, although the evaluation was performed on a set of news.

Automatic summarization is an area that has explored different methods for the automatic generation of summaries of multiple documents, such as: (1) machine learning technique approaches [4, 5] using training data to identify the characteristics that have the greatest impact on the selection of the sentences that make up the summary; (2) approaches based on text connectivity [6], with lexical strings using lexical databases such as WordNet to find relationships between different words. The chains are classified by their length and homogeneity, and the strongest lexical strings are selected. After each of these chains, sentences are selected to create the summary. Most recently the focus of rhetorical roles has been employed [7]; (3) graph-based approaches [8-10], which represent units of text (key words or sentences) in the vertices of the graph, and the similarity between the text units by means of the edges, then an iterative process is carried out and the summary with sentences of the first vertices is obtained; (4) based on algebraic reduction [11, 12] through LSA (Latent Semantic Analysis ) and NMF (Non-negative Matrix Factorization), which make use of matrix decomposition to find the sentences that best represent the document; (5) based on clustering and probabilistic models [13, 14], in which the priority is to generate sets of documents or sentences associated with a particular topic; and (6) based on metaheuristics that seek to optimize an objective function to find the sentences that will be part of the summary [15-17].

Of these methods, those based on algebraic reduction, clustering, probabilistic models and metaheuristics are language independent and unsupervised, aspects on which more emphasis is being placed in recent research so as to avoid dependence on language and training groups. Although these methods have achieved good results over other methods, recent research based on memetic algorithm for single document [18], have shown better results, making research in this area promising, and leaving the possibility of exploring the application of the memetic algorithms for multiple documents that are not currently being used. Further, memetic algorithms have contributed in solving problems of discrete combinatorial optimization obtaining very good results [19]; nevertheless, they have not yet been used to solve the problem of automatic generation of summaries from multiple documents.

In this paper a memetic algorithm based on CHC (Cross-generational elitist selection, Heterogeneous recombination, Cataclysmic mutation) algorithm and greedy search (local search) is proposed, for automatic generation of extractive and generic summaries from multiples documents, in which objective function is optimized by the lineal combination of two factors: coverage that exists between all candidate sentences in the summary and the document collection sentences; and redundancy that exists between the sentences in the summary.

The rest of the paper is organized as follows: Section 2 introduces the document representation and characteristics of the objective function proposed in the algorithm. Section 3 describes the proposed algorithm; while the results of evaluation using data sets, along with a comparison and analysis with other state-of-the-art methods, are presented in Section 4; finally, Section 5 presents conclusions and future work.

## 2    Problem Statement and Its Mathematical Formulation

The representation of a document is made based on the vector space model proposed by Salton [20]. Thus, a document is represented by the sentences that compose it, in this case, it is represented as the set of all the sentences that the collection of documents contains, i.e. $D=\{S_1, S_2, \ldots, S_n\}$, where $S_i$ corresponds to the $i$-th sentence of the document collection and $n$ is the total number of sentences in this collection. Likewise, a sentence is represented by the set $S_i = \{t_{i1},t_{i2},\ldots,t_{ik},\ldots,t_{io}\}$, where $t_{ik}$ is the $k$-th term of the sentence $S_i$ and $o$ is the total number of terms in the sentence. Thus, the vector representation of a sentence of the document is a vector containing the weights of the terms, as shown in Eq. (1).

$$s_i = \{w_{i1}, w_{i2}, \ldots, w_{ik}, \ldots, w_{im}\}$$

Where $m$ is the number of distinct terms in the document collection, $w_{i1}$ is the weight of term $t_1$ in sentence $S_i$ and $w_{ik}$ is the weight of term $t_k$ in sentence $S_i$. $\qquad$ (1)

The component $w_{ik}$ is calculated as the relative frequency of the term in the document [20]. The scheme assigns the weight as shown in Eq. (2).

$$w_{i,k} = (f_{i,k}/MaxFreq)\times\log(n/(1+n_t))$$

Where $f_{i,k}$ represents the frequency of term $k$ in sentence $S_i$, $MaxFreq_i$ is an adjustment factor that indicates the number of occurrences of the most frequent term in the sentence $S_i$, $n_k$ denotes the number of sentences in which the term $t_k$ appears, and $n$ is the number of sentences in the document collection. $\qquad$ (2)

Thus the aim of generating a summary of multiple documents is to obtain a subset of $D$ with the sentences that contain the main information of the document collection. To do this, features are used whose purpose is to evaluate the subset of sentences to determine the extent to which they cover the most relevant information of the document collection. These features are based on measures of similarity between sentences. The similarity between two sentences $S_i$ and $S_j$, according to the vector representation described, is measured in the same way as the cosine similarity [20] which relates to the angle of the vectors $S_i$ and $S_j$.

In a memetic algorithm, the objective function is in charge of guide the search of the best summaries based on sentences features. In this paper an objective function based on maximum coverage and minimum redundancy is introduced, taking into account that research that includes these factors in the objective function have shown good results in relation to the state of the art methods [15, 21].

**Coverage Factor**: A summary ought to contain the main aspects of the documents with the least loss of information. The sentences selected should therefore cover the largest amount of information contained within the set of sentences in the document collection. As such, coverage factor is calculated taking into account the cosine similarity between the text of the candidate summary and the sentences of the entire collection of documents as shown in Eq. (3).

$$Fc = sim_{cos}(R,D)$$

Where $R$ represents the text with all the candidate summary sentences; $D$ represents all the sentences of the document collection (in this case, it is the centroid of the collection). This factor therefore takes values between zero and one.                                                                (3)

**Redundancy Factor**: Managing redundancy is a very important factor, because the generated summary should avoid containing repeated information in it, that is, have the least redundancy as possible, especially when dealing with the problem of generating summaries of multiple documents covering the same topic. To eliminate redundancy in the sentences of the summary, this factor is calculated based on what was stated in [15], but carrying out a normalization so that this factor takes values between zero and one, as with the coverage factor (See Eq. (4)).

$$Fr = \frac{2}{r \times (r-1)} \sum_{i=1}^{r-1} \sum_{j=i+1}^{r} sim_{cos}(S_i, S_j)$$                                    (4)

Where $S_i$ and $S_j$ are sentences in the candidate summary and $r$ is the number of sentences in the summary.

Thus the objective function to maximize is defined as the linear combination of the coverage (Fc) and redundancy (Fr) factors (See Eq. (5)). The latter is subtracted in the equation to prevent the generated summary containing identical or similar sentences. A lambda coefficient ($\lambda$) is introduced, which gives flexibility to the objective function allowing more or less weight to be given to each factor. The coefficient $\lambda$ varies between zero and one. Eq. (6) includes a restriction to maximize the information included in the summary by selecting sentences containing relevant information but few words.

Maximize

$$f(x) = \lambda Fc - (1-\lambda)Fr = \lambda(sim_{\cos}(R,D)) - (1-\lambda)\frac{2}{r\times(r-1)}\sum_{i=1}^{r-1}\sum_{j=i+1}^{r}sim_{\cos}(S_i,S_j)$$

(5)

subject to

$$\sum_{i=1}^{r}l_i x_i \leq L$$

(6)

Where $x_i$, indicates one if the sentence $S_i$ is selected and zero otherwise; $l_i$ is the length of the sentence $S_i$ (measured in words) and $L$ is the maximum number of words allowed in the generated summary.

## 3    The Proposed Memetic Algorithm: MA-MultiSumm

In Fig. 1, the general outline of the proposed memetic algorithm for automatically generating extractive summaries based on CHC [22] and greedy search, MA-MultiSumm, is shown. The most important modifications as regarding to the original CHC algorithm, are: (1) the initial value of $d$ is smaller ($d_o=0.025\times L$) than CHC original (0.25×L), because the agent is represented in this problem by many zeros and few ones, therefore the agents are very similar to each other; (2) local search is applied to the agents to find local optimal; and (3) in the cataclysm, the two best individuals are preserved, the remaining individuals are created randomly, and threshold $d$ takes the initial value $d_o$. In section 3.1 is described the local search strategy used in MA-MultiSumm algorithm.

**Population initialization.** The initial population is composed of $p$ agents, generated randomly taking into the constraint of the maximum number of words allowed in the summary (the number of sentences in the agent is controlled by means Eq. (6)). Each agent represents the presence of the sentence in the summary by means of a one, and absence with a zero. The most common strategy for initializing the population ($t=0$) is to randomly generate each agent. So that all the sentences in the document have the same probability of being part of the agent, a random number between one and $n$ (number of sentences in the document collection) is defined, the gene corresponding to this value is chosen and a value of one is given, so that this sentence will become part of the summary in the current agent. Thus, the $c$-th agent of the initial population is created as shown in Eq. (7).

$$X_c(0) = [x_{c,1}(0), x_{c,2}(0),...,x_{c,n}(0)], \quad x_{c,s}(0) = a_s$$

Where $a_s$ is a random value in $\{0,1\}$, $c=1,2,...,p$ and $s=1,2,...,n.$, $p$        (7)

is the population size and $n$ is the number of sentences.

**Evaluation and optimization of the initial population.** After generating the initial population randomly, the fitness value of each agent is calculated using Eqs. (5)-(6). Then a percentage $op$ of the population is optimized using greedy local search, which will be explained later. Finally the fitness is recalculated, and the resulting population is ordered from highest to lowest based on this new fitness value.

```
L: agent length; p: population size; d: difference threshold; op: optimization probability;
dh: hamming distance; nofe: number of objective function evaluations;
mnofe: maximum number of objective function evaluations;

t = 0;
d = d_o                              // Minimum of different genes (sentences), the value of d_o is 0.025×L.
Initialize (P(t));                   // Random initialization, each gen represents the absence or presence
                                     // of the sentence on the summary.
Evaluate (P(t));                     // Calculate fitness for each agent in the population P(t).
Optimization (P(t));                 // Only a percentage of P(t) is optimized.
While nofe < mnofe do
    For i= 1... p/2 do
        Selection (p1, p2, P(t));           // Select parent1 (p1) and parent2 (p2) from current population.
        If (dh (p1, p2) < d) Then Continue; // Incest prevention mechanism using the hamming distance.
        HUX_Crossover (p1, p2);             // HUX Crossover among p1 and p2 to obtain offspring.
        For each offspring do               // With two offspring that were created.
            Evaluate (offspring);           // Calculate fitness for the offspring.
            If (U(0,1) < op) Optimization (offspring);    // Only a percentage op of the
                                                          // current population is optimized.
            P(t+1)=Add(offspring);          // Add offspring to the new population.
        End For each;
    End For;
    If (P(t+1) = empty) Then d = d – 1;     // It permits great similarity among the parents.
    P(t+1) = P(t+1) ∪ P(t);                 // Merge the members of the current population
                                            // with the generated offspring.
    Preserve best agents from P(t+1);       // When parent and offspring have the same fitness value,
                                            // the offspring is selected.
    If (d = 0) Cataclysm();                 // The two best individuals are preserved and the remaining
                                            // individuals are generated randomly.
    t = t +1;
End while;
Return (BestAgent);    // The agent with best fitness in last population is returned;
```

**Fig. 1.** Scheme of the MA-MultiSumm memetic algorithm

**Selection.** The generation step starts with the selection operator and is repeated $p/2$ times. The two parent agents are selected randomly from the current population ensuring that they are not repeated.

**Incest prevention.** This mechanism calculates the Hamming distance between the two parent agents to validate that the total number of distinct genes among them is greater than a threshold $d$ (minimum allowable different genes) and thus avoid incest. If this threshold is not met, new parents are selected.

**HUX crossover.** To produce the two offspring, HUX crossover strategy is used between the two parents selected. Thus, the genes found in both parents will also part of the offspring and half of the genes that are not equal are exchanged randomly.

**Optimization the offspring.** A uniform random number between zero and one is generated. If this value is less than the probability of optimization ($op$), the offspring generated by HUX crossing is optimized using a greedy local search operator. If the fitness value of the optimized agent is better than the fitness value of the agent without optimization, the current agent is replaced by the optimized agent.

**Replacement.** If in the new generation there are no offspring, the value of $d$ is decreased to allow the agents selected as parents to become more similar and generate offspring. Replacement is carried out when the population of agents generated is already full, joining with the current population, which has been sorted previously according to the fitness value. Then, the new population is formed with the $p$ best agents from the union of the two populations, giving priority to the offspring when they have fitness equal to that of the parents.

**Cataclysm.** On generating a new population, whether or not cataclysm occurs in the population is evaluated. For this, whether the minimum number of different genes to prevent incest is less than or equal to zero is checked. When cataclysm occurs, the two agents with the highest fitness value of the current generation are kept and the remaining agents are generated completely randomly according to the process explained in the generation of the initial population.

**Stopping criterion.** The running of the memetic algorithm terminates when the stop condition is met. The stop condition was established earlier as a maximum number of evaluations of the objective function.

## 3.1   Greedy Search

Regarding local search, MA-MultiSumm uses a Greedy approach [23], taking into account *op*. The agent is optimized a defined number of times (*Maxnumop*), adding and removing a sentence from the summary, and controlling the number of sentences in the agent by means Eq. (6). If the fitness value of the new agent improves previous agent, the replacement is made. Otherwise, the previous agent is retained. A movement is then made again in the neighborhood, repeating the previous steps (Fig. 2).

| |
|---|
| *Lss*: a list of sentences sorted for similarity with the documents collection;<br>*Maxnumop*: maximum number of optimizations;  *OriginalAgent*: original agent (agent to optimize); |
| For *i*=1 … *Maxnumop* do<br>    *CurrentAgent* = Copy (*OriginalAgent*);<br>    Add_sentence (*CurrentAgent*);          // A sentence with the highest value of similarity of<br>                                                             // the list *Lss* is activated in the agent.<br>    Delete_sentence (*CurrentAgent*);       // A sentence with the lowest value of similarity of<br>                                                             // the list *Lss* is turned off in the agent.<br>    Length_restriction (*CurrentAgent*);    // The restriction of the summary length is executed.<br>    Evaluate (*CurrentAgent*);                  // Calculate fitness for current agent.<br>    If (Fitness(*CurrentAgent*) > Fitness(*OriginalAgent*)) Then *OriginalAgent* = *CurrentAgent*;<br>End For |

**Fig. 2.** Procedure of greedy search

The neighborhood is generated based on a scheme of elitism, in which the sentence that is placed in one (i.e. included in the candidate summary) is selected from a list sorted according to the similarity of the sentence to the entire document collection; and the sentence that is placed in zero (thereby being removed from the candidate summary) is the one with least similarity to the entire document collection. This means that the coverage factor is the criterion used to include or remove a sentence from the candidate summary.

## 4    Experiment and Evaluation

To evaluate the MA-MultiSumm algorithm, Document Understanding Conference (DUC) datasets for the years 2005 and 2006 were used. The DUC2005 collection is comprised of fifty topics, each containing between 25 and 50 documents; and the DUC2006 comprises fifty topics, each with 25 documents. Furthermore the summary generated should be less than 250 words and have several reference summaries for each topic. For each topic the algorithm was run thirty (30) times to obtain the average of each measure for each data set.

Pre-processing of the documents involves linguistic techniques such as segmentation of sentences or words [20], removal of stop words, removal of capital letters and punctuation marks, stemming and indexing [20]. This process is carried out before starting to run the algorithm for the automatic generation of multiple documents.

The segmentation process was done using an open source segmentation tool called "splitta" (available at http://code.google.com/p/splitta). The stop words removal process was done based on the list built for the SMART information retrieval system (ftp://ftp.cs.cornell.edu/pub/smart/english.stop). The Porter algorithm was used for the stemming process. Finally, Lucene (http://lucene.apache.org) was used to facilitate the entire indexing and searching in information retrieval tasks.

Evaluation of the quality of the summaries generated by the MA-MultiSumm method was performed using metrics provided by the assessment tool ROUGE (Recall-Oriented Understudy for Gisting Evaluation) [24], version 1.5.5 (available on internet), which has been widely handled by DUC in evaluating automatic summaries. ROUGE is accepted by DUC as the official metric for the evaluation of automatic summarization of texts.

The comparison of the proposed algorithm was made against DESAMC+DocSum [16], PLSA [13], LFIPP [25], MCMR [15], HybHSum [26], LEX [27], SVR [5], iRANK [28], HierSum [29], Centroid [10], SNMF +SLSS [30], TMR [31], and MMR [32].

### 4.1    Parameter Tuning

Parameter tuning was carried out based on the Meta Evolutionary Algorithm (Meta-EA) [33], using a version of harmony search [34]. The configuration of parameters for the MA-MultiSumm algorithm is as follows: population size $ps = 70$, optimization probability $op = 0.25$, summary length maximum $slm = 275$ (during the evolutionary process), lambda $\lambda = 0.84$ and maximum number of optimizations $maxnumop = 20$ (maximum number that an agent is optimized). A further parameter handled in the pre-processing stage is known as the sentence threshold, which ensures that each sentence of the summary has a minimum similarity to the document collection. The number of evaluations of the objective function was set at 15000. The algorithm was implemented on a PC Intel Core I3 2.99GHz CPU with 3GB of RAM in Windows 7.

Regarding the objective function, the process of tuning the weights of the MA-MultiSumm objective function was divided into two stages. In the first, a genetic algorithm (GA) was designed in order to obtain various weight ranges with which the objective function was then evaluated with the MA-MultiSumm algorithm to determine the best combinations of weights. In the second stage, the best set of weights obtained in the first stage is used as a reference to generate new sets of weights that are evaluated in order to obtain a better performance of the objective function.

## 4.2   Results

Table 1 presents the results obtained in ROUGE-1, ROUGE-2 and ROUGE-SU4 measures, for MA-MultiSumm and other state-of-the-art methods for the DUC2005 and DUCC2006 data sets. The best solution is represented in bold type. The number in parenthesis in the table shows the ranking of each method. As shown in this table, MA-MultiSumm improves upon the others methods in all ROUGE measures for DUC2005. MA-MultiSumm improves performance of DESAMC+DocSum by 1.63% for ROUGE-1, 5.72% for ROUGE-2 and 1.13% for ROUGE-SU4.

**Table 1.** ROUGE values of the methods on DUC2005 and DUC2006

| Method | DUC2005 | | | | | | DUC2006 | | | | | |
|---|---|---|---|---|---|---|---|---|---|---|---|---|
| | ROUGE-1 | | ROUGE-2 | | ROUGE-SU4 | | ROUGE-1 | | ROUGE-2 | | ROUGE-SU4 | |
| DESAMC+DocSum | 0.3937 | (2) | 0.0822 | (2) | 0.1418 | (2) | **0.4345** | **(1)** | **0.0989** | **(1)** | **0.1569** | **(1)** |
| MA-MultiSumm | **0.4001** | **(1)** | **0.0868** | **(1)** | **0.1434** | **(1)** | 0.4195 | (5) | 0.0986 | (2) | 0.1526 | (4) |
| PLSA | 0.3913 | (3) | 0.0811 | (3) | 0.1389 | (5) | 0.4328 | (2) | 0.0970 | (3) | 0.1557 | (2) |
| LFIPP | 0.3905 | (4) | 0.0804 | (4) | 0.1403 | (3) | 0.4209 | (4) | 0.0934 | (4) | 0.1534 | (3) |
| MCMR | 0.3891 | (5) | 0.0790 | (6) | 0.1392 | (4) | 0.4184 | (6) | 0.0928 | (5) | 0.1512 | (5) |
| HybHSum | 0.3812 | (8) | 0.0749 | (8) | 0.1354 | (7) | 0.4300 | (3) | 0.0910 | (10) | 0.1510 | (6) |
| LEX | 0.3760 | (10) | 0.0735 | (10) | 0.1316 | (10) | 0.4030 | (9) | 0.0913 | (8) | 0.1449 | (10) |
| SVR | 0.3849 | (7) | 0.0757 | (7) | 0.1335 | (8) | 0.4018 | (10) | 0.0926 | (6) | 0.1485 | (8) |
| iRANK | 0.3880 | (6) | 0.0802 | (5) | 0.1373 | (6) | 0.4032 | (8) | 0.0912 | (9) | 0.1450 | (9) |
| HierSum | 0.3753 | (11) | 0.0745 | (9) | 0.1324 | (9) | 0.4010 | (11) | 0.0860 | (11) | 0.1430 | (11) |
| Centroid | 0.3535 | (12) | 0.0638 | (12) | 0.1198 | (12) | 0.3807 | (13) | 0.0785 | (13) | 0.1330 | (13) |
| SNMF +SLSS | 0.3501 | (13) | 0.0604 | (13) | 0.1172 | (13) | 0.3955 | (12) | 0.0855 | (12) | 0.1429 | (12) |
| TMR | 0.3775 | (9) | 0.0715 | (11) | 0.1304 | (11) | 0.4063 | (7) | 0.0913 | (7) | 0.1504 | (7) |
| MMR | 0.3479 | (14) | 0.0601 | (14) | 0.1134 | (14) | 0.3716 | (14) | 0.0757 | (14) | 0.1308 | (14) |

With the DUC2006 dataset, the results of the evaluation show that the DESAMC+DocSum method is the only one that outperforms the proposed MA-MultiSumm algorithm in the ROUGE-2 measure. In the ROUGE-1 measure, MA-MultiSumm is outperformed by DESAMC+DocSum, PLSA, HybHSum and LFIPP. In the case of ROUGE-SU4, it is outperformed by the DESAMC+DocSum, PLSA and LFIPP methods. In summary, DESAMC+DocSum exceeds MA-MultiSumm by 3.67% for ROUGE-1. For ROUGE-2, the difference between these two methods is 0.30%, and for ROUGE-SU4 it better by 2.82%.

Because the results do not identify which method gets the best results on both data sets, a unified ranking of all methods is presented, taking into account the position each method occupies for each measure. Table 2 shows the unified ranking. The resultant rank in this table (last column) was computed according to the formula in Eq. (8).

$$Ran(method) = \sum_{r=1}^{14} \frac{(14 - r + 1)R_r}{14}$$

(8)

Where $R_r$ denotes the number of times the method appears in the $r$-th rank. The denominator 14 corresponds to the number of methods with which the comparison was made.

**Table 2.** The resultant rank of the methods

| Methods | $R_r =$ | | | | | | | | | | | | | | Rank |
|---|---|---|---|---|---|---|---|---|---|---|---|---|---|---|---|
| | 1 | 2 | 3 | 4 | 5 | 6 | 7 | 8 | 9 | 10 | 11 | 12 | 13 | 14 | |
| DESAMC+DocSum | 3 | 3 | 0 | 0 | 0 | 0 | 0 | 0 | 0 | 0 | 0 | 0 | 0 | 0 | 5.8 |
| MA-MultiSumm | 3 | 1 | 0 | 1 | 1 | 0 | 0 | 0 | 0 | 0 | 0 | 0 | 0 | 0 | 5.4 |
| PLSA | 0 | 2 | 3 | 0 | 1 | 0 | 0 | 0 | 0 | 0 | 0 | 0 | 0 | 0 | 5.1 |
| LFIPP | 0 | 0 | 2 | 4 | 0 | 0 | 0 | 0 | 0 | 0 | 0 | 0 | 0 | 0 | 4.9 |
| MCMR | 0 | 0 | 0 | 1 | 3 | 2 | 0 | 0 | 0 | 0 | 0 | 0 | 0 | 0 | 2.9 |
| HybHSum | 0 | 0 | 1 | 0 | 0 | 1 | 1 | 2 | 0 | 1 | 0 | 0 | 0 | 0 | 2.6 |
| LEX | 0 | 0 | 0 | 0 | 0 | 0 | 0 | 1 | 1 | 4 | 0 | 0 | 0 | 0 | 2.4 |
| SVR | 0 | 0 | 0 | 0 | 0 | 1 | 2 | 2 | 0 | 1 | 0 | 0 | 0 | 0 | 2.1 |
| iRANK | 0 | 0 | 0 | 0 | 1 | 2 | 0 | 1 | 2 | 0 | 0 | 0 | 0 | 0 | 2.1 |
| HierSum | 0 | 0 | 0 | 0 | 0 | 0 | 0 | 0 | 2 | 0 | 4 | 0 | 0 | 0 | 2.0 |
| Centroid | 0 | 0 | 0 | 0 | 0 | 0 | 0 | 0 | 0 | 0 | 0 | 3 | 3 | 0 | 1.1 |
| SNMF +SLSS | 0 | 0 | 0 | 0 | 0 | 0 | 0 | 0 | 0 | 0 | 0 | 3 | 3 | 0 | 1.1 |
| TMR | 0 | 0 | 0 | 0 | 0 | 0 | 3 | 0 | 1 | 0 | 2 | 0 | 0 | 0 | 1.0 |
| MMR | 0 | 0 | 0 | 0 | 0 | 0 | 0 | 0 | 0 | 0 | 0 | 0 | 0 | 6 | 0.4 |

Considering the results of Table 2, the following can be observed:

— The DESAMC+DocSum method takes first place in the ranking, focusing optimization on a sentence clustering problem. During the evolutionary process it carries out 50000 evaluations of the objective function.

— The MA-MultiSumm method takes second place in the ranking, but, DESAMC+DocSum used more than thirty times evaluations of the objective function than MA-MultiSumm. MA-MultiSumm outperforms methods based on clustering and probabilistic models such as PLSA (third place in the ranking) - a probabilistic model that applies the clustering technique - and HybHSum (sixth) that uses a probabilistic model to obtain the topics and then machine learning to train with a linear regression model; it outperforms evolutionary models such as LFIPP (fourth) that is based on a differential evolution model that represents the problem with the sentences of the summary and carries out 50000 evaluations of the objective function; and it outperforms MCMR (fifth) that is based on the binary particle swarm optimization model that also carries out 15000 evaluations of the objective function, but this function is more expensive because uses the Google and cosine similarity measures.

- LEX is a method that uses clustering of terms and outperforms some probabilistic, algebraic reduction, and ranking-based methods.
- The SVR and iRank methods occupy an identical position in the ranking despite the fact that SVR is a method of algebraic reduction and iRank combines two methods of ranking that provide feedback for each other.
- The Centroid and SNMF+SLSS methods are placed equal in the rankings with a very similar performance in both data sets, despite the fact that Centroid carries out centroid-based clustering. SNMF+SLSS carries out sentence level semantic analysis (SLSS) and then symmetric non-negative matrix factorization (SNMF).
- TMR outperforms only MMR, although uses a probabilistic model for estimating the distribution of the topics and then machine learning for multinomial estimation, similar to HybHSum that ranks sixth.
- MMR comes last in the rankings, obtaining the worst results for the two sets of data in all the ROUGE measures used.

The experimental results indicate that optimization that combines global search based on population (CHC) with a heuristic local search for some of the agents (greedy search) - as is the case with the MA-MultiSumm memetic algorithm - is a promising area of research for the problem of generating summaries for multiple documents. This is because although the proposed algorithm takes second place in the ranking, the method that outperforms it (DESAMC+DocSum) involves 50000 evaluations of the objective function, exceeding at 30 times the evaluations of MA-MultiSumm (50000 vs 1500). So, given that the objective functions used are quite similar for the two methods, this implies a longer running time for the algorithm when compared with the MA-MultiSumm method.

In the proposed method, representation of the solutions is binary, indicating the presence or absence of the sentence in the summary, while in the case of the DESAMC+DocSum method, representation is real, indicating the group to which the sentence belongs. A process is then undertaken for the selection of sentences that make up the summary. This requires the DESAMC+DocSum method to carry out an additional process to obtain the summary, a process not required in the case of MA-MultiSumm.

## 5     Conclusions and Future Work

This paper proposes a memetic algorithm for automatically generating extractives summaries of multiple documents (MA-MultiSumm) based on CHC and greedy search, which prevents incest in calculating the hamming distance between the agent father and the agent mother. This it does by means of a threshold, whose value is smaller than that of the original CHC algorithm. It is noted that in this problem the agent is represented using many zeros and few ones, therefore the agents are similar to one another. The cross is made by means of the HUX scheme and optimization of the agents generated is done using local search. When cataclysm occurs, the two best individuals are preserved and the remaining individuals are created randomly.

The MA-MultiSumm method proposed was evaluated by means of ROUGE-1, ROUGE-2, and ROUGE-SU4 measures. When compared against other state of the art evolutionary methods on the data set DUC2005, the MA-MultiSumm method surpasses all methods in all measures. The DESAMC+DocSum method that takes second place is outperformed by 1.63% with ROUGE-1, 5.72% with ROUGE-2, and 1.13% with ROUGE-SU4. As regards the DUC2006 dataset, DESAMC+DocSum exceeds all methods in all measures. MA-MultiSumm with ROUGE-2 is outperformed by 0.30%; with ROUGE-1 is outperformed by 3.67%; and ROUGE-SU4 is outperformed by 2.82%.

In the unified ranking performed with all methods, the MA-MultiSumm method ranks second, behind only DESAMC+DocSum. However, this result is promising, given that the difference is minimal and, since the first makes 1500 evaluations of the objective function while the latter carries out 50000, runtime of MA-MultiSumm is shorter than for DESAMC+DocSum. In addition, while the latter represents a clustering problem and a subsequent process must be gone through to choose the sentences for the summary, in the case of MA-MultiSumm the sentences of the summary are taken directly from the best solution obtained following the running of the memetic algorithm. The MA-MultiSumm algorithm performed better in all measures with respect to the different methods used in automatic text summarization, such as graph-based, algebraic reduction, probabilistic, machine learning, and centroid.

Regarding results obtained in the task of automatically generating summaries using memetic algorithms, the use of these in this type of problem is promising, but it is necessary to continue to conduct research in order to achieve better results than those obtained in this article. Considering possible future work, it is necessary to carry out experiments on other data sets, to include other characteristics in the objective function that allow sentences relevant to the content of the documents and a summary that is closer to the reference summaries to be obtained and taking account other similarity measures like soft cosine measure [35]. Furthermore local search algorithms should also be explored, taking into account the specific characteristics of the automatic generation of summaries and thus enabling better results to be obtained.

**Acknowledgments.** The work in this paper was supported by a Research Grant from the Vicerrectoría de Investigaciones of the Universidad del Cauca and the Universidad Nacional de Colombia. We are especially grateful to Colin McLachlan for suggestions relating to English text.

# References

1. Lloret, E., Palomar, M.: Text summarisation in progress: a literature review. Artificial Intelligence Review 37(1), 1–41 (2012)
2. Nenkova, A., McKeown, K.: A Survey of Text Summarization Techniques. In: Aggarwal, C.C., Zhai, C. (eds.) Mining Text Data, pp. 43–76. Springer, US (2012)

3. Miranda, S., Gelbukh, A., Sidorov, G.: Generación de resúmenes por medio de síntesis de grafos conceptuales. Revista Signos. Estudios de Lingüística 47(86) (2014)
4. Amini, M.-R., Usunier, N.: Incorporating prior knowledge into a transductive ranking algorithm for multi-document summarization. In: Proceedings of 32nd Annual ACM SIGIR Conference on Research and Development in Information Retrieval, Boston, USA, pp. 704–705. ACM (2009)
5. Ouyang, Y., et al.: Applying regression models to query-focused multi-document summarization. Information Processing & Management 47(2), 227–237 (2011)
6. Chen, Y.-M., Wang, X.-L., Liu, B.-Q.: Multi-document summarization based on lexical chains. In: Proceedings of 2005 International Conference on Machine Learning and Cybernetics, Guangzhou, China, pp. 1937–1942. IEEE (2005)
7. Atkinson, J., Munoz, R.: Rhetorics-based multi-document summarization. Expert Systems with Applications 40(11), 4346–4352 (2013)
8. Otterbacher, J., Erkan, G., Radev, D.R.: Biased LexRank: passage retrieval using random walks with question-based priors. Information Processing and Management 45(1), 42–54 (2009)
9. Wei, F., et al.: Query-sensitive mutual reinforcement chain and its application in query-oriented multi-document summarization. In: Proceedings of the 31st Annual International ACM SIGIR Conference on Research and Development in Information Retrieval, Singapore, pp. 283–290. ACM (2008)
10. Radev, D.R., et al.: Centroid-based summarization of multiple documents. Information Processing & Management 40(6), 919–938 (2004)
11. Steinberger, J., Křišťan, M.: LSA-Based Multi-Document Summarization. In: Proceedings of 8th International PhD Workshop on Systems and Control, Balatonfured, Hungary (2007)
12. Sun, P., ByungRae, C.: Query-Based Multi-Document Summarization Using Non-Negative Semantic Feature and NMF Clustering. In: Proceedings Fourth International Conference on Networked Computing and Advanced Information Management, NCM, Gyeongju, pp. 609–614. IEEE (2008)
13. Hennig, L.: Topic-based Multi-Document Summarization with Probabilistic Latent Semantic Analysis. In: Proceedings International Conference RANLP, Borovets, Bulgaria, pp. 144–149 (2009)
14. Mei, J.-P., Chen, L.: SumCR: a new subtopic-based extractive approach for text summarization. Knowledge and Information Systems 31(3), 527–545 (2012)
15. Alguliev, R.M., et al.: MCMR: Maximum coverage and minimum redundant text summarization model. Expert Systems with Applications 38, 14514–14522 (2011)
16. Alguliev, R.M., Aliguliyev, R.M., Isazade, N.R.: DESAMC+DocSum: Differential evolution with self-adaptive mutation and crossover parameters for multi-document summarization. Knowledge-Based Systems 36(0), 21–38 (2012)
17. Abuobieda, A., Salim, N., Kumar, Y.J., Osman, A.H.: An Improved Evolutionary Algorithm for Extractive Text Summarization. In: Selamat, A., Nguyen, N.T., Haron, H., et al. (eds.) ACIIDS 2013, Part II. LNCS, vol. 7803, pp. 78–89. Springer, Heidelberg (2013)
18. Mendoza, M., et al.: Extractive single-document summarization based on genetic operators and guided local search. Expert Systems with Applications 41(9), 4158–4169 (2014)
19. Neri, F., Cotta, C.: Memetic algorithms and memetic computing optimization: A literature review. Swarm and Evolutionary Computation 2(0), 1–14 (2012)
20. Manning, C., Raghavan, P., Schütze, H.: Introduction to Information Retrieval. Cambridge University Press, Cambridge (2008)

21. Hachey, B., Murray, G., Reitter, D.: The Embra System at DUC 2005: Query-oriented Multi-document Summarization with a Very Large Latent Semantic Space. In: Proceedings of the Document Understanding Conference (DUC), Vancouver, Canada (2005)
22. Silla, C.N., Pappa, G.L., Freitas, A.A., Kaestner, C.A.A.: Automatic text summarization with genetic algorithm-based attribute selection. In: Lemaître, C., Reyes, C.A., González, J.A. (eds.) IBERAMIA 2004. LNCS (LNAI), vol. 3315, pp. 305–314. Springer, Heidelberg (2004)
23. Ochoa, G., Verel, S., Tomassini, M.: First-improvement vs. Best-improvement local optima networks of NK landscapes. In: Schaefer, R., Cotta, C., Kołodziej, J., Rudolph, G. (eds.) PPSN XI. LNCS, vol. 6238, pp. 104–113. Springer, Heidelberg (2010)
24. Lin, C.-Y.: Rouge: a package for automatic evaluation of summaries. In: Proceedings of the ACL-04 Workshop on Text Summarization Branches Out, Barcelona, Spain (2004)
25. Alguliev, R.M., Aliguliyev, R.M., Mehdiyev, C.A.: Sentence selection for generic document summarization using an adaptive differential evolution algorithm. Swarm and Evolutionary Computation 1(4), 213–222 (2011)
26. Celikyilmaz, A., Hakkani-Tur, D.: A Hybrid Hierarchical Model for Multi-Document Summarization. In: Proceedings 48th Annual Meeting of the Association for Computational Linguistics, Uppsala, Sweden, pp. 815–824. Association for Computational Linguistics (2010)
27. Lei, H., et al.: Modeling Document Summarization as Multi-objective Optimization. In: Third International Symposium on Intelligent Information Technology and Security Informatics (IITSI), China, pp. 382–386. IEEE (2010)
28. Wei, F., Li, W., Liu, S.: iRANK: a rank-learn-combine framework for unsupervised ensemble ranking. American Society for Information Science and Technology 61(6), 1232–1243 (2010)
29. Haghighi, A., Vanderwende, L.: Exploring content models for multi-document summarization. In: Proceedings of Human Language Technologies: The 2009 Annual Conference of the North American Chapter of the Association for Computational Linguistics, Boulder, Colorado, pp. 362–370. Association for Computational Linguistics (2009)
30. Wang, D., et al.: Multi-Document Summarization via Sentence-Level Semantic Analysis and Symmetric Matrix Factorization. In: Proceedings of the 31st Annual International ACM SIGIR Conference on Research and Development in Information Retrieval, Singapore, pp. 307–314 (2008)
31. Tang, J., Yao, L., Chen, D.: Multi-topic based query-oriented summarization. In: Proceedings of the Ninth SIAM International Conference on Data Mining, Nevada, USA, pp. 1148–1159 (2009)
32. Carbonell, J., Goldstein, J.: The use of MMR, diversity-based reranking for reordering documents and producing summaries. In: Proceedings of the 21st Annual International ACM SIGIR Conference on Research and development in Information Retrieval, Melbourne, Australia, pp. 335–336. ACM (1998)
33. Eiben, A.E., Smit, S.K.: Evolutionary Algorithm Parameters and Methods to Tune Them. In: Hamadi, Y., Monfroy, E., Saubion, F. (eds.) Autonomous Search, pp. 15–36. Springer, Heidelberg (2012)
34. Cobos, C., Estupiñán, D., Pérez, J.: GHS + LEM: Global-best Harmony Search using learnable evolution models. Applied Mathematics and Computation 218(6), 2558–2578 (2011)
35. Sidorov, G., et al.: Soft Similarity and Soft Cosine Measure: Similarity of Features in Vector Space Model. Computación y Sistemas 18(3) (2014)

# How Predictive Is Tense for Language Profiency? A Cautionary Tale

Alexandra Panagiotopoulos and Sabine Bergler

CLaC Laboratory, Concordia University, 1515 Ste. Catherine St. West Montreal,
Quebec, Canada, H3G 1M8

**Abstract.** The role of language proficiency in second language(L2) writing has been widely discussed in English as Second Language(ESL) research. The literature suggests that syntactic as well as lexical choices are influenced by their writer's language proficiency. Exactly which linguistic indices are related to the writing performance (and to what degree) is a central topic in the ESL literature. This paper reexamines *tense* and the related concepts *voice* and *aspect* as well as the syntactic complexity measure *level of embedding*. Tense has variously been reported as useful and as not useful for predicting proficiency. We analyze its correlation to proficiency levels in ICNALE and contrast this with the performance of different feature combinations and for different learner groups.

**Keywords:** language proficiency, tense, aspect, voice, correlated features.

## 1 Introduction

The role of language proficiency in second language(L2) writing has been widely discussed in English as Second Language(ESL) research [10,27]. The literature suggests that syntactic as well as lexical choices are influenced by their writer's language proficiency [5]. Exactly which linguistic indices are related to the writing performance (and to what degree) is a central topic in the ESL literature. This paper reexamines *tense* and the related concepts *voice* and *aspect* as well as the syntactic complexity measure *level of embedding*. Tense has variously been reported as useful and as not useful for predicting proficiency. We analyze its correlation to proficiency levels in ICNALE and contrast this with the performance of different feature combinations.

Tense is one of the many features associated with writing proficiency of L2 authors, yet accounts of its usefulness for proficiency determination conflict. Ferris [13] analyzed a corpus of 160 texts written by ESL students of different origin (Chinese, Japanese, Spanish, Arabic). She experimented on 62 quantitative, lexical and syntactic features (such as word length, relative clauses and pronouns) and observed that only 23 of those were directly related with the level of proficiency of the ESL writers and suggested that the use of tense and more specifically the use of present and past tense were not related to the writing performance. Bardovi-Harlig and Reynolds [2], on the other hand, performed

A. Gelbukh et al. (Eds.): MICAI 2014, Part I, LNAI 8856, pp. 139–150, 2014.

a cross-sectional investigation of 182 adult learners of English as a second language at six levels of proficiency and showed that the acquisition of past tense in English proceeds in stages.

Because intuitively, usage of tense and especially aspect often allow even non-experts to identify non-native speakers and their proficiency, we undertook to reevaluate the potential for tense, aspect, and selected other grammatical features and simple lexical choice to predict learner proficiency in a machine learning context.

We limit our investigation here to the verb phrase (VP), because we do not aim to present the best possible proficiency predictor, but rather to explain the seeming contradictions in the literature regarding the effectiveness of tense for proficiency prediction. We surmised that the assumed independence of tense as a feature might be at the root of the puzzle. We comprehensively analyzed performance of groupings of the selected grammatical features and report on the non-linear performance differences for different groupings of interdependent features. In particular, we investigate the relation between L2 proficiency and the verb phrase characteristics *aspect, voice, degree of embedding* and *embedding types*, as well as simple n-gram features to assess lexical choice.

In this paper,we use the International Corpus of Network of Asian Learners of English (ICNALE)[1]. It contains writing samples of university students on two topics: "It is important for college students to have a part time job?" and "Smoking should be completely banned at all the restaurants in the country". The essays are divided into three levels of proficiency according to The Global Standard for English Language Testing (TOEIC)[2] rating guidelines, Beginner (-500), Intermediate (500+), and Advanced (700+).

## 2  Related Work

Many traditional writing proficiency metrics use statistics on syllables, words, sentences and documents. These surface features include the average number of syllables per word, the number of words per sentence, or word frequency in different text segments. However, McNamara et al. [21] used a corpus of expert-graded essays as gold standard to automatically distinguish between essays rated to have high vs low proficiency using complex linguistic features. These included linguistic indices of cohesion (coreference and connectives), syntactic complexity (number of words before the main verb, sentence structure overlap), lexical diversity, and characteristics of words (frequency, concreteness, imaginability). They report that the three indices most predictive of essay quality were syntactic complexity, lexical diversity and word frequency. Ortega [24] studied syntactic complexity in relation to second language (L2) proficiency by categorizing university student's essays into more than two proficiency groups, concluding that the most indicative measures are words per T-unit (minimal clause constituting a complete sentence), words per sentence, words per clause and number of clauses per T-unit.

---

[1] http://language.sakura.ne.jp/icnale/
[2] http://www.etscanada.ca/toeic

Other attempts to define which linguistic indicators associate with writing proficiency assess L2 text in terms of grammatical and lexical means. Min [23] studied the relation between tense and aspect for Chinese and Korean learners of English as a second language. His study focused on examining English verb tense and aspect combinations in 120 argumentative essays corresponding to three proficiency levels (intermediate L2, advanced L2, and native speakers). His findings suggested that patterns of using English verb tense and aspect was relevant to the students' L2 writing proficiency because advanced students showed their grammatical knowledge in the paper's purpose, contents, and discourse register. Hinkel [16], concentrating on advanced learners of English and native speakers only, reported on the use of English tenses, aspects and passive voice in academic texts. He reported that advanced L2 writers showed lower frequency of present perfect and high frequency of simple past in their papers compared with L1 writers. Moreover, L2 writers showed reduced use of passive voice constructions, possibly due to lack of familiarity.

Crossley et al. [9] studied 100 writing samples from 100 L2 learners of different cultural backgrounds. The samples were analyzed for lexical indices such as word frequency and correctness by the computational tool Coh-Metrix. The L2 writing samples were categorized into beginning, intermediate, and advanced groupings based on the TOEFL and ACT ESL Compass scores of the writer. The results indicated that automated, lexical indices can be used to predict the language proficiency levels of second language learners based on their writing samples. In a more recent study, Crossley et al. [8] underline the importance of multiword units for proficiency, using n-gram indices that encode rhetorical, syntactic, grammatical, and cohesion markers in different sections (introduction, body, and conclusion paragraphs) and entire essays. They proved that n-grams' association with the writing proficiency increased when combined with other variables.

# 3    Methodology

We study and contrast the combination of features with single indices, focusing on grammatical verb phrase features (namely tense, aspect, voice, type and degree of embedding) and n-grams. We show that while a single feature can be a proficiency indicator, aggregation with other features obtains better performance.

## 3.1    Corpus

The writing conditions of most existing learner corpora are not strictly controlled, meaning it is not always clear whether the observed difference is really due to the difference in writing ability or the variation in topics of the essays. For the purpose of this analysis we used the International Corpus Network of Asian Learners of English(ICNALE) [18]. It contains data from eight countries and areas in Asia, as well as essays of native speakers of English (N). University students were asked to write argumentative essays on two topics: "It is important for college students to have a part time job" and "Smoking should be completely banned at all the restaurants in the country". Students had twenty to forty minutes at their disposal to write essays no more than 300 words without the use of a dictionary. The learners were classified into three writing proficiency levels based on CERF[3] levels, A2(Waystage), B1(Threshold) and B2$^+$(Vantage or Higher). The placement of each essay to the respective category is based on its score and following the TOEIC scoring system: A2 ($<$500), B1 ($>=$ 500) and B2$^+$ ($>=$ 700). This proficiency-based subdivision makes it possible to compare Non Native Speakers (NNS) at different L2 proficiency levels, as well as different NNS writer groups to L1 authors. Table 1 shows the size of the datasets.

**Table 1.** Size of Categories in ICNALE

|              | A2      | B1      | B2$^+$  | N      |
|--------------|---------|---------|---------|--------|
| # of Essays  | 960     | 3776    | 465     | 402    |
| # of Tokens  | 211,168 | 867,100 | 111,333 | 89,057 |

The control of writing conditions is crucial when compiling learner corpora. For both topics, writers were required to show clearly whether they agreed or disagreed with the proposed statements and also support their claims with appropriate examples. Limiting the number of topics makes the content of the corpus lexically more homogeneous, which enables us to conduct a robust comparison among different writer groups [17].

### 3.2  Features

We model the student essays with a support vector machine (SVM) [7] over the following features:

**Word level n-grams** are all possible continuous groupings of n words in a text [6], see Example 1 from ICNALE

(1) "Having a part-time job is beneficial for university students."
    **unigrams**= {*Having, a, part-time, job, is,...*}
    **bigrams**= {*Having a, a part-time, part-time job,...*}
    **trigrams**= {*Having a part-time, a part-time job,...*}

Whether in first or second language, writers make use of specific lexical choices which reflect in part their proficiency [22,15]. We include unigrams, bigrams and trigrams to assess the effectiveness of those specific lexical indices.

**Verb phrase** components constitute one of the most essential parts of the sentence structure [25]. Following Quirk et al. [25] a verb phrase consists of a finite or a non-finite verb. Finite verbs carry tense, aspect, mood and voice, non-finite verbs does not.

---

[3] http://www.coe.int/t/dg4/linguistic/liam/levels/levels_EN.asp

*Tense* in English localizes an action as taking part in the *present, past* or *future*.

*Grammatical aspect* refers to the manner in which the action is regarded or experienced, *progressive* for protracted, habitual, or on-going events, *perfective* for completed events, and *indefinite* for reports of factive statements that are not clearly specified as being either progressive or perfective.

*Voice* determines whether the grammatical subject semantically functions as an agent or a patient, *active* or *passive* voice [25].

*Levels of embedding* indicates a verb's position in the parse tree. Hinkel [16] states that an advanced learner of English constructs less complex sentences than a beginner. We use the Penn Treebank Tagset [20] for sentence structure derived by the Stanford parser [11]. The suitability of automatic parsing for language learner data and the effect of learner errors on the parser has been reported by Geertzen et al. [14].

*Type of embedding (constituent)* English grammar [25] stipulates a sentence as simple or complex. A simple sentence contains only one verb, the main verb of the sentence. A complex sentence consists of a main verb and one or more subordinate verbs. A subordinate verb is part of a subordinate clause. We distinguish three types of embedding :Verbs that belong to clauses that contain a subject(*sbarverb*), such as relative clauses, verbs that occur in subordinate clauses without subject, such as purpose clauses(*subverb*), and verbs that occur outside subordinate clauses(*other*).

### 3.3    Implementation

We analyze every essay of ICNALE corpus in terms of verb phrase features and word level n-grams. For our word level n-grams, we split every essay into sentences, remove punctuation marks, and create sequences of n words. For our verb phrase features we identify *tense, aspect* and *voice*, using Stanford parser [11] and in-house verb phrase analysis(Example 2).

*Example*

(2) Smoking *is allowed*, but only in *designated* areas.
   *is allowed* : present tense, indefinite aspect, passive voice
   *designated* : non-finite

We report a verb's level and type of embedding, by observing the position of the clause containing it. For example the verb *act* of Figure 1 is a subordinate verb(*sbarverb*) with level of embedding 6 because it's immediate verb phrase ancestor(VP) is part of a subordinate clause(SBAR) with a tree hight of value 6.

For our text classification task, we represent every essay by building a vector of binary inputs indicating whether an n-gram or a verb phrase feature exists in the text or not. To illustrate, if we had only 4 feature values *present, active,*

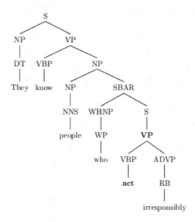

**Fig. 1.** Embedding features of *act*: level of embedding: 6, constituent (type of embedding): SBAR

*sbarverb, subverb*, the vector *1 1 0 0* represents that the text contains present tense and active voice but no subordinate verbs.[4]

Every essay belongs to one of the four classes: A2, B1, B2 ,N. To avoid selection bias we perform random undersampling in the categories A2 and B1 which contained more essays than B2 and N. Overall we used 1280 essays (320 from each class) for training our model and 320 (80 from each class) for testing. In the training phase, we do feature selection by applying the Information Gain(IG) metric[5], which resulted in discarding those feature values not relevant to the target classes we wanted to predict.

The machine learning algorithm of our choice is SVM with Gaussian RBF kernel. To find the optimal values for cost ($c$=10) and gamma ($\gamma$=6) parameters, we apply Grid search and 10-fold-cross validation.

Finally, we measure the performance of all feature combinations using the area under the ROC curve (ROC area) [12]. The ROC area is a widely used measure of performance of supervised classification rules. Its advantage is that the performance of a classifier is measured independently of its chosen threshold [12]. To assess the validity of our results we perform a two tailed t-test on the obtained ROC area values and we compare the obtained $p - value$ to significance level $\alpha = 0.05$ [19].

## 4   Experiments and Results

Our basic question is: to what extent are grammatical features like tense predictive of language proficiency? Given the apparent contradictions in the literature, we surmised that the underlying issue is the fact that tense is not a free-standing

---

[4] This radically binary scheme outperformed a more nuanced vector of fractions or counts.

[5] Information Gain Ratio results are identical to IG on our corpus.

feature, but is only one grammatical feature of the VP, in English largely coextensive with aspect. We compiled a comprehensive series of statistics on ICNALE in order to contrast the predictive potential of tense, aspect, voice, level of embedding, and type of subordinate clause in single feature predictors or in various combinations[6]. Because all of these "features" are necessarily coextensive with words, we contrast and combine the grammatical features with traditional unigram, bigram, and trigram statistics. The tables below indicate the area under the ROC curve as a performance measure to evaluate the predictive power of our features for writing proficiency.

## 4.1   Predictive Potential of Single Features

Table 2 presents the performance of each of our eight features in isolation, as a set of baselines. *Tense* and *level of embedding(le)* exceed the performance of the other features. The strongest lexical feature is trigram[7], presumably because proper use of phrases such as *the fact that* distinguishes learners of different levels. The ROC area values indicate that constituent (type of embedding) does not look like a good predictor of writing proficiency of L2 authors($<0.5$).

**Table 2.** Individual features in ICNALE

| Features | ROC Area |
|----------|----------|
| tense | 0.559 |
| le | 0.551 |
| aspect | 0.540 |
| trigram | 0.536 |
| voice | 0.521 |
| unigram | 0.517 |
| bigram | 0.515 |
| constituent | 0.498 |

## 4.2   Combinations of Features

When we consider all possible combinations of features, verb phrase features dominate. Table 3 shows the 15 best feature combinations. The feature combinations which are statistically significant are *tense* (p-value 0.028), *tense aspect* (p-value 0.039), and *tense constituent* (p-value 0.045).

That the top three combinations include *tense* by itself and that as a single feature it is statistically significantly above chance seems to validate our initial intuition that it is predictive, outdone only by the combination with *aspect*, which mirrors a grammatical constellation for English verbs. To further probe

---

[6] This is identical the same procedure as forward feature selection, except that we analyzed and compared feature bundles from the human grammarian's point of view.

[7] Note that statistically the difference between the different baselines is not significant.

**Table 3.** Performance of top 15 feature combinations

| Feature Combination | ROC Area |
| --- | --- |
| tense aspect | 0.563 |
| tense | 0.559 |
| tense constituent | 0.557 |
| | |
| tense aspect constituent | 0.555 |
| tense voice | 0.553 |
| tense voice aspect | 0.553 |
| tense voice aspect constituent | 0.553 |
| constituent le | 0.551 |
| tense voice constituent | 0.551 |
| le | 0.546 |
| tense voice trigram | 0.546 |
| voice aspect trigram | 0.544 |
| aspect constituent trigram | 0.544 |
| tense voice constituent trigram | 0.544 |
| voice aspect constituent trigram | 0.544 |

why the ESL literature reports conflicting usefulness of tense, we analyze the data to arrive at a much more tentative conclusion, namely volatility even in well understood and very homogeneous data.

Intriguingly, among the top three is the combination of *tense* with the lowest scoring single feature, *constituent*, demonstrating an unsettling nonlinearity. Assessing a feature in isolation does not provide enough insight to predict its potential in combination. While we accept this as a given mathematically for non-independent features, still in most machine learning applications generalizations are drawn from few probes and if automatic feature selection is applied it is not usually analyzed in detail by the application user. We probe a little deeper, to better reconcile grammatical intuition with statistical properties of a corpus.

Surprisingly, *n-grams* here do not reach the top performance combinations with the exception of *trigram* when combined with *tense* and *voice*. Note the performance progression, *tense* 0.559, *tense voice* 0.553, *tense voice trigram* 0.546 illustrates the main point of this paper: features with good individual performance and supposedly well understood correlation properties behave in surprising ways and are not cumulative.

The low performance of ngrams, usually the top performer in most applications, is partially explained by the corpus style. Since ICNALE contains essays on only two topics and students did not have access to a dictionary, the vocabulary is unusually restricted and homogeneous. Similarly, the performance of *tense* and *aspect* might well decrease on a wider variety of text types with greater variability. Opinion essays are not expected to show much variation in tense and aspect. Writers of argumentative essays typically support their arguments by describing specific events and by providing generalizations and generalizable statements or describing events that are considered general truths [1]. According to Beason and Lester [3], *present tense* should be used to make statements of facts or generalizations and *past tense* should be used to narrate a story or an event that happened in the past. Hinkel [16] supports the previous statement by reporting that students tend to use present tense and indefinite aspect more when they write argumentative essays.

**Table 4.** Percent occurrence of tense, aspect, voice features in essays

| Tense | A2 | B1 | B2 | N | Aspect | A2 | B1 | B2 | N | Voice | A2 | B1 | B2 | N |
|---|---|---|---|---|---|---|---|---|---|---|---|---|---|---|
| present | 51 | 47 | 44 | 44 | indefinite | 68 | 66 | 61 | 58 | active | 67 | 64 | 58 | 60 |
| past | 3 | 4 | 4 | 5 | progressive | 2 | 2 | 2 | 3 | passive | 4 | 4 | 5 | 6 |
| modal_present | 8 | 8 | 7 | 4 | perfective | 1 | 1 | 1 | 3 | novoice | 29 | 31 | 36 | 36 |
| modal_past | 5 | 6 | 7 | 7 | noaspect | 29 | 31 | 36 | 36 | | | | | |
| future | 3 | 3 | 3 | 4 | | | | | | | | | | |
| notense | 29 | 31 | 36 | 36 | | | | | | | | | | |

Table 4 shows that all four proficiency groups mainly make use of *present tense* and *indefinite aspect*. The table reports the percentage of essays that contain the given feature value. We observe that there is an increasing use of past tense, also of progressive and perfective aspect from the low (A2) second language learner to the native (N) speakers of English. Aspect is a grammatical feature that differs greatly even in closely related languages and is difficult to acquire. Because this is a well-known fact, ESL teachers are taught to advise their students to avoid errors by avoiding both perfective and progressive aspect [4,26] in essay writing, as seen in Table 4.

*Tense* and *aspect* as a feature combination is foreshadowed in grammar books and is consistently strong when we augment our existing corpus with essays of different topics written by second language learners of English (Gachon Learner Corpus[8]): there *voice le* is the best feature combination, while *tense aspect* is a close second before *voice le constituent*(0,602, 0.609, 0.598). *Tense* by itself ranks only 35th in that augmented corpus.

### 4.3   Language of Origin

The satisfying results we get for the ICNALE corpus are shaken up when we perform the same analysis on a subset, namely the CEEAUS, the seed corpus including only Japanese NNSs. Table 5 shows the performance of the single features on that subcorpus.

Here, the n-gram features dominate by a large margin and *tense* as a single feature does not appear in the top combinations. Table 5 shows the top ten feature combinations for CEEAUS. We note that this volatility across corpora

---

[8] http://koreanlearnercorpusblog.blogspot.be/p/corpus.html

**Table 5.** Feature performance in CEEAUS

| Features | ROC Area | Top Combinations | ROC Area |
|---|---|---|---|
| unigram | 0.762 | tense le unigram bigram trigram | 0.781 |
| bigram | 0.729 | tense constituent le unigram bigram trigram | 0.781 |
| trigram | 0.640 | tense voice le unigram bigram trigram | 0.779 |
| aspect | 0.630 | tense voice constituent le unigram bigram trigram | 0.779 |
| le | 0.617 | constituent le unigram bigram trigram | 0.778 |
| tense | 0.582 | le unigram bigram trigram | 0.778 |
| voice | 0.580 | voice constituent le unigram bigram trigram | 0.775 |
| constituent | 0.498 | voice le unigram bigram trigram | 0.775 |
| | | voice aspect constituent unigram | 0.771 |
| | | voice aspect unigram | 0.771 |

can only be appreciated when studying the various ranks of feature combinations, a task that to date still has to be done manually.

## 5   Conclusion

The literature reports conflicting usefulness for *tense* as a feature for the prediction of proficiency in English as a Second Language research. A comprehensive analysis of tense and related grammatical notions (*aspect, voice, level of embedding, type of embedding*) on ICNALE, a corpus of essays written by Asian learners of English, conclusively shows that *tense* by itself is a good predictor, outperformed only by the combination of *tense* and *aspect*.

However, more detailed analysis shows that the subset of the corpus written by students of Japanese origin, CEAAUS, shows drastically different results. Here, *n–gram* features dominate.

In addition, we showed that care has to be taken when projecting individual feature performance onto feature combinations, where low performing features like *voice* in our case, may well participate in the top combinations. The conclusion is thus that feature combinations have to be carefully assessed across the full set of forward feature selection results. Moreover, even on very similar datasets, the conclusions do not necessarily carry over, as the strikingly different performance of our features on the larger corpus and its Japanese subcorpus demonstrate. This volatility points to the need for larger learner corpora and also for greater variation of text types contained.

The puzzle from the literature can, however, be tentatively answered: *tense* is a predictor of proficiency alone or in combination with *aspect*, but the particularities of a specific dataset greatly influence its perceived utility.

## References

1. Baker, J., Brizee, A., Angeli, E.: Essay writing: The argumentative essay (2013)
2. Bardovi-Harlig, K., Reynolds, D.W.: The role of lexical aspect in the acquisition of tense and aspect. TESOL Quarterly 29(1), 107–131 (1995)

3. Beason, L., Lester, M.: A Commonsense Guide to Grammar and Usage with 2009 MLA Update. Bedford/St. Martin's (2010)
4. Biber, D., Johansson, S., Leech, G., Conrad, S., Finegan, E.: Longman Grammar of Spoken and Written English. Pearson ESL (1999)
5. Canale, M., Swain, M.: Theoretical bases of communicative approaches to second language teaching and testing. Applied Linguistics 1(1) (1980)
6. Cavnar, W.B., Trenkle, J.M.: N-gram-based text categorization. In: Proceedings of SDAIR-94, 3rd Annual Symposium on Document Analysis and Information Retrieval, pp. 161–175 (1994)
7. Cortes, C., Vapnik, V.: Support-vector networks. Machine Learning 20(3), 273–297 (1995)
8. Crossley, S.A., Defore, C., Kyle, K., Dai, J., McNamara, D.S.: Paragraph specific n-gram approaches to automatically assessing essay quality. In: Proceedings of the 6th Educational Data Mining (EDM,) Conference, pp. 216–220. Springer, Heidelberg (2013)
9. Crossley, S.A., Salsbury, T., McNamara, D.S., Jarvis, S.: Predicting lexical proficiency in language learner texts using computational indices. Language Testing 28(4), 561–580 (2011)
10. Cumming, A.: Theoretical perspectives on writing. Annual Review of Applied Linguistics 18, 61–78 (1998)
11. de Marneffe, M.-C., MacCartney, B., Manning, C.D.: Generating typed dependency parses from phrase structure parses. In: LREC, pp. 449–454 (2006)
12. Fawcett, T.: An introduction to ROC analysis. Pattern Recognition Lettters 27(8), 861–874 (2006)
13. Ferris, D.R.: Lexical and syntactic features of ESL, writing by students at different levels of L2 proficiency. TESOL Quarterly 28(2), 414–420 (1994)
14. Geertzen, J., Alexopoulou, T., Korhonen, A.: Automatic linguistic annotation of large scale L2 databases: The EF-Cambridge Open Language Database (EFCamDat). In: Second Language Research Forum: Building Bridges between Disciplines, Cascadilla Proceedings Project, Somerville, MA, USA, pp. 240–254 (2014)
15. Hinkel, E.: Simplicity without elegance: Features of sentences in L1 and L2 academic text. TESOL Quarterly 37(2), 275–301 (2003)
16. Hinkel, E.: Tense, aspect and the passive voice in L1 and L2 academic texts. Language Teaching Research 8(1), 5–29 (2004)
17. Ishikawa, S.: A corpus-based study on Asian learners' use of English linking adverbials. Themes in Science and Technology Education. Special Issue on ICT in language learning 3(1-2), 139–157 (2010)
18. Ishikawa, S.: A new horizon in learner corpus studies: The aim of the ICNALE project. In: Weir, G.R.S., Ishikawa, S., Poonpon, K. (eds.) Corpora and Language Technologies in Teaching, Learning and Research, pp. 3–11. University of Strathclyde Press, Glasgow (2011)
19. Liu, H., Li, G., Cumberland, W.G., Wu, T.: Testing statistical significance of the area under a receiving operating characteristics curve for repeated measures design with bootstrapping. Journal of Data Science 3, 257–278 (2005)
20. Marcus, M.P., Marcinkiewicz, M.A., Santorini, B.: Building a large annotated corpus of English: The Penn Treebank. Computational Linguistics 19(2), 313–330 (1993)
21. McNamara, D.S., Crossley, S.A., McCarthy, P.M.: Linguistic features of writing quality. Written Communication 27(1), 57–86 (2010)
22. Meara, P., Jacobs, G., Rodgers, C.: Lexical signatures in foreign language free-form texts. ITL Review of Applied Linguistics, 85–96, 135–136 (2002)

23. Min, K.E.: How grammar matters in NNS academic writing: The relationship between verb tense and aspect usage patterns and L2 writing proficiency in academic discourse. Ph.D. thesis, University of Illinois at Urbana-Champaign (2013)
24. Ortega, L.: Syntactic complexity measures and their relationship to L2 proficiency: A research synthesis of college-level L2 writing. Applied Linguistics 24(4), 492–518 (2003)
25. Quirk, R., Greenbaum, S., Geoffrey, Leech, S.: A Comprehensive Grammar of the English Language. Longman, London (1985)
26. Rutherford, W.E.: Second language grammar: learning and teaching. Applied linguistics and language study, Longman (1987)
27. Sasaki, M., Hirose, K.: Explanatory variable for ESLstudents' expository writing. Language Learning 46, 137–174 (1996)

# Evaluating Term-Expansion
# for Unsupervised Image Annotation

Luis Pellegrin, Hugo Jair Escalante, and Manuel Montes-y-Gómez

Computer Science Department,
Instituto Nacional de Astrofísica, Óptica y Electrónica (INAOE),
Tonantzintla, Puebla, 72840, Mexico
{pellegrin,hugojair,mmontesg}@inaoep.mx

**Abstract.** Automatic image annotation (AIA) deals with the problem of automatically providing images with labels/keywords that describe their visual content. Unsupervised AIA methods are often preferred because they can annotate (virtually) any possible concept to images and do not require labeled data as their supervised counterparts. Unsupervised AIA methods use a reference collection of images with associated (unstructured, freeform) text to annotate images. Thus, this type of methods heavily rely on the quality of the text in the reference collection. With the goal of improving the annotation performance of unsupervised AIA methods, we propose in this paper a term expansion strategy that expands the text associated with images from the reference collection. The proposed method is based on term co-occurrence analysis. We evaluate the impact that the proposed expansion has in the annotation performance of a straight unsupervised AIA method using a benchmark for large scale image annotation. Two types of associated text are used and several image descriptors are considered. Experimental results show that, by using the proposed expansion, better annotation performance can be obtained, where the improvements depend on the type of associated text that is considered.

## 1 Introduction

Since the last decade, the development of multimedia devices has facilitated the generation of vast amounts of images and videos which are stored locally by users or shared via the internet; for instance, only in Facebook about 300 million images are uploaded every day [1]. The availability of such amounts of data makes necessary the development of methods and tools that can allow users to access the images they are interested on. In this context, a relevant task is that of Automatic Image Annotation (AIA), i.e., the task of assigning labels/keywords to images that describe their visual content [1]. The importance of AIA lies in that these type of methods allow users to search for images by using keywords [2].

---

[1] http://gigaom.com/2012/10/17/
facebook-has-220-billion-of-your-photos-to-put-on-ice/

A. Gelbukh et al. (Eds.): MICAI 2014, Part I, LNAI 8856, pp. 151–162, 2014.

The AIA task has been traditionally faced with two main approaches: supervised and unsupervised ones [3]. The difference between these two approaches lies on whether they use manually labeled data or not, and on how the annotation process is performed. Supervised methods require a training data set with labeled images to learn the correspondence between images and labels. This type of methods have reported competitive performance, see e.g., [4]. However, an important limitation of these methods is that new images can be labeled only with concepts available in the training set, besides, they require of manually labeled data and have been applied in scenarios with a few labels (typically a few tens).

Unsupervised methods, on the other hand, assign concepts to images by processing the text available in a reference collection of images, where each image is associated to a free and unstructured text[2]. For labeling an image, unsupervised AIA methods apply text mining techniques to the texts associated to images (in the reference collection) that are most similar to the test/query image [5,6]. By working with unsupervised AIA it is possible to consider a larger diversity of labels for annotation than with supervised methods, besides, no manually-labeled data is required and more scalable systems can be developed [7]. Since reference collections for unsupervised AIA are not "curated", the quality of text plays a key role on the performance of AIA.

This paper aims at improving the scope that images in the reference collection have into annotation process for unsupervised AIA. Specifically, we aim at expanding the textual information associated to images in such a way that not only concepts/labels present in original text can be used for annotation, but also, related terms. Our hypothesis is that by using term co-occurrence information we can discover related terms that can be used to label images. This working hypothesis has been proved to be helpful in related tasks [4,8]. However, to the best of our knowledge, this form of expansion has not been used in the context of AIA. We introduce a term-expansion strategy based on co-occurrence statistics and evaluate the benefits of using the expanded text for unsupervised AIA. We report experimental results in a large scale image annotation benchmark and show that term expansion can be very helpful for improving the annotation performance of unsupervised AIA.

The rest of this paper is organized as follows. The next section reviews related work. Section 3 describes the considered AIA method and introduce the proposed expansion strategy. Section 4 presents experimental results using two different types of associated text. Finally, Section 5 presents conclusions and discusses directions for future work.

## 2   Related Work

In unsupervised AIA one has access to a reference collection of images with associated texts. Although this text is somehow related to images, it is important to emphasize that images are not labeled with and therefore supervised learning

---

[2] For instance, a reference collection might be a subset of images in the Web, where images are associated to the text in the webpage they are contained in.

is not an option. Instead, standard unsupervised AIA methods annotate images in two steps as follows. Given an image to annotate, first a content-based image retrieval (CBIR) module is used to obtain the $k-$most similar images to the query image; next, the texts associated to these $k$ images are processed to obtain a set of keywords to annotate the image.

The works of Makadia et al. [5] and Villegas et al. [6] are two representative methods of unsupervised AIA, where the main difference between them is the way in which associated text is processed to obtain labels for an image. In [5] the authors propose a greedy strategy, where the most frequent terms in the first text are used as labels, if the number of desired labels is reached the method stops, otherwise, it keeps assigning label to images greedily. The method described in [6], on the other hand, assign to images the labels that mostly co-occur with terms in the retrieved texts[3]. In this paper, we consider an AIA method similar to that proposed in [6], however, we expand the terms associated to images before applying the annotation strategy. In this way, not only terms appearing in the text can be used for annotation, but also related terms.

Other interesting techniques have been proposed to obtain the annotation for images. For instance, in [9] it is proposed a measure to estimate the relevance of labels to images; this estimate is based on the difference of the distribution of the label to annotate in the $k$ images returned by the CBIR and its distribution in a reference collection of images. In [10] BM25 (Okapi best matching 25) is used to assign weights to labels, and images are annotated with labels having the greatest scores. Both methods could be used in combination with our proposal, however, in this work we focused on the straight annotation process and postpone the use of more elaborated methods for future work.

## 3  Textual Expansion for Unsupervised Annotation

This section describes the proposed term expansion technique and how we use it for AIA, see Figure 1. Before introducing the expansion method we describe the considered method for unsupervised AIA, which resembles the method in [6].

### 3.1  Unsupervised Image Annotation

Figure 1 shows the considered AIA method. Given an image to annotate: first a CBIR module is used to retrieve $k-$most similar images from a reference collection. Next, using the associated text of these $k$ images, a text mining module is used to derive the labels to annotate. A standard AIA method (e.g., those in [6,5]) comprises the modules within the box; the improvement reported in this paper comprises the modules below the box (see the next subsection).

The CBIR module involves the extraction of visual features for representing images and using a similarity/distance function to compare query and reference images [2]. We considered standard visual descriptors such as SIFT and color

---

[3] In [6] a set of reference labels is considered, in such a way that only labels in the reference set can be used for labeling images.

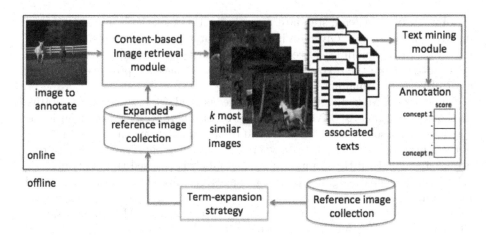

**Fig. 1.** Unsupervised AIA with the proposed term-expansion strategy. *Without expansion follows a traditional unsupervised AIA.

histograms, as provided with the considered data set (see Section 4). As distance function we used the L1 distance:

$$L1(\mathbf{x}, \mathbf{y}) = \frac{1}{D} \sum_{i=1}^{D} |x_i - y_i| \tag{1}$$

where $\mathbf{x}, \mathbf{y} \in \mathbb{R}^D$ are vectors of visual descriptors representing two images, $x_i$ is the $i^{th}$ element of vector $\mathbf{x}$, and $D$ is the dimensionality of the input space.

Once that $k-$images have been retrieved, the annotation process consists of mining the text associated to these images to extract the terms to label the query image. For this process we considered a straightforward strategy that accounts for the frequency of terms in the $k$ retrieved texts. Candidate terms to be used as labels for the query image are sorted in descending order of their frequency, and we assign to the image the top $q-$concepts with highest scores.

We have described a standard/basic AIA method. One should note that this AIA strategy can be used to label images with both: the standard setting, i.e., without term expansion, (the modules in the box in Figure 1) and the proposed term-expansion approach (the whole approach depicted in Figure 1).

## 3.2 Term-expansion Strategy

This section describes the proposed term expansion technique, which aims at improving the quality of the reference collection, see Figure 1. Our approach aims to associate images with similar contexts to each other, i.e., images that are associated to terms that co-occur with similar terms across the reference collection. Thus, the text associated to images is augmented with related terms;

or, from a different perspective, one can see this expansion as expanding the set of images that contain each term, see Figure 4.

More formally, let $\mathcal{C}$ denote the reference collection formed by image-text pairs, i.e., $\mathcal{C} = \{(I_i, T_i)\}_{1,\ldots,M}$, where each image $I_i$ is represented by a vector of visual features $\mathbf{x}_i \in \mathbb{R}^D$ and its associated text $T_i$ is represented by a bag-of-words $\mathbf{a}_i \in \mathbb{R}^{|V|}$, that is, $\mathbf{a}_i = \langle a_{i,1}, \ldots, a_{i,|V|} \rangle$ is a $|V|-$dimensional vector of reals where the $j^{th}$ element indicates the (normalized) frequency of occurrence of term $t_j$ in text $T_i$, where $V$ is the vocabulary in the reference collection (i.e., the set of different terms in texts from the reference collection). The proposed method expands each $T_i$ component (i.e., the vector $\mathbf{a}_i$), resulting in an expanded collection $\mathcal{C}^* = \{(I_i, T_i^*)\}_{1,\ldots,M}$, where $T_i^*$ is a modified version of $T_i$ that entails the expanded information (i.e., some terms in $\mathbf{a}_i^*$ that were zero in $\mathbf{a}_i$ can have now non-zero values). The rest of this section describes the way in which bag-of-words vectors are expanded.

The expansion strategy relies on term co-occurrence analysis. As a first step, we quantify the degree of association between terms by estimating co-occurrence statistics in the texts from the reference collection. Specifically, we consider the following term-relatedness measure which aims at approximating the conditional probability of occurrence of a term given another one:

$$P(t_k|t_j) \approx \frac{O(t_j, t_k)}{O(t_j)} \tag{2}$$

where $O(t_k, t_j)$ is the number of documents[4] in which terms $t_k$ and $t_j$ co-occur, and $O(t_j)$ is the number of documents in which term $t_j$ appears. Let $\mathbf{a}_i^* = \langle a_{i,1}^*, \ldots, a_{i,|V|}^* \rangle$ denote the expanded textual representation $T_i^*$ associated to image $I_i$. Then, the expansion for term $a_{i,k}^*$ is given by:

$$a_{i,k}^* = \sum_{j=1}^{n} a_{i,j} \cdot P(t_k|t_j) \tag{3}$$

where $t_j, j = \{1, \ldots, n\}$, denote the terms that appear in the original text $T_i$ and $P(t_k|t_j)$ expresses the relatedness of the term $t_j$ to the term $t_k$. This expansion is performed over the whole vocabulary (e.g., every element $a_{i,k}$ of $\mathbf{a}_i$ is expanded). In this way, the whole vector of terms is expanded by looking at the context of the corresponding associated text. One should note, that the expanded textual vector increases the number of terms associated to each image, which latter is used for AIA.

Although it is important to expand every term in the vocabulary in terms of the context of the associated text, it is often possible to introduce noisy information that may degrade the annotation performance. Hence, we considered a more controlled form of expansion in which only terms that co-occur with high frequency will be expanded. We use Equation (4) to obtain the $P(t_k|t_j)$

---

[4] We consider as a document the pair of image and associated text in the reference collection.

component in Equation (3), to expand only a subset of terms as determined by a threshold $u$.

$$P(t_k|t_j) = \begin{cases} 0 & \text{if } P(t_k|t_j) < u \\ P(t_k|t_j) & \text{if } P(t_k|t_j) \geq u \end{cases} \qquad (4)$$

In order to define $u$ we took into consideration several options and we found that, in general, it is difficult to fix an optimal cutoff value for every possible situation. Therefore, instead of using a fixed threshold we adopted a dynamic value that depends on the mean and standard deviation on the co-occurrence values of each term:

$$u = \mu(P(t_{1,\ldots,n}|t_j)) + \sigma(P(t_{1,\ldots,n}|t_j)) \qquad (5)$$

The next section presents an experimental study that aims at evaluating the benefits offered by the proposed expansion strategy.

## 4   Experimental Results

This section reports results of experiments that evaluate the proposed expansion strategy in the task of unsupervised AIA. First we describe the considered data set, next we present the experimental settings, then we report the experimental results.

### 4.1   Scalable Concept Annotation Data Set

For the evaluation of the proposed expansion strategy we considered a benchmark used in the scalable concept annotation subtask at ImageCLEF2013 [11,6]. It was created by filtering out over 31 million images that were obtained by querying three popular search engines; a subset of 250,000 images (together with the webpages that contained the images) was selected to be used as the reference collection. A subset of 1000 images was manually selected and labeled with $n$ concepts, taken from a vocabulary of 107 possible concepts that are used for the evaluation of the annotation performance. The reference collection includes the 250,000 images and their corresponding associated texts. For the associated text we have used two resources: the complete WebPage that contained each image and the keywords that were used to retrieve the image. Images are represented by 7 variants of visual descriptors: SIFT, color histogram, GETLF, GIST and three subtypes of color SIFT descriptors (C, RGB and OPPONENT SIF), all of them are histograms that account for the occurrence of representative visual descriptors taken from a codebook (bag-of-visual words). These descriptors were made available by the owners of the data set [11,6].

### 4.2   Experimental Settings

The text in the reference collection was indexed[5] to obtain the bag-of-words representations, $\mathbf{a}_i$, for each text $T_i$. This indexing procedure was applied separately for the two types of textual information (i.e., keywords and WebPages).

---

[5] We used the Text to Matrix Generator (TMG 5.0) in Matlab [12].

In order to make more manageable the vocabulary of terms from the WebPages stop words and terms with very low/high frequency were removed.

For the evaluation of our method we adopted the same protocol from the scalable concept annotation task [6]: given an input image and a set of $c-$specific concepts the system decides which of them are present in the image and which ones are not. In fact, the annotation methods provide a ranking of the $c-$concepts in descending order of their relevance to describe the query image. The evaluation is performed by estimating the Average Precision (AP) of the ranked list of concepts as follows:

$$AP = \frac{1}{|G|} \sum_{g=1}^{|G|} \frac{t}{rank(g)} \tag{6}$$

where $G$ is the ordered set of the ground truth annotations, and $rank(g)$ is the ordered position, in the ranked list provided by the AIA system, of the $g^{th}$ ground truth annotation. Thus, lager values of AP indicate better annotation performance. For all of our experiments we associate each image with the top-10 concepts/terms with higher frequency (see Section 3). Hence, our system always return a list of 10 concepts, sorted in descending order of relevance.

### 4.3   Experiment 1: WebPages vs. Keywords Annotation

The aim of this experiment was to evaluate the annotation performance before applying the expansion strategy by using two different types of associated text in the reference collection: 1) WebPages, and 2) keywords. We considered all of the visual descriptors for the CBIR module and compare the annotation performance for different values of $k$ (the number of nearest images considered for AIA, see Section 3.). The results of this experiment are shown in Figure 2.

We can clearly observe that better annotation performance was obtained with WebPages using any of the seven visual descriptors (see Figure 2 (a)). We believe that the WebPages include more information that can be used to describe the visual content of images, so that the WebPages offer better annotation performance than keywords, which only include few words. Thus, despite being cleaner, keywords do not contain enough useful-information and, therefore, it seems this type of information is more appropriate to be expanded with our proposed technique. On the other hand, it can be seen that, in terms of visual descriptors (see Figure 2 (b)), better results were obtained with SIFT descriptors and its color-variants. Also, it is clear that, in general, better performance is obtained with larger values of $k$, this can be due to the fact that, in this way, more term-frequency is accumulated, which can be beneficial for AIA.

### 4.4   Experiment 2: Direct vs. Expanded Annotation

In a second experiment we evaluated the annotation performance when using the expanded text and compared this performance with the traditional AIA approach. For clarity, and because of results from the previous section, we only show results obtained with the OPPONENT-SIFT visual descriptor.

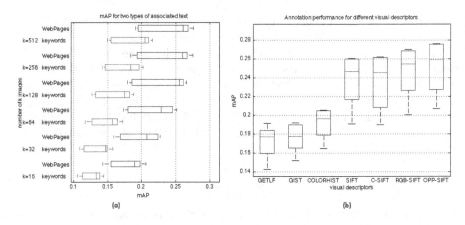

**Fig. 2.** mean Average Precision (mAP): (a) using keywords and WebPages as associated text in the reference collection using all the 7 different visual descriptors, and (b) the 7 different visual descriptors using keywords and WebPages

The results of this experiment are shown in Figure 3; we compare performance without expansion, with expansion of all terms (*exp-total*), and with controlled expansion (*exp-(M+std)*), see Section 3, for WepPages and keywords.

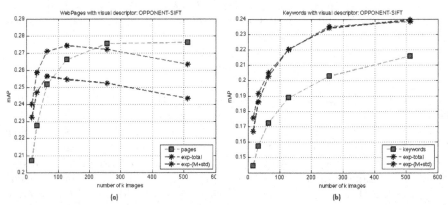

**Fig. 3.** mAP using the original text in the reference collection vs. expanded variants for WebPages (a) and keywords (b); OPPONENT-SIFT was used as visual descriptor

Without expansion, we can observe that by using keywords the annotation performance tends to increase slowly up to $k \approx 512$ (Figure 3 (b)), and the performance using WebPages has a lapse of convergence after $k \approx 256$ images are used (Figure 3 (a)). We believe that the convergence in these two cases is due to a saturation of information, that is, there exist a majority of images that contain the concepts to annotate. On the other hand, using a complete expansion, we can observe that the performance with the keywords improved, whereas the performance with WebPages started to drop as the number of images increased. This behavior is somewhat expected as: (1) having rich enough information (WebPages) suggests an expansion will not may have an impact (instead, noise removal mechanisms may be helpful for this type of data); and (2) having scarce information (keywords) is indicative of the need for an expansion.

Finally, we can observe that if we perform a controlled expansion we can improve the annotation performance of WebPages using a less images ($k$) for the CBIR module. In fact, we can achieve similar performance when using $k = 512$ (without expansion) and $k = 128$ (with controlled expansion). This is an interesting result because we can use 4-times less images and still obtain quite competitive performance. One should note that when considering larger values of $k$ the annotation performance decreases. This can be due to the fact that when estimating the threshold $u$ for too many texts, non-relevant/noisy terms may be the more frequent ones.

In order to give insights into the quality of the expansion that can be generated with our method we show in Figure 4 some images with their associated keywords before and after applying the expansion procedure. For each image, we show at most the top-10 words most relevant from the expansion strategy.

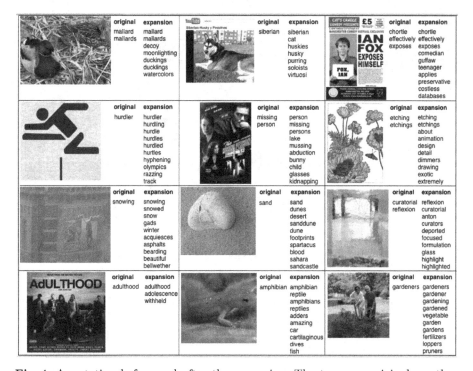

**Fig. 4.** Annotation before and after the expansion. The terms as original are those extracted from the keywords.

It is interesting that we can find in the expanded text many related terms to the original keywords that can be used to label images. For example, using as original 'chortle', 'effectively' and 'exposes' (refer to third image in the first row in Figure 4), in the expansion we can see terms like 'comedian' and 'guffaw' that are related terms to 'chortle'. Another observation is that some terms are ambiguous like 'siberian' and these can express different concepts, as consequence the expansion includes different concepts (like 'cat' or 'purring') and not all are related to the visual content of the image (refer to second image of the first row).

On the other hand, we evaluate qualitatively the images related to a given concept before and after the expansion. In Figure 5, we present the 10-top related images to the concept 'cloud'; we can observe that before the expansion there are images not related to the concept but after the expansion we can find three related topics: 1) 'cloud' like meteorology definition, 2) 'cloud' related to computation and, 3) 'cloud' related to a video game.

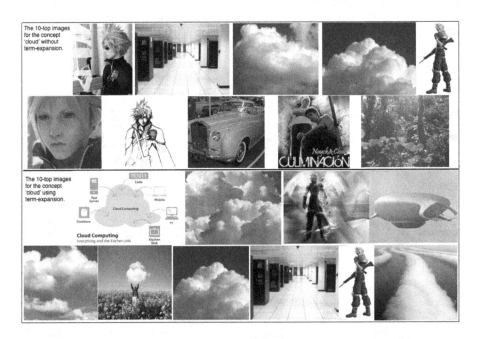

**Fig. 5.** 10-top related images to the concept 'cloud' before and after the expansion

In the Figure 6 we present another example of the expansion; we show 10-top related images to the concept 'traffic', we can observe an increase in the number of images related to 'traffic' like transportation definition as well as an increase in the number of images in 'traffic' related to information at the Internet.

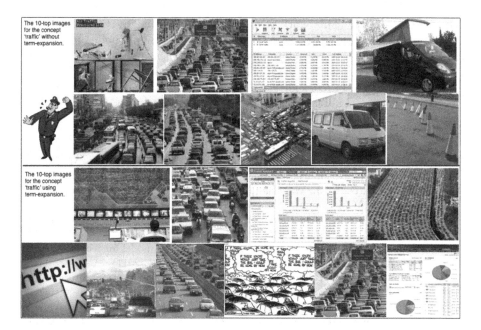

**Fig. 6.** 10-top related images to the concept 'traffic' before and after the expansion

## 5   Conclusions

In this paper we have introduced a new term expansion strategy for unsupervised image annotation. This strategy is based on term co-occurrence analysis; it aims to expand the text associated to images from the reference collection with related terms that could contribute to improve the annotation performance.

Our research on the expansion strategy is ongoing and requires an in depth evaluation and analysis with a larger pool of concepts/labels. However the results presented are encouraging. The set of experiments we discussed showed that, by using the proposed expansion, better annotation performance can be obtained, where the improvements depend on the type and amount of associated text that is considered. Particularly our results suggest that the expansion will not may have an impact when original textual information is rich enough (as in the case of full web pages), but that it could be really useful when this information is scarce (such as in the case of having a bunch of keywords).

For future work we are interested in expanding not only the textual information associated to images from the reference collection but also their visual representation. The idea is to enhance the performance of the CBIR module by allowing the retrieval of relevant images having related (although not equal) visual features.

**Acknowledgments.** This work was partially supported by CONACyT under scholarship No. 214764 and by the LACCIR programme under project ID R1212LAC006. Hugo Jair Escalante was supported by the internships programme of CONACyT under grant No. 234415. The authors would like to thank Mauricio Villegas and Roberto Paredes for their support on the considered data set.

# References

1. Barnard, K., Duygulu, P., de Freitas, N., Forsyth, D., Blei, D., Jordan, M.: Matching words and pictures. Journal of Machine Learning Research 3, 1107–1135 (2003)
2. Datta, R., Joshi, D., Li, J., Wang, J.: Image retrieval: Ideas, influences, and trends of the new age. ACM Computing Surveys (CSUR) 40 (2008)
3. Hanbury, A.: A survey of methods for image annotation. Journal of Visual Languages and Computing 19, 617–627 (2008)
4. Escalante, H.J., Montes, M., Sucar, E.: An energy-based model for region labeling. Computer Vision and Image Understanding 115, 787–803 (2011)
5. Makadia, A., Pavlovic, V., Kumar, S.: Baselines for image annotation. International Journal of Computer Vision 90, 88–105 (2010)
6. Villegas, M., Paredes, R., Thomee, B.: Overview of the imageclef 2013 scalable concept image annotation subtask. In: CLEF 2013 Evaluation Labs and Workshop, Online Working Notes, 1–19 (2013)
7. Carneiro, G., Chan, A., Moreno, P., Vasconcelos, N.: Supervised learning of semantic classes for image annotation and retrieval. IEEE Transactions on Pattern Analysis and Machine Intelligence 29, 394–410 (2007)
8. Escalante, H.J., Montes, M., Sucar, E.: Multimodal document indexing based on semantic cohesion for image retrieval. Information Retrieval 15, 1–32 (2012)
9. Uricchio, T., Bertini, M., Ballan, L., Del Bimbo, A.: MICC-UNIFI at ImageCLEF 2013 scalable concept image annotation. In: Working Notes for CLEF 2013 Conference, Valencia, Spain, September 23-26 (2013)
10. Reshma, I., Ullah, M., Aono, M.: KDEVIR at ImageCLEF 2013 image annotation subtask. In: Working Notes for CLEF 2013 Conference, Valencia, Spain, September 23-26 (2013)
11. Villegas, M., Paredes, R.: Image-text dataset generation for image annotation and retrieval. In: Berlanga, R., Rosso, P. (eds.) II Congreso Español de Recuperacion de Informacion, CERI 2012, pp. 115–120 (2012)
12. Zeimpekis, D., Gallopoulos, E.: TMG: A MATLAB toolbox for generating term-document matrices from text collections. In: Grouping Multidimensional Data: Recent Advances in Clustering, pp. 187–210. Springer (2010)

# Gender Differences in Deceivers Writing Style

Verónica Pérez-Rosas and Rada Mihalcea

University of North Texas, University of Michigan
{vrncapr,mihalcea}@umich.edu

**Abstract.** The widespread use of deception in written content has motivated the need for methods to automatically profile and identify deceivers. Particularly, the identification of deception based on demographic data such as gender, age, and religion, has become of importance due to ethical and security concerns. Previous work on deception detection has studied the role of gender using statistical approaches and domain-specific data. This work explores gender detection in open domain truths and lies using a machine learning approach. First, we collect a deception dataset consisting of truths and lies from male and female participants. Second, we extract a large feature set consisting of n-grams, shallow and deep syntactic features, semantic features derived from a psycholinguistics lexicon, and features derived from readability metrics. Third, we build deception classifiers able to predict participant's gender with classification accuracies ranging from 60-70%. In addition, we present an analysis of differences in the linguistic style used by deceivers given their reported gender.

**Keywords:** deception, linguistics, machine learning.

## 1 Introduction

The increasing presence of deceit in written content has motivated the need for automatic methods able to identify deceptive behavior. Particularly, the identification of deception based on demographic data such as gender, age, education, and religion among others, has become of importance due to ethical and security concerns. Online date websites, forums, and social media, have reported multiple cases of strategic misrepresentation, with people lying mainly about their gender, age, and physical attributes such as height and weight [15,17,6]. Among these aspects, we focus on the identification of gender in deception, which can also be associated with gender imitation or gender misrepresentation.

We start by collecting a deception dataset consisting of truths and lies from male and female participants. Unlike other studies, where authors established a specific domain, the domain of our dataset is not pre-determined as we hypothesize that when lying in an open domain setting deceivers will show natural bias towards specific topics related to gender.

Using this dataset, we extract a large feature set consisting of n-grams, shallow and deep syntactic features, semantic features derived from a psycholinguistics

A. Gelbukh et al. (Eds.): MICAI 2014, Part I, LNAI 8856, pp. 163–174, 2014.

lexicon, and features derived from readability metrics. Most of these features have been previously found to be effective for the prediction of deceptive behavior.

We perform a set of experiments to explore three research questions. First, can we build deception classifiers using short open domain truths and lies? Second, given a deceptive corpus from female and male deceivers, can we build deception classifiers able to predict deceiver's gender? Third, what are the topics more frequently discussed by male and female deceivers? Finally, we discuss our main findings and future work directions.

## 2   Related Work

Several efforts have been presented to approach the automatic identification of deceivers in written sources using computational linguistic approaches. Lie detection has been explored in different domains such as e-mail communication, dating websites, blogs, forums, chats, and social network websites.

Research in this area has shown the effectiveness of features derived from text analysis, including n-grams, sentence counts, and sentence length. More recently, features derived from syntactic Context Free Grammar (CFG) parse trees, and part-of-speech (POS) tags have also been used to aid the deceit detection [4,18]. Syntactic complexity has been also found to be correlated with deception [19] as related research suggests that deceivers might create less complex sentences in an effort to conceal the truth and being able to recall their lies more easily [2].

A widely used resource for incorporating semantic information is the Linguistic Inquiry and Word Count (LIWC) dictionary [13]. LIWC is a lexicon of words grouped into semantic categories relevant to psychological processes. Several research works have relied on the LIWC lexicon to build deception models using machine learning approaches [10,1] and showed that the use of semantic information is helpful for the automatic identification of deceit.

Deception detection has usually been applied to discriminate true-tellers from liars. For instance, Ott et al. [12] identified spam producers by analyzing deceptive reviews. Also, Fornaciari and Poesio [5] analyzed transcripts of court cases to identify deceptive testimonies.

Despite the fact that gender imitation and misrepresentation has been reported as one of the main forms of deception in online sources [7], very little attention has been paid to address the identification of deception based on demographic data using computational approaches. It is however worth mentioning important efforts in the field of psychology to analyze demographics influence during the deception process. Studies have revealed interesting findings regarding the role of gender during deception. For instance, according to Kaina et al. [8], females are more easily detectable when lying than their male counterparts. On the other hand Tilley et al. [14] reported that females are more successful in deception detection than male receivers. Furthermore, gender perception has an important effect on the receiver and it can lead to important implications. For instance, gender perception can have an impact on trustworthiness, as females are perceived as more cooperative and less dominant than males [3].

Finally, it is important to point out that the scarcity of resources for this task so far made it difficult to approach the problem using machine-learning techniques. We are aware of only one other resource for deception detection where demographic data is available [16]. The lack of standard datasets for this task motivated us to build our own dataset, which is publicly available at http://lit.eecs.umich.edu and represents an additional contribution of this work.

## 3   Dataset

In order to collect a deception dataset, we set up a task on Amazon Mechanical Turk where we asked workers to provide seven lies and seven truths, each consisting of one sentence, on topics of their choice. Participants were asked to provide plausible lies and avoid non-commonsensical statements such as "A cat can bark." We also collected demographic data for the contributors, such as gender, age, and education level. The final dataset consists of 3584 truths and lies provided by 512 contributors. The dataset distributions for gender, truths, and lies are presented in Table 2. Sample one-liners containing truths and lies are presented in Table 2.

**Table 1.** Dataset distribution

| Gender | Lies | Truths | Total |
|--------|------|--------|-------|
| Female | 2086 | 2086 | 4172 |
| Male | 1498 | 1498 | 2996 |
| Total | 3584 | 3584 | 7168 |

**Table 2.** Sample open domain lies and truths provided by a male and a female participant

| Female | |
|--------|--------|
| Lie | Truth |
| I'm allergic to alcohol | Giraffes are taller than zebras. |
| I am missing a toe on my left foot. | Humans are not able to fly. |
| My shoes cost me over a hundred dollars. | The meat industry is cruel to animals. |
| Male | |
| Lie | Truth |
| I own two Ferraris, one red and one black | I love to play soccer with my friends |
| I wake up at 11 o clock every day | I wake up at 6 am because I have to work at 7 am |
| I have a jumping bed in my backyard | I own a 2003 white lancer and a 2008 silver Toyota 4runner |

## 4   Features

We extract a large number of features, consisting of several features that have been previously found to correlate with deception cues.

**Unigrams:** We extract unigrams derived from the bag of words representation of the one-liners present in our dataset. Our unigrams features are encoded as term frequency inverse document frequency (tf-idf) values.

**Shallow and deep syntax:** Following Feng et al. [4] we extract a set of features derived from POS tags and production rules based on CFG trees. We use the Berkeley parser to obtain both POS and CFG features. Our POS features are encoded as the tf-idf values of each POS tag occurring in the dataset. The CFG derived features consist of all lexicalized production rules combined with their grandparent node and are also encoded as tf-idf values.

**LIWC derived features:** We use features derived from the LIWC lexicon, except for the paralinguistic classes. These features consist of word counts for each of the 80 semantic classes present in the LIWC lexicon.

**Syntactic complexity and readability score features:** To extract these features we use a tool provided by Lu et al. [9], which generates fourteen indexes representing sentence syntactic complexity including: mean length of sentence (MLS), mean length of T-unit (MLT), mean length of clause (MLC), clauses per sentence (C/S), verb phrases per T-unit (VP/T), clauses per T-unit (C/T), dependent clauses per clause (DC/C), dependent clauses per T-unit (DC/T), T-units per sentence (T/S), complex T-unit ratio (CT/T), coordinate phrases per T-unit (CP/T), coordinate phrases per clause (CP/C), complex nominals per T-unit (CN/T), and complex nominals per clause (CP/C). In addition, we also incorporate standard readability metrics such as Flesch-Kincaid and Gunning Fog.

## 5   Experiments

We perform several experiments to answer the research questions formulated at the beginning of this paper.

### 5.1   Is It Possible to Build Accurate Deception Classifiers for Short Open Domain Truths and Lies?

To answer this question, we build deception classifiers using each set of features described in section 4, and also using a combination of unigrams and each of the remaining feature sets. All classifiers were created using the Support Vector Machine (SVM) algorithm as implemented in the Weka toolkit with the default parameter configuration. Results are obtained using a ten-fold cross-validation.

First, we evaluate the deception detection task. We build classifiers using all truths and lies present in the dataset, regardless of gender. The purpose of this experiment is to evaluate the deception detection task when using short deceptive and truthful statements and also to explore which feature set is more suitable for these data sets. Figure 1 presents the overall and per-class accuracies obtained by each classifier.

As the graph shows, the individual use of unigrams and features derived from POS and CFG leads to similar classification accuracies. Also, the classifier built with features representing syntactic complexity and readability scores is the worst performing classifier. However, when combined with unigrams, this turns out to lead to the best classifier with the highest overall accuracy values. In

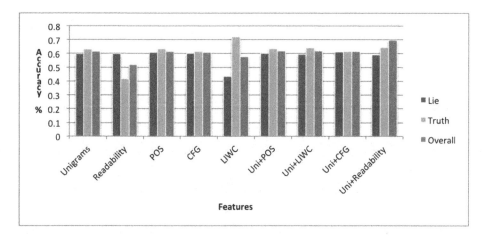

**Fig. 1.** Deception classification results in terms of accuracy percentages using different feature sets

general, from this graph we can observe that given the various classifiers, the deceptive class is always more difficult to predict than the truthful one. Interestingly, the LIWC-based classifier shows the best performance for the truthful class.

Second, we explore the deception detection within gender. We split our dataset based on reported gender and obtain two datasets. One dataset consists of truths and lies from males (male dataset), while the other consists of truths and lies from females (female dataset). As before, we build deception classifiers for each dataset using the different feature sets. Classification results are reported in Table 2 and 3 respectively.

From these figures we notice that combining unigrams with readability and syntactic complexity features seem to help the most while predicting deception. We can observe also interesting differences in the classification accuracy per class. For instance, the classification accuracies obtained for the truth and lie classes on the male dataset are very similar, thus suggesting that truths and lies are equally difficult to predict. However, for the female dataset, the detection of truths seems easier than the detection of lies.

## 5.2 Can We Build Deception Classifiers Able to Predict Deceiver's Gender?

To answer this question we focus on predicting the gender of an author of a deceptive sentence. Thus, in these experiments, we use a subset from our deception dataset consisting of only lies.

Using this deception corpus, we build several deception classifiers using the each of feature sets described in section 4. As before, our experiments are performed using the SVM algorithm and using 10-fold cross-validation. Note that the class distribution for this deceptive corpus is unbalanced as we have 2086 fe-

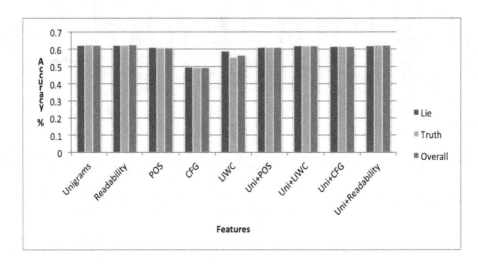

**Fig. 2.** Deception classification of female truths and lies for several feature sets

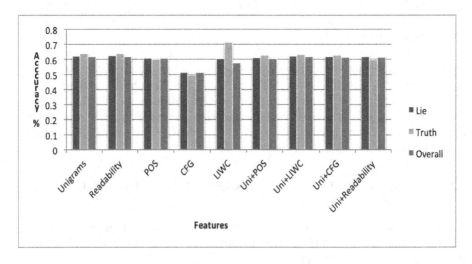

**Fig. 3.** Deception classification of male truths and lies for several feature sets

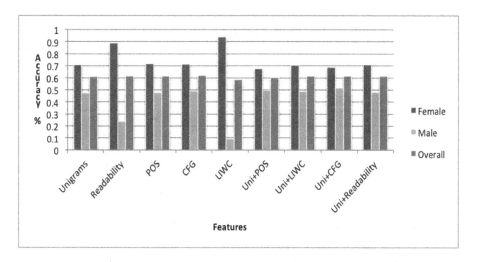

**Fig. 4.** Gender classification results in terms of accuracy percentage using different feature sets

male and 1498 male instances. Thus, the baseline, corresponding to the majority class is 58.2%.

Figure 4 shows the accuracy results for female and male classes, and overall accuracy. From this figure, we can observe that the female class is more easily predicted than the male class. While this can be in part attributed to the dataset imbalance, these results are also in line with the findings reported in Ho et al. [7], where female deceivers were more easily identifiable than the males ones. Among the different classifiers presented in this graph, we can observe that overall accuracy values are very similar to each other and the male class is always more difficult to predict. This time the combination of unigrams and CFG features seems to provide the best performance.

### 5.3   What Are the Topics More Frequently Discussed by Male and Female Deceivers?

To answer this question, we initially attempted to automatically identify topics from lies generated by male and female deceivers. We further split our deception corpus into male and female sets and applied Latent Dirichlet Allocation (LDA) topic modeling to identify which topics are associated to each gender. However, this approach generated a very large number of topics and we were unable to identity specific topics that allowed us to make such comparisons.

In order to provide some insight about word usage differences, we opted instead for applying the method proposed by Mihalcea et al. [11] and obtained the most dominant semantic word classes, extracted using the LIWC lexicon, associated to each gender. Table 3 shows the most dominant words classes used by both female and male deceivers as well as only female and only male.

**Table 3.** Results from LIWC word class analysis. Top ranked semantic classes associated to truths and lies generated by both female and males (Male+Female), male only (Male), and female only (Female).

| Lies | | | | | |
|---|---|---|---|---|---|
| Male+Female | | Male | | Female | |
| Class | Score | Class | Score | Class | Score |
| Certain | 1.94 | Other | 2.22 | **Certain** | 1.87 |
| Negate | 1.79 | **Negate** | 2.08 | **Negate** | 1.63 |
| You | 1.68 | **Certain** | 2.06 | **You** | 1.59 |
| Anger | 1.64 | Death | 2.04 | Motion | 1.47 |
| Down | 1.42 | **Anger** | 2.03 | **Down** | 1.45 |
| Motion | 1.41 | **You** | 1.77 | **Money** | 1.35 |
| Money | 1.38 | **Friends** | 1.71 | **Anger** | 1.28 |
| Friends | 1.37 | **Othref** | 1.67 | Future | 1.20 |
| Othref | 1.35 | **Down** | 1.47 | **Othref** | 1.19 |
| Death | 1.28 | **Money** | 1.44 | Sports | 1.15 |
| Other | 1.26 | Sleep | 1.41 | **Eating** | 1.15 |
| Eating | 1.22 | **Eating** | 1.36 | **Friends** | 1.14 |
| Truths | | | | | |
| Male+Female | | Male | | Female | |
| Incl | 0.87 | Leisure | 0.82 | Number | 0.85 |
| Number | 0.86 | Posemo | 0.82 | Music | 0.85 |
| Discrep | 0.85 | Sports | 0.79 | Tentat | 0.83 |
| Posemo | 0.85 | Occup | 0.75 | We | 0.83 |
| School | 0.83 | Job | 0.73 | Tv | 0.76 |
| Family | 0.82 | **Posfeel** | 0.72 | Metaph | 0.75 |
| Sexual | 0.81 | **Relig** | 0.70 | **Posfeel** | 0.75 |
| Tv | 0.79 | Sexual | 0.70 | Anx | 0.74 |
| See | 0.75 | School | 0.64 | Discrep | 0.72 |
| Music | 0.74 | Music | 0.60 | See | 0.67 |
| Posfeel | 0.73 | Groom | 0.59 | **Relig** | 0.62 |
| Relig | 0.65 | Family | 0.59 | Sleep | 0.61 |

To provide a more comprehensive analysis, this table also shows the most dominant classes used by true-tellers. To facilitate the comparisons based on gender, we show in bold the overlapping classes taken from the top twelve ranking classes for both deceptive and truthful categories.

From this table, we can observe that, regardless of their gender, deceivers make use of negation, negative emotions, and references to others. On the other hand, when telling the truth, more positive emotion (Posemo) and positive feeling (Posfeel) words are used. Also, some word classes suggest topics associated with truths, such as religion, family, and school.

Regarding the differences between genders, we first observe that the overlap of semantic word classes associated with deception is greater than the overlap of classes associated with true-telling. One possible explanation for this is that

**Table 4.** Sample lies from male and female participants for overlapping semantic classes

| Class | Male | Female |
|-------|------|--------|
| Negate | I don't have a steady job.<br>I do not work out at gym.<br>I don't own a cellphone. | I do not lie.<br>Sports are not dangerous.<br>I do not love shopping very much. |
| Anger | I hate polygamy<br>I killed someone last night.<br>I hate my little brother and think he is annoying. | I hate dogs.<br>I have never told a lie.<br>Blue eyed people are dangerous |
| Friends | I like the neighbors.<br>Ricky martin has a lovely girlfriend.<br><br>I don't care about my friends. | I have three boyfriends.<br>The neighbors across the street have twelve children.<br>I have never made friends over the Internet. |
| Eating | I woke up this morning and had breakfast in bed.<br>Eating a mushroom every morning in empty stomach helps to reduce weight<br>You can lose weight without exercising or changing your diet. | You will lose weight if you buy my diet chocolate pies.<br>I am going to eat at a restaurant that pays me to eat there.<br><br>People eat breakfast at night. |

lies are told about similar topics while truths seem to be more diverse. Tables 4 and 5 show sample lies from male and female participants for four overlapping and non-overlapping semantic classes. As observed, both male and female share some commonalities on the words used when deceiving. For instance, the use of negation and anger words, and words referring to friends and eating. On the other hand, in Table 5 we can see that females lie more about sports and future actions, while males lie about topics such as death and sleep.

To further analyze the word usage by gender, we also obtain the most dominant words per gender using the same method we used before for the semantic classes, but this time applied to the most frequent words used by deceivers. Results from this analysis are reported in Table 6.

From this table, we can observe significant differences in the word usage by each gender. Interestingly, the word safe is present in lies being told by both males and females. From a closer look at the deceptive corpus, we can frequently observe lies such as: "Drinking and driving is a winning and safe combination," "The internet is a totally safe way for children to spend their day, "East los Angeles is a safe place," or "Your privacy is safe on the internet."

## 6   Conclusions

In this paper, we presented a set of experiments where we explored the gender detection task in deceptive content. We collected a deception dataset consisting of one-liners truths and lies. Through several experiments, we showed that this

**Table 5.** Sample lies from male and female participants for non-overlapping semantic classes

| Class | Sample lies |
|-------|-------------|
| | Male |
| Dead | My girlfriend committed suicide yesterday. |
| | Drinking cyanide doesn't kill humans. |
| Sleep | The kids go to bed without any trouble |
| | I will go to sleep early today. |
| Other | Superman has the letter "m" on his chest. |
| | My friend can smell with the help of his fingers. |
| | Female |
| Future | I am excited about going to work tomorrow. |
| | Obamacare may be obtained after extensive genetic testing. |
| Sports | I love to watch football, i have never missed a game. |
| | Shaq o'neill is a famous tennis player. |
| Motion | I learned driving and used to drive at the age of 5. |
| | I am able to fly a plane. |

**Table 6.** Top dominant words used per gender in the deception corpus

| Male | | Female | |
|------|------|------|------|
| Word | Score | Word | Score |
| Woman | 12.39 | Dollars | 9.93 |
| Really | 10.48 | Government | 6.46 |
| Night | 5.40 | Times | 5.46 |
| Safe | 5.24 | Never | 4.56 |
| he | 5.08 | Everyone | 3.97 |
| Think | 4.76 | Know | 3.97 |
| Always | 4.44 | Won | 3.72 |
| Drinking | 4.13 | Safe | 3.31 |
| His | 4.13 | Million | 2.9 |
| Never | 4.08 | Always | 2.98 |
| They | 3.40 | Car | 2.88 |

data can be used to build deception classifiers able to discriminate between truths and lies. We also explored the gender detection on a fraction of the data consisting of only lies. Our results showed that the female deceivers are more easily detected than males and that classifiers based on unigrams show robust performance. We provided also an analysis of the differences in topics and words used by deceivers from each gender. Our results showed that is more difficult to identify lies than truths. Also, when it comes to gender, lies being told by females are more easily identifiable than lies being told my males. In the future, we are planning to conduct a more detailed analysis where we will study differences related to age and gender perception.

**Acknowledgments.** This material is based in part upon work supported by National Science Foundation awards #1344257 and #1355633, by grant #48503 from the John Templeton Foundation, and by DARPA-BAA-12-47 DEFT grant #12475008. Any opinions, findings, and conclusions or recommendations expressed in this material are those of the authors and do not necessarily reflect the views of the National Science Foundation, the John Templeton Foundation, or the Defense Advanced Research Projects Agency.

# References

1. Almela, A., Valencia-García, R., Cantos, P.: Seeing through deception: A computational approach to deceit detection in written communication. In: Proceedings of the Workshop on Computational Approaches to Deception Detection, pp. 15–22. Association for Computational Linguistics, Avignon (2012), http://www.aclweb.org/anthology/W12-0403
2. De Paulo, B., Lindsay, J., Malone, B., Muhlenbruck, L., Charlton, K., Cooper, H.: Cues to deception. Psychological Bulletin 129(1) (2003)
3. Dreber, A., Johannesson, M.: Gender differences in deception. Economics Letters 99(1), 197–199 (2008)
4. Feng, S., Banerjee, R., Choi, Y.: Syntactic stylometry for deception detection. In: Proceedings of the 50th Annual Meeting of the Association for Computational Linguistics: Short Papers, ACL 2012, vol. 2, pp. 171–175. Association for Computational Linguistics, Stroudsburg (2012), http://dl.acm.org/citation.cfm?id=2390665.2390708
5. Fornaciari, T., Poesio, M.: Automatic deception detection in italian court cases. Artificial Intelligence and Law 21(3), 303–340 (2013), http://dx.doi.org/10.1007/s10506-013-9140-4
6. Guadagno, R.E., Okdie, B.M., Kruse, S.A.: Dating deception: Gender, online dating, and exaggerated self-presentation. Comput. Hum. Behav. 28(2), 642–647 (2012), http://dx.doi.org/10.1016/j.chb.2011.11.010
7. Ho, S.M., Hollister, J.M.: Guess who? an empirical study of gender deception and detection in computer-mediated communication. Proceedings of the American Society for Information Science and Technology 50(1), 1–4 (2013)
8. Kaina, J., Ceruti, M.G., Liu, K., McGirr, S.C., Law, J.B.: Deception detection in multicultural coalitions: Foundations for a cognitive model. Tech. rep., DTIC Document (2011)

9. Lu, X.: Automatic analysis of syntactic complexity in second language writing. International Journal of Corpus Linguistics 15(4), 474–496 (2010)
10. Mihalcea, R., Strapparava, C.: The lie detector: Explorations in the automatic recognition of deceptive language. In: Proceedings of the Association for Computational Linguistics (ACL 2009), Singapore (2009)
11. Mihalcea, R., Pulman, S.: Linguistic ethnography: Identifying dominant word classes in text. In: Gelbukh, A. (ed.) CICLing 2009. LNCS, vol. 5449, pp. 594–602. Springer, Heidelberg (2009)
12. Ott, M., Choi, Y., Cardie, C., Hancock, J.: Finding deceptive opinion spam by any stretch of the imagination. In: Proceedings of the 49th Annual Meeting of the Association for Computational Linguistics: Human Language Technologies, HLT 2011, vol. 1, pp. 309–319. Association for Computational Linguistics, Stroudsburg (2011), http://dl.acm.org/citation.cfm?id=2002472.2002512
13. Pennebaker, J., Francis, M.: Linguistic inquiry and word count: LIWC. Erlbaum Publishers (1999)
14. Tilley, P., George, J.F., Marett, K.: Gender differences in deception and its detection under varying electronic media conditions. In: Proceedings of the Proceedings of the 38th Annual Hawaii International Conference on System Sciences (HICSS 2005) - Track 1, vol. 1, p. 24.2. IEEE Computer Society, Washington, DC (2005), http://dx.doi.org/10.1109/HICSS.2005.284
15. Toma, C., Hancock, J., Ellison, N.: Separating fact from fiction: An examination of deceptive self-presentation in online dating profiles. Personality and Social Psychology Bulletin 34(8), 1023–1036 (2008), http://psp.sagepub.com/content/34/8/1023.abstract
16. Verhoeven, B., Daelemans, W.: Clips stylometry investigation (csi) corpus: A dutch corpus for the detection of age, gender, personality, sentiment and deception in text. In: Calzolari, N., Choukri, K., Declerck, T., Loftsson, H., Maegaard, B., Mariani, J., Moreno, A., Odijk, J., Piperidis, S. (eds.) Proceedings of the Ninth International Conference on Language Resources and Evaluation (LREC 2014), European Language Resources Association (ELRA), Reykjavik (2014)
17. Warkentin, D., Woodworth, M., Hancock, J.T., Cormier, N.: Warrants and deception in computer mediated communication. In: Proceedings of the 2010 ACM Conference on Computer Supported Cooperative Work, pp. 9–12. ACM (2010)
18. Xu, Q., Zhao, H.: Using deep linguistic features for finding deceptive opinion spam. In: Proceedings of COLING 2012: Posters, The COLING 2012 Organizing Committee, Mumbai, India, pp. 1341–1350 (December 2012), http://www.aclweb.org/anthology/C12-2131
19. Yancheva, M., Rudzicz, F.: Automatic detection of deception in child-produced speech using syntactic complexity features. In: Proceedings of the 51st Annual Meeting of the Association for Computational Linguistics (Volume 1: Long Papers), pp. 944–953. Association for Computational Linguistics, Sofia (2013), http://www.aclweb.org/anthology/P13-1093

# Extraction of Semantic Relations from Opinion Reviews in Spanish

Sofía N. Galicia-Haro[1] and Alexander Gelbukh[2]

[1] Faculty of Sciences UNAM Universitary City, Mexico City, Mexico
sngh@fciencias.unam.mx
[2] Centro de Investigación en Computación, Instituto Politécnico Nacional, Mexico
www.Gelbukh.com

**Abstract.** We report research on semantic relations extraction to build taxonomies. The state of the art approaches are based on text corpus or on domain texts acquisition to accurately characterize the domain of interest. We analyzed the application of unsupervised methods for ontology building using a collection of opinion reviews in Spanish and the Web. We present some results and discuss the obtained relations.

**Keywords:** semantic relations, opinion reviews, linguistic patterns, ontology.

## 1 Introduction

The motivation of this work is analyze if the general methods actually applied to scientific and specialized documents to extract semantic relations are the methods to obtain very basic semantic relations. Nowadays it is possible to obtain high quantity of documents related to daily life knowledge in forums, social networks and product reviews. However, those texts have personal experiences, personal thoughts, opinions about anything, etc. The challenge to extract information from them is hard since the treatment of this kind of texts have to cope with unstructured text, lower linguistic quality, information not related to the main topic (noise), and deceptive reviews (spam). Opinion reviews on common daily life products could be obtained from Internet and they include knowledge from a basic domain.

Concept hierarchies allow to structure information into categories for example: *a washing machine is a home appliance, a washing machine is a kind of white goods,* the semantic field of washing machine is included within that of home appliance and within that of white goods. Concept hierarchies are crucial for ontology construction that has been contemplated in research activities such as machine translation, information retrieval, question-answering, information systems in general, etc. to represent knowledge. Ontology formalizes the relationships among the concepts, with the interpretation of the semantic relationships among the concepts the implicit knowledge could be inferred. Ontologies, in general, are composed by *classes*, concepts of a specific domain, *relations*, binary associations between concepts, and *instances*, real world examples.

A. Gelbukh et al. (Eds.): MICAI 2014, Part I, LNAI 8856, pp. 175–190, 2014.

Making explicit the knowledge implicitly contained in texts is a great challenge. Knowledge is found in texts at different levels of explicitness. For example, dictionaries contain explicit knowledge in form of definitions such as *a whale is a mammal*. However, the more technical and specialized the texts are, the less basic knowledge is explicit. The same could be inferred for texts using everyday language: humans are not interested in explicit the basic knowledge that they shared.

In this paper we thus examine the possibility of extracting semantic relations by applying techniques that do not require labeled examples (unsupervised techniques) which have been utilized in ontology construction. We were concerned with the extraction of concept relations from opinion reviews in Spanish and the Web. We analyzed the appropriateness of diverse linguistic patterns for the Spanish domain we worked.

The remainder of this paper is organized as follows: Section 2 describes the acquisition and characteristics of the opinion reviews collection and the methods to obtain the terms associated to the concepts. Section 3 describes the applied approaches to extract taxonomic relations from the Web. In this section we also describe the method to assign relations to more general concepts. Section 4 describes the heuristics to obtain instances and subclasses. In Section 5, we present the current results and their discussion. Finally we present the conclusions.

## 2     Corpus

The first step for this work was the compilation of opinion reviews. We were interested in texts whose topic was related to ordinary things or commonplaces, for example: washing machine opinions in Spanish. Opinion reviews are texts containing concepts and some relations related to the specific domain, specific products in general.

We automatically gathered 2,580 washing machine opinions from the site *ciao*[1]. The average size per file in tokens was 345. The total number of tokens in the collection was 854,280. The total collection named COM has been annotated with lemma and part of speech (PoS) information using FreeLing [16], an open source library. We randomly selected 500 opinion reviews to compare concepts extraction and to analyze the type of texts they are, this collection was named SOM. The collection SOM has 5,696 sentences, 179,768 tokens and 16,897 words with different PoS.

We found that errors in PoS assignments are due to lack of punctuation, for example, *Para* 'of' (in English) was tagged as personal noun (PE) because of missing a previous point. Some nouns were tagged PE since the reviewers wrote capitalized words after semicolon and comma. Other words marked as PE correspond to adverbs, nouns, prepositions and words with all uppercase letters. Some common nouns were incorrectly tagged because of missing accent marks. We did not consider spelling correction in any form because of the diversity of errors and the kind of grammatical and orthographic rules that reviewer authors violate. The only processing that was

---

[1]  http://www.ciao.es/

applied to the tagged opinion reviews collection was to change upper case letters to lower case for all POS except personal nouns.

The advantage of these text reviews is their closed domain in general, i.e. the specific domain they are dedicated to, excluding the spam opinions and some text parts related to the reviewer's life or other descriptions surrounding their opinions. All opinions were considered even we know they include these portions of texts not relevant to the main topic. Another advantage is the reduced sense ambiguity of words if it is compared with open domains.

## 2.1    Terms and Concepts

Term recognition has been performed based on diverse criteria, assigning a score to each term candidate to evaluate its termhood. The score has been based on (1) The distributional properties of term candidates, such as frequency, for example [13] to extract terms from specific domain, (2) The linguistic knowledge, for example, rules describing naming structures for protein names [7], and (3) The combination of the above criteria, for example, C/NC-value [6], merging statistical and linguistic knowledge for the extraction of compound terms.

In our collection, review authors know the product and all the terms related to the product which were the targets of their opinions, so a good part of the vocabulary associated to the domain concepts was included in such reviews. Due to their purpose, the reviews share the main terms, those that could be used to categorize the product, so we decided to use distributional properties of term candidates in the collection. For this reason, the terms should appear in most of the reviews.

Since term refers to a specific concept of a domain, and in general, terms are formed by noun phrases, the recognition of relevant terms was based on three steps: (1) All words tagged as common nouns were extracted, (2) The large list of term candidates was ranked by frequency, and (3) The candidates with frequencies in the lower range were eliminated.

For the SOM collection the initial list had 3931 common nouns, the frequency range to filter out candidates was $1 \leq freq < 10$ and the possible terms extracted were 469. For the COM collection the initial list had 9472 common nouns, the frequency range to filter out candidates was $1 \leq freq < 50$ and the possible terms extracted were 427. The most frequent term candidate was precisely *lavadora* 'washing machine, in English' with 1563 occurrences in SOM and 7361 in COM.

In addition to frequency, TF-IDF is a well-known useful quantity in Information Retrieval to distinguish words with similar frequency in a collection, for example *something* and *revolutions*. TF-IDF is a way to combine word term frequency and document frequency into a single weight. Table 1 shows the ten top terms in COM considering the frequency value and the TF-IDF value.

The Pearson correlation coefficient between term frequencies in SOM and term frequencies in COM was 0.98 and the correlation coefficient between TF-IDF values in SOM and TF-IDF values in COM was 0.94 These results show that a small collection, one fifth of the complete collection is sufficient to obtain the base terms.

In [20], the building process of a taxonomy was based on analyzing a considerable amount of web sites to find candidates of concepts and relationships for a domain defined by an initial keyword which should be representative enough for a domain. In our case such initial keyword is the most frequent noun: *lavadora* 'washing machine'. However due to the specific domain a set of terms should be linked by semantic relations. Since we do not have reference data to compare the possible terms, we set a threshold by looking for a significant drop in the scores and we selected 15% of the top candidates for the rest of the work. Although we could not define the utility of the selected terms, there is an intuition that they are useful for the extraction of semantic relations and deserve to be taken in account.

**Table 1.** Distributional properties of term candidates: frequency and tf-idf in COM

| Term | Freq | Term | TF-IDF |
|------|------|------|--------|
| *lavadora* 'washing machine' | 7361 | *lavado* 'washing' | 3317.3 |
| *ropa* 'cloth' | 4396 | *ropa* 'cloth' | 3266.8 |
| *lavado* 'washing' | 3349 | *programa* 'program' | 3016.7 |
| *agua* 'water' | 2221 | *agua* 'water' | 2965.3 |
| *carga* 'load' | 2083 | *carga* 'load' | 2587.7 |
| *marca* 'brand' | 2011 | *centrifugado* 'spinning' | 2415.2 |
| *programa* 'program' | 1789 | *marca* 'brand' | 2283.0 |
| *precio* 'price' | 1722 | *tiempo* 'time' | 2198.0 |
| *tiempo* 'time' | 1547 | *lavadora* 'washing machine' | 2185.1 |
| *centrifugado* 'spinning' | 1533 | *casa* 'house' | 2145.8 |

## 2.2    Multiword Terms

The C-value [6] is a well-known statistical measure that combines statistical and linguistic information for the extraction of multi-word and nested terms. C-value has been applied to different languages including Spanish [2]. This measure assigns a termhood to a candidate string, based on: the total frequency of occurrence of the candidate string in the corpus, on the frequency of the candidate string as part of other longer candidate terms, on the number of these longer candidate terms, and on the length of the candidate string (in number of words).

The first step in this method is the definition of linguistic patterns for Spanish terms. Authors explained that they depend on the decision to balance precision and recall. Preference on recall would require an open filter (one that permits more types of strings.) We decided to use this filter only excluding PE's, since in general they correspond to *real world examples* (model names, brand names, etc.) and errors of the POS tagger. The only preposition considered was "*de*" 'of' that is required to join nouns and adjectives although it has other uses that caused errors in the extraction of term candidates. The linguistic patterns are the following:

Noun [Noun]+
[Noun | Adjective]+ [Preposition$_{DE}$ Noun]+
Noun Preposition$_{DE}$ [[Noun Adjective] | [Adjective Noun]]+

We automatically obtained with these patterns 24,755 multiword term candidates.

The next step in the method proposed by [6] was obtaining the C-value whose aim was to improve the extraction of nested terms, it was specially built for extracting multi-word terms. The C-value is calculated as follows:

$$
C\_value(a) = \begin{cases} \log_2|a| \cdot f(a) & a \text{ is not nested} \\ \log_2|a| \left( f(a) - \dfrac{1}{P(T_a)} \displaystyle\sum_{b \in T_a} f(b) \right) & \text{otherwise} \end{cases}
$$

Where $a$ is the candidate string, $f(\bullet)$ is its frequency of occurrence in the corpus, $T_a$ is the set of extracted candidate terms that contain $a$, $P(T_a)$ is the number of these candidate terms.

Table 2 shows the results obtained for the ten top multiword term candidates by C-value and frequency. We could note that *prendas delicadas* 'delicate garments' and *ropa delicada* 'delicate clothes' could be considered variants of the same term referred to a common program in washing machines but we know that they could also be used for other purposes. We could observe in these multiword terms that some of them correspond to concepts and others correspond to characteristics of concepts.

**Table 2.** Candidate terms according to their C-value and frequency

| C-value | Term Candidates | Frequency |
| --- | --- | --- |
| 101 | *acero inoxidable* 'stainless steel' | 111 |
| 109 | *prendas delicadas* 'delicate garments' | 117 |
| 114.9 | *ropa delicada* 'delicate clothes' | 117 |
| 118.3 | *consumo de agua* 'water consumption' | 120 |
| 134.5 | *tiempo de lavado* 'washing time' | 136 |
| 151.7 | *velocidad de centrifugado* 'spin speed' | 154 |
| 153 | *eficiencia energética* 'energy efficiency' | 165 |
| 237.3 | *capacidad de carga* 'load capacity' | 243 |
| 258.5 | *carga frontal* 'front load' | 293 |
| 334.5 | *programa de lavado* 'washing program' | 337 |

We found an interesting problem whose solution we have now postponed. There are concepts that have several possible candidates, for example: *inicio diferido* 'delayed start' have several multiword elements related to the same concept. The variants include: *inicio retardado* 'retarded start', *encendido programable* 'programmable switch on', *control de inicio* 'control start', *inicio programado* 'scheduled start', *inicio automático* 'auto start', *preselección de inicio* 'start time-preselection', *opción de inicio* 'start time option', *temporizador de encendido* 'start timer', and other variants in word order of previous examples.

We supposed that such variants should be assumed by the authors of the opinion reviews and by translators of the washing machine instruction manuals from English to Spanish, but we found that those variants also have an origin in the instruction manuals of the manufacturers. We downloaded several washing machine instruction manuals in Spanish of different brands and we found that for the same function they used the following terms: *encendido programado* 'scheduled switch on', *lavado diferido* 'delayed washing', *inicio diferido, retraso tiempo* 'delay time'. We confirmed in washing machine instruction manuals in English that the variants of definitions appeared in them.

We also found variants due to expressions of human nature, where not only synonyms were found but diminutives and other forms, for example: *botón* 'switch' and *tecla* 'button', *botoncito de encendido* 'little on switch'. All variants should be analyzed in context to determine if they strictly refer to the term or to other aspect.

To improve the precision of their results, the authors used a stop list and the NC-value. The stop list contained words which are not expected to occur as term words in the domain. We manually made the stop-list according to such criteria, it consists of 67 words, mainly prepositions (excepting "*de*") and adjectives, for example: *alto* 'high', *amplio* 'wide', *anterior* 'previous', *bonito* 'pretty', *bueno* 'good', etc.

The adjectives were taken from the top high word frequencies in the COM collection. However they could not be taken automatically since there are terms of the domain that contain adjectives with high frequency like *frontal* 'front' in *carga frontal* 'front load' and *delicada* 'delicate' in *ropa delicada* 'delicate clothes'.

The NC-value [6] incorporated context information into the C-value method for the extraction of multi-word terms. The NC-value was only useful in our work to eliminate rare candidates that have a fix context, for example: garbage (e.g. "*abcd abcd abcd*" in a SPAM review), and fixed phrases (e.g. "*punto de vista*" 'point of view'.) We found that term candidate's contexts in these opinion reviews were, with high percentage, adjectives, prepositions, articles and punctuation signs. For this reason, the stop list was more effective than the NC-value.

## 3    Linguistic Patterns and Taxonomical Relations

Construction of a taxonomy of concepts, consisting of hyponym relations, i.e. *is-a* relations, has been based on statistical analysis, on natural language analysis techniques applied to texts, on acquisition methods from complex resources and on combinations of them. Statistical analysis have included to model the data, for example [14] calculated the marginal distribution of data including weighted features that consist of concepts and contexts to represent the data. Natural language analysis include lexico-syntactic patterns, for example, for German language [22]; linguistic parsing, for example [5] modeled the context of a certain term as a vector representing syntactic dependencies. Methods requiring complex resources included WordNet-based approaches, for example, [10] integrated semantic information using WordNet as external knowledge source for semantic relation extraction between nominals. Recently methods for heuristic identification of concepts based on dependency parsing were introduced [3, 17, 18, 19].

Due to the interest to work with unsupervised methods, small collection of texts and because of the limited contexts in the opinion reviews in Spanish we decided to use lexico-syntactic patterns to acquire taxonomic relations from other resources as the Web.

## 3.1    Matching Patterns in the Web for Hypernyms

In unsupervised methods, Hearst's linguistic patterns [11] are very well known to extract taxonomic relations. The taxonomic relations or concepts hierarchies include the *is-a* (kind of) relation where the *hyponym* is the word or phrase whose semantic field is included within that of another word, its *hypernym*. For the example: *washing machine is a home appliance, washing machine* is the hyponym and *home appliance* is the *hypernym*.

These linguistic patterns have widely been applied on English texts. However, as far as we know little work has been done to test that such linguistic patterns are suitable for diverse languages and domains. We were interested in the analysis of such patterns for Spanish. We considered lexico-syntactic patterns according to Hearst but to match in the Web instead of a corpus, by means of the snippets.

For other languages, these patterns have been modified, for example [22] obtained domain specific patterns for German language that define reliable domain specific relations. In Spanish language according to its grammar the patterns should be modified to include gender and number. For the previous reason and as also was considered by [4] we used plural forms of NP's since the general writing forms are common in plural instead of singular. We also extended the patterns to include gender in both feminine and masculine.

The Spanish versions of the Hearst patterns are:

a) $NP_0$ *tales como* $\{NP_1, NP_2, ..., (y \mid o)\}$ $NP_n$
b) $NP \{, NP\} * \{,\}$ *u (otros $\mid$ otras)* $NP_0$
c) *tales* $NP_0$ *como* $\{NP,\}* \{(o \mid y)\}$ $NP$
d) $NP \{, NP\}* \{,\}$ *y (otros $\mid$ otras)* $NP_0$
e) $NP_0 \{,\}$ *incluyendo* $\{NP,\}* \{o \mid y\}$ $NP$
f) $NP_0 \{,\}$ *especialmente* $\{NP,\}* \{o \mid y\}$ $NP$

They imply that for all $NP_i$, $1 \leq i \leq n$ hyponym($NP_i$, $NP_0$) where NP means noun phrase, $NP_0$ is the hypernym, * indicates repetition of cero or more times, the elements in brackets {...} are meant to be optional and the elements separated by | are meant to be either one or another. The words *incluyendo* 'including', *especialmente* 'especially', *y* 'and', *o/u* 'or', *tales como* 'such as', *otras/otros* 'others', were the Spanish versions of the specific English words.

We employed these lexico-syntactic patterns to obtain the taxonomic relations for *lavadoras* 'washing machines' to more general classes and to more detailed classes, i.e. we placed in *lavadoras* as a hyponym in the patterns to obtain their hypernyms and also we placed in *lavadoras* as the hypernym in the patterns to obtain their hyponyms. The former case is described in the rest of this section and the second one is explained in Section 4.

The main idea of obtaining more examples from the Internet was based on searching for variants by including Google's asterisk facility [8]. For the example phrase *electrodomésticos tales como lavadoras, secadoras y refrigeradores* 'appliances such as washing machines, dryers or refrigerators' the string becomes in the search "* tales como lavadoras, *, * y *" using the Google search engine tool limited to the Spanish language where the asterisk substitutes for the eliminated noun phrases.

Google returns hits where there is a string of words initiated by different words, then the sequence *tales como lavadoras* 'such as washing machines', ending with a series of words but not by force include commas and conjunctions.

According to the google guide the use of * will match one or more words in a phrase and could be expected that as more asterisks the search have more hits will return Google, however each asterisk will return other sequences and not precisely those we expected. The search "* *tales como lavadoras, *, * y *" gives different results than the search "* *tales como lavadoras, * y *". The quantity of hits is the same in both searches but at least the order is diverse. The results for the searches: "*, *especialmente lavadoras, * o *" and "*, especialmente lavadoras, *, * o *" give different quantity of hits. Also commas and accent marks could appear or not.

We wrote a program that generated the patterns for each term candidate, then it launched the Google search for each one and it extracted the sequenced words that contained the pattern. The quantity of pages automatically obtained was limited to obtain 30 pages (300 snippets maximum). The results were registers with the pattern, the quantity of hits, and the sequenced words that contain the pattern.

Based on these results we manually analyzed at most the first 100 hits of each pattern for the term *lavadoras* 'washing machines' to determine the performance of the Hearst's patterns in Spanish for this domain and to analyze the use of asterisks to retrieve the possible hypernyms. For these reasons we consider two types of searches: one with the above defined patterns following the series of NP and with a simplified version of asterisks quantity (Table 3). There were a slightly better results with the simplified version.

Table 3 shows the analysis of the first 100 hits for the simplified Hearst's patterns in Spanish. The column "Pattern" corresponds to the Internet search string, the second column presents the quantity of hits, and the third column shows the percentage of the first 100 hits that matched the patterns, excluding those of the "Noise" column. The fourth column shows the percentage of the first 100 hits corresponding to a bad examples of hypernyms mainly due to a bigger context that gives different meaning of the relation between hyponym and possible hypernym. The fifth column corresponds to the percentage of the useless snippets due to retrieval of strings that not matched with the pattern, or due to absence of the pattern in the snippet.

**Table 3.** Examples of the first 100 hits for the simplified Hearst's patterns

| Pattern | Hits | Possible candidates | Noise | Useless |
|---|---|---|---|---|
| (a) "* *tales como lavadoras, * y *" | 859,000 | 51% | 9% | 40% |
| (b) "*, *lavadoras u otros *" | 32,900 | 77% | 3% | 23% |
| "*, *lavadora u otras *" | 37 | 81% | – | 19% |
| (c) "*tales * como lavadoras, * y *" | 8 | – | – | 100% |
| (d) "*, *lavadoras y otros *" | 225000$^+$ | 41% | 5% | 54% |
| "*, *lavadoras y otras *" | 52,900 | 28% | 26% | 46% |
| (e) "*, *incluyendo lavadoras, * o *" | 6 | 17% | 50% | 33% |
| (f) "*, *especialmente lavadoras, * o *" | 2 | – | – | 100% |

We chose to retrieve examples from the Web since it is the option allowed us to find phrases generated by native speakers more quickly. Nevertheless, it is known that searching the Internet has drawbacks but we decided to do so on the basis that we did not know how the results were classified [12], the snippets contains linguistic errors, the results of the use of asterisks not exact match the patterns, and the quantity of hits changes every day.

However, although we assume that these results are mere indicative of specific performance, we based the selection of the adequate Spanish patterns on such percentages and on observations made during the manual analysis. For example, the pattern "*tales * como lavadoras*" retrieved many snippets without matching words with the asterisk, we suppose that due to much less examples. Such behavior then resulted in the pattern "*\* tales como lavadoras*". The patterns (e) and (f) are related to the meanings: part-of, containing-something that could be useful for other semantic relations extraction.

In order to use more patterns we analyzed in the same form the patterns obtained by Ortega [15] excluding the patterns that exactly included diverse forms of the string "is-a" since it requires the selection of the suitable article that could give the highest quantity of results, the appropriate article according to countable and mass nouns and a context that permits to determine that the complement is related to the term. The best results were obtained with the pattern "*lavadora es el único \**" 'washing machine is the only \*' that retrieved 29% of possible candidates from 28 hits.

Following the suggestions of [11] in how to obtain new patterns we obtained the patterns shown in Table 4, where the results correspond to their test with $NP_0$ being the main term: *lavadoras* 'washing machines'.

**Table 4.** Results of the first 100 hits for the proposed patterns

| Pattern | Hits | Possible candidates | Noise | Useless |
|---|---|---|---|---|
| (g) NP {,} *entre otros* $NP_0$ | 196,000 | 26% | 2% | 72% |
| NP {,} *entre otras* $NP_0$ | 14,500 | 37% | 7% | 56% |
| (h) $NP_0$ {,} *ya sea la* NP | 8,910 | 13% | 12% | 75% |
| $NP_0$ {,} *ya sea una* NP | 80 | 32% | 7% | 61% |
| (i) $NP_0$ {,} *en particular la* NP" | 28 | – | 15% | 85% |
| $NP_0$ {,} *en particular una* NP" | 20 | 45% | 5% | 50% |

As we could note these new patterns are less productive than those already selected. A greater recall could be obtained at the cost of a lower precision since the results correspond to the very general resource that is the Web including all domains. Another factor that should be considered is that patterns gives different quantity of hits depending on singular or plural form, for example: "*\* tales como lavadoras, \* y \**" retrieved more hits than the corresponding singular form.

To obtain the taxonomic relations we decided to use the patterns (a), (b) and (g).

## 3.2    Hypernym Ranking

To obtain automatically the possible hypernyms we wrote a program that extracted from the results of the previous step with the three selected patterns those words sequences that exactly match the patterns generated, where the rules to identify the possible hypernyms were a simplification of the linguistic patterns applied in getting C-value: those noun phrases limited to only one prepositional group with "*de*" 'of'. This task was performed using the system obtained by [9] to assign the corresponding POS.

To discriminate the possible hypernyms from noise one general method is ranking them to determine the correct and most domain related hypernyms. Several statistical measures have been considered in unsupervised methods and the Web is one of the main sources to obtain such data. We tested the results using conditional probability, point-wise mutual information but the best results were obtained with the measure of Cimiano *et al* [4]. They used the sum of number of Google hits over all patterns for a certain pair (hyponym, hypernym) and normalized by dividing through the number of hits returned for the hyponym. Table 5 shows some results for the ranking of the possible hypernyms. These examples were selected to show how a figurative sense was low ranked (animals as hypernym) and also a candidate obtained due to lack of context (industrial purposes).

**Table 5.** Possible hypernyms ranking

| hyponym | Possible hypernym | Cimiano et al |
|---------|-------------------|---------------|
| *lavadoras* | *electrodomésticos* 'home appliances' | 2.303e-5 |
| *lavadoras* | *aparatos* 'appliances' | 1.498e-5 |
| *lavadoras* | *artefactos* 'artifacts' | 6.151e-6 |
| *lavadoras* | *bienes duraderos* 'durable goods' | 1.104e-6 |
| *lavadoras* | *fines industriales* 'industrial purposes' | 4.732e-7 |
| *lavadoras* | *animales* 'animals' | 1.578e-7 |

For the best results obtained from the previous step we again applied the same process to obtain their corresponding hypernyms. Table 6 shows some examples of the quantity of possible hypernyms (PH) obtained among the three linguistic patterns applied. All the examples shared possible hypernyms, although the third column only presents the first examples in alphabetical order. For example, the hyponym *equipo* 'equipment' has as possible hypernym the term *dispositivos* 'devices'. The examples showed in Table 6 are some of the members of one group automatically obtained from the term *washing machines* clustering terms sharing possible hypernyms.

To define which member is parent of which other, we wrote a program to compare two cases for each pair of hypernyms: *A is hypernym of B* and *B is hypernym of A*. The process comprised: 1) obtainment of the corresponding three patterns for each case, 2) acquisition of the hits for each search, and 3) calculation of the ranking measure. The examples in Table 7 were obtained from the group above described, we show some of the top results obtained, where the first column correspond to the compared pair terms, the second shows the value of the ranking measure.

**Table 6.** Examples of the quantity of possible hypernyms extracted

| Hyponym | # PH | Examples |
|---------|------|----------|
| *aparato* 'appliance' | 62 | *accesorios* 'accessories', *alimentación* 'feeding', ... |
| *artefacto* 'artifact' | 42 | *acciones* 'actions', *amenidades*, 'amenities', *armas explosivas* 'explosive weapons', .. |
| *electrodoméstico* 'home appliance' | 60 | *accesorios*, *aparatos* 'appliances', *aparatos indispensables* 'essential appliances', ... |
| *equipo* 'equipment' | 58 | *activos fijos* 'fixed assets', *actividades* 'activities', ... |
| *lavadora* 'washing machine' | 58 | *animales* 'animals', *aparatos*, *aparatos de alta energía* 'high energy appliances', ... |

The taxonomic relations obtained were:

*lavadoras* 'washing machines'→*electrodomésticos* 'home appliances' → *aparatos* 'appliances' → *artículos* 'consumer goods' → *productos* 'products'
*aparatos* 'appliances' → *dispositivos* 'devices' → *artículos* 'consumer goods'
*aparatos* 'appliances' → *equipos* 'equipments'→ *artículos* 'consumer goods'
*objetos* 'objects' → *cosas* 'things'
*equipos* 'equipments' → *dispositivos* 'devices' → *productos* 'products'
*productos* 'products' → *bienes* 'goods'→ *cosas* 'things'

**Table 7.** Examples of the top results for the relations among hypernyms

| Hyponym – Hypernym | Ranking measure |
|--------------------|-----------------|
| *objetos – cosas* 'objects – things' | 0.002387 |
| *mercancías – cosas* 'merchandises – things' | 0.002002 |
| *dispositivos – cosas* 'devices – things' | 0.001532 |
| *máquinas – equipos* 'machines – equipments' | 0.001273 |
| *artefactos – cosas* 'artifacts – things' | 0.000994 |
| *aparatos – objetos* 'appliances – objects'' | 0.000740 |

# 4    Instances and Subclasses

In this section we describe the work that we made to obtain the taxonomic relations to more detailed classes, placing in *lavadoras* 'washing machines' as the hypernym in all the Hearst's patterns to obtain their hyponyms. First, we followed the same process developed in the previous section. However we found that only two patterns obtained results but no about hyponyms of washing machines.

The pattern "*lavadoras tales como * y *"* returned 21 hits: 6 for washing machine brands (5 identical snippets), 7 hits for automatic washing machines, 1 for spare parts of washing machines, and 1 for digital washing machines. The pattern "*, * y otras lavadoras*" returned 52 hits: 4 for washing machine brands, 2 for other kind of washers and 1 for a superior load washing machine.

We could observe that automatic washing machines, digital washing machines and superior load washing machine are hyponyms or subclasses in this domain but very few examples were obtained with the Hearst's patterns. So in this section we describe other methods to obtain instances and subclasses.

## 4.1   Instances

To obtain the instances of this domain we used the COM collection and we defined a heuristic to select the personal nouns (PE's) that users included in the reviews as the instances of the previous noun phrases that they followed. We wrote a program to obtain the possible instances by four steps:

1.  Extraction of noun phrases including PE's by means of the pattern: Noun+[PE]+ Clustering the results with a frequency greater than one that share the same nouns and also the longest sequences of Noun+ PE.  For example: *marca Fago*r 'Fagor brand' and *marca Bosch* 'Bosch brand' share the same noun *marca* 'brand'.
2.  Elimination of the results whose shared strings  do not correspond to terms, applying a filter based on the terms extracted in section 2.1
3.  Ranking of the results to eliminate writing style and orthographic errors by means of a cohesion measure calculated from the hits retrieved by searches on the Web.

**Table 8.** Some results for instance extraction

| Hyponym - Hypernym | Instance |
|---|---|
| *lavadora LG* 'LG washing machine' | LG |
| *marca Fagor* 'Fagor brand' | Fagor |
| *lavadora marca fagor* 'fagor brand washing machine' | Fagor |

## 4.2   Subclasses

In [1], the authors analyzed the language used for classification relations in Spanish and collected the most common ways in it to express the *subclass-of* relation. The *subclass-of* relation patterns were obtained from a Science and Technology corpus for the following verbs: *clasificar* 'classify', *distinguir* 'distinguish', and *divider* 'divide'. The patterns are the following:

1.  *Los/las* NP<superclass> *se clasifican en* |*como* | *se dividen en* [CD] [*los/las siguientes*] [CN] [PARA] [(NP<subclass>,)* *y*] NP<subclass>
2.  *Se distinguen* CD CN *de* NP<superclass> : [(NP<subclass>,)* *y*] NP<subclass> CD CN *de* NP<superclass> *se distinguen* : [(NP<subclass>,)* *y*] NP<subclass>

Here, CN stands for Class Name, and includes the generic names: group, type, class; CD stands for Cardinal Number; PARA stands for Paralinguistic Sign. *Los/las* 'the', *siguientes* 'following', *y* 'and', *se* (reflexive pronoun), *en* 'in', *de* 'of'

We transformed such patterns in the same manner described in section 3 to obtain strings from Web searches. The best results were obtained for the simplified versions shown in Table 8. Where the third column (#SC) shows the subclass-of relations obtained and the third column indicates the quantity of hits of noise snippets.

From the subclasses obtained only the multiword term *carga frontal* 'front load' correspond to a subclass.

**Table 9.** Result of linguistic patterns for *subclass-of* relation

| Subclass (SC) Pattern | #hits | #SC | Noise | Example |
|---|---|---|---|---|
| "lavadoras se clasifican en * y *" | 11 | 2 | 1 | *carga frontal y carga superior* 'front loading and top loading' |
| "lavadoras se dividen en *" | 15 | 2 | 8 | *automáticas o semiautomáticas* 'automatic or semiautomatic |
| "se distinguen * lavadoras: * y * " | 2 | 1 | 1 | *carga frontal y carga superior* 'front loading and top loading' |

# 5    Results and Discussion

In ontology building a general evaluation method for domain taxonomies is based on comparison with manually created taxonomies by experts in the domain or by comparison with complex resources as WordNet. In the washing machines domain, there is no a created taxonomy by experts. The more related work is that of Shah et al [21] that was intended to develop an ontology for Home Energy Management Domain, their interest is devoted to energy consumption, to obtain the detailed specification of the attributes that contributes towards the overall energy consumption. However their work was made manually, they started with the study of general classifications of home electrical appliances provided by various home appliances vendors and manufacturers and included definitions of concepts and properties adopted in part from a general ontology.

We divided the evaluation in two parts, one for the single word and multiword terms, and a second evaluation for the semantic relations. The evaluation of the terms was made using washing machine manuals. We extracted titles and information appearing in single lines assuming that they contain important concepts. The terms resulting after this comparison were 45% of the list obtained in section 2. However for the same list three human evaluators considered that the 65% were thought interesting of the domain.

The evaluation of the semantic relations was a comparison among the hierarchies obtained by tools accessed by the Web, for example WordNet[2], BabelNet[3] and Multilingual Central Repository[4] (MCR). From all of them we obtained the results for *lavadora, centrifugado,* and other 8 concepts.

We observed that although all the tools included the concept *washing machine* the quantity of relations is diverse. For example in WordNet there is the hierarchy:

---

[2]  http://wordnetweb.princeton.edu/perl/webwn
[3]  http://babelnet.org/explore.jsp
[4]  http://adimen.si.ehu.es/cgi-bin/wei/public/wei.consult.perl

*washing machine* → *white goods* → *home appliance* → *appliance* → *durables* → *consumer goods* → *commodity* → *artifact* → *whole unit* →*object*

The MCR has the following structure for *lavadora*:

*lavadora* → *electrodoméstico* 'home appliance' → *aparato* 'appliance' → *artículo* 'consumer goods', *bien* 'goods', *mercancía* 'merchandise' →*artefacto* 'artifact' →*unidad completa* 'whole unit' → *objeto* 'object'

Although there was not an ontology to make a real evaluation, the experimental results shows that the generated relations have the basic qualities of a concept hierarchy. In addition, there are other concepts included in our results: *equipment, machine, device, product*, and others. Table 10 shows some of the results on which we based the taxonomic relations obtained and described in section 3.2 The strongness of the taxonomic relationship was indicated by the higher value rank. We included some results at the bottom of Table 10 to compare the values of the relationships, for example *bienes – cosas* 'goods – things' versus *cosas – bienes* 'things – goods'.

**Table 10.** Results for the hyponym-hypernym relations

| Hyponym - Hypernym | Ranking measure |
|---|---|
| *objetos – cosas* 'objects - things' | 0.002387 |
| *dispositivos – cosas* 'devices - things' | 0.001532 |
| *máquinas – equipos* 'machines - equipments' | 0.001273 |
| *artefactos – cosas* 'artifacts - things' | 0.000994 |
| *aparatos – dispositivos* 'appliances - devices' | 0.000339 |
| *bienes – cosas* 'goods - things' | 0.000213 |
| *electrodomésticos – aparatos* 'home appliances -appliances' | 0.000127 |
| *equipos – dispositivos* 'equipments - devices' | 0.000119 |
| *artículos – productos* 'consumer goods - products' | 0.000115 |
| *equipos – artículos* 'equipments – consumer goods'' | 0.000029 |
| *lavadoras – electrodomésticos* 'washing machines – home appliances' | 0.000023 |
| *dispositivos – aparatos* 'devices - appliances' | 0.000001240 |
| *aparatos – equipos* 'appliances - equipments' | 0.000002276 |
| *dispositivos – productos* 'devices - products' | 0.000001971 |
| *aparatos – artículos* 'appliances – consumer - goods' | 0.000001961 |
| *dispositivos – artículos* 'devices- consumer goods | 0.000000572 |
| *cosas – bienes* 'things - goods' | 0.000000067 |

## 6     Conclusions

In this paper we presented a non-supervised, web-based approach to the automatic extraction of semantic relations: *is-a* and *instances* in the domain of *washing machines*. The methods we considered were: (1) statistics of the collection, (2) extraction of concepts and relations by linguistic patterns for Spanish, (3) Web-based ranking of the results for extraction of useful examples, and (4) clustering of syntactic constructions: noun compounds and prepositional phrases for determination of detailed relations.

The sources were opinion reviews in Spanish and searches to the Web. The extraction of terms and instances was difficult due to the reduced context of the reviews and the tagging mistakes because of lower linguistic quality, noise and spam in the reviews. We analyzed the appropriateness of diverse linguistic patterns for the Spanish domain we worked. We obtained results that were contrasted with several materials in the absence of a created taxonomy with which to compare.

**Acknowledgment.** Work partially supported by Mexican Government: CONACYT, SNI, PAPIIT-UNAM, SIP-IPN 20144534.

# References

1. Aguado de Cea, G., Álvarez de Mon, I., Montiel-Ponsoda, E.: From linguistic patterns to ontology structures. In: Proceedings of the 8th International Conference on Terminology and Artificial Intelligence (2009), http://ceur-ws.org/Vol-578/paper15.pdf
2. Barrón-Cedeño, G., Sierra, P., Drouin, S.: Ananiadou. An Improved Automatic Term Recognition Method for Spanish. Proceeding of Computational Linguistics and Intelligent Text Processing, 125–136 (2009)
3. Cambria, E., Poria, S., Gelbukh, A., Kwok, K.: Sentic API: A Common-Sense Based API for Concept-Level Sentiment Analysis. In: Proceedings of the 4th Workshop on Making Sense of Microposts (#Microposts2014), co-located with the 23rd International World Wide Web Conference (WWW 2014), Seoul, Korea. CEUR Workshop Proceedings, vol. 1141, pp. 19–24, CEUR-WS.org (April 7, 2014)
4. Cimiano, P., Pivk, A., Schmidt-Thieme, L., Staab, S.: Learning Taxonomic Relations from Heterogeneous Sources of Evidence. In: Buitelaar, P., Cimiano, P., Magnini, B. (eds.) Ontology Learning from Text: Methods, Evaluation and Applications. Frontiers in Artificial Intelligence, vol. 123, pp. 59–73. IOS Press, Amsterdam (2005a)
5. Cimiano, P., Hotho, A., Staab, S.: Learning Concept Hierarchies from Text Corpora using Formal Concept Analysis. J. Artif. Intell. Res. (JAIR) 24, 305–339 (2005b)
6. Frantzi, K., Ananiadou, S., Mima, H.: Automatic recognition of multi-word terms: the C-value/NC-value method. International Journal on Digital Libraries 3(2), 115–130 (2000)
7. Gaizauskas, R., Demetriou, G., Humphreys, K.: Term recognition and classification in biological science journal articles. In: Proceedings of Workshop on Computational Terminology for Medical and Biological Applications, pp. 37–44 (2000)
8. Gelbukh, A.F., Bolshakov, I.A.: Internet, a true friend of translator: the Google wildcard operator. International Journal of Translation 18(1-2), 41–48 (2006)
9. Gelbukh, A., Sidorov, G.: Approach to construction of automatic morphological analysis systems for inflective languages with little effort. In: Gelbukh, A. (ed.) CICLing 2003. LNCS, vol. 2588, pp. 215–220. Springer, Heidelberg (2003)
10. Giuliano, C., Lavelli, A., Pighin, D., Romano, L.: FBK-IRST: Kernel Methods for Semantic Relation Extraction. In: Proceedings of the 4th International Workshop on Semantic Evaluations (SemEval-2007), pp. 141–144 (2007)
11. Hearst, M.: Automatic acquisition of hyponyms from large text corpora. In: 14th International Conference on Computational Linguistics, France, pp. 539–545 (1992)
12. Kilgarriff, A.: Googleology is bad science. Computational Linguistics 33, 147–151 (2007)

13. Kim, S.N., Baldwin, T., Kan, M.-y.: An Unsupervised Approach to Domain-Specific Term Extraction. In: Proceedings of the Australasian Language Technology Association Workshop (ALTW:B), pp. 94–98 (2009)

14. Liu, X., Song, Y., Liu, S., Wang, H.: Automatic Taxonomy Construction from Keywords. In: Proceedings of the 18th ACM SIGKDD International Conference on Knowledge Discovery and Data Mining, pp. 1433–1441 (2012)

15. Ortega, R., Aguilar, C., Villaseñor, L., Montes, M., Sierra, G.: Hacia la identificación de relaciones de hiponimia/hiperonimia en Internet. Revista Signos. Estudios de Lingüística 44(75), 68–84 (2011)

16. Padró, L., Collado, M., Reese, S., Lloberes, M., Castellón, I.: FreeLing 2.1: Five Years of Open-Source Language Processing Tools. In: Proceedings of 7th Language Resources and Evaluation Conference (LREC 2010), ELRA La Valletta, Malta (2010)

17. Poria, S., Agarwal, B., Gelbukh, A., Hussain, A., Howard, N.: Dependency-Based Semantic Parsing for Concept-Level Text Analysis. In: Gelbukh, A. (ed.) CICLing 2014, Part I. LNCS, vol. 8403, pp. 113–127. Springer, Heidelberg (2014)

18. Poria, S., Cambria, E., Winterstein, G., Huang, G.-B.: Sentic patterns: Dependency-based rules for concept-level sentiment analysis. Knowledge-Based Systems 69, 45–63 (2014)

19. Poria, S., Ofek, N., Gelbukh, A., Hussain, A., Rokach, L.: Dependency tree-based rules for concept-level aspect-based sentiment analysis. In: Presutti, V., Stankovic, M., Cambria, E., Cantador, I., Di Iorio, A., Di Noia, T., Lange, C., Reforgiato Recupero, D., Tordai, A. (eds.) SemWebEval 2014. CCIS, vol. 475, pp. 41–47. Springer, Heidelberg (2014)

20. Sánchez, D., Moreno, A.: A methodology for knowledge acquisition from the web. KES Journal 10(6), 453–475 (2006)

21. Shah, N., Chao, K.-M., Zlamaniec, T., Matei, A.: Ontology for Home Energy Management Domain. DICTAP (2), 337–347 (2011)

22. Xu, F., Kurz, D., Piskorski, J., Schmeier, S.: A Domain Adaptive Approach to Automatic Acquisition of Domain Relevant Terms and their Relations with Bootstrapping. In: Proceedings of the 3rd International Conference on Language Resources an Evaluation, LREC 2002 (2002)

# Evaluating Polarity
# for Verbal Phraseological Units*

Belém Priego Sánchez[1,2], David Pinto[2], and Salah Mejri[1]

[1] LDI, Université Paris 13, Sorbonne Paris Cité,
99 avenue Jean-Baptiste Clément, Paris, France
{abpriegosanchez,smejri}@ldi.univ-paris13.fr
[2] FCC, Benemérita Universidad Autónoma de Puebla,
Av. San Claudio y 14 Sur, Col. San Manuel, Puebla, México
dpinto@cs.buap.mx

**Abstract.** Fixation in linguistic expressions is an inherent property of natural language that plays a central role in their description. Verbal phraseological units are phrases made up of two or more words characterized for presenting certain degree of fixation or idiomaticity (at least one of these words is a verb that plays the role of the predicate).

Phraseological units do not appear so frequently in manually constructed lexical resources as they do in real-word text, and this problem of coverage may impact the performance of many natural language processing tasks. Therefore, the construction of automatic understanding systems for these types of linguistic structures is very important, since they are a standard way of expressing a concept or idea. In this paper we present a set of experiments towards the automatic identification of the polarity of verbal phraseological units. We obtained a maximum performance of 80% for this particular task when the contextual information of a phraseological unit is considered, in comparison with a 62% when the VPU alone is only used. These results highlight the importance of analyzing automatically this type of linguistic structures. It should be stressed at the outset that these experiments are intended as a preliminary study rather than as a comprehensive analysis or solution of the aforementioned problem.

**Keywords:** Verbal phraseological units, Text polarity, Machine learning.

## 1   Introduction

Phraseological Units (PU), also known as phrasemes or fixed expressions, are basically multi-word lexical units that are characterized for presenting certain degree of fixation or idiomaticity. In other words, PU's are a combination of words whose meaning are not necessarily deduced from the meaning of its components, i.e., the words together can mean more than their sum of parts [1].

---

* This paper has been partially supported by the CONACYT grant #218862.

A. Gelbukh et al. (Eds.): MICAI 2014, Part I, LNAI 8856, pp. 191–200, 2014.
© Springer International Publishing Switzerland 2014

Thus, PU's almost never presents the following criteria: compositionality, substitutability and modifiability, therefore, avoiding any modification to its structure. A phraseological unit is a lexicalized, reproducible bilexemic or polylexemic word group in common use, which has a relative syntactic and semantic stability. This type of linguistic structure may be idiomatized, may carry connotations, and may have an emphatic or intensifying function in a text.

Phraseological units are a stable group of words with partially or fully transferred meanings, for example, "Greek gift" (a gift given with the intention of tricking and causing harm to the recipient), "to kick the bucket" (to die) or "it is raining cats and dogs" (it is raining very hard).

Phraseological Units (PU) belong to what Coseriu [2] called "repeated discourse", and they are mainly characterized by the following three features:

1. Their poly-lexical behaviour that distinguish them from isolated words of the language, either simple or compound words.
2. Their fixation degree, that presents them as they were atomic units (inseparables) just like simple units are.
3. Their idiomaticity or lexical opacity, a feature that sometimes may be missing, as it occurs in the so-called collocations, a type of phrases that we will describe in the following paragraphs.

The study of this type of linguistic expressions has a growing importance in recent years, in part because the linguistic and computational linguistic community has understood that this phenomenon covers all the sentence components [3], a fact that involves different dimensions of the natural language: linguistics, pragmatics, culturals, among others [4]. PU's are not nearly as frequent in lexical resources as they are in real-word text, and this problem of coverage may impact the performance of many natural language processing tasks.

In this paper we focus our experiments on detecting the polarity of Verbal Phraseological Units (VPU's). For this purpose, we have executed several experiments using various supervised classifiers, so that we can have an idea of the best performance we can obtain for determining the polarity of such linguistic expressions. The experiments were carried out using a corpus of VPU's manually tagged with three possible classes (positive, negative and neutral).

The remaining of this paper is structured as follows. Section 2 presents the state of the art in determining polarity of verbal phraseological units. Section 3 describes the experiments carried out in this paper towards the automatic identification of the polarity of VPU's. Finally, in Section 4 we give the conclusions and findings of this research work.

## 2    Verbal Phraseological Units

In this research work, we are particularly interested in studying spanish phraseological units containing one verb as the grammar nucleus, i.e., verbal phraseological units which present a high degree of fixation in comparison with other phraseological units [5], for example, *Leer entre líneas (To read between the lines)*.

There are several studies that primarily focus their approaches on the stable group of phraseological units made up of two or more words that function as a lexical unit with its own meaning, not derived from the sum of its components, i.e., the study is based on a sentence as a basic linguistic unit. As mentioned by Mejri [6], fixed expressions are similar to mono-lexical predicates due to their syntactic-semantic behaviour, its linguistic description is done with the help of the same tools used to describe simple lexical units.

In collocations, the syntactic positions are lexically unsaturated, but verbal phraseological units perfectly illustrate the overall saturation as indicated in [6,7]. Taking this characteristic into account together with the fact that verbal phrases have a paradigmatic rupture, we can focus our attention in this type of phraseological units.

As many other authors, Mogorron [8] has mentioned that the whole meaning of VPU's cannot be deduced from the meaning of their components. Additionally, we remark that these units have the idiomaticity as their main property. This author concentrates his effort in constructing dictionaries of VPU's, a very time consuming task which highlights the interest of the linguistic community in this field.

In this paper, we assume that the VPU has already been identified into the raw text, and therefore, we can evaluate their polarity. This task is not easy, since the polarity of a VPU may vary in function of its context. However, the experiments will show that we can obtain a reasonable performance by using only the VPU itself.

Polarity detection is a basic task of sentiment analysis which aims to automatically identify whether the expressed opinion in a document, a sentence or an entity feature/aspect is positive, negative, or neutral. To our knowledge, there are not related works for the automatic identification of polarity for VPU's, but there are some other works dealing with the polarity of phrases or sentences in general. Turney [9] and Pang [10] are two early works in this research line who applied different methods (at document level) for detecting the polarity of product reviews and movie reviews, respectively. Other authors such as Hu et al. [11] have attempted to identify polarity for adjectives using some linguistic resources such as Wordnet. This very fast approach does not need of training data necessary for obtain a good predictive accuracy (around 69%), but the main disadvantages is that it does not deal with multiple word sense, context issues, and it does not work for multiple word phrases (or non-adjective words).

The rise of social media such as blogs and social networks has fueled interest in sentiment analysis. In particular, there exist a number of works in literature associated to the automatic identification of emotions in Twitter, mainly due to the massification of this social network around the world and the easy manner we can access to the Tweets from API's provided by Twitter itself. Some of these works have focused on the contribution of some particular features, such as Part of Speech (PoS) tags, emoticons, etc. on the aforementioned task. In [12], for example, the a priori likelihood of each PoS is calculated. They use up to 100 additional features that include emoticons and a dictionary of positive and negative words. They have reported a 60% of accuracy in the task. On the other hand, in [13], a strategy based on discursive relations, such as conectiveness and conditionals, with low number of lexical resources is proposed. These relations are integrated in classical models of representation like bag of words with the aim of improving the accuracy values obtained in the process of classification. The influence of semantic operators such as modals and negations are analyzed, in particular, the degree in which they affect the emotion present in a given paragraph or sentence.

One of the major advances obtained in the task of sentiment analysis has been done in the framework of the SemEval competition. In 2013, several teams have participated with different approaches [14,15,16,17,18,19,20,21,22,23,24,25,26]. Most of these works have contributed in the mentioned task by proposing methods, techniques for representing and classifying documents towards the automatic classification of sentiment in Tweets.

Thus, the sentiment analysis algorithms reported in literature mostly use simple terms to express sentiment about a product or service. However, cultural factors, linguistic nuances and differing contexts make it extremely difficult to turn a string of written text into a simple pro or con sentiment. The fact that humans often disagree on the sentiment of a given text, illustrates how difficult this task should be for computers to get it right. The shorter the string of text, the harder it becomes. In particular, detecting polarity for VPU's is assumed to be a high complex task.

## 3   Detecting the Polarity of VPU's

In this paper we present a set of experiments towards the automatic identification of the polarity for verbal phraseological units. We have selected an approach based on machine learning, thus a set of samples manually tagged were constructed. The description of the dataset used for training is given in Section 3.1. Thereafter, in Section 3.2 we describe the classifiers used in the experiments. Finally, in Section 3.3 we present the results and findings of the experiments carried out.

### 3.1   Data Set

The data set employed in the experiments is made up of two corpora: 1) A list of verbal fixed expressions manually tagged with a particular class of polarity (positive, negative and neutral), and 2) A set of sentences in which appear one verbal fixed expression, i.e., a VPU with its corresponding context.

We have extracted the verbal fixed expressions from a dictionary named "Dictionary of Mexicanisms (Diccionario de Mexicanismos)". This dictionary was constructed by the Mexican Academy of the Language[1] and it has the following three essential features:

---

[1] http://www.academia.org.mx/

a) Synchronic. It represents the current use of lexical elements (the second half of the twentieth century and early twenty-first century).

b) Contrastive. The dictionary was constructed having in mind a comparison of how something is said in Mexico with respect to the manner it is expressed in other countries that speak variations of the spanish language, in particular, with Spain.

c) Descriptive. It describes each entry of the dictionary without normative criteria, i.e., indicating the real use of the words, taking into consideration words coming from other languages and neologisms.

**Corpus 1.** In particular, we have collected 1,219 different verbal fixed expressions from this dictionary, and all of them have been tagged with one of the following polarity classes: positive, negative or neutral.

In Table 1 we can see an example of some VPU's that occur frequently. Actually, the Mexican VPU "quedar bien" (to look good) is a very frequent VPU in Mexico, which regularly may have a negative connotation suggesting a degree of insincerity or something more superficial and "dishonest" than, for example, "to make an impression".

**Table 1.** Example of Mexican verbal phraseological units

| VPU | Polarity |
| --- | --- |
| quedar bien (to look good) | negative |
| dar de alta (to discharge) | neutral |
| ponerse las pilas (get up to speed) | positive |
| remar contra corriente (to go against the tide) | negative |
| dar el grito (screaming blue murder) | negative |
| poner en su lugar (to put in his/her place) | neutral |
| dejar así (to let matters take their course) | neutral |

**Corpus 2.** The second corpus is a set of texts in which exist at least one VPU inside. As we mentioned before, the aim is to evaluate whether or not the words in the VPU context may leverage or harm the prediction of the VPU polarity. In this preliminary experiments, the dataset is made up of only 256 texts, but we are working to increase the number of contexts for each VPU. In Table 2 we can see some examples of these texts written in Mexican spanish, whereas in Table 3 we can see the meaning of the VPU in English and the corresponding polarity associated. The following section describes the classifiers used in the experiments.

**Table 2.** Example of texts with one Mexican VPU. The English translation of the verbal phraseological units together with its polarity mark is given in Table 3.

| #   | Text containing one VPU inside |
| --- | --- |
| 1 | Se vendieron **como pan caliente** los 8 Ferrari 458 Speciale. |
| 2 | El Papa **toma el toro por los cuernos.** |
| 3 | Mi cell **valió queso.**!! |
| 4 | En la escuela ya me **agarraron de su puerquito.** Todos me dicen apodos. |
| 5 | Europa tiene dificultades para **abrir paso** a nuevas industrias de alta tecnología. |

**Table 3.** Example of texts with one Mexican VPU (cont...)

| #   | meaning of the VPU | Polarity |
| --- | --- | --- |
| 1 | Selling like hotcakes | positive |
| 2 | To take the bull by the horns | positive |
| 3 | Broke down | negative |
| 4 | you kick me when I am down | negative |
| 5 | to make way/to push | neutral |

### 3.2   Description of the Classifiers Employed

In order to have a perspective of the type of classifier that can best deal with the problem of automatic detection of VPU polarity, we have selected one learning algorithm from four different types: Bayes, Lazy, Functions and Trees. The following four learning algorithms were chosen:

**J48:**   This is the C4.5 decision tree learner which implements the revision 8 of C4.5.

**SMO:**   This is a sequential minimal optimization algorithm for support vector classification.

**K-Star:**   This is the $k$-nearest neighbor classifier with a generalized distance function.

**NaïveBayes:**   This is the standard probabilistic Naïve Bayes classifier.

All the texts were represented by means of a vector of $n$-grams frequencies, with $n = 1, 2$ and 3. Frequencies greater than two for the $n$-grams were only considered for the vector features. The results obtained in the experiments follows.

### 3.3   Experimental Results

We have carried out two different experiments. Firstly, we have calculated the polarity of the verbal phraseological units itself, i.e., without any other words surrounding the VPU. The aim of this experiment is to determine the maximum value of accuracy that may be obtained when none other classification feature but the VPU components are used. Secondly, we have executed an experiment with a set of texts that contain each one at least one VPU. In this case, we are interested in evaluating whether or not the context of the VPU may help or damage the accuracy when predicting their polarity.

In Table 4 we can see the results obtained when classifying the polarity of VPU's using only their components. As we can see, the maximum percentage of accuracy obtained is around 62% with both, the lazy K-Star classifier, and the support vector machine classifier.

**Table 4.** Results obtained when classifying VPU's (without context)

| Classifier | Type | Correct | Incorrect |
|---|---|---|---|
| Naïve Bayes | Bayes | 61.44 | 38.55 |
| K-Star | Lazy | 62.67 | 37.32 |
| SMO | Functions | 62.75 | 37.24 |
| J48 | Trees | 52.33 | 47.66 |

In Table 5 we can see the results obtained when classifying the polarity of VPU's using their components together with their context. As we can see, the maximum percentage of accuracy obtained is around 80% with the support vector machine classifier. The lowest value obtained was with the lazy K-Star classifier, but even so, it has obtained a much better performance than the best result obtained when the VPU alone has been considered. Thus, we can verify that, indeed, the context may help to improve the performance when classifying the polarity of VPU's. We consider that this result is derived from the fact that the context is well defined (a small number of related words).

**Table 5.** Results obtained when classifying VPU's (with context)

| Classifier | Type | Correct | Incorrect |
|---|---|---|---|
| Naïve Bayes | Bayes | 78.57 | 21.42 |
| K-Star | Lazy | 77.03 | 22.93 |
| SMO | Functions | 80.45 | 19.54 |
| J48 | Trees | 78.94 | 21.05 |

## 4    Conclusions

In this paper we have presented experiments towards the automatic identification of polarity for verbal phraseological units. Two different experiments were carried out: firstly we have evaluated the performance of different classifiers when the training data consider only the VPU. Secondly, we have considered to include the context of the VPU in order to determine whether or not such contextual words may help or harm the performance of the classification process.

The experiments show that the contextual words help indeed to improve the accuracy of the polarity classification of VPU's. Even the worse result obtained when using the VPU with their contexts outperformed the best result when the context is not considered.

As future work we are planning to include more samples for each VPU in order to validate the results obtained in these experiments.

# References

1. Martinez-Blasco, I.: Verbos soporte y fijació lexica. In: Las construcciones verbo-nominales libres y fijas, 47–59 (2008)
2. Coseriu, E.: Principios de semántica estructural. Gredos, Madrid, 113 (1977)
3. Mejri, S.: Le figement lexical. descriptions linguistiques et structuration sémantique. Publications de la faculté des lettres de Manouba, Tunis (1997)
4. Mejri, S.: Catégories linguistiques et étiquetage de corpus. In: L'information Grammaticale, Peeters, Paris (2007)
5. Sfar, I.: Polylexicalite et continuite prédicative: le cas des locutions verbales figées. In: Las construcciones verbo-nominales libres y fijas. Aproximación contrastiva y traductológica, 213–221 (2008)
6. Mejri, S.: Constructions à verbes supports, collocations et locutions verbales. In: La traduction des MEJRI Salah (2008)
7. Gelbukh, A., Sidorov, G., Han, S.-Y., Hernández-Rubio, E.: Automatic enrichment of very large dictionary of word combinations on the basis of dependency formalism. In: Monroy, R., Arroyo-Figueroa, G., Sucar, L.E., Sossa, H. (eds.) MICAI 2004. LNCS (LNAI), vol. 2972, pp. 430–437. Springer, Heidelberg (2004)
8. Huerta, P.M.: Estudio contrastivo lingüístico y semántico de las construcciones verbales fijas diatópicas mexicanas/española. In: Las construcciones verbo-nominales libres y fijas, 179–198 (2010)
9. Turney, P.D.: Thumbs up or thumbs down?: Semantic orientation applied to unsupervised classification of reviews. In: Proceedings of the 40th Annual Meeting on Association for Computational Linguistics, ACL 2002, pp. 417–424. Association for Computational Linguistics, Stroudsburg (2002)
10. Pang, B., Lee, L., Vaithyanathan, S.: Thumbs up? sentiment classification using machine learning techniques. In: Proceedings of EMNLP, pp. 79–86 (2002)
11. Hu, M., Liu, B.: Mining and summarizing customer reviews. In: Proceedings of the Tenth ACM SIGKDD International Conference on Knowledge Discovery and Data Mining, KDD 2004, pp. 168–177. ACM, New York (2004)
12. Agarwal, A., Xie, B., Vovsha, I., Rambow, O., Passonneau, R.: Sentiment analysis of twitter data. In: Proceedings of the Workshop on Language in Social Media (LSM 2011), Portland, Oregon, pp. 30–38 (2011)
13. Mukherjee, S., Bhattacharyya, P.: Sentiment analysis in Twitter with lightweight discourse analysis. In: Proceedings of COLING 2012, Mumbai, India, pp. 1847–1864. The COLING 2012 Organizing Committee (2012)
14. Becker, L., Erhart, G., Skiba, D., Matula, V.: Avaya: Sentiment analysis on twitter with self-training and polarity lexicon expansion. In: Second Joint Conference on Lexical and Computational Semantics (*SEM), Volume 2: Proceedings of the Seventh International Workshop on Semantic Evaluation (SemEval 2013), Atlanta, Georgia, USA, vol. 2, pp. 333–340 (2013)

15. Han, Q., Guo, J., Schuetze, H.: Codex: Combining an svm classifier and character n-gram language models for sentiment analysis on twitter. In: Second Joint Conference on Lexical and Computational Semantics (*SEM), Volume 2: Proceedings of the Seventh International Workshop on Semantic Evaluation (SemEval 2013), Atlanta, Georgia, USA, pp. 520–524 (2013)
16. Chawla, K., Ramteke, A., Bhattacharyya, P.: Iitb-sentiment-analysts: Participation in sentiment analysis in twitter semeval 2013 task. In: Second Joint Conference on Lexical and Computational Semantics (*SEM), Volume 2: Proceedings of the Seventh International Workshop on Semantic Evaluation (SemEval 2013), Atlanta, Georgia, USA, pp. 495–500 (2013)
17. Balahur, A., Turchi, M.: Improving sentiment analysis in twitter using multilingual machine translated data. In: Proceedings of the International Conference Recent Advances in Natural Language Processing RANLP 2013, Hissar, Bulgaria, pp. 49–55. INCOMA Ltd, Shoumen (2013)
18. Balage Filho, P., Pardo, T.: Nilc_usp: A hybrid system for sentiment analysis in twitter messages. In: Second Joint Conference on Lexical and Computational Semantics (*SEM), Volume 2: Proceedings of the Seventh International Workshop on Semantic Evaluation (SemEval 2013), Atlanta, Georgia, USA, pp. 568–572 (2013)
19. Moreira, S., Filgueiras, J.A., Martins, B., Couto, F., Silva, M.J.: Reaction: A naive machine learning approach for sentiment classification. In: Second Joint Conference on Lexical and Computational Semantics (*SEM), Volume 2: Proceedings of the Seventh International Workshop on Semantic Evaluation (SemEval 2013), Atlanta, Georgia, USA, pp. 490–494 (2013)
20. Reckman, H., Baird, C., Crawford, J., Crowell, R., Micciulla, L., Sethi, S., Veress, F.: teragram: Rule-based detection of sentiment phrases using sas sentiment analysis. In: Second Joint Conference on Lexical and Computational Semantics (*SEM), Volume 2: Proceedings of the Seventh International Workshop on Semantic Evaluation (SemEval 2013), Atlanta, Georgia, USA, pp. 513–519 (2013)
21. Tiantian, Z., Fangxi, Z., Lan, M.: Ecnucs: A surface information based system description of sentiment analysis in twitter in the semeval-2013 (task 2). In: Second Joint Conference on Lexical and Computational Semantics (*SEM), Volume 2: Proceedings of the Seventh International Workshop on Semantic Evaluation (SemEval 2013), Atlanta, Georgia, USA, pp. 408–413 (2013)
22. Marchand, M., Ginsca, A., Besançon, R., Mesnard, O.: [lvic-limsi]: Using syntactic features and multi-polarity words for sentiment analysis in twitter. In: Second Joint Conference on Lexical and Computational Semantics (*SEM), Volume 2: Proceedings of the Seventh International Workshop on Semantic Evaluation (SemEval 2013), Atlanta, Georgia, USA, pp. 418–424 (2013)
23. Clark, S., Wicentwoski, R.: Swatcs: Combining simple classifiers with estimated accuracy. In: Second Joint Conference on Lexical and Computational Semantics (*SEM), Volume 2: Proceedings of the Seventh International Workshop on Semantic Evaluation (SemEval 2013), Atlanta, Georgia, USA, pp. 425–429 (2013)
24. Hamdan, H., Béchet, F., Bellot, P.: Experiments with dbpedia, wordnet and sentiwordnet as resources for sentiment analysis in micro-blogging. In: Second Joint Conference on Lexical and Computational Semantics (*SEM), Volume 2: Proceedings of the Seventh International Workshop on Semantic Evaluation (SemEval 2013), Atlanta, Georgia, USA, pp. 455–459 (2013)

25. Martínez-Cámara, E., Montejo-Ráez, A., Martín-Valdivia, M.T., Ureña López, L.A.: Sinai: Machine learning and emotion of the crowd for sentiment analysis in microblogs. In: Second Joint Conference on Lexical and Computational Semantics (*SEM), Volume 2: Proceedings of the Seventh International Workshop on Semantic Evaluation (SemEval 2013), Atlanta, Georgia, USA, pp. 402–407 (2013)
26. Levallois, C.: Umigon: sentiment analysis for tweets based on terms lists and heuristics. In: Second Joint Conference on Lexical and Computational Semantics (*SEM), Volume 2: Proceedings of the Seventh International Workshop on Semantic Evaluation (SemEval 2013), Atlanta, Georgia, USA, pp. 414–417 (2013)

# Restaurant Information Extraction (Including Opinion Mining Elements) for the Recommendation System

Ekaterina Pronoza, Elena Yagunova, Svetlana Volskaya, and Andrey Lyashin

Saint-Petersburg State University, Saint-Petersburg, Russian Federation
{katpronoza,iagounova.elena,svetlana.volskaya}@gmail.com
Scicon Ltd, Saint-Petersburg, Russian Federation
andrey.lyashin@scicon.com

**Abstract.** In this paper information extraction method for the restaurant recommendation system is proposed. We aim at the development of an information extraction (IE) system which is intended to be a module of the recommendation system. The IE system is to gather information about different aspects of restaurants from online reviews, structure it and feed the recommendation module with the obtained data. The analyzed frames include service and food quality, cuisine, price level, noise level, etc. In this paper service quality, cuisine type and food quality are considered. As part of corpus preprocessing phase, a method for Russian reviews corpus analysis (as part of information extraction) is proposed. Its importance is shown at the experimental phase, when the application of machine learning techniques to aspects extraction is analyzed. It is shown that the ideas obtained at the corpus preprocessing stage can help to improve machine learning models performance.

**Keywords:** corpus analysis, restaurant reviews, information extraction, recommendation system, machine learning.

## 1 Introduction

In this paper information extraction (IE) method for the Russian restaurant recommendation system is proposed. It is based on the application of linguistic information gathered from corpus analysis and can be used for similar domains and under-resourced languages. Our information extraction framework is a part of the project which aims at implementing restaurants recommendation system, and in this paper we consider two tasks: reviews corpus analysis and the application of machine learning techniques to the problem in question. During the latter task we use the information obtained at the corpus analysis phase. Our approach includes opinion mining since restaurant characteristics are both objective and subjective.

Our corpus analysis method is based on non-contiguous bigrams and part of speech (POS) distribution analysis. Trigger words dictionaries are learnt using the bootstrapping method.

A. Gelbukh et al. (Eds.): MICAI 2014, Part I, LNAI 8856, pp. 201–220, 2014.

The frames to be extracted include service quality, food quality, cuisine type, price level, noise level, etc. Each frame has its own set of aspects. We suppose that the most important characteristics of a restaurant are service and food quality and cuisine type and therefore we only consider these three frames and focus on the extraction of their aspects. Such an assumption is proved by the distribution of the aspects in the data.

We also suppose that the proposed IE system can be highly effective despite the difficulties imposed by the structure of a typical Russian restaurant review. Although the key information about restaurant characteristics does not always lie on the surface, tuning machine learning models according to the results of corpus analysis can help to improve the performance of an IE system.

## 2    Related Work

Information extraction (IE) task as part of recommendation system development is discussed in [21]. The authors propose a rule-based approach to the extraction of key words from user's email. These keywords are put into a car recommendation system which is using content-based filtering approach with Jaccard Coefficient method.

In [16] a tag extraction algorithm for web pages entering a recommendation system is presented. The algorithm is based on semi-supervised document classification.

An approach to key words extraction for a learning recommendation system is described in [11]. The algorithm employs TF-IDF measure and a combination of collaborative filtering (see [27], [31]) and content-based filtering strategies (see [26], [27], [34]).

The bootstrapping approach has been successfully applied in web page classification [17], text classification ([13], [18]), named entity classification ([7], [15], [19], [22]), parsing ([28], [36]) and IE ([6], [12] , [29], [37]).

As some of restaurant aspects are quite subjective and represent users' opinion or sentiment, our task becomes similar to sentiment classification. In our research we experiment with such classification models as Naive Bayes, Logistic Regression and Linear Support Vector Machines. These models are commonly used both in sentiment analysis and opinion mining ([2], [4], [10], [14], [20], [23], [30], [35], [39]), and typical tasks usually include classifying movie or product reviews or attitudes toward a political figure/event (in a blog, tweet, etc.) into positive and negative ones.

When it comes to applying machine learning techniques to sentiment classification, it is crucially important to identify relevant features, and we pay special attention to it.

In sentiment classification n-grams (contiguous ones) are certainly the most commonly used features ([2], [10], [23], [38], [39]).

Sometimes words in n-grams are substituted with their semantic classes [10].

In [33] syntactic n-grams composed of syntactically related words are considered. However, such an approach requires syntactic parsing which is problematic for the Russian language at the moment.

There are also experiments with part-of-speech (POS) tags and POS-tagged n-grams [2]. POS information, (namely, adverb-adjective pairs) is used in [3]. They classify adverbs of degree into five categories and propose a scoring method of adverb-adjective combination. It is shown that adverb features improve model performance with respect to the identification of sentiment degree.

Negation handling techniques (e.g., adding "not_" to a negated word) are described in [9], [10], [2] and [20].

In [14] valence shifters (intensifiers and diminishers) are included in the bigram features.

In this paper we use contiguous n-grams as a baseline. We further extend this baseline feature set with non-contiguous n-grams and with the features obtained from the corpus analysis (predicative attributive words and modifiers). The latter ones generalize the adverb-adjective combination idea described in [3] and are similar to the notion of valence shifters in [14]. The former ones (non-contiguous bigrams) help to deal with negations which can be expressed in different ways in Russian. Following [23] we construct n-gram occurrence feature vectors which are reported to be more effective than n-gram frequency ones.

As far as corpus analysis is concerned, we use the bootstrapping method for trigger words dictionary learning as part of restaurant information extraction. A simple semi-supervised scheme is applied to the identification of new trigger words from the list of non-contiguous bigrams. At the corpus analysis phase our focus is on the estimation of trigger words and patterns coverage of users' reviews, and at the experimental phase we show the importance of preliminary corpus analysis.

## 3    Data

Our corpus consists of 32525 users' reviews about restaurants (and 4.2 millions of words). The data is represented by a collection of texts in the Russian colloquial language from a review site where users post their reviews about different products and services. Review lengths vary from 1 to 96 sentences, with average value equal to about 10 sentences.

There is also a part of this corpus which was annotated in a semi-supervised way. It includes 1025 reviews about 206 restaurants located in the centre of Saint-Petersburg.

This subcorpus was annotated with the aspects which are shown in Table 1. The aspects related to food quality, cuisine type and service quality frames, are given in bold.

Thus, the task of information extraction with respect to food and service quality frames can be reformulated as sentiment analysis with respect to the corresponding aspects.

**Table 1.** Restaurant aspects

| Aspect | Value domain | Aspect | Value domain |
|---|---|---|---|
| Restaurant type | String | Price level | $\{-2; -1; 0; 1; 2\}$ |
| **Cuisine type** | String(s) | Average cheque | Integer or Interval |
| **Food quality** | $\{-2; -1; 0; 1; 2\}$ | Smoking room | $\{yes; no; area; room\}$ |
| Company | $\{large; small\}$ | Children | $\{yes; no\}$ |
| Audience | String(s) | Children's room | $\{yes; no\}$ |
| **Service quality** | $\{-2; -1; 0; 1; 2\}$ | Dancefloor | $\{yes; no\}$ |
| **Service speed** | $\{-2; -1; 0; 1; 2\}$ | Bar | $\{yes; no\}$ |
| **Staff politeness** | $\{-2; -1; 0; 1; 2\}$ | Parking place | $\{yes; no\}$ |
| **Staff amiability** | $\{-2; -1; 0; 1; 2\}$ | VIP room | $\{yes; no\}$ |
| Noise level | $\{-2; -1; 0; 1; 2\}$ | Dancefloor | $\{yes; no\}$ |
| Cosiness | $\{yes; no\}$ | A railway station (nearby) | $\{yes; no\}$ |
| Romantic atmosphere | $\{yes; no\}$ | A hotel (nearby) | $\{yes; no\}$ |
| Cramped (or not) | $\{yes; no\}$ | A shopping mall (nearby) | $\{yes; no\}$ |

## 4    Machine Learning Models

### 4.1    Naive Bayes

The Naive Bayes Model uses Bayes' theorem which states

$$P(y \mid x_1,...,x_n) = \frac{P(y)P(x_1,...x_n \mid y)}{P(x_1,...x_n)},$$

where $y$ is a class variable and $(x_1,...,x_n)$ is a dependent feature vector. With the naive independence assumption stating that $P(x_i \mid y, x_1,...,x_{i-1}, x_{i+1},...,x_n) = P(x_i \mid y)$ (i.e., that features are independent), Bayes' theorem relationship can be rewritten as follows:

$$P(y \mid x_1,...,x_n) = \frac{P(y)\prod_{i=1}^{n} P(x_i \mid y)}{P(x_1,...,x_n)}.$$

Since the denominator is constant given the input training data $(x_1,...,x_n)$, the $\hat{y}$ estimation of $y$ is calculated as follows: $\hat{y} = \arg\max_y P(y)\prod_{i=1}^{n} P(x_i \mid y)$.

Despite its simplicity, Naive Bayes model has proved to be efficient for linearly separable and even non-linearly separable problems.

## 4.2    Logistic Regression

Logistic Regression (Logit Regression) is a probabilistic statistical classification model.

Given class variable $y$ and training data $(x_1,...,x_n)$, we assume that $P\{y = 1 \mid x_1,...,x_n\} = f(z)$, where $z = \theta_1 x_1 + ... + \theta_n x_n, \theta_1,...,\theta_n$ are feature weights and $f(z) = \dfrac{1}{1+e^{-z}}$ is a logistic (sigmoid) function.

Following the expectation maximization procedure $\theta$ aspects are chosen to maximize the function

$$\sum_{i=1}^{m} y^{(i)} \log f(\theta^T x^{(i)}) + (1 - y^{(i)}) \log(1 - f(\theta^T x^{(i)})).$$ To avoid overfitting, logistic regression is regularized. In this case, the optimization problem can be formulated as follows:

$$\max_{\theta} (\sum_{i=1}^{m} \log P\{y^{(i)} \mid x^{(i)}, \theta\} - \lambda \|\theta\|_1)$$ (L1 regularized Logistic Regression)

or

$$\max_{\theta} (\sum_{i=1}^{m} \log P\{y^{(i)} \mid x^{(i)}, \theta\} - \lambda \|\theta\|^2)$$ (L2 regularized Logistic Regression).

In our research Logistic Regression (a randomized version) is also used for penalizing unimportant features at the feature selection stage.

## 4.3    Support Vector Machine

Support Vector Machines (SVM), introduced in [8] are supervised learning models used in many classification problems. An SVM constructs hyperplanes in a high-dimensional space of training data points, and the best separation between the classes is achieved by the hyperplane with the largest distance to the nearest training data point of any class (a linear SVM finds a linear separating hyperplane with the maximal margin).

More formally, a linear SVM model requires the solution of the following problem:

$$\begin{cases} \min_{w,b,\zeta} (\frac{1}{2}\|w\|^2 + C\sum_{i=1}^{n} \zeta_i) \\ c_i(w \bullet x_i - b) \geq 1 - \zeta_i, 1 \leq i \leq n \\ \zeta_i \geq 0, 1 \leq i \leq n \end{cases}$$

where $\{(x_i, c_i)\}, i = 1..n$ is a set of training examples, with each $x_i$ representing a multi-dimensional vector, • denotes the dot product, $w$ is the normal vector to the hyperplane, $b$ refers to the offset of the hyperplane from the origin along the normal vector $w$, variables $\zeta_i$ measure the degree of misclassification of the data and $C$ is a regularization aspect.

SVM models have been widely used in many natural language applications and have proved to be a powerful classification method.

# 5 Corpus Analysis

## 5.1 Main Phases of Analysis

In our research, corpus analysis procedure can be divided into the following phases:

- Corpus preprocessing (tokenization, lemmatization, normalization and sentence splitting). We also include unigrams and bigrams extraction here (see 5.2);
- Trigger words dictionaries construction (see 5.3). In this paper, such procedure is described for service quality and food quality & cuisine type frames (with one dictionary for service quality frame and another one for the other two frames). Besides, three predicative-attributive dictionaries are built for the three frames mentioned (one dictionary per frame). The words from these dictionaries are further used in the patterns (see 5.5);
- The estimation of trigger words dictionaries coverage of the reviews corpus (see 5.4);
- Patterns construction based on the POS-distribution of trigger words' context (see 5.5);
- The estimation of patterns coverage of the reviews corpus (see 5.6). NP patterns (which dominate in the corpus according to the statistics in 5.5) are given a detailed attention.

## 5.2 Corpus Preprocessing

The corpus is tokenized, then lemmatized using pymorphy2[1] tool and split into sentences. Taking into account our data characteristics (Russian colloquial language), we also normalize the corpus by reducing multiplied vowels and some consonants (which are often used to express author's strong emotions) to single ones (e.g., in words like "ооооочень" /veeeery/ or "оччченъ" /verrry/ which refer to "очень" /very/).

Having adopted a (lexeme, POS) pair as an element of analysis, we compute unigram and bigram frequencies. We extract contiguous bigrams as well as non-contiguous ones, with no more than two words between bigram components. Our

---

[1] Russian and English morphological analyser for Python:
http://pymorphy2.readthedocs.org/

motivation is that at the primary stage of an information extraction task we should look at the context of words. It can further help us during both trigger words dictionaries construction and patterns development.

## 5.3    Dictionary Construction

At the primary stage of information extraction, our task is to construct a dictionary of trigger words, which indicate the presence of a certain frame in a review, and to develop patterns for frame aspects extraction. This stage (as well as the other stages) of corpus analysis is described in [25] and therefore we shall not go into details here, only paying attention to the key issues.

All trigger words dictionaries described in this paper (each of them consisting of a set of lexemes with a given POS) are constructed using the bootstrapping method.

The seed for service quality frame consists of a small set of nouns which Russian native speakers presumably use to refer to service (e.g., "персонал" /staff/, "официант" /waiter/, "официантка" /waitress/, "обслуживание" /service/, etc.). We use our bigrams list during the bootstrapping iterations to get the context of the trigger words. Context words are restricted to adjectives and participles (in short or full form). During each of the iterations we look into the list of new words and put out the ones which do not refer to the subject in question. We also compute scores of the words and range the words according to their scores so that the words we are most confident in would be at the top.

For example, having a seed word "персонал" /staff/ with score X and a bigram "гостеприимный, П персонал, С" (hospitable, Adjective staff, Noun) with score Y we should record "гостеприимный" /hospitable/ into our current trigger words list with X*Y score. The initial scores for all the seed words are chosen to be equal to 1. In our research, new trigger words no longer emerged after 5 iterations and there were 73 lexemes in the dictionary.

A predicative-attributive dictionary for service quality frame is also constructed. It includes 226 lexemes (namely, adjectives and participles) which are revealed during the bootstrapping procedure as the neighbours of the trigger words. Finally we construct two predicative-attributive dictionaries for food quality and cuisine type (including 112 and 48 lexemes respectively).

## 5.4    Dictionary Coverage Estimation

We consider it important to estimate our dictionary coverage, i.e., the percentage of reviews which contain words from the dictionaries. Estimation results are presented in Table 2. Thus, it turns out that in 66% of reviews people use at least one of the trigger words to describe service quality.

**Table 2.** Dictionary coverage estimation

| Frame | Dictionary coverage percent |
|---|---|
| Service quality | 66% |
| Food quality | 71% |
| Cuisine type | 25% |

As far as food quality and cuisine type are concerned, their common dictionary covers 96% of reviews. We also estimate their coverage separately by calculating the portion of reviews where a corresponding trigger word occurs in the context of a word from the corresponding predicative-attributive dictionary. The reason of such a low value for the cuisine type frame (25%) is, on the one hand, the limited amount of cuisine type predicative-attributive words and, on the other hand, the vast amount of the cuisine trigger words.

### 5.5     Patterns Construction

Having estimated trigger words dictionary and justified the use of a standard pattern scheme for the reviews, we proceed to patterns development.

We adopt an approach to pattern development based on the POS-distribution of the neighbours of the trigger words.

We consider top 5 trigger words with maximum frequency in the corpus and retrieve POS-distribution of their context from the non-contiguous bigrams list. We only consider POS-distribution for "обслуживание" /service/ neighbours (see Table 3) in this paper as for the other four words it appears to be similar.

**Table 3.** POS-distribution for "обслуживание" /service/ and "кухня" /cuisine/ left (see POS Left column) and right (see POS Right column) neighbour words (top-10)

| Обслуживание /Service/ | | | | | Кухня /Cuisine/ | | | | |
|---|---|---|---|---|---|---|---|---|---|
| POS Left | Freq | % | POS Right | Freq | % POS Left | Freq | % | POS Right | Freq | % |
| Noun | 1409 | 21 | Noun | 1941 | 19 Adjective | 3576 | 23 | Noun | 2085 | 17 |
| Conjunction | 1306 | 20 | Preposition | 1552 | 15 Noun | 3010 | 20 | Adjective | 1633 | 13 |
| Adjective | 822 | 12 | Adjective | 1457 | 14 Conjunction | 1638 | 11 | Conjunction | 1405 | 11 |
| Preposition | 757 | 11 | Adverb | 1034 | 10 Preposition | 1560 | 10 | Preposition | 1377 | 11 |
| Verb | 546 | 8 | Conjunction | 1004 | 10 Verb | 1415 | 9 | Verb | 1289 | 11 |
| Pronoun | 493 | 7 | Verb | 909 | 9 Pronoun | 1036 | 7 | Pronoun | 1101 | 9 |
| Adverb | 331 | 5 | Particle | 573 | 6 Adverb | 663 | 4 | Adverb | 941 | 8 |
| Particle | 311 | 5 | Pronoun | 562 | 6 Adjective pronoun | 635 | 4 | Particle | 610 | 5 |
| Adjective pronoun | 233 | 4 | Adjective (short) | 370 | 4 Infinitive | 472 | 3 | Adjective (short) | 610 | 5 |
| Adjective (short) | 171 | 3 | Adjective pronoun | 309 | 3 Particle | 441 | 3 | Adjective pronoun | 437 | 4 |

According to the POS-distribution of the neighbours of the trigger words, service trigger nouns are mostly used together with nouns both to the left and to the right. Phrases like "В этом ресторане обслуживание ..." /In this restaurant the service is.../ or "Обслуживание ресторана..." /The service of the restaurant is.../ are quite common in the Russian language when restaurant reviews are concerned. Prepositions and conjunctions take the $2^{nd}$ place, but we are interested in the characteristics of service, and looking further at the $3^{rd}$ place we have adjectives and, later on, verbs.

As in the service quality case, we consider top trigger words (with maximum frequency in the corpus) of food quality and cuisine type frames. The word "кухня" /cuisine/ is one of the most frequent trigger words of the corresponding frames, and its neighbouring words POS-distribution is shown in Table 3.

POS-distribution shown in Tables 1–2 suggests that trigger words of the frames in question occur mostly as parts of noun phrases (NPs) and then, less frequently, as parts of verbal phrases (VPs).

As part of the research a tool for trigger words context extraction was implemented. It consists of grammar rules and query language based on parts of speech patterns. Thus, a query like "ADV* ADJ+ ПЕРСОНАЛ" corresponds to all text fragments where "ПЕРСОНАЛ" /staff/ lexeme is preceded with one or more adjectives and with zero or more adverbs. This is an example of a simple NP for the "ПЕРСОНАЛ" /staff/ target lexeme.

For the service quality, cuisine type and food quality extraction we consider a more complex NP structure, where a target lexeme can be represented by any of the words from the corresponding trigger words dictionary, and both left and right descriptions consist of zero or more adjectives or participles probably preceded by negations or modifiers (e.g., "очень" /very/, "вполне" /quite/, "немного" /slightly/, etc.) and repeated one or more times. Adjectives and participles are not restricted to the predicative-attributive dictionaries.

## 5.6    Patterns Coverage Estimation

To estimate patterns coverage, i.e., the percentage of reviews which contain patterns described in the previous section, we use the same scheme as in the case of dictionaries in section 5.4. In this paper we only consider NP patterns with respect to service quality, food quality and cuisine type.

It appears that NP patterns constructed for service quality frame cover 38% of reviews (unannotated ones), food quality NP patterns covered 71% and cuisine type NP patterns covered 25% of reviews (see Table 4).

It is easy to see that for food quality and cuisine type NP patterns coverage percent is identical to that of trigger dictionary coverage. Therefore, the application of NP patterns to the extraction of the two aspects in question seems to be a successful strategy.

NP patterns coverage results for cuisine type and service and food quality on the annotated data are also presented in Table 4.

**Table 4.** NP patterns coverage estimation (on the whole corpus)

| Aspect | Unannotated Corpus: Coverage | Annotated Corpus: Coverage |
|---|---|---|
| Service quality | 41% | 39% |
| Cuisine type | 25% | 57% |
| Food quality | 71% | 59% |

It should be mentioned that, were we to implement a rule-based (namely, NP-patterns-based) aspects extraction system, such an estimation could be considered an upper bound for the recall score. Therefore, to compare the performance of such hypothesized system to that of the models which we are going to introduce in Section 6, we also estimate NP patterns coverage on the annotated subcorpus (precisely, on the reviews where the corresponding aspect values are not missing). The results of the estimation are given in Table 4. It is shown in Section 7 that machine learning models performance scores for food and service quality aspects are higher than those presented in Table 4.

## 5.7    Aspect Values Distribution

Having annotated our training subcorpus, we found out that while some of the restaurant aspects are quite often mentioned by users in their reviews (e.g., food quality), the others are almost never spoken of (e.g., the availability of a railway station or hotel). As our annotated subcorpus is limited at the moment, we must ensure that there is enough training data to extract aspects using machine learning. Thus, our aspects can be divided into two groups:

- frequent ones, which are going to be extracted using machine learning techniques, and
- rare ones, for which a list of hand-crafted rules is going to be used.

To classify all the aspects into these two groups, we calculate the frequencies of their values in the annotated subcorpus. The obtained distribution is given in Table 5 (with groups labels listed in the last column).

In Table 5 NaN stands for a missing value (in case an aspect is not mentioned in the review at all), and "non-NaN" in the average cheque field stands for any value different from NaN (as there are too many possible values of the average cheque aspect in the training data). The aspects which, in our opinion, can be extracted using machine learning techniques (i.e., the "Frequent" group in our classification), are given in bold. They were chosen according to their NaN value portion (which does not exceed 90%).

As it can be seen from Table 5, restaurant characteristics such the availability of a bar or a dancefloor are seldom mentioned and some (e.g., the availability of a

**Table 5.** Aspect values distribution

| Aspect | Value | Frequency | Group | Aspect | Value | Frequency | Group |
|---|---|---|---|---|---|---|---|
| Staff amiability | -2 | 2% | | Noise level | -2 | 1% | |
| | -1 | 5% | | | -1 | 2.6% | |
| | 0 | 1% | Frequent | | 0 | 0.2% | Frequent |
| | 1 | 16% | | | 1 | 8.5% | |
| | 2 | 10% | | | 2 | 1.7% | |
| | NaN | 66% | | | NaN | 86% | |
| Average cheque | non-NaN | 8% | Rare | Parking place | yes | 0.7% | |
| | NaN | 92% | | | no | 0.5% | Rare |
| Bar | yes | 5% | Rare | | NaN | 98.8% | |
| | NaN | 95% | | Staff politeness | -2 | 2.6% | |
| Children's room | yes | 2% | | | -1 | 2% | |
| | no | 1% | Rare | | 0 | 0.1% | Frequent |
| | NaN | 97% | | | 1 | 13% | |
| Children | yes | 7% | | | 2 | 9% | |
| | no | <1% | Rare | | NaN | 73.3% | |
| | NaN | >92% | | Service quality | -2 | 5% | |
| Company | large | 7% | | | -1 | 8% | |
| | small | 3% | Frequent | | 0 | 2% | Frequent |
| | NaN | 90% | | | 1 | 19% | |
| Cosiness | yes | 32% | | | 2 | 21% | |
| | no | 5% | Frequent | | NaN | 45% | |
| | NaN | 63% | | Railway station | yes | <1% | Rare |
| Cramped (or not) | yes | 5% | | | NaN | >99% | |
| | no | 7% | Frequent | Romantic atmosphere | yes | 9% | |
| | NaN | 88% | | | no | 2% | Frequent |
| Dancefloor | yes | 2% | Rare | | NaN | 89% | |
| | NaN | 98% | | Food quality | -2 | 4% | |
| Hotel | yes | 1% | Rare | | -1 | 6% | |
| | NaN | 99% | | | 0 | 4% | Frequent |
| Price level | -2 | 4% | | | 1 | 30% | |
| | -1 | 10% | | | 2 | 42% | |
| | 0 | 3% | Frequent | | NaN | 14% | |
| | 1 | 17% | | Shopping mall | yes | 1% | Rare |
| | 2 | 4% | | | NaN | 99% | |
| | NaN | 62% | | Smoking room | area | <1% | |
| Service speed | -2 | 6% | | | no | 1% | Rare |
| | -1 | 6% | | | room | 4% | |
| | 0 | 1% | Frequent | | yes | 1% | |
| | 1 | 11% | | | NaN | >93% | |
| | 2 | 8% | | | | | |
| | NaN | 68% | | | | | |
| VIP room | yes | 1% | Rare | | | | |
| | NaN | 99% | | | | | |

railway station) are almost never mentioned at all with respect to the restaurants in the centre of Saint-Petersburg. The aspects in bold are, on the contrary, quite often spoken of.

Some aspect values represent sentiment (e.g., food quality, staff amiability and staff politeness values) and are absolutely subjective, while others refer to a particular restaurant quality (e.g., the availability of a bar) and are more objective. All sentiment-related aspects are categorized into five different classes. These classes represent five degrees of sentiment, from highly-negative ("-2") to highly positive ("2").

## 6    Feature Representation

In our experiments we use scikit-learn[2]: an efficient machine learning library for Python.

For the aspects chosen as the most frequent ones, we try the following models: Logistic Regression, Support Vector Machine and Naive Bayes. As we have already mentioned, in this paper we are taking a closer look at service and food quality and cuisine type aspects, but since the latter suggests a multi-label task, we shall only consider machine learning models with respect to food and service quality at the moment.

Since the annotated corpus includes a large amount of missing values (NaNs), we divide our classification task into two parts: first, a classifier is trained to tell between the missing and present values, and then, if the value is present, it should be classified. In this paper the second classification task (for non-NaN values) is considered.

Our baseline feature set consists of unigrams and bigrams (only contiguous ones). We also tried trigrams but, since they did not improve performance much while making feature space larger, we decided not to include them in the feature set.

We experiment with two extended features sets. First, we only add non-contiguous bigrams (with window size equal to 3 as it appeared to perform best). Then, in the second set, we add emoticons and exclamations, predicative-attributive words and key words and expressions instead.

All the three feature sets and their detailed descriptions are presented in Table 6.

As far as n-grams are concerned, we use lemma occurrence vectors instead of lemma count vectors as it was proved to be a better strategy for sentiment analysis [23].

Since the number of features described in Table 6 is more than one and half a million, we also use feature selection to remove irrelevant or unimportant features.

We tried feature selection methods implemented in scikit-learn: linear SVM and Logistic Regression for penalizing irrelevant features and chose Randomized Logistic

---

[2] http://scikit-learn.org

Regression (Logistic Regression model re-estimated many times so that having a group of correlated features it would not always select only one of them) as it demonstrated best performance scores on our sparse data.

**Table 6.** Feature sets

| Feature | Description | Baseline | Extended1 | Extended2 |
|---|---|---|---|---|
| Unigrams | 1, if a unigram occurs in the review, else 0 | + | + | + |
| Contiguous bigrams | 1, if a bigram occurs in the review, else 0 | + | + | + |
| Non-contiguous bigrams | 1, if a bigram occurs in the review, else 0 | | + | |
| Emoticons & Exclamations | 1, if any emoticon occurs in the review in the same sentence with some trigger word, else 0 | | | + |
| | 1, if an exclamation mark occurs in the review in the same sentence with some trigger word, else 0 | | | |
| Predicative-attributive words | 1, if a predicative-attributive word occurs in the review within 4 words to the left from some trigger word, else 0 | | | + |
| | 1, if a predicative-attributive word occurs in the review within 4 words to the left from some trigger word AND a modifier occurs in the review within 4 words to the left this predicative-attributive word, else 0 | | | |
| Key words and expressions | 1, if a key word or expression occurs in the review, else 0 | | | + |

## 7    Evaluation

As it was stated earlier in this paper, the results of reviews corpus analysis help us to improve the performance of our machine learning models, and it refers not only to the dictionaries learned at the preprocessing stage but also to the idea of using non-contiguous bigrams.

To evaluate our models, we use cross-validation procedure. A 90-10% shuffle 10-fold cross-validation (samples are shuffled and randomly split into training and test sets, with test set size equal to 10% of the whole annotated corpus) is chosen due to the fact that for "negative" classes there are less examples than for "positive" ones for each of the aspects in question.

Precision, recall and F1 scores for the food quality aspect are given in Tables 7 (baseline), 8 and 9 (extended).

**Table 7.** Food Quality: Baseline Performance (best average weighted score in bold)

| Model | -2 | -1 | 0 | 1 | 2 | AVG |
|---|---|---|---|---|---|---|
| Naive Bayes | | | | | | |
| Precision | 47,50 | 43,67 | 26,67 | 69,56 | 81,14 | |
| Recall | 34,33 | 54,92 | 16,25 | 64,25 | 87,74 | |
| F1 | 35,19 | 45,78 | 18,88 | 66,50 | *84,11* | **69,45** |
| Logistic Regression | | | | | | |
| Precision | 51,67 | 31,76 | 0,00 | 64,02 | 75,38 | |
| Recall | 16,50 | 27,25 | 0,00 | 66,37 | 84,92 | |
| F1 | 24,36 | 27,63 | 0,00 | *64,93* | *79,77* | 64,24 |
| SVM | | | | | | |
| Precision | 39,00 | 28,50 | 6,67 | 63,69 | 76,38 | |
| Recall | 29,00 | 30,17 | 3,75 | 63,51 | 81,27 | |
| F1 | 31,94 | 28,15 | 4,68 | 63,41 | *78,65* | 63,99 |

In these tables, class labels "-2", "-1", "0", "1" and "2" represent five degrees of sentiment with respect to food quality, from highly negative ("-2") to highly positive ("2").

In each of the tables the values in the last column correspond to the average weighted F1. The weights are calculated as relative frequencies of class labels in the annotated subcorpus. We consider F1 the most important measure for our system and therefore choose it as an aggregated score.

F1 scores which are higher than their respective average weighted score are given in italics. It is not surprising that such F1 scores mostly occur in "2" or "2" and "1" categories because these classes, being the most frequent ones in the annotated sub-corpus, have the largest weights. Whichever feature set is chosen, the winning Naive Bayes model shows the largest bias to the "2" class as only "2" class F1 scores appear to be above the aggregated F1 score level for this model. However, this is not consi-dered a drawback since for our restaurant recommendation system reviews with "2" (highly positive) food quality grade are the most important ones when food quality is concerned.

According to the results in Tables 7, 8 and 9, Naive Bayes appears to be the best of the three classifiers considered. Its baseline and extended versions show similar scores while SVM and Logistic Regression with extended feature sets improve upon the corresponding baselines.

Moreover, for all the three models both extended versions achieve more or less the same performance score, while the second feature set evidently takes less space than the first one. It means that having learnt the necessary dictionaries, we can do without

**Table 8.** Food Quality: Extended (1) (best average weighted score in bold)

| Model | -2 | -1 | 0 | 1 | 2 | AVG |
|---|---|---|---|---|---|---|
| Naive Bayes | | | | | | |
| Precision | 71,83 | 49,07 | 26,86 | 66,90 | 80,15 | |
| Recall | 51,00 | 43,80 | 28,92 | 70,03 | 82,33 | |
| F1 | 50,46 | 45,24 | 25,91 | 68,29 | *81,13* | **70,08** |
| Logistic Regression | | | | | | |
| Precision | 75,00 | 51,83 | 25,00 | 64,67 | 78,12 | |
| Recall | 33,50 | 29,08 | 12,50 | 75,24 | 84,05 | |
| F1 | 42,40 | 36,41 | 16,00 | *69,21* | *80,83* | 68,77 |
| SVM | | | | | | |
| Precision | 51,67 | 36,51 | 29,17 | 62,72 | 76,04 | |
| Recall | 34,33 | 22,68 | 15,17 | 71,25 | 79,59 | |
| F1 | 38,00 | 25,69 | 19,22 | *66,38* | *77,65* | 65,57 |

**Table 9.** Food Quality: Extended (2) (best average weighted score in bold)

| Model | -2 | -1 | 0 | 1 | 2 | AVG |
|---|---|---|---|---|---|---|
| Naive Bayes | | | | | | |
| Precision | 65,71 | 60,83 | 38,33 | 62,82 | 80,77 | |
| Recall | 49,67 | 57,19 | 18,67 | 67,31 | 85,34 | |
| F1 | 53,71 | 55,69 | 24,13 | 64,59 | *82,80* | **70,26** |
| Logistic Regression | | | | | | |
| Precision | 72,50 | 54,56 | 20,00 | 62,64 | 78,08 | |
| Recall | 45,33 | 33,27 | 5,00 | 71,67 | 85,62 | |
| F1 | 53,78 | 37,00 | 8,00 | 66,48 | *81,46* | 68,64 |
| SVM | | | | | | |
| Precision | 39,29 | 51,51 | 10,00 | 62,45 | 78,38 | |
| Recall | 38,67 | 39,11 | 9,17 | 69,55 | 81,09 | |
| F1 | 37,11 | 40,66 | 9,50 | 65,36 | *79,35* | 66,21 |

non-contiguous bigrams in the feature set and thus reduce its size. Therefore dictionaries-based approach seems to be more effective when food quality aspect extraction is concerned.

As our second extended feature set (dictionary-based one) includes several different features we test each of them separately to find those which contributes most to the overall performance. It was found out that both SVM and Logistic Regression are most sensitive to emoticons and exclamation marks, less sensitive to predicative-attributive dictionaries and least sensitive to key words and expressions.

Precision, recall and F1 scores for service quality are shown in Tables 10 (baseline), 11 and 12 (extended).

**Table 10.** Service Quality: Baseline Performance (best average weighted score in bold)

| Model | -2 | -1 | 0 | 1 | 2 | AVG |
|---|---|---|---|---|---|---|
| Naive Bayes | | | | | | |
| Precision | 56,58 | 64,70 | 10,00 | 60,82 | 72,78 | |
| Recall | 64,82 | 59,55 | 3,33 | 65,76 | 77,99 | |
| F1 | 57,89 | 59,56 | 5,00 | 62,89 | *74,98* | **64,37** |
| Logistic Regression | | | | | | |
| Precision | 62,40 | 51,15 | 10,00 | 51,76 | 64,98 | |
| Recall | 43,27 | 39,67 | 3,33 | 59,59 | 75,00 | |
| F1 | 48,23 | 42,42 | 5,00 | 54,12 | *69,22* | 56,14 |
| SVM | | | | | | |
| Precision | 53,33 | 40,84 | 0,00 | 51,69 | 65,74 | |
| Recall | 49,76 | 36,30 | 0,00 | 55,30 | 71,32 | |
| F1 | 48,16 | 37,60 | 0,00 | 51,86 | *68,13* | 54,30 |

As in the case of food quality, the last column of each table corresponds to the average weighted F1 score. All the denotation (class labels from -2 to 2, scores in bald or in italics) is similar to that of the Tables 7–9.

According to the Tables 10–12, the Naive Bayes models demonstrate the best performance for the service quality aspect as well as for the food quality aspect.

However, in the service quality case the scores of extended models differ: extended (1) is better than extended (2) while both of them are better than baseline. It means that the best strategy for service quality extraction involves including non-contiguous bigrams in the feature set. In fact, such an assumption conforms to the results of corpus analysis. We have already shown that NP patterns coverage is quite low for service quality (39%) on the annotated data, especially when compared to that of food quality (59%). These NP patterns are indirectly included in the feature set by using predicative-attributive words preceded by modifiers. It is caused by the fact that the service quality characteristic can be expressed in a review in wide variety of ways which are better captured by non-contiguous bigrams than by patterns or dictionaries.

**Table 11.** Service Quality: Extended (1) (best average weighted score in bold)

| Model | -2 | -1 | 0 | 1 | 2 | AVG |
|---|---|---|---|---|---|---|
| Naive Bayes | | | | | | |
| Precision | 68,33 | 50,32 | 15,00 | 69,19 | 77,09 | |
| Recall | 70,99 | 44,54 | 15,00 | 71,88 | 81,08 | |
| F1 | 67,58 | 45,47 | 15,00 | 70,10 | *78,95* | **68,77** |
| Logistic Regression | | | | | | |
| Precision | 73,03 | 57,51 | 20,00 | 63,98 | 71,05 | |
| Recall | 52,96 | 40,17 | 10,00 | 68,65 | 84,47 | |
| F1 | 57,68 | 46,04 | 13,33 | *65,70* | *76,97* | 65,05 |
| SVM | | | | | | |
| Precision | 58,75 | 51,87 | 25,00 | 63,91 | 72,28 | |
| Recall | 51,85 | 40,65 | 18,33 | 67,98 | 80,35 | |
| F1 | 52,46 | 44,86 | 20,00 | *65,28* | *75,75* | 63,80 |

**Table 12.** Service Quality: Extended (2) (best average weighted score in bold)

| Model | -2 | -1 | 0 | 1 | 2 | AVG |
|---|---|---|---|---|---|---|
| Naive Bayes | | | | | | |
| Precision | 71,71 | 44,01 | 10,00 | 68,94 | 73,93 | |
| Recall | 60,36 | 50,22 | 2,50 | 67,16 | 77,69 | |
| F1 | 63,32 | 45,59 | 4,00 | 67,11 | *75,27* | **65,33** |
| Logistic Regression | | | | | | |
| Precision | 62,55 | 38,78 | 0,00 | 59,18 | 67,25 | |
| Recall | 39,79 | 39,03 | 0,00 | 57,30 | 80,27 | |
| F1 | 47,76 | 38,29 | 0,00 | 57,41 | *72,63* | 57,90 |
| SVM | | | | | | |
| Precision | 48,55 | 37,10 | 25,00 | 60,52 | 66,35 | |
| Recall | 37,60 | 37,31 | 10,00 | 55,55 | 76,85 | |
| F1 | 41,06 | 36,21 | 14,00 | *56,87* | *70,63* | 56,27 |

Thus, according to the results of the experiments, a conclusion can be made that using dictionaries (see extended-2) in the feature set allows for more precise models taking less memory and therefore seems to be a perspective approach. In this case, the evident possible ways of system performance improvement include more elaborate dictionaries learning (e.g., for food quality). However, when for some reasons thorough corpus analysis cannot be conducted or size and quality of dictionaries are insufficient (e.g., for service quality at the moment), non-contiguous bigrams (see extended-1) offer a good corpus independent alternative.

# 8     Conclusion and Future Work

This paper presents restaurant information extraction method implemented as a part of the restaurant recommendation system project and a part of the master's thesis devoted to information extraction and opinion mining.

We demonstrate an approach for reviews corpus analysis based on non-contiguous bigrams and POS-distribution of the neighbours of the trigger words. We also experiment with machine learning models with respect to restaurant aspect extraction and show that their performance can be improved by the results and ideas derived from corpus analysis thus proving the importance of the latter.

In particular, it is shown that using trigger words and predicative-attributive words dictionaries is an effective approach for food quality extraction while the service quality aspect, which is harder to deal with, demands a wider range of features (in our research, non-contiguous bigrams are used).

We should note that our corpus consists of Russian colloquial texts, and Russian is known for its rich morphology and free word order which complicates its automatic processing. Another complicating factor which makes information extraction difficult is the fact that the use of recommendation systems is not yet widespread in Russia, and therefore the reviews are often not what one would expect them to be (e.g., free narratives are quite common).

However, according to the results, ideas from corpus analysis can improve the performance of our system. Our further work directions include detailed analysis of service quality aspect and expansion of the training data.

**Acknowledgement.** The authors acknowledge Saint-Petersburg State University for a research grant 30.38.305.2014.

# References

1. Almazro, D., Shahatah, G., Albdulkarim, L., Kherees, M., Martinez, R. and Nzoukou, W.: A Survey Paper on Recommender Systems. Arxiv preprint, arXiv:1006.5278 (2010)
2. Bakliwal, A., Patil., A., Arora, P. and Varma, V.: Towards Enhanced Opinion Classification using NLP Techniques. In: Proceedings of the Workshop on Sentiment Analysis where AI meets Psychology (SAAIP), IJCNLP, Chiang Mai, Thailand, November 13, 2011, pp. 101–107 (2011)
3. Benamara, F., Cesarano, C., Picariello, A., Reforgiato, D. and Subrahmanian, V. S.: Sentiment analysis: Adjectives and adverbs are better than adjectives alone. In: Proceedings of the International Conference on Weblogs and Social Media (ICWSM) (2007)
4. Bermingham, A. and Smeaton, A.: Classifying Sentiment in Microblogs: Is Brevity an Advantage? CIKM'10, Toronto, Ontario, Canada, October 26–29, 2010 (2010)

5. Bodapati, A.V.: Recommendation Systems with Purchase Data. Journal of Marketing Research, Volume 45 (1), pp. 77–93 (2008)
6. Carlson, A., Betteridge, J. and Wang, R. C.: Coupled Semi-Supervised Learning for Information Extraction. Third ACM international conference on Web search and data mining, New York, USA, pp. 101–110 (2010)
7. Collins, M., Singer, Y.: Unsupervised models for named entity classification. In: Proceedings of the Joint SIGDAT Conference on Empirical Methods in Natural Language Processing and Very Large Corpora (EMNLP), pp. 100–110 (1999)
8. Cortes, C. and Vapnik, V.: Support-vector Network. Machine Learning, Volume 20, pp. 273-297 (1995)
9. Das, S. R., and Chen, M. Y.: Yahoo! for Amazon: Sentiment parsing from small talk on the web. Management Science, Volume 53 (9), September 2007, pp. 1375–1388 (2007)
10. Dave, K., Lawrence, S. and Pennock, D. M.: Mining the Peanut Gallery: Opinion Extraction and Semantic Classification of Product Reviews. In: Proceedings of the 12th International Conference on World Wide Web, New York, USA, 2003, pp. 519–528 (2003)
11. Emadzadeh, E., Nikfarjam, A., Ghauth, K. I. and Why, N. K.: Learning Materials Recommendation Using a Hybrid Recommender System with Automated Keyword Extraction. In: World Applied Sciences Journal, Volume 9 (11), pp. 1260–1271, ISSN: 1818–4952 (2010)
12. Huang, R. and Riloff, E.: Multi-faceted Event Recognition with Bootstrapped Dictionaries. NAACL-HLT 2013, Atlanta, Georgia, USA, 9–14 June 2013, pp. 41–51 (2013)
13. Joorabchi, A. and Mahdi, A. E.: A New Method for Bootstrapping an Automatic Text Classification System Utilizing Public Library Resources. 19th Irish Conference on Artificial Intelligence and Cognitive Science (AICS-2008) (2008)
14. Kennedy, A. and Inkpen, D.: Sentiment Classification of Movie Reviews Using Contextual Valence Shifters. In: Computational Intelligence (2006)
15. Lee, S. and Lee, G. G.: G.B.: A bootstrapping Approach for Geographic Named Entity Annotation. Asia Information Retrieval Symposium (2004)
16. Leksin V. and Nikolenko S. I.: Semi-supervised Tag Extraction in a Web Recommender System. Proceedings of the 6th International Conference on Similarity Search and Applications (SISAP 2013), Lecture Notes in Computer Science, pp. 206–212 (2013)
17. Lim, E. P., Sun, A. and Marissa, M.: Conceptual Classification of Web Pages using Bootstrapping and Co-Training Strategies. In: Cyberscape Journal, Volume 4 (1). Research Collection School of Information Systems, ISSN: 1675-9281 (2006)
18. Lin, F. and Cohen, W. W.: The MultiRank Bootstrap Algorithm: Semi-Supervised Political Blog Classification and Ranking Using Semi-Supervised Link Classification. Language Technologies Institute, School of Computer Science, Carnegie Mellon University. Retrieved from: http://www.lti.cs.cmu.edu. Access date: October 9, 2013 (2008)
19. Murphy, T and Curran, J. R.: Experiments in Mutual Exclusion Bootstrapping. Australasian Language Technology Workshop 2007, pp. 66–74 (2007)
20. Narayanan, V., Arora, I. and Bhatia, A.: Fast and Accurate Sentiment Classification Using an Enhanced Naive Bayes Model. In: arXiv:1305.6143 (2013)
21. Naw, N. and Hlaing, E. E.: Relevant Words Extraction Method for Recommendation System. In: International Journal of Emerging Technology and Advanced Engineering, Volume 3 (1), January 2013, ISSN: 2250–2459 (2013)
22. Niu, C., Li, W., Ding, J. and Srihari, R. K.: A Bootstrapping Approach to Named Entity Classification Using Successive Learners. 41st Annual Meeting of the ACL (2003)

23. Pang, B., Lee, L. and Vaithyanathan, S.: Thumbs up? Sentiment classification using machine learning techniques. In: Proceedings of the Conference on Empirical Methods in Natural Language Processing (EMNLP), pp. 79–86 (2002)
24. Park D. H., Kim H. K. and Kim J. K.: A Literature Review and Classification of Recommender Systems Research. Social Science, Volume 5, pp. 290–294 (2011)
25. Pronoza, E., Yagunova, E., Lyashin, A.: Restaurant Information Extraction for the Recommendation System. In: Proceedings of the 2nd Workshop on Social and Algorithmic Issues in Business Support: "Knowledge Hidden in Text", LTC'2013, (2013)
26. Pazzani, M. J. and Billsus, D.: Content-Based Recommendation Systems. In: Brusilovsky P., Kobsa A., and Nejdl W. (Eds.) The Adaptive Web, Lecture Notes in Computer Science 4321, pp. 325–341. Heildelberg: Springer-Verlag (2007)
27. Ricci F., Rikach L., Shapira B. and Kantor, P.: Recommender Systems Handbook. US: Springer. p. 62 (2010)
28. Richardson, S. D.: Bootstrapping Statistical Processing into a Rule-based Natural Language Parser. Microsoft Research, One Microsoft Way, Redmond, WA 98052. Retrieved from: http://research.microsoft.com/apps/pubs/default.aspx?id=69572. Access date: October 9, 2013 (1994)
29. Riloff, E. and Jones, R.: Learning Dictionaries for Information Extraction by Multi-Level Bootstrapping. Sixteenth National Conference on Artificial Intelligence (AAAI-99), Orlando, Florida, USA (1999)
30. Saif, H.: Sentiment Analysis of Microblogs. Mining the New World. Technical Report KMI-12-2, March 2012 (2012)
31. Schafer, J. B., Frankowski, D., Herlocker, J. and Sen. S.: Collaborative Filtering Recommender Systems. In: Brusilovsky P., Kobsa A., and Nejdl W. (Eds.) The Adaptive Web, Lecture Notes in Computer Science 4321, pp. 291–324. Heildelberg: Springer-Verlag (2007)
32. Schafer, J.B., Konstan, J. and Riedi, J.: Recommender systems in e-commerce. 1st ACM conference on Electronic commerce EC 99, pp. 158–166 (1999)
33. Sidorov, G., Velasquez, F., Stamatatos, E., Gelbukh, A. and Chanona-Hernández, L.: Syntactic N-grams as machine learning features for natural language processing. In: Expert Systems with Applications, Volume 41 (3), 2014, pp. 853–860, doi: 10.1016/j.eswa.2013.08.015 (2014)
34. Semeraro, G.: Content-based Recommender Systems: problems, challenges and research directions. 8th Workshop on Intelligent Techniques for Web Personalization & Recommender Systems (2010)
35. Shah, K., Munshi, N. and Reddy, P.: Sentiment Analysis and Opinion Mining of Microblogs. May 5, 2013 (2013)
36. Smith, A. D. and Eisner, J. Bootstrapping Feature-Rich Dependency Parsers with Entropic Priors. 2007 Joint Conference on Empirical Methods in Natural Language Processing and Computational Natural Language Learning, Prague, June 2007, pp. 667–677 (2007)
37. Thelen, M. and Riloff, E.L.: A Bootstrapping Method for Learning Semantic Lexicons Using Extraction Pattern Contexts. Empirical Methods in NLP (EMNLP) (2002)
38. Turney, P.: Thumbs up or Thumbs Down? Semantic Orientation Applied to Unsupervised Classification of Reviews. Proceedings of the 40th Annual Meeting of the Association for Computational Linguistics (ACL), Philadelphia, July 2002, pp. 417-424 (2002)

39. Wang, S. and Manning, Ch.D.: Baselines and Bigrams: Simple, Good Sentiment and Topic Classification. In: Proceedings of the 50th Annual Meeting of the Association for Computational Linguistics (ACL'2012): Short Papers - Volume 2, pp. 90–94 (2012)
40. Yangarber, R., Grishman, R., Tapanainen P. and Huttunen, S.: Automatic Acquisition of Domain Knowledge for Information Extraction. 18th conference on Computational linguistics (COLING '00), Volume 2, pp. 940–946 (2002)

# Aggressive Text Detection for Cyberbullying

Laura P. Del Bosque and Sara Elena Garza

Facultad de Ingeniería Mecánica y Eléctrica,UANL
San Nicolás de los Garza, Nuevo León, México
{laura.delbosquevg, sara.garzavl}@uanl.edu.mx

**Abstract.** Aggressive text detection in social networks allows to identify offenses and misbehavior, and leverages tasks such as cyberbullying
detection. We propose to automatically map a document with an aggressiveness score (thus treating aggressive text detection as a regression
problem) and explore different approaches for this purpose. These include lexicon-based, supervised, fuzzy, and statistical approaches. We
test the different methods over a dataset extracted from Twitter and
compare them against human evaluation. Our results favor approaches
that consider several features (particularly the presence of swear or profane words).

**Keywords:** Twitter, sentiment analysis, fuzzy logic, supervised
learning.

## 1 Introduction

The way in which people communicate has changed and evolved during the last
decades [12]. Even though technology offers several benefits for young people
(12-25 years old), it has also several negative effects [4]; for instance, e-mail, tex-
ting, chats, smart phones, web cams, and web sites might be used to hurt other
people [3]. In fact, the continuous intentional aggression over an indefense victim via electronic media is known as *cyberbullying* [7]. For several reasons (e.g.
allowing people to hide behind an alias), this kind of virtual stalking is actually
more pernicious than traditional bullying [12]. Unfortunately, phenomena such
as these could ultimately end in violence and suicide. Needless to say, it is important to address this problem—for example, by using information technologies
to identify cases of cyberbullying.

We believe that the first step towards cyberbullying automatic identification
concerns *aggressive text detection*, where we consider as aggressive any text or
document that intends to offend a person or group of persons. To tackle this
issue, we define a simple aggressiveness scale (0-10, where 10 is strongly aggressive) and propose several methods to score a document in terms of aggression;
these methods have been selected and designed by assuming that aggressive text
detection is a sub-task of *sentiment analysis*, and thus include lexicon-based,
supervised, fuzzy, and statistical approaches.

A. Gelbukh et al. (Eds.): MICAI 2014, Part I, LNAI 8856, pp. 221–232, 2014.
© Springer International Publishing Switzerland 2014

To evaluate the proposed approaches, we extracted two comment datasets from Twitter, a popular microblog where users are free to express their opinions and address other users (presumably without censorship). We compared the automatically-generated scores with the manual scores from a group of evaluators. Our results, in general, show that several of the approaches are feasible, particularly those that combine different features.

The remainder of this document is organized as follows: Section 2 provides a brief background on sentiment analysis, and Section 3 presents related work. Section 4 introduces the different approaches that were employed for aggressive text scoring, and Section 5 describes experiments and results. Finally, Section 6 presents conclusions and future work.

## 2    Sentiment Analysis

Sentiment analysis studies subjective expressions (reviews, comments, views, emotions, etc.) that are usually found on media such as blogs, discussion boards, and news [9]. This discipline is inherently complex and involves an assortment of other disciplines, such as NLP, text mining, NER, and machine learning. Sentiment analysis includes several tasks:

**Document Sentiment Classification.-** Consists of determining whether a document is positive or negative. This is also known as *polarity detection*.

**Aspect-Based Analysis.-** Consists of detecting which specific aspect is being liked or disliked.

**Opinion Lexicon Generation.-** Consists of collecting words or phrases that express sentiment.

**Comparative Opinion Mining.-** Consists of analyzing opinions that compare items or aspects.

With respect to sentiment classification, there are two main forms to fulfill this task. One of these concerns *lexicon-based methods* (also referred to as unsupervised or semantic approaches) and the other concerns *supervised learning methods*; both of these exhibit pros and cons. Lexicon-based methods usually involve searching for the document's words in a given lexicon (vocabulary) and retrieving their polarity; the document's polarity is generally determined with a *term counting* strategy [8], i.e. a strategy in which a document is classified as positive when there are more positive than negative words and vice-versa. Supervised approaches, on the other hand, learn a model that predicts the document's polarity given a set of training examples; common supervised methods for classification include naïve Bayes, neural networks, and support vector machines (SVM).

## 3    Related Work

State-of-the-art methods for aggressive text detection within the framework of cyberbullying are oriented towards binary text classification using supervised approaches; these works—which also tend to explore different alternatives—are strongly committed towards finding an adequate set of features for performing the classification. The work by Dinakar et al. [5], for example, considers that a hurtful comment (document) covers *sensitive topics*, such as physical appearance, sexuality, race and culture, and intelligence. Their approach, consequently, trains both binary and multi-class classifiers to detect comments exhibiting these topics (separate binary classifiers are trained to decide whether a comment covers or does not cover one of the sensitive topics); the features they take into account are varied and include tf-idf unigrams (i.e., text frequency-inverse document frequency with single words), the presence of swear words (obtained from a lexicon), frequent POS bigrams (i.e., part-of-speech tag pairs) in hurtful messages, and topic-specific unigrams and bigrams. The approach is tested using JRip, J48, SVM, and naïve Bayes over a set of Youtube comments; results are compared against a manual classification. The JRip binary classifier was the best.

A similar approach is followed by Dadvar et al. [4]; these authors propose to consider gender information for aggressive document detection; for this reason, they train two separate classifiers (one per gender). Their features include second-person pronouns, swear words (take the most frequent also by gender), and tf-idf values. This approach is tested using an SVM to classify MySpace posts; their results (also compared vs. a manual annotation) show that taking gender into account, in fact, does increase precision.

Another outstanding work is the one by Nahar et al. [10]; this work extracts *semantic features* using Latent Dirichlet Allocation (LDA), and utilizes the lexicon of noswearing.com, tf-idf values, and second-person pronouns also as features for training an SVM. They test their approach over a dataset provided by the workshop of Content Analysis for the Web, which comprises comments from Twitter, Slashdot, and MySpace.

Sood et al. [11], following a similar line, detect profanity in text by employing Amazon's Mechanical Turk to label a set of comments from a social news site. The labeled dataset (represented as a *bag-of-words* where order is not important) is used to extract features such as bigrams and stems, which are used, in turn, to train an SVM. The rationale behind employing a supervised approach consists of overcoming the limitations of lexicon-based approaches, since these can fail to detect foul language by missing variations and invented or mispelled words. The authors do experiment, though, with the Levensthein distance to leverage the accuracy of the noswearing.com lexicon.

We attempt to go beyond binary classification by treating the aggressive text detection task as a *regression problem* and by using lexicons that, to the best of our knowledge, have not been tested for this particular task.

## 4   Aggressive Text Detection

The problem we tackle consists of automatically mapping a document $d_i$ to an aggressiveness score $sc_i$. The first step towards attempting to solve this problem is defining a bounded range for the score to fall in. We consider the range $[0, 10]$ to be appropriate for this context, since it is neither extremely coarse nor extremely granular; for this range, 0 indicates no aggression and 10 indicates a strong aggression.

The second step (and probably the most difficult) concerns finding a suitable technique to produce the scoring. Because an aggressive text could be seen as intrinsically negative, we conceive aggressiveness scoring as a sub-task of *sentiment analysis*, specifically of *polarity detection*. Furthermore, given that polarity detection is mostly either lexicon-based or supervised, exploring these kinds of approaches seems reasonable; in addition, since our specific problem regards *regression*, it also seems valid to explore statistical approaches such as linear regression. Let us describe each of these candidates.

## 4.1   Lexicon-Based Approaches

Our lexicon-based approaches are, to some extent, similar to term counting using a bag-of-words model— i.e. word ordering in the text is unimportant; however, we mainly focus on detecting negative terms (or the absence of positive ones). Let us briefly provide a background on each particular approach and then describe how the aggressiveness score is generated for that approach.

**Swear Words.** Our first lexicon (which we shall refer to as "NS") is extracted from the noswearing.com site, which comprises a collection of offensive words and their meanings, as well as a list of variants for these words; by being open to submissions from anyone, the site resembles a wisdom-of-crowds resource, thus offering a vocabulary that appears to be well suited for our purposes. To derive a score using this lexicon, we obtain the relative frequency of offensive words for the document and normalize this frequency using the maximum that has been found in the document collection. The relative frequency $f_i$ of offensive words for a document $d_i$ is calculated as the proportion of swear words in $d_i$, such that

$$f_i = \frac{o_i}{n_i}, \tag{1}$$

where $o_i$ and $n_i$ are, respectively, the total of offensive words and the total of words (both for $d_i$). The score $sc_i$ is finally calculated by normalizing this relative frequency with the maximum $f_{\max}$ found and multiplying the result by ten, as the normalized frequency yields a value within $[0, 1]$:

$$sc_i = (10) \left( \frac{f_i}{f_{\max}} \right). \tag{2}$$

So, for example, assume that $w_1$ and $w_2$ are swear words in a document $d_i = \{w_1, w_2, w_3, w_4\}$. In this case, $f_i = \frac{2}{4} = 0.5$; if $f_{\max} = 0.6$, then $sc_i = \frac{0.5}{0.6} = 0.83$.

**ANEW.** This lexicon, which stands for "Affective Norms for English Words" [2], is an affective resource that has been used for measuring happiness [6]. ANEW comprises a set of 1,034 words manually scored according to three aspects or *semantic differentials* (i.e. scales whose extremes are two opposite adjectives):

1. Pyschological valence (bad-good)
2. Motivation (passive-active)
3. Domain (weak-strong)

The overall affective value for a given word (as well as the value for each of the differentials) lies within the range $[1, 9]$, where 9 is the closest to happiness. To calculate the score using ANEW, we take the overall values for the document words found in the lexicon and average them; for example, given document $d_i = \{w_1, w_2, w_3, w_4\}$, if $w_2$ and $w_4$ were found and their respective overall values turned out to be 5.0 and 8.5, the average overall value would be $\frac{(5.0+8.5)}{2} = 6.75$. Since this value reflects a degree of happiness that increases with larger values (on the contrary of our scale, where greater values are more negative) and ANEW's range slightly differs from ours, we translate the resulting averages using

$$sc_i = \frac{(b - a)\left[(d - v_i) - c\right]}{d - c} + a$$

$$= \frac{(10)\left[(9 - v_i) - 1\right]}{8}$$

(3)

where $a = 0$, $b = 10$, $c = 1$, $d = 9$, and $v_i$ is the average value obtained from document $d_i$; note that $[a, b]$ is our range of aggressiveness and $[c, d]$ is ANEW's range of happiness. For the example provided above, the average value $v_i = 6.75$ would be translated into an aggressiveness score $sc_i = 1.56$.

**SentiWordNet.** The third lexicon used is SentiWordNet, which is a WordNet-based[1] tool for opinion mining. As the original WordNet, SentiWordNet contains English nouns, verbs, adjectives, and adverbs that are grouped into "synsets", i.e. sets cognitive synonyms, each expressing a distinct concept. The synsets are, as well, interlinked by means of conceptual semantic and lexical relations. SentiWordNet assigns each synset three classifications with respect to confidence, negativity, positivity, and objectivity [1]. Each synset is, therefore, associated to three numerical values: Pos(s), Neg(s), and Obj(s). These values, respectively, indicate positive, negative or objective (neutral) polarities and fall within the range $[0, 1]$; let us note that the sum of the three associated values is necessarily 1.0, which means that each synset has a value other than zero in at least one category [1].

To calculate the aggressiveness score with SentiWordNet, we averaged the negative polarities of the document words found in the lexicon—similar to the approach followed with ANEW. However, in contrast with ANEW, the resulting average is already negative and could easily be converted to our scale by multiplying the average by ten.

---

[1] WordNet is available at http://wordnet.princeton.edu

An important issue to consider, though, with SentiWordnet is the presence of ambiguity; in our case, the type of ambiguity that could potentially affect our scoring is *polisemy*, i.e. words with multiple meanings. Our first attempt to handle this kind of ambiguity consists, simply, of discarding those words that have multiple negative polarities; searching for a finer disambiguation process is left for future work.

### 4.2    Other Approaches

We also explore fuzzy, statistical, and supervised approaches. This second handful of approaches aims to combine different features or variables and is, to some extent, leveraged by the previous lexicon-based methods.

**Fuzzy Systems.** A *fuzzy system* is an expert system that works with imprecise, vague knowledge and is based, as the name suggests, on *fuzzy logic* [13]. This kind of system maps a set of given inputs to an output by means of an *inference engine* that uses a fuzzy *rule base*. To perform inferences with this rule base, the inputs are *fuzzified* and the fuzzy result is *defuzzified*; the latter process yields a "crisp" output. Fuzzy rules have an "if-then" structure that contains *linguistic variables*. A *linguistic variable* is a variable associated with a numeric variable $x$ and whose values are *fuzzy sets*. A fuzzy set, in turn, is a set whose elements have a membership value within the range $[0, 1]$—as opposed to crisp sets where elements are either present or absent. Membership values are given by *membership functions*.

Using the brief previous framework, let us describe the design of our fuzzy system for aggressiveness scoring. While several designs have been explored, the one presented here—as we will see later—has achieved, so far, the best results for the fuzzy approach. This design considers two inputs: the document's length (total words) and the number of swear words. The output is an aggressiveness value between 0 and 1. The system, therefore, contains three linguistic variables, each defined to have five possible values or fuzzy sets (see Table 1). All fuzzy sets are represented with triangular membership functions whose parameters (start, peak, end) are determined according to the mean and standard deviation of the particular dataset being used; while the former implies redefining the function parameters for each dataset (which seems reasonable when dealing with different document collections), we believe that this criterion is better than arbitrarily defining the functions. With respect to the system's rule base, it consists of 25 rules extracted from our prior experience on the subject (see Table 2 for some examples). Fuzzification and defuzzification are, respectively, carried out with the singleton and centroid methods.

Since the value returned by the fuzzy system lies within the range $[0,1]$, we only multiply this value by ten to place it in the range of our aggressiveness score.

**Supervised Learning and Linear Regression.** Supervised learning approaches, in contrast to fuzzy systems, act as black boxes. While this

**Table 1.** Fuzzy sets

| Document length | Number of swear words | Aggressiveness |
|---|---|---|
| Too short | None | Very positive |
| Short | Very few | Positive |
| Moderate | Few | Tends to be aggressive |
| Long | Many | Aggressive |
| Very long | Too many | Very aggressive |

**Table 2.** Inference rules examples

IF document is too short and has a few swear words THEN document is positive.
IF document is short and has too many swear words THEN document is very aggressive.
IF document is moderated and has none swear words THEN document is very positive.
IF document is long and has too many swear words THEN document is very aggressive.

hinders their capability of explaining why a certain output was obtained, it is also true that we do not have to build an expertise-demanding knowledge base. A supervised approach, however, requires a set of *labeled examples*. Each example consists of an input (represented by a number of *features*) and its corresponding output (label). A determined amount of examples is used for *training* (learning the function that maps an input to an output) and another amount is used for *testing* (validating that the function generalizes well by using unseen examples). Neural networks are a strong representative for supervised learning; such networks aim to mimic the human brain by considering a set of *neurons* (usually spread into *layers*) connected by synaptic *weighted edges*. Neural networks learn by repeatedly adjusting these weights.

Linear regression—a classical statistics-oriented technique–also learns a model that predicts outputs based on inputs with multiple features; the model is a *linear* function (hence the name) that best fits the data.

For predicting the aggressiveness score via supervised learning or linear regression, the following set of features is considered:

1. Document length (number of words)
2. Number of offensive words (using the **noswearing** lexicon)
3. Frequency of the word "you"
4. NS score
5. ANEW score (using the 1-9 original scale)
6. SentiWordNet score

## 5 Experiments and Results

The aim of our experiments is two-fold: on one hand, we wish to compare our candidate approaches, and on the other hand, we also wish to have a notion of which features better support aggressive text detection. For this matter, we test each approach with a set of comments extracted from *Twitter*; not only is this social network/microblogging service important and popular, but also (according to our point of view) prone to cyberbullying and harassment.

## 5.1  Setup

Our Twitter repository was gathered by crawling comments containing words such as "school", since this is the typical environment for cyberbullying and conversations leading to it; the collected comments belong to the English language, since the lexicons we use were made for this language (working with Spanish, which is our native tongue, is left for now as future work). From the obtained repository, we solely selected those comments that were directed towards one or more users, assuming that personal references potentially build cyberbullying attempts as well; in Twitter, directed comments are called *mentions* and are depicted with @username, where username represents the recipient of the comment. With this filtered repository, we furtherly generated two datasets: one with comments containing the word "f*ck"[2] and another containing the word "b*tch". To avoid using these words over and over again, let us refer to these datasets as, respectively, the *f-dataset* and the *b-dataset*. The reason for choosing comments with swear words obeys the intuition of finding aggression in these types of comments, while also acknowledging that both words have a certain degree of ambiguity. A summary of the repository is given in Table 3, and Table 4 presents some comment examples.

**Table 3.** Twitter repository used for this research

| Classification | Number of comments |
|---|---|
| Dataset | 111,381 |
| Directed comments | 12,705 |
| f-dataset | 281 |
| b-dataset | 110 |

**Table 4.** Examples of comments (swear words are partly censored)

| Comments |
|---|
| @F*ckCrystal i gotta go to school at 5 so idk if you wanna chill after that?? |
| @ParishRory @Sh4niqua pffffft hah no way shes a f*cking bully. I'm actually scared of her |

Both datasets were manually scored by four evaluators, who were instructed to place a number between zero and ten according to the perceived aggressiveness in each particular comment (zero being not aggressive and ten being very

---

[2] For respect, we do not show the complete swear word. The reader might guess the word we are referring to.

aggressive). To verify that these human judgments were similar—and, therefore, useful to our purposes—, we carried out ANOVA (see Table 5). Comments were discarded until the test was past, leaving the f-dataset with 174 comments and the b-dataset with 69 comments; let us note that the comments removed were the ones where there was no uniform judgment (e.g. one evaluator placed a mild aggression score and another placed a strong aggression score). This reveals the degree of complexity for the task, since not even humans agree in a percentage of the cases.

**Table 5.** Results for analysis of variance

| ANOVA | f-dataset | b-dataset |
|---|---|---|
| Population (n) | 174 | 69 |
| Evaluators (a) | 4 | 4 |
| Independent evaluator subtotal [A] | 4610.2 | 1946.1 |
| Sum of [A] [T] | 4275 | 1685.2 |
| Individual value [Y] | 14271 | 3868 |
| Square sum between groups | 334.9 | 260.9 |
| Square sum within groups | 9660.8 | 1921.9 |
| Degree of freedom between groups | 3 | 3 |
| Degree of freedom within groups | 692 | 272 |
| Mean square between groups | 111.6 | 86.9 |
| Quadratic mean in group | 13.9 | 7.1 |
| F Ratio (F) | 7.9 | 12.3 |
| Comparison between observed F vs. Distributed F | 2.6 / 3.8 | 2.7 / 3.8 |

The final comments on both datasets were pre-processed by eliminating punctuation marks, changing every word to lower case, and utilizing *regular expressions* to: correct misspelled words (for instance, "biatch" or "biotchhh"), expand acronyms such as "OMFG", and separate words with swearing (e.g. the username @muppyb*tch would be broken down into @muppy and b*tch). We also translated emoticons such as :), :(, and :@ to affective terms like "happy", "sad", or "angry".

Before showing and discussing results, let us note that we selected the *multilayer perceptron* neural network as our supervised learning approach; the parameters for this neural network (as well as for linear regression) were the default used by the WEKA toolkit. Training and testing were performed using a cross-validation of ten folds. In addition, different runs were performed using all attributes, all atributes minus no. 3 (you's), only attributes 1,2, and 4 (length, badwords, and NS score), and only attributes 1 and 2. Let us respectively refer to these variants as *6-attribute*, *5-attribute*, *3-attribute*, and *2-attribute*.

## 5.2 Results and Discussion

Each approach was evaluated using the two datasets. For comparison, we employed the Mean Squared Error (MSE), which is calculated as $(x-y)^2$, where $x$ is the average human score and $y$ is the score obtained using a particular approach. To have a clearer view of results, we also introduced a baseline method, which consisted of randomly-generated scores; such random scores were generated 30 times and then averaged.

Our results are shown in Figures 1 and 2; Table 6, more precisely, depicts all errors. The overall best approach (lowest MSE) was the 2-attribute linear regression, followed by the 3-attribute neural network, the fuzzy system, the NS lexicon, SentiWordNet, and finally ANEW. Interestingly, this last approach was worse than the baseline; we believe this may be due to the presence of slang and informal text, as well as to some kind of ambiguity. If we contrast single-source approaches (lexicons) vs. multiple-source approaches (supervised, statistical, and fuzzy), there is also an important difference; in that sense, those methods combining different variables or features seem to work better than methods with a single type of information. Furthermore, if we contrast the results obtained per dataset, we may note that the f-dataset in general obtained smaller errors than the b-dataset; for statistical and supervised approaches, this could be due to the size of the dataset (more examples available to train). Within the lexicon-based methods, not surprisingly, the best results were obtained by the NS approach; while this could be partly due to the datasets (chosen by searching for swear words), we believe that the strength of the approach rather lies on the close relationship that exists between aggressiveness and profane language. We could also question whether aggressiveness could be conceived without taking into account this kind of language. In that sense, the presence and number of swear words in the text could act as a key feature.

**Table 6.** MSE Results

| Approach | f-dataset | b-dataset | Average |
|---|---|---|---|
| NS | 5.2 | 7.2 | 6.23 |
| ANEW | 16.1 | 33.9 | 24.95 |
| SentiWordNet | 11.2 | 8.4 | 9.8 |
| Fuzzy system | 4.8 | 6.1 | 5.5 |
| Neural network | 4.2 | 6.2 | 5.2 |
| Linear regression | **3.6** | **5.9** | **4.8** |
| Baseline | 15.6 | 20.1 | 17.9 |

By drilling down the obtained results, it is also important to note that the hardest cases for all approaches were the ones with a high degree of aggressiveness; we believe this is due to several reasons. On one hand, these comments are more scarce than the rest, which implies less examples to train or characterize. On the other hand, there could be aspects in those comments that need to be considered, such as the underlying emotions, intentions, and context. It would also be interesting to include weight assignment for swear words and evaluate if this change impacts some of the results.

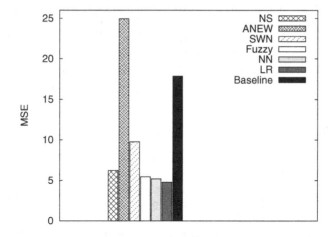

**Fig. 1.** Average mean squared error (MSE). NS= `noswearing.com` lexicon, SWN= SentiWordNet, NN= Neural Network, LR= Linear Regression.

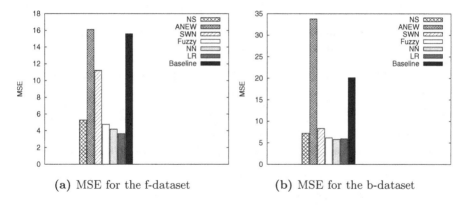

(a) MSE for the f-dataset          (b) MSE for the b-dataset

**Fig. 2.** Mean squared error by dataset

## 6   Conclusions and Future Work

In the present work, we have tackled aggressive text detection as a regression problem that consists of mapping a document to an *aggressiveness score*; to the best of our knowledge, state-of-the-art methods tend to cast this issue as a binary classification problem. We have defined a simple scale that ranges from zero to ten (where ten is the most aggressive) and assumed, as well, that aggressive text detection is a sub-task of sentiment analysis that is closely related to document polarity detection. Taking the former into account, we proposed and explored lexicon-based, supervised, fuzzy, and statistical approaches, which were tested over a Twitter repository. Our results show that linear regression seems to be a solid candidate for scoring the documents, and that the use of profane language (swear words) seems also to be a key feature for the task.

Future work includes refining our approaches to better handle difficult cases (e.g. creating other designs for the fuzzy system), testing more supervised approaches (SVM, for instance), using a larger dataset, working with documents in Spanish, and building a framework for cyberbullying automatic identification.

# References

1. Análise de sentimentos no Twitter utilizando SentiWordNet, Proposta de Trabalho de Graduação (2011)
2. Bradley, M.M., Lang, P.J.: Affective norms for English words (ANEW): Instruction manual and affective ratings. Technical report, Center for Research in Psychophysiology, University of Florida (1999)
3. Campbell, M.A.: Cyber bullying: An old problem in a new guise? Australian Journal of Guidance and Counselling 15(1), 68–76 (2005)
4. Dadvar, M., de Jong, F.M.G., Ordelman, R.J.F., Trieschnigg, R.B.: Improved cyberbullying detection using gender information. In: Proceedings of the Twelfth Dutch-Belgian Information Retrieval Workshop (DIR 2012), Ghent, pp. 23–26. University of Ghent (2012)
5. Dinakar, K., Reichart, R., Lieberman, H.: Modeling the detection of textual cyberbullying. In: The Social Mobile Web (2011)
6. Dodds, P.S., Danforth, C.M.: Measuring the happiness of large-scale written expression: Songs, blogs, and presidents. Journal of Happiness Studies 11(4), 441–456 (2010)
7. Dorothy, L.: Espelage and Susan M Swearer. Research on school bullying and victimization: What have we learned and where do we go from here? School Psychology Review (2003)
8. Kennedy, A., Inkpen, D.: Sentiment classification of movie reviews using contextual valence shifters. Computational Intelligence 22(2), 110–125 (2006)
9. Liu, B.: Sentiment analysis and opinion mining. Synthesis Lectures on Human Language Technologies 5(1), 1–167 (2012)
10. Nahar, V., Xue, L., Chaoyi, P.: An effective approach for cyberbullying detection. Communications in Information Science and Management Engineering (2012)
11. Sood, S., Antin, J., Churchill, E.: Using crowdsourcing to improve profanity detection. In: AAAI Spring Symposium Series, pp. 69–74 (2012)
12. Sticca, F., Perren, S.: Is cyberbullying worse than traditional bullying? Examining the differential roles of medium, publicity, and anonymity for the perceived severity of bullying. Journal of Youth and Adolescence, pp. 1–12 (2012)
13. Zadeh, L.A.: Fuzzy sets. Information and Control 8(3), 338–353 (1965)

# A Sentiment Analysis Model: To Process Subjective Social Corpus through the Adaptation of an Affective Semantic Lexicon

Guadalupe Gutiérrez[1,2], Lourdes Margain[1], Carlos de Luna[1], Alejandro Padilla[3], Julio Ponce[3], Juana Canul[2], and Alberto Ochoa[4]

[1] Universidad Politécnica de Aguascalientes, México
[2] Universidad Juárez Autónoma de Tabasco, México
[3] Universidad Autónoma de Aguascalientes, México
[4] Universidad Autónoma de Ciudad Juárez, México

**Abstract.** The social networks proliferation over the Internet has generated an interest from the users to express communicate and make opinions about different topics, services or people. This has led the creation of tools, methods, techniques and models that are enable to obtain information from the web in order to analyze and identify the emotion that is shown by the users in their opinions, this has given the key to the development and improvement of sentimental semantic lexicons to the emotional analysis in opinions. This paper shows the proposal of the Model to Analyze Emotions in subjective social corpus through the adaptation of an affective semantic lexicon, focused on the extension of an affective lexicon in order to adequate to the Spanish spoken in Mexico considering the linguistic variations.

**Keywords:** Affective semantic lexicon, opinion mining, sentiment analysis.

## 1 Introduction

The development and innovation of different information technologies has allowed to establish a global communication without limits, for example the social networks (e.g. Facebook, Twitter) and other ways of social communication have established both pc and mobile devices (e.g. Whatsapp, Telegram, Wechat). The social networks expansion has made an interest from the users to not only share objective information, also subjective information, commenting and making opinions about diverse kinds of interest topics[1, 2]. This has caused an exponential growth about the opinions from the users regarding services, products and even public figures, this has called the attention from the companies, government, and science education institutions as a potential opportunity to analyze, structure, process this information in order to identify emotions form the users.

A report published by Nielsen [3], manifests that 70% from the social networks users pay attention to other users comments, 65% look for information before making a decision, 50% make use of the social networks to complain or make a claim. Due to

A. Gelbukh et al. (Eds.): MICAI 2014, Part I, LNAI 8856, pp. 233–244, 2014.

this Balahur [4] commented "this new reality has led a place to important changes in the form, and speed of flow of the news and their related opinions, giving a place to new challenging social, economic and psychological phenomena".

This paper describes the proposal for a Model designed to analyze subjective social corpus applied to opinion mining. This work organization begins with the state of the art about the existing lexicons for the emotions analysis, the problematic of the research, the semantic model proposal for the analysis of emotions in Subjective Social Corpus applied to opinion mining (denominated in this paper as ASES Model), the description of the process of adequacy lexicon SentiSense, the preliminary results, the conclusions and the future work.

# 2    Lexicon

The lexicon is the most important resource to work with algorithms applied to the emotions analysis. Feldman [5] describes three possible options to work with lexicons, the first is about a manual approach where all codification is manual, which makes a laborious process and not feasible. The second is an approach based on dictionaries, using a set of adequate seed words to a specific domain gets expanded by combining with other resources for example WordNet[1], however the disadvantage of the approach based on dictionaries is that the resources with the ones that are mixed are independent and do not capture specific particularities from the specific domain. The third option is about the approach based on the corpus in which one set of seed words gets expanded through the extensive use of documents in only one domain.

## 2.1    WordNet, a Lexical Database

The Royal Spanish Academy dictionary[2] defines that a lexicon is a vocabulary or set of words from a language that reside in the usage from a region. WordNet was created in 1985 by George A. Miller, is an extended lexicon database designed specifically for the English language, despite in the beginning emerge as a combination between lexicon and a simple thesaurus to understand, actually it is considered a basic tool for the development of complex textual analysis applications and the processing of the Natural Language Processing (NLP). WordNet is organized into four basic lexicon categories: names, verbs, adjectives and adverbs. It's based on concepts that their representation inside the database is made through the denominated synonym sets or synsets. The WordNet database is free and available for research or project development without any profit. Because at the present WordNet has been used as an standard for the automated semantic disambiguation at word level it is decided to apply as a lexical database in the ASES Model as well as the big interest that has been shown by the scientific community from the NLP area it is also has been made up to the Spanish language and it's most recent version offers an morphosyntactic and semantic annotation.

---

[1] http://www.wordnet-online.com/
2 http://www.rae.es/

## 2.2     Affective Lexicons

An affective lexicon can be understood as a set of words associated with a tag that has emotional kind information. In this kind of lexicon are two types that differ:

- Lexicon based on words (terms), where the word is tagged with the emotional information.
- Lexicon based in concepts, which is based on the meaning of the words to tag the concept according to the emotion that expresses.

Both kind of lexicon are based on two theories, the psychological theory of the emotional categories and the psychological theory of the emotional dimensions. The psychological theory of the emotional categories seeks for tagging the entries with the basic emotions like sadness or fear, while the ones based on emotional dimensions

**Table 1.** WordNet Affect and SentiWordNet characteristics

| Lexicon | Characteristics | Weakness |
|---|---|---|
| WordNet Affect | • Tag based on an emotional hierarchy, the concepts of WordNet that have an affective meaning.<br><br>• WordNet Affect has been developed through a process semi-automated, where in the first step was manually tagged with the emotional categories, one initial set of synsets, automatically expanding through the relation of these. | • Although it is designed for emotional categories usage, these are extensive and not based on the psychological theories.<br><br>• Has concepts tagged with more than one emotional category, which cause situations where is not possible to determinate the right emotion without a specific disambiguation process, also could cause that the recovered emotional category is not the most appropriated.<br><br>• There is no an updated version due to the WordNet latest version for Windows is the 2.1, while WordNet Affect is based on the version 1.6. |
| SentiWordNet | • Every synset has been tagged with three numerical values in the categories Pos(s), Neg(s) and Obj(s), representing the positive polarity, the negative polarity and the neutrality of the concept.<br>• Has been developed through the automated classification of the synsets of WordNet. | • SentiWordNet has an advantage of covering all the synsets of WordNet, even thought is also a weakness because in some cases, the concepts that are not properly related with the initial set of manually tagged synsets will not get the adequate ratings. |

tag the entries by popularity. Most lexicons are based on these theories are at word level which stands out the LIWC Dictionary[3] (Linguistic Inquiry and Word Count Dictionary) for those based on the psychology theory of the emotional categories and the General Inquirer [6] for those based on the theory of emotional dimensions. Nevertheless for those lexicons based on the concepts stand out WordNet Affect[4] and SentiWordNet[5]. The table 1 shows some outstanding characteristics from these lexicons.

As we can observe on the table 1, WordNet Affect and SentiWordNet have some weaknesses related with updates, disambiguation and some others, also one really important point is that they are not available on Spanish language, therefore their usage on the ASES Model is not convenient due to is needed to use dictionaries, and then verify and validate that the translations are accurate, causing more dedication on the translating process leaving behind other tasks form the ASES Model. For this reason is decided to adequate one Spanish emotional lexicon considering the Carrillo work[7], which is a lexicon based on concepts and supporting psychological theory of the emotional categories, to capture the polarity and also the intensity associated to every category at evaluating one text emotionally.

For adapting SentiSense is important consider a lexical in Spanish created by Díaz[8] is a dictionary, tagged with six basic emotions, which considers probability percentages with an emotional sense; called: probability factor affective use to assign a weight factor to potentially emotional words. Also the study of Sidorov[9] is considered important because present best settings of parameters for application to opinion mining in Spanish considering the dictionary of the six basic emotions by Díaz.

# 3     ASES Model: Proposal

Although the analysis of emotions is actually addressed by researchers and companies around the world, there is a problematic that there is no standard or methodology to follow [5] and the most of the resources are for the English language and even if translators are been implemented for working in other languages; the adaptation of these resources is complicated due to the language nature and the linguistic variations form each region or country. For this reason it is considered important to design a Semantic Model for the Emotions Analysis in Subjective Social Corpus applied to opinion mining, which considers the adaptation of resources to Spanish language (lexicons) in consideration of the language variations from some Mexico regions. The adaptation of a lexicon will contribute in a future that it could be complemented with other different languages to shape one standard lexicon with the purpose that will be available for other researchers in the emotional analysis.

## 3.1     Definitions to Consider in the ASES Model

Before starting with the description of the ASES Model architecture, is important to introduce some terms.

---

[3] http://www.liwc.net/

[4] http://wndomains.fbk.eu/

[5] http://sentiwordnet.isti.cnr.it/

- **Social Web Object.** Is denominated to the opinion resource form the web or that is available in one corpus form the social web. For example the figure 6 shows a new shared on Facebook through the news channel CNN[6] about the strategy that has been implemented by some hotels to attract clients offering Internet service. This news is liked by 694 users, it has been shared 32 times and there are different opinions from the users, nevertheless there is a chance of spam existence. (Observe the comment 2 enclosed in a rectangle form the figure 1).

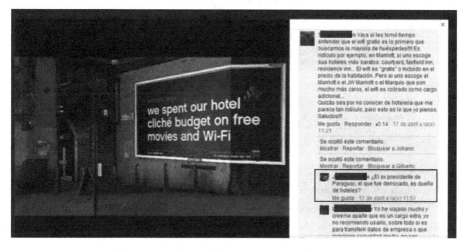

**Fig. 1.** An example of subjective opinions and spam

- **Object Semantic.** It is denominated object semantic to the object form a social web that contains three basic components according to Balahur [4, 10] should contain an opinion: titular, one opinion and the object on which the opinion is being done. The classification process of semantic objects is another way to ensure an object cleaning process form the social web, because is possible that it has misspelling or even with emoticons[7].

- **Emotive object.** Is denominated to the semantic object that is classified by an emotive effect, in this paper emotive effect is a positive emotion, negative or neutral.

---

[6] CNN.- Cable News Network, es una cadena de televisión estadounidense en cubrir noticias las 24 horas del día.

[7] Graphic symbol used in communications through email and serves to express the mood of the sender. Dictionary of the Real Spanish Academy.

## 3.2    ASES Model Architecture Diagram

The proposed architecture from ASES model is shown in the figure 2 and is based on six phases, each one responsible for carrying out a specific task, which are described below the figure.

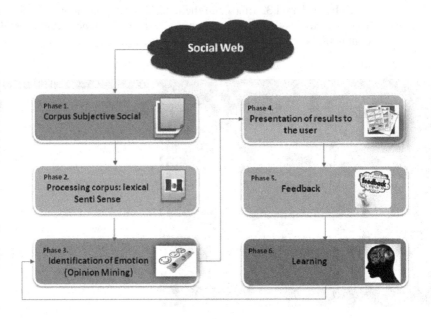

**Fig. 2.** ASES model architecture

**Phase 1. Subjective Social Corpus**

In this phase is going to be chosen the corpus to analyze with the ASES Model, on the web there is a corpus variety in different languages (e.g TASS[8], AnCora[9]), the advantage of these is that they have passes through a cleaning process, they do not contain spam, misspelling and most of them contain the three basic opinion elements, also there are some in Spanish. This kind of corpus comes from social networks like Facebook, Twitter or movie suggestion application (Netflix). Right now for this phase is working with a corpus form the mobile application Foursquare, because it has been found less spam on the opinions from the users that make "check-in" and comment about the service, product, location and the place's environment. Other possible corpus that could be used to analyzed is the comments made by the Strategic Information Systems engineering students from the Aguascalientes Polytechnic University about their teachers, according to [11] there has been good results applying the emotional analysis in the education. The figure 3 shows the three phases that a corpus must pass through in order to use the ASES Model those phases are described below:

---

[8] www.daedalus.es/TASS2013/about.php
[9] http://clic.ub.edu/corpus/en

- It must contain subjective opinions from users, and it can be downloaded through a social network.
- It must undergo a cleaning process to avoid spamming.
- It has to be processed along with the lexicon (which was determined in the ASES model); therefore, both must be contextually related.
- Subsequently the corpus has to be classified into two emotional dimensions enlisted as follows: very positive, positive, very negative, negative and neutral.

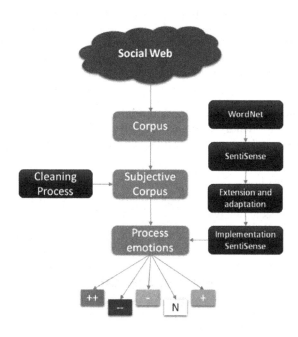

**Fig. 3.** Social subjective corpus process

**Phase 2. Processing Corpus: lexical SentiSense**

Due to WordNet consideration as the main standard for lexicon development, an investigation has been launched with the main purpose of finding affective lexicons that were generated via WordNet. The following lexicon (SentiSense) [7] developed by Carrillo will be used to adequate and extend the process into the Spanish (Mexico) language. Also, this lexicon has the peculiarly of being based in concepts. For the SentiSense implementation into the ASES model it is necessary to follow the steps portrayed on figure 4. With SentiSense support on this phase, it is possible to make object processing from social web to a later conversion into semantic objects.

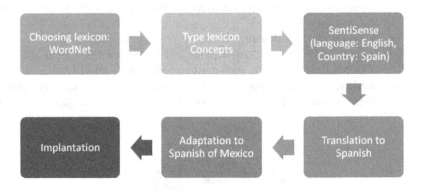

**Fig. 4.** Work steps for SentiSense implantation in ASES model

## Phase 3. Emotions Identification (Opinion mining)

Phase 3 is intended to identify emotions throughout opinion mining technique. This works by converting each semantic object into an emotive object.

## Phase 4. Results Display

This phase is addressed towards two types of users, user A and user B. In figure 5 user A is portrayed as an analyst capable of using ASES to evaluate users opinions about services or products provided. On the other hand, user B is depicted as a customer who reviews user opinions in order to acquire a product or a service.

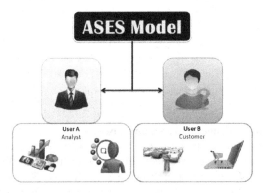

**Fig. 5.** Users ASES Model

## Phase 5. Feedback

In every system that possess any artificial intelligence technique it is important to check user's feedback. This phase allows users to perform feedbacks to the ASES model with the objective to evaluate effectiveness in emotive objects classification; besides, it is also capable of evaluating utility degree.

**Phase 6. Learning**

In this phase ASES model feedback is reviewed aiming to evaluate effectiveness in classifications as well as utility degree. Data generated through these means presents utility as a comparison model with other preexisting models.

# 4    Lexicon Implementation Process

SentiSense [12, 13] is selected as the lexicon which will undergo a process of extension, adequacy and implementation into the ASES model. It is based on labeling WordNet concepts instead of words. For example, if we assign such an emotion as fear to a word like cancer (meaning tumor), and the search engine finds cancer (meaning constellation) this word will be mislabeled. Hence, it is quite necessary to analyze each word until emotional labeling is properly assigned (WSD Word Sense Disambiguation algorithm will be used).

Freeling software tool will be used to extend and adequate SentiSense. This software tool is specially designed for Spanish processing texts and it provides enough plugins to obtain WordNet 3.0 concepts in Spanish (WordNet included in Multilingual Central Repository[10]). Also, another advantage of Freeling is that it uses WSB as a UKB algorithm (Graph Based Word Sense Disambiguation and Similarity). This algorithm it is considered as a very accurate one.

In figure 6 an example of Synsets WordNet association and the associated SentiSense lexicon into a text are portrayed. It is important to emphasize that synsets can only be classified as names, verbs, adjectives and adverbs (as illustrated on the figure). Each synset in the text is related to SentiSense to identify the associated emotion. In this case the analyzer will find the word cancer and it will properly classify as a negative emotion such as fear.

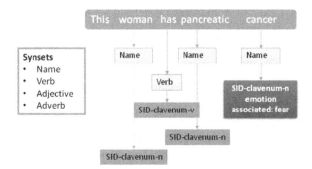

**Fig. 6.** Example of WordNet synsets and SentiSense association into a text

It is important to highlight that SentiSense was created to identify words in English language as default. It is composed of 5,496 words and 2190 synsets labeled under an emotional category.

To extend and adequate SentiSense into Spanish (Mexico) language the following methodology was proposed: it consists into an automatic emotions labeling (e.g. SentiWordNet) following the original steps according to SentiSense creation. Two XML data files were designed. The first contains emotional categories (see fig. 7) as well as counter emotions within case. The second XML file contains synsets related to WordNet (see fig. 8).

```
<?xml version="2.0"?>
<SentiSenseCategoriasEmocion>
<CategoriasEmocion name="alegría' antonym="tristeza" />
<CategoriasEmocion name="miedo' antonym="calma" />
<CategoriasEmocion name="amor' antonym="odio" />
<CategoriasEmocion name="esperanza' antonym="desesperación"/>
</SentiSenseCategoriasEmocion>
```

**Fig. 7.** XML extract of emotional categories

```
<SentiSenseCorpus>
<Concept synset="SID-00152712-A" pos="adjective"
gloss="carente de cordialidad..." emotion="disgusto"/>
<Concept synset="SID-00050667-R" pos="adverb"
gloss="de una manera graciosa..." emotion="alegría"/>
<Concept synset="SID-03430539-N" pos="noun"
gloss="el arma se disparó..." emotion="miedo"/>
<Concept synset="SID-02571914-V" pos="verb"
gloss="ella tendrá un bebé..." emotion="sorpresa"/>
...
</SentiSenseCorpus>
```

**Fig. 8.** XML extract of SentiSense in Spanish (Mexico)

In figure 8 it can be observed that each concept contains a key related to WordNet in order to identify its meaning and emotion based on the considered POS. It could be an adjective, adverb, substantive or verb. In table 2 emotion-synset relation is enlisted.

**Table 2.** Emotional category and corresponding synset

| Emotion | Key | Similar Emotion |
|---------|-----|-----------------|
| Disgust | SID-00152712-A | "disgust, revolt ..." |
| Joy | SID-00050667-R | "exultation, jubilance ..." |
| Fear | SID-03430539-N | "fearful, frightful" |
| Surprise | SID-02571914-V | "amazingly, surprisingly ..." |

Currently SentiSense lexicon is ruled by 14 emotional categories, which are: ambiguous, anger, calmness, despair, disgust, anticipation, fear, hate, hope, joy, like, love, sadness and surprise.

## 5    Conclusions and Future Work

The emotional analysis has been implemented at different levels and perspectives, not only by researchers also by the companies that implement it in marketing in order to make profit. Even that is a recent area and is completely new and nowadays there are not standard nor methodologies to be implemented and follow, the creation of the ASES Model presume a contribution for the companies or researchers from Mexico to be implemented, also the extension and adjustment from the SentiSense lexicon will contribute based on Carrillo [12] as an useful resource for the emotional analysis in other countries beside Spain.

As future work we plan to develop a tool for automatic labeling, that applying the technique of case-based reasoning, construct based on successful cases: corpus correctly classified and labeled for use in different contexts.

## References

1. Bing, L.: Sentiment Analysis and Opinion Mining (Synthesis Lectures on Human Language Technologies). Morgan & Claypool Publishers (May 23, 2012) ISBN-13: 978-1608458844
2. Pang, B.L.: Opinion mining and sentiment analysis. Foundations and Trends in Information Retrieval 2(1-2) (2008)
3. Nielsen, State of the Media: The Social Media Report 2012. NM Incite (2012)
4. Balahur, A.: Methods and Resources for Senttiment Analysis in Multilingual Documents of Different Text Types. Tesis de Doctorado. Departamento de Lenguajes y Sistemas Informáticos. Universidad de Alicante (2011)
5. Feldman, R.: Techniques and applications for sentiment analysis. Communications ot the ACM 56(4), 82–89 (2013)
6. Stone, P., Dumphy, D., Smith, M., Ogilvie, D.: The General Inquirer: A Computer Approach to Content Analysis. The MIT Press, Cambridge (1966)
7. Carrillo de Albornoz, J.: Un Modelo Lingüístico-Semántico Basado en Emociones para la Clasificación de Textos según su Polaridad e Intensidad. Tesis doctoral. Departamento de Ingeniería del Software e Inteligencia Artificial. Facultad de Informática. Universidad Complutense de Madrid (2011)
8. Díaz, I., Sidorov, G., Suárez, S.: Creación y Evaluación de un Diccionario Marcado con Emociones Ponderado para el Español. Onomazein (May 29, 2014) doi:10.7764/onomazein
9. Sidorov, G., Miranda-Jiménez, S., Viveros-Jiménez, F., Gelbukh, A., Castro-Sánchez, N., Velásquez, F., Díaz-Rangel, I., Suárez-Guerra, S., Treviño, A., Gordon, J.: Empirical Study of Machine Learning Based Approach for Opinion Mining in Tweets. In: Batyrshin, I., González Mendoza, M. (eds.) MICAI 2012, Part I. LNCS, vol. 7629, pp. 1–14. Springer, Heidelberg (2013)

10. Wiebe, J., Riloff, E.: Creating Subjective and Objective Sentence Classifiers from Unannotated Texts. In: Gelbukh, A. (ed.) CICLing 2005. LNCS, vol. 3406, pp. 486–497. Springer, Heidelberg (2005)
11. Ortigosa, A., Martín, J., Carro, R.: Sentiment Analysis in Facebook and its application to e-learning. Computers in Human Behavior (2013),
    http://dx.doi.org/10.1016/j.chh.2013.05.034
12. Carrillo de Albornoz, J., Plaza, L., Gervás, P.: SentiSense: An easily scalable concept-based affective lexicon for Sentiment Analysis. In: The 8th International Conference on Language Resources and Evaluation, LREC 2012 (2012)
13. Carrillo de Albornoz, J., Chugur, I., Amigó, E.: Using an Emotion-based Model and Sentiment Analysis Techniques to Classify Polarity for Reputation. In: Proceedings CLEF 2012 Labs and Workshop Notebook Paper (2012)

# Towards Automatic Detection of User Influence in Twitter by Means of Stylistic and Behavioral Features*

Gabriela Ramírez-de-la-Rosa, Esaú Villatoro-Tello,
Héctor Jiménez-Salazar, and Christian Sánchez-Sánchez

Departamento de Tecnologías de la Información,
Universidad Autónoma Metropolitana Unidad Cuajimalpa. México D.F.
{gramirez,evillatoro,hjimenez,csanchez}@correo.cua.uam.mx

**Abstract.** Online communities are filled with comments of loyal readers or first-time viewers, that are constantly creating and sharing information at an unprecedented level, resulting in millions of messages containing opinions, ideas, needs and beliefs of Internet users. Therefore, businesses companies are very interested in finding influential users and encouraging them to create positive influence. Influential users represent users with the ability to influence individual's attitudes in a desired way with relative frequency. We present an empirical analysis on *influential* users identification problem in Twitter. Our proposed approach considers that the influential level of users can be detected by considering its communication patterns, by means of particular writing style features as well as behavioral features. Performed experiments on more that 7000 users profiles, indicate that it is possible to automatically identify influential users among the members of a social networking community, and also it obtains competitive results against several state-of-the-art methods.

**Keywords:** Opinion Leaders, User Influence, Author Profiling, Machine Learning, Natural Language Processing.

## 1 Introduction

According to [14], it was in 1995 when the first noteworthy social networking Web site appears, namely Classmates.com. Nowadays, almost 20 years later, such type of Web sites, *e.g.* Facebook, Twitter, YouTube, Flickr, etc., constitute a considerable portion of Internet use [6], and represent companies valued at millions of dollars. Such online communities are fulled with comments of loyal readers or first-time viewers, that are constantly creating and sharing information at an unprecedented level, resulting in millions of messages, photos, or videos, but more importantly opinions, ideas, needs and beliefs of the massive audience that makes up the Internet [7].

---

* This work was partially supported by CONACyT México Project Grant CB-2010/153315, and SEP-PROMEP UAM-PTC-380/48510349. We also thank to UAM Unidad Cuajimalpa and SNI-CONACyT for their support.

A. Gelbukh et al. (Eds.): MICAI 2014, Part I, LNAI 8856, pp. 245–256, 2014.

As established by [14] the business model followed by most of the social networking sites is based on advertising. Hence, when users surf through a site, some advertisements are displayed on the Web pages delivered to the users. Accordingly, social networking firms earn money from either just showing advertisements to users, or for each click made by users in response to an advertisement. Such marketing strategy is called viral advertisement [13], given that an appropriate (well directed) advertisement can produce a snow-ball effect, since the influence of users on their friends can increase or decrease sales. Therefore, businesses companies are very interested in finding influential people and encouraging them to create positive influence.

Influence has long been studied in the fields of sociology, communication, marketing, and political science [2]. As we mention before, the notion of influence plays a vital role in how businesses operate and how a society functions. Traditional communication theory states that a minority of users, called *influentials*, surpass in persuading others [2]. This theory predicts that by means of targeting these *influentials* in the social networking sites, it would be possible to achieve a large-scale chain-reaction of influence driven by word-of-mouth, with a very small marketing cost. Such *influentials* are also known as *opinion leaders* or just *leadership*, that according to [3] represent users with the ability to informally influence individual's attitudes or behavior in a desired way with relative frequency.

In this article we present an empirical analysis on *opinion leaders* identification problem in a popular social networking medium, *i.e.*, Twitter. As it is known, from its inception in 2006, Twitter has become one of the most important platform for microblog posts. Recent statistics reveal that there are more that 250 million users that write more than 500 million posts every day[1], talking about a great diversity of topics. As a consequence, several entities such as companies, celebrities, politicians, etc., are very interested in using this type of platform for increasing or even improving their influence among Twitter users, aiming at obtaining good reputation values.

Our proposed approach for *opinion leaders* identification is based on the idea that the leadership/influential level of an author can be detected by considering its writing style, and its behavior within the Twitter's community. Accordingly, we propose several stylistics attributes (lexical richness, language complexity, etc), as well as different behavioral features (posts' frequency, directed tweets, etc.), that are computed directly from users twitter accounts. Once all features are computed, we train a classification model for identifying opinion leaders through machine learning algorithms. Performed experiments on more that 7000 users profiles, indicate that it is possible (to some extent) automatically identify influential users among the members of a social networking community. In order to compare our obtained results among the state-of-the-art methods, we replicate the methodology proposed in the RepLab 2014 [1] workshop, where such task was evaluated this year. From this exercise, we show that our proposed method obtains competitive results against participant systems in the RepLab 2014.

---

[1] https://about.twitter.com/company

The rest of this document is organized as follows. Section 2 present some related work concerning to the leadership classification task. Section 3 describes our proposed method; particularly it details the proposed *stylistics* and *behavioral* features. Then, Section 4 describes used datasets, experimental setup and shows obtained results by our proposed approach. Finally, Section 5 depicts our conclusions and some future work directions.

## 2   Related Work

Leadership identification can be seen as a particular problem of Author Profiling, which consists in discovering those users that could represent an opinion leader among a community, *i.e.*, finding those users who are the most influential (opinion makers) within a community of users. One of the challenges here is to identify an author or authors that are influential to a particular community. For Twitter, some methods [10] use a variation of the PageRank algorithm, taking advantage of the following-followers schema on Twitter. Some others methods [8], set the influential level of an author according to the number of tweets that are categorized as important. However, in a very dynamic environment, some of these methods may have some difficulties updating the influential level for every user or even more, for every tweet.

Nevertheless, there are several approaches that have been proposed to tackle the problem of identifying leadership in social network. From variants of Pagerank [10,12] to supernetwork algorithms [11] where proposed solutions had taking into account diverse kind of information. Perhaps we have to go back to works on Social Sciences to adopt a framework and give a more sustainable approach.

In this sense the work of David Huffaker [7] may be a good instance. This work examines leadership behavior defined accordingly to replies trigger, conversation creation, and language diffusion. The author used a sample of 33,540 users, comprising 632,622 messages from Google Groups ranging from June 2003 to January 2006. For each approach defining the leadership behavior, he analyzed how much it is characterized using three models compose by some independent variables, namely: i) Communication Activity, represented by number of posts, number of replies, tenure in community; ii) Social Network, as expansiveness, reciprocity, and brokering; and iii) Language Use, through of talkativeness, linguistic diversity, assertiveness, and affect. The results of this study were: on communication activity dimension tenure is related to influence others; on social network dimension may be expressed as expansiveness and reciprocity but brokering was not related to the ability to influence communication; and for language use, the talkativeness, linguistic diversity, assertiveness and affect are relevant to this dimension.

In other direction, it is important to mention a work which tries to solve the problem in a hybrid manner, namely tweet-centric [9]. The tweet-centric approach considers tweet-value as well as users at Micro-blog. Authors proposed a user-tweet interaction model which measures author ranking through a weighted and directed graph whose nodes are users and tweets; edges are defined considering references either user-tweet, or tweet-user, according to user re-tweet with/without comments (tweet readers), or in-degree of the tweet, respectively. They applied measures in order to find relevant tweets considering topic-specific and relevant users (tweet authors). The two measures, tweet-score and user-score (readers), are based on convergence of an iterative formula applied to each node. Then scores are combined aiming to rank tweet authors which represents influence of an author on a topic giving by the quality of tweets he/she wrote. Authors of [9] report results of the later scores used on three topics, which have identified more influential users on four months of information collected from Tenence Micro-blog, a 200 million users social network. Besides, they applied Pagerank and HITS in order to compare the results of identifying most influential user obtaining the best average rating score for the top 5 users on such topics.

Notice that most of the techniques focus on connections between users. However, we must be aware that if there is no communication, there is no possible influence. In the real world (*i.e.*, offline world), connection among users usually means communication, but in online world, people are often connected and not necessarily communicating with each other. Hence, our proposed approach for *opinion leaders* identification considers that the influential level of users can be detected by considering its communication patterns (new posts, direct messages, etc.), by means of particular writing style features as well as behavioral features.

## 3    Influence Features

In this section we present and describe the proposed characteristics for identifying influential users on Twitter. As we have mentioned before, our proposed approach for *opinion leaders* identification is based on the idea that the leadership/influential level of an author can be detected by considering its writing style, and its behavior within the Twitter's community. Accordingly, we propose 9 stylistics attributes (**S**), as well as 23 different behavioral features (**B**), that are computed directly from users twitter accounts.

Before describing our proposed features, it is important to mention how each profile holder was treated for our performed experiments. Each user's profile contained in the employed data set (See section 4.1), was considered as a two different information sources: *i)* information contained in user's public profile,*i.e.*, user's self description and user's public statistics; *ii)* user's posts, *i.e.*, user's written tweets. Following sections describe in detail the given name for each proposed feature and the intuitive idea of each one.

### 3.1    Features Extracted from Users' Public Profile

*Usernames at Description* (B). Usernames are identified by the pattern *@SomeUsername*. We account for how often users employ usersnames on the description of their public profile. Some users use their profile description to indicate others accounts about themselves that can be relevant to their followers. Our intuition indicates that influential users might have greater number of other related usernames.

*Number of Hashtags* (B). This feature shows the average frequency of hashtags ( indicated in Twitter by the symbol #) used by some person on their description profile. We believe that influential users will use hashtags more often.

*Employed URLs* (B). With this attribute we account the number of external links used on the public profile description. Our intuition is that influential users try to guide their followers to websites related with their profession, company, product, etc., so they can have more exposure.

*Self-mentions* (B). We account every time the user employs part of their Twitter's username on the profile description. We believe that one difference between influential/non-influential users might be these self-mentions.

*Tenure* (B). This feature compute the antiquity of an user, in number of months, since their account was created on Twitter (not since their first post) until July 2014. Our intuition is that users with more tenure are more influential.

*Number of Tweets* (B). This is the number of tweets posted by an user since the creation of their account. May be possible that influential user have more tweets than non-influential users.

*Number of Followings* (B). With this attribute we account for the number of other Twitter's account this user follows. The intuition behind this feature is that an influential user tends to follow very few account.

*Number of Followers* (B). Similarly, this attribute account for the number of other Twitter's accounts follow this user. Our intuition here is that influential users tends to be more followed than non-influential users.

*Number of Media Shared* (B). Media is both a video or a photo share on posts. Number of media shared is the total number of media shared considering the entire user's history on Twitter. Might be that influential users tends to share more media than non-influential users.

*Number of Favorites* (B). This feature indicates how often the user in revision marks favorites from other users. We believe that non-influential user are more likely to mark more favorites posts from others.

*Following per Followers* (B). This feature counts the number of following accounts for each follower that a particular user has. A big number for this attribute might indicate that we are facing a non-influential user.

*Followers per Following* (B). On the contrary to the previous feature, this one accounts for the number of followers an user has for every other account this user follows.

*Tweets per Follower* (B). Indicates the number of tweets posted (in average) for each follower. We believe that one difference between influential/non-influential users might be this ratio.

*Tweets per Month* (B). Similarly, this feature shows the average tweets posted in a month. As we will describe below, we believe that the frequency of posting is a good indication for finding influential/non-influential users.

*Media per Month* (B). This attribute counts how often an user shared media to their followers by month. We believe that influential user tends to share media to show evidence that might give them reliability.

*User's category* (B). Each user can be categorized by type of author, for instance journalist, professional, authority, activist, investor, celebrity, etc. Such category was given in the employed dataset.

## 3.2   Features Extracted from Users' Posts

*Employed URLs* (B). Indicates how often (in average) users appeal for external links within their posts. We believe that one difference between influential/non-influential users might be the frequency of use of URLs.

*Number of Hashtags* (B). Similarly, this feature shows the average frequency of hashtags (indicated in Twitter by the symbol #) used by some person. Our intuition is that influential users will use hashtags more often.

*Direct Messages* (B). Direct messages are identified by the pattern *@SomeUser-Name*. We account for how often users employ direct messages. Our intuition indicates that non-influential users might have greater number of direct messages interactions.

*Words per Post* (S). This feature indicates the number of employed words (in average) for each tweet. This feature does not counts external links, hashtags neither direct messages. We believe that it is more probable that influential users tend to use more words within their posts.

*Words' Size* (S). This feature measures for the length in characters of employed words by some user in their posts. Our intuition indicates that influential users would use more complex (larger) words in their tweets.

*User Name Length* (S). Indicates the length in characters of the username on Twitter of some person. We believe that influential users might have a more descriptive username, hence a more large username.

*Vocabulary Richness* (S). Vocabulary richness is often used in quantitative stylistics. It measures the number $n$ of different words in the vocabulary $V$ used in a text. We expect that influential users, might have a more rich vocabulary across their posts.

*Number of Hapax* (S). As known, *hapax* is a word that occurs only once within a context. We believe that there must be a difference between influential and non-influential users with respect to the number of employed hapaxes.

*Number of Retweets* (B). This feature indicates how often external users make *retweet* to the produced content by the user in revision. Our idea is that if some user is in fact an influential user, their produced content will have a greater number of retweets.

*Number of Favorites* (B). Similar to the previous, this feature indicates how often the content produced by the user in revision has been marked as favorite. Accordingly, if some user is in fact an influential user, their produced content will have a greater number of favorites.

*Characters per Tweet* (S). As known, tweets must contain at most 140 characters including urls, hashtags, user mentions and the text itself. Our idea was that it is more probable that influential users tend to use the top allowed number of characters every time they write a post.

*Special Symbols* (S). This features was intended to account for every special symbol used by some user, *e.g.*, emoticons. We expect that non-influential users might use with a higher frequency these symbols than an influential user.

*Size of User Mentions* (S). This features determines the average size (in characters) of the mentioned users across the tweets of the user in revision. Our intuition is that, if the user is an influential person, the average size of users related to him/his must be of similar characteristics.

*Size of Hashtags* (S). Similar to the previous, this feature computes the average size (in characters) of the used hashtags across the tweets of the user in revision. We believe that, if the user is in fact influential, he/she must employ similar hashtags across their posts.

*Update Frequency* (B). It indicates the time taken by the user in revision for writing a new post. Our idea is that influential users must be more active/dynamic within the community.

*Update Frequency SD* (B). This feature complements the previous one, since it refers to the standard deviation (SD) of the update frequency time. Similar to previous feature, we believe that there must be a difference between influential and non-influential users when it refers to their update frequency time.

It is worth mentioning that all proposed features, *i.e.*, both those extracted from the public profile and those extracted from published tweets were normalized for the performed experiments.

### 3.3  Classifiers

Since our proposal for *opinion leaders* representation does not dependent of a particular learning algorithm we can use any classifier to face the influentials classification problem. For our experiments we selected 6 different learning algorithms representative of the wide diversity of methods available in the machine learning field [5]. Specifically, we considered the following classifiers:

- **Naïve Bayes(NB).** A probabilistic-based method that assumes attributes are independent among them given the class.
- **Support vector machine (SVM).** A linear discriminant that aims to find an optimal separating hyperplane, a linear kernel was used for this work.
- **J48.** An algorithm used to generate a decision tree, which select most discriminating features based on its entropy measure.
- **BayesNet.** A probabilistic graphical model that reflects the states of some part of a world that is being modeled and it describes how those states are related by probabilities.
- **RBFNet.** An artificial neural network that is able to predict the output by means of using a linear combination of radial basis functions of the inputs and neuron parameters.
- **IBK.** A non-parametric method where objects are classified by a majority vote of its neighbors, with the objects being assigned to the class most common among its $k$ nearest neighbors

We used the Weka implementation of the above described algorithms, where default parameters were considered for all of the classifiers [4].

# 4    Experiments and Results

## 4.1    Datasets

For our experiments we employed the data set from RepLab 2014 [1]. The data set consists of more than 7,000 Twitter profiles (all with at least 1,000 followers) related to the automotive, banking and miscellaneous domains. This data set was manually labeled by reputation experts, hence each user's profile is labeled as *influential* and *non-influential*. Additionally, each user has been categorized as journalist, professional, authority, activist, investor, company, or celebrity, *i.e.*, users have been assigned to their role/activity within the community.

**Table 1.** Training and test sets statistics in terms of number of users profiles; for each user's profile the last 600 tweets were retrieved

| Split/Num. of | Influentials | Non-influential | Automotive | Banking | Miscellaneous | Profiles |
|---|---|---|---|---|---|---|
| Training set | 796 | 1,704 | 1,186 | 1, 314 | 0 | 2,500 |
| Test set | 1,541 | 3,399 | 2,323 | 2,487 | 130 | 4,940 |

Table 1 shows how the data set was split into training and test set in terms of users profiles. Notice that for the training set in the miscellaneous domain, none users profiles were given. Additionally, it is worth mentioning that the total number of tweets that were processed was approximately of 4.5 millions, divided into 1.5 million for training and 3 million for test.

## 4.2    Experimental Results

The main goal of our experiments was to find if proposed attributes are discriminative enough for identifying influential users from non-influential users on Twitter.

Since we have a data set divided in several domains (See Section 4.1), we follow a *in-domain* and a *cross-domain* methodology for performing our experiments. That is, for the *in-domain* experiments we trained and test with Automotive domain, and we trained and test with Banking domain respectively. Table 2 shows obtained performance in terms of the F-measure (based on Precision and Recall values) for the *in-domain* experiments.

**Table 2.** In-domain obtained performance of classification with six different learning algorithms in the Automotive and Banking domains respectively

| | NB | BayesNet | SVM | RBFNet | IBK | J48 |
|---|---|---|---|---|---|---|
| **Automotive** | 0.648 | 0.695 | **0.696** | 0.611 | 0.632 | 0.636 |
| **Banking** | 0.582 | 0.664 | **0.693** | 0.650 | 0.652 | 0.668 |

As we can see from Table 2 the performance across classifiers are similar, thus the results are not dependent to a particular learning algorithm, on the contrary are caused by the discriminative power of our proposed attributes.

Since the data set we used provides a third domain (Miscellaneous) only for testing, we have no data to train an adequate model such as we did with Automotive and Banking. In order to test our proposed attributes in this third domain we use Banking, Automotive and a combination of both data sets for training, then we evaluate the constructed model on the Miscellaneous domain. Obtained performance of this experiment is shown in Table 3.

**Table 3.** Classification of *Miscellaneous* domain using three different sets for training, *i.e.*, cross-domain methodology

| Training with | NB | BayesNet | SVM | RBFNet | IBK | J48 |
|---|---|---|---|---|---|---|
| Automotive | 0.441 | 0.443 | 0.424 | 0.435 | **0.530** | 0.329 |
| Banking | 0.503 | 0.578 | 0.554 | 0.539 | **0.609** | 0.563 |
| Automotive & Banking | 0.518 | 0.557 | 0.563 | 0.533 | **0.580** | 0.515 |

Table 3 shows a decrement on F-measure for miscellaneous in comparison to the previous two domain. This low performance can be caused by the fact that we have very few profiles for this domain, but also may indicate that the users from different domain behave and write in a particular manner. To investigate this hypothesis deeply, we propose to use a model trained on Automotive and Banking and test with the contrary domain (we refer to this experiment as cross-domain experiment). Results of these set of experiments are shown in Table 4.

**Table 4.** Performance of classification cross-domain. The last column shows the best result obtained when we train with data from the same domain as testing (see Table 2).

| Training - Testing | NB | BayesNet | SVM | RBFNet | IBK | J48 | In-domain |
|---|---|---|---|---|---|---|---|
| Banking - Automotive | 0.531 | 0.526 | **0.559** | 0.500 | 0.451 | 0.554 | 0.696 |
| Automotive - Banking | 0.485 | 0.392 | **0.513** | 0.362 | 0.423 | 0.374 | 0.693 |

The Table 4 shows a decrements in F-measure of 13% and 19% approximately for Automotive and Banking respectively in comparison to the best result (*i.e.*, In-domain column) obtained when training with data from the same domain (See Table 2). As we mentioned before, these results may indicate that users from specific domains behave and write different than users writing about other domains. In order to see which of the proposed attributes are the most relevant for each domain we apply information gain and we show the list of these most informative attributes in Table 5.

Table 5 supports our hypothesis since the best attributes for each domain are very different, only 53% of all relevant attributes for Automotive are shared

**Table 5.** List of attributes with more information gain by domain. Stylistics attributes are marked with *. Shared attributes across domains are marked in bold.

| | From profile user's information | From user's tweets |
|---|---|---|
| Automotive | Usernames at Description, **Number of Tweets**, Tweets per Month, and **User's Category**. | Number of Hashtags, **Employed URLs**, Words' Size*, Vocabulary Richness*, Number of Hapax*, **Number of Retweets, Number of Favorites**, Special Symbols*, Size of Hashtags*, Update Frequency, and Update Frequency SD. |
| Banking | Number of Hashtags, **Number of Tweets**, Number of Followers, Number of Media Shared, Number of Favorites, Followers per Following, Tweets per Follower, Media per Month, and **User's Category**. | **Employed URLs**, Words per Post*, **Words' Size*, Number of Hapax*, Number of Retweets, Number of Favorites**, Characters per Tweet*, and **Special Symbols***. |

with Banking, and 44% of the total relevant attributes for Banking are shared with Automotive. From the list we can say a few things. Firstly, the *number of hashtags* on the user's profile are better for Banking than Automotive, but the *number of hashtag* in the user's posts are better for Automotive than Banking. The *update frequency* is more important for Automotive domain than Banking domain. In general, several attributes related with the update frequency is important for Automotive but not for Banking. Also, more attributes extracted from the public user's profile say more about the influence of users on Banking. Further experimentation must be done to investigate the attributes' relevance for each class (*i.e.* influential and non-influential users) rather than domains.

### 4.3   Comparison against RepLab 2014 Best Systems

One of the challenges proposed in this year RepLab campaign [1] was to identify an author or authors that are influential to a particular community. Such task was named as the *author ranking* subtask, and was evaluated as a traditional ranking information retrieval problem. In other words, systems' output will be a ranking of profiles, where the most influential users must appear at the first positions of the resultant list of users' profiles.

In order to compare our obtained results against participant systems in the *author ranking* subtask, we employed the confidence level of used classifiers in order to provide an ordered list of influential users. Figure 1 shows the interpolated precision graphs obtained by our method using the proposed features.

The baseline proposed for the RepLab organizers corresponds to rank authors according to the number of followers they have. As can be noticed, such baseline works (to some extent) just in the Miscellaneous domain.

It is important to mention, that experiments showed in Figure 1 we used our best classification results, *i.e.,* for the Automotive and Banking domain we employed the output produced by the SVM classifier whilst for the Miscellaneous the IBK classifier.

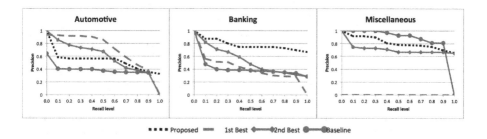

**Fig. 1.** Comparison of influentials ranking using our proposed features against the two top best systems in the RepLab 2014 and the Followers baseline

In general, obtained results are very competitive against those obtained by the participant systems in this year's RepLab campaign, specially for the Banking domain, our proposed method was able to outperform current methods.

## 5   Conclusions and Future Work

In this paper, we have described a method for addressing the problem of author profiling, particularly, a method intended to help discovering which author have more influence (opinion leaders) and which of those are less influential or have no influence at all (non opinion leaders) among a social network community.

The main contribution of this paper are the proposed characteristics, which aim at capturing stylistic and behavioral features from authors. Our intuitive idea for proposing such features is that *influential* users would have similar writing styles as well as similar posting behaviors. Some of the advantages of our proposed method is that it represents a fast and not expensive technique to determine influential users. Performed experiments demonstrate that proposed features allow to obtain similar results across several classification methods, indicating that obtained performance do not depend on any particular classification model.

Additionally, in order to compare our proposed method against state-of-the-art methods, we replicate the methodology followed by the RepLab 2014 campaign. Obtained results indicate that our method reach a competitive performance, and for particular domains is also able to outperform to all participant systems from the RepLab 2014.

In the light of the results we presented, our future work intents to perform an attribute' relevance analysis to focus on the impact of each attribute for classes (i.e. influential and non-influential users) rather than domains.

## References

1. Amigó, E., Carrillo-de-Albornoz, J., Chugur, I., Corujo, A., Gonzalo, J., Meij, E., de Rijke, M., Spina, D.: Overview of repLab 2014: Author profiling and reputation dimensions for online reputation management. In: Kanoulas, E., Lupu, M., Clough, P., Sanderson, M., Hall, M., Hanbury, A., Toms, E. (eds.) CLEF 2014. LNCS, vol. 8685, pp. 307–322. Springer, Heidelberg (2014)

2. Cha, M., Haddadi, H., Benevenuto, F., Gummadi, K.P.: Measuring User Influence in Twitter: The Million Follower Fallacy. In: Proceedings of the 4th International AAAI Conference on Weblogs and Social Media (ICWSM), Washington DC, USA, May 2010. AAAI Press, Menlo Park (2010)
3. Chakravarthy, S., Prasad, G.V.B.: The impact of opinion leader on consumer decision making process. International Journal of Management and Business Studies 1(3), 61–64 (2011)
4. Stephen, R.: Garner. Weka: The waikato environment for knowledge analysis. In: Proc. of the New Zealand Computer Science Research Students Conference, pp. 57–64 (1995)
5. Hastie, T., Tibshirani, R., Friedman, J.: The Elements of Statistical Learning: Data Mining, Inference, and Prediction. Springer (2009)
6. Horrigan, J.: Online communities: Networks that nurture long-distance relationships and local ties. PEW Internet and Family Life Project, Washington, DC (2001)
7. Huffaker, D.: Dimensions of leadership and social influence in online communities. Human Communication Research 36(4), 593–617 (2010)
8. Kong, S., Feng, L.: A tweet-centric approach for topic-specific author ranking in micro-blog. In: Tang, J., King, I., Chen, L., Wang, J. (eds.) ADMA 2011, Part I. LNCS, vol. 7120, pp. 138–151. Springer, Heidelberg (2011)
9. Kong, S., Feng, L.: A tweet-centric approach for topic-specific author ranking in micro-blog. In: ADMA (1), pp. 138–151 (2011)
10. Liu, D., Wu, Q., Han, W.: Measuring micro-blogging user influence based on user-tweet interaction model. In: Tan, Y., Shi, Y., Mo, H. (eds.) ICSI 2013, Part II. LNCS, vol. 7929, pp. 146–153. Springer, Heidelberg (2013)
11. Ma, N., Liu, Y.: Superedgerank algorithm and its application in identifying opinion leader of online public opinion supernetwork. Expert Systems with Applications 41(4, pt 1), 1357–1368 (2014)
12. Page, L., Brin, S., Motwani, R., Winograd, T.: The pagerank citation ranking: Bringing order to the web. Technical Report 1999-66, Stanford InfoLab (November 1999)
13. Afrasiabi Rad, A., Benyoucef, M.: Towards detecting influential users in social networks. In: Babin, G., Stanoevska-Slabeva, K., Kropf, P. (eds.) MCETECH 2011. LNBIP, vol. 78, pp. 227–240. Springer, Heidelberg (2011)
14. Trusov, M., Bodapati, A.V., Bucklin, R.E.: Determining influential users in internet social networks. Journal of Marketing Research XLVII, 643–658 (2010)

# Multisensor Based Obstacles Detection in Challenging Scenes

Yong Fang, Cindy Cappelle, and Yassine Ruichek

IRTES-SET, UTBM, 90010 Belfort Cedex, France

**Abstract.** Obstacle detection is a significant task that an Advanced Driving Assistance System (ADAS) has to perform for intelligent vehicles. In the past decade, many vision-based approaches have been proposed. The majority of them use color, structure and texture features as clues to group similar pixels. However, motion blur generated by the movement of obstacles during exposure is not taken into account in most of the approaches. Generally, many visual clues could fail due to this problem. In this paper, we propose a method, which is independent to the visual clues of target obstacles, to deal with this problem. The proposed approach integrates fisheye image, laser range finder (LRF) measurements and global positioning system (GPS) data. Firstly, the road is detected in fish-eye image by a classification algorithm based on illumination-invariant grayscale image. Secondly, the corresponding geometrical shape of the road is estimated using a geographical information system (GIS). Based on the road geometrical shape, the possible regions of obstacles are then located. Finally, LRF measurements are used to check if there exist obstacles in the possible regions. Experimental results based on real road scenes show the effectiveness of the proposed method.

**Keywords:** Obstacles detection, Motion blur, Road model, GPS, LRF.

## 1 Introduction

For autonomous or intelligent vehicles, an important task is to keep the vehicle traveling in a safe region and prevent collisions. To meet that requirement, the vehicle must have the ability to perceive the obstacles around itself. Generally, obstacles detection is a challenging work for intelligent vehicles in outdoor scenarios due to background changement with the traveling of the vehicle and the appearance of obstacles is hard to predict. For the past decade, many solutions have been proposed to deal with these problems in the intelligent vehicle research community. According to adopted equipments, these solutions can be divided into three types: passive sensors based, active sensors based and both of them based. In papers [1]-[8], camera based methodologies are used to detect obstacles. Among these approaches, some of them employ a priori knowledge of obstacles such as color [2], vertical and horizontal edges [3][4], texture [5], and symmetry of objects [1] to separate the obstacles from the background.

A. Gelbukh et al. (Eds.): MICAI 2014, Part I, LNAI 8856, pp. 257–268, 2014.
© Springer International Publishing Switzerland 2014

Although these methods are simple and efficient, they are easily influenced by illuminance and weather changes. Some of them utilize stereo vision to estimate the position of obstacles in 3D space. In paper [6], the authors construct a V-disparity image based on stereo image pair to detect obstacles on the road. In paper [7], the authors compute the inverse perspective mapping (IPM) of both the right and left images, and take the difference between them. Based on the flat-road assumption, the left and right boundaries of each obstacle are contained into two triangles in the difference image. The location of the two triangles is performed by a polar histogram. In spite of advantages over priori knowledge

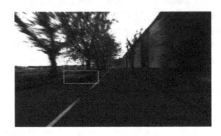

**Fig. 1.** The challenging case: motion blur effect for the red vehicle in the image

solutions, the approaches based on stereo vison are computationally expensive. Other researchers use motion based method to detect obstacles. In paper [8], assuming a calibrated camera and known ego-motion, the authors cluster optical flow estimated from spatio-temporal derivatives of gray value images to eliminate outliers, and then detect both moving and stationary objects. This method can compute the relative speed between the vehicle and objects. However, the used optical flow is sensitive to vehicle movements.

In paper [9], A LRF is utilized for obstacles detection task. LRF is an active sensor which can provide reliable and high accuracy range measurements and is not likely affected by the illumination change. The authors use lines to represent vehicles, and predict their location using an extended Kalman filter (EKF). However, in practise, it's not sufficient to meet our requirements in complex outdoor scenarios that obstacles are described merely by a few simple geometries in a specific plane. In paper [10], obstacle is represented in an occupancy grid map that is divided into regularly spaced grid of cells. Nevertheless, the resolution of obstacles depend on the grid map. The higher resolution grid map is, the more memory it takes.

In paper [11], LRF and camera are combined to detect and recognize objects in front of the vehicle. The LRF is used to locate regions of interest (ROI), and then a classifier based on support vector machine (SVM) is applied to classify the content of the ROI. Our research is belonging to this line.

Nevertheless, all of the methods described above don't take motion blur into account. Most of motion blur cases stem from objects movement in a scene during exposure. In weak lighting scene, motion blur often appears and severely limits image quality. In this paper, a novel approach based on a fisheye camera, a 2D LRF, a GPS receiver and a 2D GIS is proposed to deal with such case (like in Fig.1). The pixels in image are firstly classified as "road" and "non-road" . Then, the corresponding geometrical shape of road area is estimated by GPS and relevant road database. By combining the road detection results and the corresponding road geometrical shape, possible regions of obstacles are located. Finally, LRF measurements are used to check if there exist obstacles in these possible regions.

The paper is organized as follows: Section 2 presents the framework of the proposed approach. Section 3 describes how to acquire road geometrical shape. Section 4 introduces how LRF measurements are used to check the presence of obstacles in potential regions extracted from the image. Comparison of the proposed approach against the methods in [12] and [13] is reported in Section 5. Conclusions are given in section 6.

## 2    Framework Overview

The general framework diagram of the proposed approach is shown in Fig.2. There are three inputs for the framework. Among these inputs, one is a fisheye

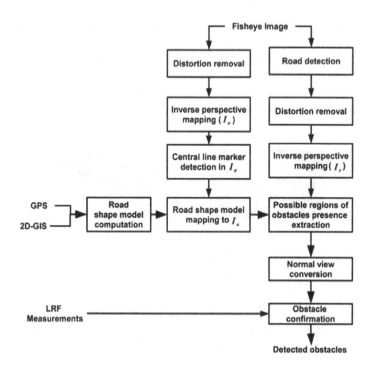

**Fig. 2.** Obstacles detection framework diagram

image. The pixels in the fisheye image are classified as "road" or " non-road" (Fig.3) by a classification algorithm based on illumination-invariant grayscale image which is robust to the variation of illumination and can be computed easily in log-chromaticity space introduced by Finlayson et al [14]. The reader who wants to know more details about the road detection can refer to the paper [15]. The next step is to remove fisheye image distortion. Compared to classic lens, fisheye lens has greater field of view (FOV). However, this leads to great distortion. These great distortions, specially for motion blur cases, make obstacles detection more complex. To simplify our work, the fisheye image and road detection results are then preprocessed to remove the distortions. After distortions removal, the next step is to determine the IPM of the two undistorted images (original fisheye image and image of road detection). Due to perspective effect, the parallel lines in a real scene will intersect in the image, and this makes the extraction of useful information more difficult. The IPM of the image can reduce the perspective effect well. In this paper, the method proposed in paper [7] is adopted to compute $I_o$ (IPM of the undistorted image of original fisheye image) and $I_r$ (IPM of the undistorted image of road detection result).

Another input of the framework is GPS data. GPS is an important positioning system used widely for localizing vehicles within a map. In our approach, it is used together with a 2D-GIS to estimate the road geometrical shape in $I_o$. Firstly, the road model is constructed from the GPS data and the relevant road database. The road geometrical shape in $I_o$ is then determined by mapping the road model into $I_o$ . The details of this step are described in Section 3.

The last input is LRF measurements. These measurements are used to confirm presence obstacles in $I_r$. Firstly, possible regions of presence of obstacles in the road are located using $I_o$ and $I_r$. Then, the LRF measurements are used to confirm the obstacles ahead the vehicle in these regions. This task is introduced in detail in section 4.

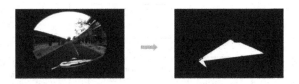

**Fig. 3.** Road detection: The left image is original image. The right image is road detection result.

## 3   Road Geometry Information

Road geometry information reflects the geometry of the road such as left turn, right run, or cross-like junction. This contextual information is a very useful clue for locating possible regions of obstacles presence on the road. The key point to determine the road geometry information is to construct a road shape model and to map it into $I_o$

## 3.1   Road Shape Model Extraction Using GPS and 2D-GIS

The road shape model consists of road skeleton and road boundary. The road skeleton consist in linking concatenates all the road nodes in the road one by one within a map database (See Fig.4). However, there often exists great gap between two adjacent road nodes. Before constructing the road skeleton, a linear interpolation is then implemented.

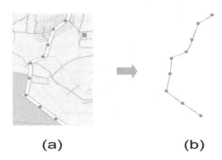

**(a)**                                                    **(b)**

**Fig. 4.** Road skeleton construction. (a) The white area represents a road within a map. The green points are the road nodes in the road. (b) The road skeleton.

Firstly, the GPS data are used to find out the road segment where the target vehicle is traveling within the map and to determine traveling direction on this road segment. Based on these road information, the road node of the road where the vehicle is traveling can be obtained from the map database (OpenStreetMap [16]). Let denote $R_c$ the road where the vehicle is traveling. Let $R_i (i = 1, 2..., N)$ represent the i-th road node of $R_c$ in the map database. The linear interpolation operation is implemented between two adjacent road nodes if the following condition is satisfied.

$$d_{R_i R_{i+1}} < \lambda \quad (i = 1, 2, ..., N - 1) \tag{1}$$

where $d_{R_i R_{i+1}}$ is the distance between $R_i$ and $R_{i+1}$ nodes, $\lambda$ is a threshold set manually. In our approach, it is set to 2 (unit meter). The result of the interpolation operation is illustrated in Fig.5.

After the linear interpolation operation, the closest node to the vehicle location is chosen among the road nodes and interpolation nodes as the starting point of road skeleton. Along the traveling orientation, the interpolation nodes and road nodes are concatenated one by one from the starting point to form the road skeleton of the road ahead the vehicle.

The road boundary is a set of lines which are piecewise parallel to the road skeleton. The distance from the skeleton to the road boundary depends on the road width which can be estimated according to the road attributes in the database and additional countries national road legislation. The road shape model is the combination of the road skeleton and the road boundary (Fig.6).

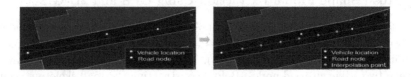

**Fig. 5.** Left image reflects the road database obtained from openstreetmap. Black area represents the road. White points denote the road nodes, yellow point indicates the vehicle location. Right image is the results of interpolation operation.

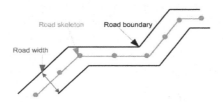

**Fig. 6.** Road shape model

## 3.2   Mapping of the Road Shape Model into Image

In paper [17], the authors map the road shape model to driver's view. However, it refers to a transformation from world coordinate system to image coordinate system, and some of transformational parameters are hard to determine. To avoid this problem, in our approach, the road shape model is mapped into the IPM image $I_o$. However, this mapping requires necessarily some marks on the road. In our method, the lane markers are used. The advantage of lane markers over the boundary of road is that the lane markers are not easily covered by other objects in the traveling journey. We make the assumption that there exists a central lane marker for the road where the vehicle is traveling. In practice, many roads can satisfy this demand directly or indirectly. Firstly, the central lane marker in $I_o$ image is detected using the method in [18]. Then, the road skeleton of the road is aligned with the detected central lane marker. Actually, only a rotation angle for the aligning operation is calculated. The above mapping process is illustrated in Fig.7.

## 4   Image Based Obstacles Detection and LRF Based Validation

The road obstacles detection process is composed of two major steps. Firstly, possible regions of presence of obstacles are located. Then, the LRF measurements are used to validate if there effectively exist obstacles in these possible regions.

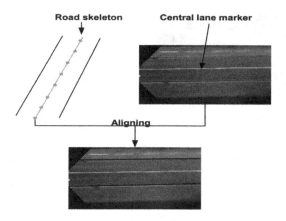

**Fig. 7.** Mapping Process. The up left image is the road shape model, the up right image is $I_o$ with detected central lane marker and the bottom image is the mapping result.

## 4.1 Regions of Obstacles Presence Extraction

The possible regions of presence of obstacles are located by combining $I_o$ image with previously described road geometry information and $I_r$ image. From the previous description, it is known that $I_r$ is actually the road detection result of $I_o$. Thus, the road geometry information in $I_r$ is the same in $I_o$. Based on the road geometry information in $I_r$, the road pixels beyond the road boundary are firstly removed. Then, the non-road pixels within the road boundary are conserved and the road pixels within the road boundary are ignored(Fig.8(a)). The non-road pixels are then assigned into different groups by using a connect-component algorithm. All the pixels in the same group are connected, and pixels in different groups are not connected. Similarly to paper [19], polar histogram (Fig.8(b)) is used to filter these groups. A group is retained if the two following conditions are satisfied:

$$\begin{cases} P_g > S_p \\ S_g > S_s \end{cases} \tag{2}$$

where $P_g$ is the peak number of the group in polar histogram, $S_g$ is the pixels number of the group, $S_p$ and $S_s$ are rough thresholds to filter the too small groups. In our experiment, $S_p$ is set to 50 and $S_s$ is set to 200. As a result, the area of the retained groups represent the possible regions of obstacles presence.

## 4.2 LRF Based Obstacles Confirmation

After determining the possible regions of obstacles presence, the IPM image containing these possible regions is converted to the normal view. Let denote $I_n$ this normal view image and $S_{pr}$ the set of the non-road pixels. From Fig.9(a), it is

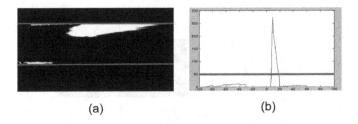

**Fig. 8.** (a) Red lines in the image $I_r$ show the boundary of the road. Non-road pixels within the road boundary are conserved (b)Corresponding polar histogram.

known that there may exist pixels in $S_{pr}$ which don't belong to obstacles (ie. belonging to the road). The LRF measurements are then applied to rule out these irrelevant pixels. Before removing the irrelevant pixels, these LRF measurements are classified into different classes. We suppose that the extrinsic parameters between the fisheye camera and LRF are known. The LRF measurements are then projected into the image $I_n$. The pixel that corresponds to each LRF measurement can then be determined. Let denote $P_i(i = 1, 2..., K)$ the corresponding pixel of the i-th LRF measurement. In our work, we find that the 8-neighbor of $P_i$ often belongs to a same object. To extend the useful information, $P_i$ and its 8-neighbor are grouped as a bigger correspondence, and the bigger correspondence shares the LRF measurement of $P_i$. Then, based on the acquired road geometry information, the bigger correspondences lying beyond the boundary of the road are removed. The remained bigger correspondences are assigned to different groups using connect-component algorithm. A cluster algorithm based on Euclid distance operation is then applied to these different groups. Let denote $G_i$ and $G_j$ the i-th and j-th group respectively. If the following two conditions are satisfied, the two groups are put in the same class:

$$\begin{cases} |C_{G_i} - C_{G_j}| < \beta \\ |M_{G_i} - M_{G_j}| < \gamma \end{cases} \tag{3}$$

where $C_{G_i}$ and $C_{G_j}$ are the centroids of the i-th and j-th groups respectively, $M_{G_i}$ and $M_{G_j}$ are the average LRF measurements of the i-th and j-th groups respectively, $\beta$ and $\gamma$ are empirical thresholds. In experiment, $\beta$ and $\gamma$ are set to 40 and 5 respectively. As a result, these different groups gathered into serval different classes (Fig.9(b)). Let denote $K_i(i = 1, 2..., M)$ the i-th class, $c^l_{K_i}$ and $c^r_{K_i}$ are the columns number corresponding to the left and right boundary of this class respectively in image $I_n$. If there does not exist any pixel belonging to the non-road pixels set $S_{pr}$ between $c^l_{K_i}$ and $c^r_{K_i}$ in image $I_n$, this class will be removed. In the opposite case, if the minimum distance between the rows to which the elements of this class correspond and the rows where these pixels are located is greater than a threshold (set to 15 in the experiment), this class is also removed. Otherwise, this class is reserved and all the pixels in $S_{pr}$ between $c^l_{K_i}$ and $c^r_{K_i}$ are checked. A pixel is identified as a pixel belonging to an obstacle

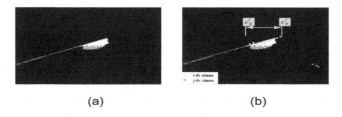

(a)                                    (b)

**Fig. 9.** (a)The image $I_n$. White points are the non-road pixels. Obviously, some of the pixels belong to the road (b) The big correspondences gathered into two classes: the yellow one and the green one.

if the two following conditions are satisfied:

$$\begin{cases} c^l_{K_i} < c_p < c^r_{K_i} \\ \min_j(|r^j_{K_i} - r_p|) < c^r_{K_i} - c^l_{K_i} \end{cases} \tag{4}$$

where $c_p$ and $r_p$ are the column and row numbers of the pixel respectively, $r^j_{K_i}$ is the row number to which the j-th elements of $K_i$ correspond.

## 5   Experiments and Results

### 5.1   Set Up

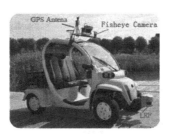

**Fig. 10.** The configuration of the used experimental platform

In experiments, image sequences are captured by a fisheye camera. The used Fujinon fisheye lens provides up to 185 degrees wide angle. The PL-B742 camera provides 1.3 megapixel ($1280 \times 1024$) RGB image and the frame rate is 15 fps. Each frame is synchronized with GPS information provided by a standard GPS antenna. The fish-eye camera is mounted on the top of the prototype vehicle to collect and record experimental data in real road scenarios. The used LRF is a LMS211 providing up to 80 meters measurement range. The layout of these devices is shown in Fig.10.

## 5.2   Results

The experimental data consist of a road database obtained from openstreetmap and 231 frames with the corresponding LRF measurements and GPS data captured when the vehicle was moving. The ground truth is labelled manually. To evaluate the performance of the proposed method, the results obtained using our method are compared with the results obtained with two other methods proposed in [13] and [12]. Public codes for the two methods are available on the internet. Some results of the three approaches are shown in Fig.11. As shown,

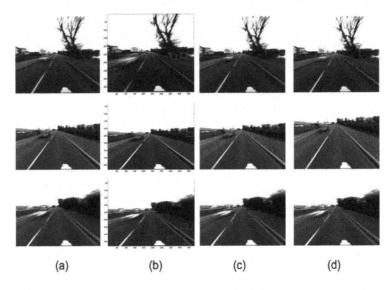

(a)         (b)         (c)         (d)

**Fig. 11.** (a) Original image (b)Results obtained with the approach of paper [13] (c)Results obtained with the approach of paper [12]. (d)Results obtained with our approach.

we can see that, from the three examples proposed in Fig.11, no obstacle is detected using the approach in paper [12]. Most of the detection results obtained by the [13] are wrong. Better results are obtained with our approach. The proposed method is also tested without LRF measurements. The results are shown in Table 1. One can notice that the LRF measurements improve the correct rate greatly. However, the hit rate declines sightly. This is caused by the loss of LRF measurements of obstacles. Fig.12 shows an example of such failure case.

## 6   Conclusion

We proposed an efficient algorithm for obstacles detection in presence of motion-blur in processed images captured in outdoor scenarios. The approach combines GPS information, fisheye image and LRF scan to detect obstacles in front of the

**Table 1.** The performance of the proposed approach with and without LRF measurements. $Hit\ Rate\ =\ \frac{The\ number\ of\ the\ correct\ detected\ obstacles}{The\ total\ number\ of\ the\ ground\ truth\ obstacles}$ $Correct\ Rate\ =\ \frac{The\ number\ of\ the\ correct\ detected\ obstacles}{The\ total\ number\ of\ the\ detected\ obstacles}$

| Condition | Hit Rate | Correct Rate |
|---|---|---|
| **Without LRF measurements** | 0.8076 | 0.5297 |
| **With LRF measurements** | 0.7255 | 0.9063 |

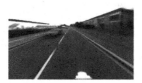 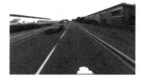

**Fig. 12.** The failure case. Left image is the undistorted one. Right image is the obstacle detection result. In this case, we lost the LRF measurements of the red vehicle

vehicle. The experimental results show that the combination of GPS information, fisheye image and LRF measurements allow to achieve some improvements for obstacle detection in hard conditions (in presence of motion blur). For further work, we intend to try to stabilize the LRF measurements and improve the road detection method to reach a higher hit rate for obstacles detection.

# References

1. Zielke, T., Brauckmann, M., Vonseelen, W.: Intensity and edge-based symmetry detection with an application to car-following. CVGIP: Image Understanding 58(2), 177–190 (1993), doi:10.1006/ciun.1993.1037
2. Guo, D., Fraichard, T., Xie, M., Laugier, C.: Color modeling by spherical influence field in sensing driving environment. In: Proceedings of the IEEE Intelligent Vehicles Symposium, pp. 249–254 (2000)
3. Jazayeri, A., Cai, H., Zheng, J.Y., Tuceryan, M.: Vehicle detection and tracking in car video based on motion model. IEEE Transactions on Intelligent Transportation Systems 12(2), 583–595 (2011)
4. Bucher, T., Curio, C., Edelbrunner, J., Igel, C., Kastrup, D., Leefken, I., Lorenz, G., Steinhage, A., Von Seelen, W.: Image processing and behavior planning for intelligent vehicles. IEEE Transactions on Industrial Electronics 50(1), 62–75 (2003)
5. Kalinke, T., Tzomakas, C., Seelen, W.V.: A texture-based object detection and an adaptive model-based classification. In: Proceedings of the IEEE Intelligent Vehicles Symposium, pp. 341–346 (1998)
6. Labayrade, R., Aubert, D., Tarel, J.P.: Real time obstacle detection in stereovision on non flat road geometry through "v-disparity" representation. In: Proceedings of the IEEE Intelligent Vehicle Symposium, vol. 2, pp. 646–651 (June 2002)
7. Bertozzi, M., Broggi, A.: GOLD: a parallel real-time stereo vision system for generic obstacle and lane detection. IEEE Transactions on Image Processing 7(1), 62–81 (1998)

8. Kruger, W., Enkelmann, W., Rossle, S.: Real-time estimation and tracking of optical flow vectors for obstacle detection. In: Proceedings of the IEEE the Intelligent Vehicles Symposium, pp. 304–309 (1995)
9. Rebai, K., Benabderrahmane, A., Azouaoui, O., Ouadah, N.: Moving obstacles detection and tracking with laser range finder. In: International Conference on Advanced Robotics, pp. 1–6 (June 2009)
10. Weiss, T., Schiele, B., Dietmayer, K.: Robust driving path detection in urban and highway scenarios using a laser scanner and online occupancy grids. In: Proceedings of the IEEE Intelligent Vehicles Symposium, pp. 184–189 (June 2007)
11. Monteiro, G., Premebida, C., Peixoto, P., Nunes, U.: Tracking and classification of dynamic obstacles using laser range finder and vision. In: Proc. of the IEEE/RSJ International Conference on Intelligent Robots and Systems, IROS (2006)
12. Felzenszwalb, P.F., Girshick, R.B., McAllester, D., Ramanan, D.: Object detection with discriminatively trained part-based models. IEEE Transactions on Pattern Analysis and Machine Intelligence 32(9), 1627–1645 (2010)
13. Negri, P., Clady, X., Hanif, S.M., Prevost, L.: A cascade of boosted generative and discriminative classifiers for vehicle detection. EURASIP J. Adv. Signal Process (2008), http://dx.doi.org/10.1155/2008/782432
14. Finlayson, G.D., Hordley, S.D., Lu, C., Drew, M.S.: On the removal of shadows from images. IEEE Transactions on Pattern Analysis and Machine Intelligence 28(1), 59–68 (2006)
15. Fang, Y., Cappelle, C., Ruichek, Y.: Road detection using fisheye camera and laser range finder. In: Elmoataz, A., Lezoray, O., Nouboud, F., Mammass, D. (eds.) ICISP 2014. LNCS, vol. 8509, pp. 495–502. Springer, Heidelberg (2014)
16. Haklay, M., Weber, P.: OpenStreetMap: user-generated street maps. IEEE Pervasive Computing 7(4), 12–18 (2008)
17. Alvarez, J.M., Lumbreras, F., Gevers, T., Lopez, A.M.: Geographic information for vision-based road detection. In: IEEE Intelligent Vehicles Symposium, pp. 621–626 (June 2010)
18. Aly, M.: Real time detection of lane markers in urban streets. In: IEEE Intelligent Vehicles Symposium, pp. 7–12 (June 2008)
19. Yang, C., Hongo, H., Tanimoto, S.: A new approach for in-vehicle camera obstacle detection by ground movement compensation. In: Conference on Intelligent Transportation Systems (ITSC), pp. 151–156 (2008)

# GP-MPU Method for Implicit Surface Reconstruction

Manuel Guillermo López[1], Boris Mederos[2], and Oscar Dalmau[1]

[1] Centro de Investigación en Matemáticas, CIMAT
[2] Universidad Autónoma de Ciudad Juárez, UACJ,
Departamento de Física y Matemáticas
{manuel.lopez,dalmau}@cimat.mx, boris.mederos@uacj.mx

**Abstract.** This work addresses the problem of surface reconstruction from unorganized points and normals that are acquired from laser scanning of 3D objects. We propose a novel technique for implicit surface reconstruction that effectively combines the trend setting method known as Multi-level Partition of the Unity (MPU) with the Gaussian Process Regression. The reconstructed implicit surface is obtained by subdividing the domain into a set of smaller sub-domains using the MPU algorithm, in each sub-domain a Gaussian Process Regression is carried out that provides accurate local approximations which are blended to obtain a global representation corresponding to the reconstructed implicit surface. The proposed algorithm is able to deal efficiently with point clouds presenting several features such as complex topology and geometry, missing regions and very low sampling rate. Moreover, we conduct some experiments with several acquired data and perform some comparisons with state of the art techniques showing competitive results.

## 1 Introduction

The development of 3D scanning technology has made possible the application of 3D object modeling to a wide range of practical applications in multimedia, entertainment, medicine, biomechanic, and cultural heritage, just to mention a few. This has trigger several computational challenges problems such as acquisition, reconstruction, and simulation, etc. In this work we will focus on the problem of surface reconstruction from unorganized point clouds which is stated formally as: *Given a finite set of point $P \subset \mathbb{R}^3$ with normal $N \subset \mathbb{R}^3$ sampled from a smooth surface $S$ find a smooth surface $F$ close to $S$.*

The surface reconstruction problem has received in the last two decades a lot of attention entailing several approaches to deal with it. The main techniques used can be generally categorized in two types:

**Delaunay Triangulation/Voronoi Diagram**: These algorithms yield a polygonal mesh filtering the Delaunay/Voronoi diagram and the resulting mesh interpolates the point clouds, some examples of this kind of methods are Ameta et al. [1], [2], Boissonat et al. [3], Dey et al. [4] and Mederos et al. [5]. It is worth

A. Gelbukh et al. (Eds.): MICAI 2014, Part I, LNAI 8856, pp. 269–280, 2014.
© Springer International Publishing Switzerland 2014

to recall that these algorithms come with the theoretical guarantees that the reconstructed surface $F$ is homeomorphic and/or homotopy equivalent to the original surface $S$ depending on the sampling density. For a deep treatment of this subject we refer to the book of Dey [4].

**Implicit Surface.** The main idea of this approach is to reconstruct the surface $F$ as the zero level set of some smooth function $g$ i.e.,

$$F = \{x \in \mathbb{R}^3 : g(x) = 0\}.$$

The function $g$ is determined based on the knowledge of the points cloud $P = \{x_1, x_2, \ldots, x_k\}$ and the set of normals $N = \{n_1, n_2, \ldots, n_k\}$. There are different methods to obtain the implicit reconstruction. Next we describe some of the most relevant.

**Radial Basis Functions (RBFs).** Carr et al [6] estimate the function $g$ as a linear combination of radial functions centered at a set of constraint points $\{c_1, c_2, \ldots, c_l\}$

$$g(x) = \sum_{i=1}^{l} w_i \phi(\|x - c_i\|), \tag{1}$$

with weights $w_i$ which are determined by imposing surface constrains at the points $c_i$ and then solving a linear system which is hard to compute for a large number of samples. One way to overcome this issue is to employ a compact support radial basis function $\phi$, this certainly improves the computational burden. On the other hand, the resulting surface is not fair especially in regions with highly irregular sampling densities. Another relevant work is the Turk and O'brien approach [7] that computes the implicit surface as a radial basis function that minimizes the thin plate energy subject to a set of off-surface constrains.

**Point Set Surface.** These kind of methods are based on moving least square and yield smooth reconstructed surfaces through the use of Levin's projection operator [8]. The reconstructed surface is obtained as the set of stationary points of the operator, i.e., $F$ is the set of points where the operator is the identity. Examples of these methods are given in Adamson and Alexa [9], Kollury [10] and Guennebaud and Gross [11].

**Poisson Method.** Kazdan et al. [12] (**Poisson**) propose to determine the indicator function of the shape $\chi_S$ whose gradient best approximates the normal vector field $N$ which is interpolated from the discrete set of normals, i.e., $\chi_S = \operatorname{argmin}_\chi \|\nabla \chi - N\|_2^2$. This minimization problem leads to solve a Poisson equation which is handled by using locally supported radial basis functions on an octree. The results of the method are very satisfactory, providing good preservation of details. The works of Kazdan et al. [13] (**Fourier**) and Manson et al. [14] improve the computational overload using Fourier and Wavelet basis respectively to solve the Poisson equation.

**Muti-level Partition of Unity (MPU).** This approach (Ohtake et al. [15] (**MPU**)) relies on performing a hierarchically decomposition of the domain in small sub-domains where a tridimensional or bidimensional polynomial is fitted to the point cloud in each sub-domain. Subsequently, Ohtake et al. [16] propose an improvement of the original MPU algorithm which combines an adaptive partition of unity with least square radial basis functions. A more detailed explanation of the MPU method will be given in Section 2.

In the last decade, in the context of machine learning, Gaussian process approaches for regression and classification [17] have had an increasing use, due to their flexibility and versatility to solve the regression problem. The Gaussian process technique has also been applied to the problem of shape estimation in several recent works. In Smith et al. [18] and Castro et al. [19] the focus is on the application in the context of Urban environments and Robotics; these methods are devoted to the reconstruction of elevation maps which is not a fully 3D approach. In the work of Dragiev et al. [20] an implicit surface reconstruction is performed in the real 3D context, although the reconstructed 3D shapes are simple since the main goal of this work is to deal with the problem of robot grasping. In Williams and Fitzgibbon [21] an implicit surface reconstruction from 3D point cloud is developed, but due to the computational complexity of the Gaussian process regression, which is of order $O(N^3)$, the method uses few sample points which leads to oversmoothed reconstructed surfaces. To overcome the drawback of the Williams and Fitzgibbon's method, we propose a reconstruction technique which relies on the combination of the Gaussian process regression, with the MPU algorithm, in this way we take advantage of the best properties of both techniques. This combination allows us to reconstruct surfaces using the complete point cloud and also enables us to carry out an implicit surface fitting that captures significant details and features that appear on the surface that when applying each method separately is hard to achieve.

The main contribution of our work is the combination of Gaussian process regression and the MPU algorithm. The proposed technique obtains good surface fitting and also is able to handle the reconstruction of regions with lack of samples, i.e., point clouds with missing regions. Additionally, the method can reconstructs surfaces from few samples of the original point cloud.

The paper is organized as follows: In section 2 we give a detailed description of the MPU method. In section 3 we give an introduction to Gaussian process regression. Section 4 explains our proposed method in detail. Section 5 presents a comparison of the results obtained with our proposed method and those obtained with some state of the art methods. The algorithms are compared visually and numerically using some acquired complex data models. Finally section 5 presents the conclusions and future directions of research.

## 2    Multi-Level Partition of Unity

The MPU algorithm computes the reconstructed surface $F$ as the zero level set $F = g^{-1}(0)$ of a smooth function $g : \Omega \subset \mathbb{R}^3 \to \mathbb{R}$. To determine $f$ the method decomposes the domain $\Omega$ in a finite collection of subdomains $\{\Omega_i\}_{i=1}^n$, i.e., $\Omega = \bigcup_{i=1}^n \Omega_i$. In each subdomains $\Omega_i$ a local approximation $\phi_i(\cdot)$ to the set $S \cap \Omega_i$ is determined using the information of the points in $P \cap \Omega_i$ and its associated normals. Once the local approximating functions $\phi_i(\cdot)$, $i = 1, \ldots, n$ are determined, the function $g$ is computed as a weighted combination of the $\phi_i(\cdot)$, $i = 1, \ldots, n$

$$g(x) = \sum_{i=1}^{n} w_i(x)\phi_i(x), \ x \in \Omega, \tag{2}$$

where $w_i(\cdot), i = 1, \ldots, n$ are compact support smooth functions satisfying

$$\Omega_i \subset \text{support}(w_i) \subset \Omega, \text{ and } \sum_{i=1}^{n} w_i(x) = 1, \forall x \in \Omega. \tag{3}$$

In that way the algorithm integrates local approximations $\phi_i(\cdot)$ into a global implicit approximation $g$. Typically, the decomposition of the domain $\Omega$ is carried out by using an octree partition technique where the leaves of the octree correspond to the subdomains $\Omega_i$. The decomposition of an octree cell $C_i$ in the subdivision process is performed whenever the two conditions are fulfilled:

- The approximation error of $\phi_i(\cdot)$ to the local points cloud is bigger that some tolerance parameter $\epsilon$.
- The depth of the cell $C_i$ in the tree is smaller than some fixed level $l$.

In [15] the function $\phi_i : \mathbb{R}^3 \to \mathbb{R}$ is a quadratic polynomial which is determined as the best approximation of the distance function in the least square sense

$$\phi_i = \text{argmin} \sum_{x_j \in P \cap \text{ support}(w_i)} w_i(x_j)\phi_i(x_j)^2 + \sum_{v_j \in V_i} (\phi_i(v_j) - d_j)^2, \tag{4}$$

where $V_i$ is the set of vertices of the cube $C_i$ and $d_i$ are the signed distances of the vertex $o_i$ to the centroid of the point set $P \cap \text{support}(w_i)$; the above problem (4) leads to solve a linear system of equations with unknowns equal to the coefficients of the polynomial $\phi_i$. In general, in low sampled region, the resulting linear system is ill posed leading to unfair approximations. Another drawback of this approach is that in order to capture the fine details and oscillations in the points cloud it is necessary to build a very deep octree which increases the memory requirements.

The support of the weight function $w_i(\cdot)$ is a sphere of radio $R_i$ with center $c_i$ which is the center of $C_i$. Sometimes the sphere does not contain enough points to perform a good fitting, in that case the radius $R_i$ is successively increased ($R_i \leftarrow R_i + \alpha d$, where $d$ is the length of the half diagonal of $C_i$ and $\alpha$ is a parameter specified by the user) until we get an appropriated number of sample points of $P$ inside the sphere, i.e., the number of points is bigger than a fixed parameter $\eta$ defined by the user.

The weight function used by the MPU method is the quadratic B-spline $b(\cdot)$

$$w_i(x) = b\left(\frac{3\|x - c_i\|_2}{2R_i}\right), \tag{5}$$

where $c_i$ and $R_i$ are the center of the cell $C_i$ and the radius of the spherical support of $w_i(\cdot)$ respectively.

# 3  Gaussian Process Regression

A Gaussian Process (GP) is a stochastic process $\{f(x)\}_{x \in \Omega}$ such that given any finite set of indexes $\{x_1, x_2, \ldots, x_m\} \subset \Omega$ the variable $(f(x_1), f(x_2), \ldots, f(x_m))$ has a joint Gaussian distribution with covariance matrix $K_{x_1, x_2, \ldots, x_m}$ which is a positive defined matrix of size $m \times m$.

The main characteristics of GP like isotropy and smoothness are determined by the covariance function $k(x, x')$ between any pair $x, x' \in \Omega$ which is a symmetric non-negative function also called kernel. The theorem [22, Theorem 3.11. p. 61] guarantees that there exists a function $\psi : \Omega \to \mathcal{H}$, where $\mathcal{H}$ is a Hilbert space, so-called nonlinear feature map, that allows to represent the kernel $k : \Omega \times \Omega \to \mathbb{R}$ as an inner product $k(x, x') = \langle \psi(x), \psi(x') \rangle$. The covariance $K_{x_1, x_2, \ldots, x_m}$ is expressed in terms of the kernel in the following way $K = K_{x_1, x_2, \ldots, x_m} = (k(x_i, x_j))_{i, j = 1, \ldots, m}$ also known as the Gram matrix.

GP has been used in Bayesian regression as a prior over functional spaces. This will be the main focus of our application of GP to surface reconstruction. Now we will present the Gaussian Process Regression (GPR). Let us consider the following data model: $y(x) = f(x) + \epsilon$, where $f(x)$, $x \in \Omega$ are considered latent variables which are modeled as a prior GP and $\epsilon$ is a Gaussian random variable with zero mean and variance $\sigma$, also the two variables $y(x_1)|f(x_1)$ and $y(x_2)|f(x_2)$ are independent for any $x_1, x_2 \in \Omega$, $x_1 \neq x_2$. From now on we will use the following notation $y_x = y(x)$ and $f_x = f(x)$ indistinctly. The problem that we are interested in is to compute the predictive distribution $P(f_x|\mathcal{D}, x)$, where $\mathcal{D} = \{(x_i, y_i) : x_i \in \Omega, y_i \in \mathbb{R}, i = 1, \ldots, n\}$ is a set of previous noisy observations at a set of points $\{x_1, x_2, \ldots, x_n\}$ that we will call of training set and $x$ is a test point.

The predictive distribution of $f_x|\mathcal{D}, x$ is computed using the Bayesian approach along with the fact that $f_x$ is a GP (Rasmussen and Williams [17]) which implies that $f_x|\mathcal{D}, x \sim \mathcal{N}(\mu_x, \sigma_x)$, where the mean and variance are given by

$$m_x = k^\top (K + \sigma I)^{-1} y, \quad \sigma_x = k(x, x) - k^\top (K + \sigma I)^{-1} k, \tag{6}$$

where $y = (y_1, y_2, \ldots, y_n)^\top$ is the observation vector, $K = (k(x_i, x_j))_{i, j = 1, \ldots, n}$ is the covariance matrix and $k = (k(x, x_1), k(x, x_2), \ldots, k(x, x_n))^\top$.

# 4  Proposed Surface Reconstruction Method

The MPU algorithm is computational simple due to the fact that the local approximations are computed using a polynomial function of degree two. On the other hand, this simple polynomial fitting entails that the quality of the reconstruction is not very accurate, especially in regions with fine details. For that reason we replace the local polynomial fitting with GPR which produces a better fitting without the need to subdivide the domain too much.

In order to perform the GPR we consider a training set $D$ decomposed in the following way: $\mathcal{D} = \mathcal{D}_{out} \cup \mathcal{D}_{cloud} \cup \mathcal{D}_{in}$. We recall that we have an oriented set of normals $N$ pointing outwards of the surface $S$. Next we describe the sets $\mathcal{D}_{out}$ , $\mathcal{D}_{cloud}$ and $\mathcal{D}_{in}$. In this sense we define the set $P_{out}$, $P_{cloud}$ and $P_{in}$ as

$$P_{out} = \{x_i^+ \in \Omega : x_i^+ = x_i + h \cdot n_i, \, x_i \in P, \, i = 1, \ldots, k\}, \, \mathcal{D}_{out} = P_{out} \times \{h\},$$
$$P_{cloud} = P, \, \mathcal{D}_{cloud} = P_{cloud} \times \{0\},$$
$$P_{in} = \{x_i^- \in \Omega : x_i^- = x_i - h \cdot n_i, \, x_i \in P, \, i = 1, \ldots, k\}, \, \mathcal{D}_{in} = P_{in} \times \{-h\},$$

where $h$ is a small positive offset. Therefore, the sets $P_{out}$ and $P_{in}$ are offset points which are outside and inside of the surface respectively, the Figure 1 depicts this fact precisely. In each node $C_i$ of the octree we determine the set $\mathcal{D}_i = \{(x, y) \in$

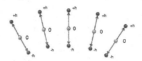

**Fig. 1.** Training set: $\mathcal{D}_{out}$ corresponds to red points, $\mathcal{D}_{in}$ corresponds to blue points and green points correspond to $\mathcal{D}_{cloud}$

$\mathcal{D} : x \in \text{supp}(w_i), \, y \in \{-h, 0, h\}\}$ which is used to compute the posterior mean $m(x) = m_x, \, x \in \text{supp}(w_i)$. The support of the weight function is a sphere with the same center of the cell $C_i$ and radius $R_i$ which is computed using the same procedure used in [15] which was explained in the previous section.

The training set defined in that way allows the GPR to determine in each cell $C_i$ a local approximation of the point cloud as the zero level set of the mean function

$$S_i^{local} = \{x \in \text{supp}(w_i) : m_i(x) = 0\} = m_i^{-1}(0). \tag{7}$$

Therefore, at the end of the octree building process we end up with a set of octree leaves $\{C_1, C_2, \ldots, C_n\}$ where in each cell the local approximations $\phi_i(\cdot)$, previously defined in (2), are given by the posterior means $m_i(\cdot)$, therefore the resulting implicit function is

$$f(x) = \sum_{i=1}^{n} w_i(x) m_i(x), \, x \in \Omega \subset \mathbb{R}^3. \tag{8}$$

The weight function $w_i(\cdot)$, with support containing the leaf $C_i$, used by our method is the same as the one employed in Ohtake et al. [15] which is the quadratic B-spline already defined in the previous section. Once the implicit function (8) is computed a triangular mesh is generated using the marching cube algorithm [23]. Observe that the learning complexity in every leaf is cubic on the number of points in that leaf, which is smaller than $N^3$.

# 5   Experimental Results

In this section we apply our algorithm to different data sets which correspond to complex shapes. We also present visual and numerical comparison of our algorithm with some state of the art methods. As we can see in the experiments, our algorithm is able to produce satisfactory reconstructions of data sets with complex topology, fine details as well as varying density, see Figure 2. In the

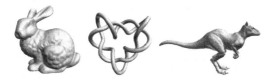

**Fig. 2.** Three reconstructed data sets: Knot, Bunny and Dino

next experiment, Figure 3, we show that our method is able to obtain good reconstructed surfaces when the data sets are sparse, i.e., point clouds sampled at low rates. Figure 5 shows a visual comparison of our method with respect to

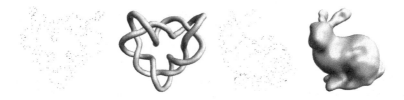

**Fig. 3.** Reconstruction using our proposed method. The first two pictures show a point cloud of 350 from 28659 points (Knot model) and its reconstruction. The next two pictures show a point cloud of 350 from 35933 points (Bunny Model) and its reconstruction.

the methods: Fourier, Poisson and MPU methods. Note that in the Dragon figure the details like the scales are well preserved, also in the Squirrel and Armadillo the surfaces are well reconstructed. Observe in Figure 4 that the Squirrel point cloud has some big missing parts. Additionally in Figure 6, we compare our algorithm using three complex point clouds: Quasimoto, Gargoyle and Dancing Children, the Figure 4 shows that the previous point clouds have missing region, nontrivial topology, moreover the Gargoyle data set contains details of varying size. In the Quasimoto model, it can be observed that the proposed method is able to reconstruct the legs better than all the other methods. The level of details of our method is similar to the Poisson reconstructed model. The Gargoyle model shows that the best reconstructions results are obtained by the Poisson method and our proposed method produces comparable results. Both

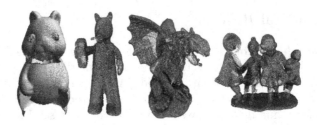

**Fig. 4.** Point Clouds corresponding to the Squirrel, Quasimoto, Gargoyle and Dacing Children Models

methods are able to obtain a better level of detail and shape preservation than the remaining methods. Figure 7 shows a zoom of the region corresponding to the black rectangle in Figure 6 that depicts details of the reconstruction of the Gargoyle model.

In the last model, the Dancing Children, the best reconstructions are obtained by the Poisson method followed by our proposal. It can be observed that in the hat region of this model, our reconstruction is not satisfactory compared with the Poisson and Fourier methods. The reason is that in regions with large holes, our algorithm tries to incorporate surrounding information, and for this purpose it needs to increase the region size used by the GP regression algorithm, which eventually could lead to include points that belong to another nearby surface component. As future work, we will try to solve this limitation by only incorporating information on the boundary of the holes.

In tables 1 and 2 we present the results of applying two error measures, the mean distance (9) and the mean angle deviation (10) respectively, proposed in Berger et al. [24] to compare the obtained mesh $M$ of each method with an implicit surface $\mathcal{I}$ which is considered as the ground truth. These implicit surfaces are obtained using the Polygonal MPU method proposed in [24], and are available in http://www.cs.utah.edu/~bergerm/recon_bench/.

The mathematical expressions for the mean distance is

$$d(\mathcal{I}, M) = \frac{1}{|S|} \left( \sum_{(x,\alpha) \in C_{\mathcal{I}}} \|x - \alpha\|_2 + \sum_{(\alpha,x) \in C_M} \|\alpha - x\|_2 \right), \qquad (9)$$

and for mean angle deviation is

$$d_N(\mathcal{I}, M) = \frac{1}{|S|} \left( \sum_{(x,\alpha) \in C_{\mathcal{I}}} \angle(x, \alpha) + \sum_{(\alpha,x) \in C_M} \angle(\alpha, x) \right), \qquad (10)$$

where $|S| = |C_M| + |C_{\mathcal{I}}|$ with $C_{\mathcal{I}} = \{(x, \alpha) : \alpha \in P_{\mathcal{I}}, x = \Phi(\alpha)\}$ and $C_M = \{(x, \alpha) : x \in P_M, \alpha = \Psi(x)\}$ are the sets of corresponding closest points, $P_{\mathcal{I}}$ and $P_M$ are a uniform sampling of the Implicit and polygonal surfaces $\mathcal{I}$ and $M$. The expression $\angle(x, \alpha)$ stands for the angle between the normals at $x$ and $\alpha$ in each model. A detailed explanation of these metrics can be found in [24].

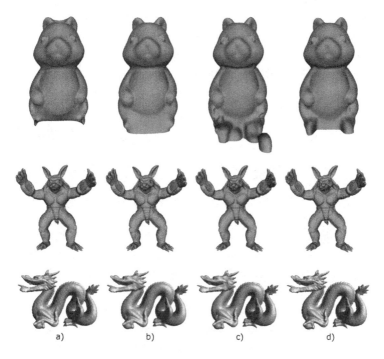

**Fig. 5.** A visual comparison of the results obtained applying the methods: a) Fourier, b) Poisson, c) MPU and d) Proposed to the three point clouds: Squirrel, Armadillo and Dragon

**Table 1.** Comparison results with the mean distance measure $d(\mathcal{I}, M)$

|                   | Fourier   | Poisson   | MPU       | Proposed  |
|-------------------|-----------|-----------|-----------|-----------|
| Quasimoto         | 0.1109327 | 0.0884068 | 0.0914109 | 0.0901929 |
| Gargoyle          | 0.1449956 | 0.1230899 | 0.1267464 | 0.1227051 |
| Dancing children  | 0.1500898 | 0.1162674 | 0.1232541 | 0.1161708 |

The kernel function $k : \Omega \times \Omega \to \mathbb{R}$ used in the GP regression of our proposed method is the thin-plate $k(x, y) = 2\|x - y\|_2^3 - 3R\|x - y\|_2^2 + R^3$ which has only one parameter $R$ determined in the same way as is proposed in [21], $R$ is set to the maximum distance between every pair the points in each subdomain. Moreover, we make experiments with other two commonly used kernel (exponential and polynomial); in which we observe a high variability in the quality of the reconstruction when we change the parameters, whereas with the thin-plate kernel we observe small variations in the reconstruction surface when we change the parameter $R$.

The data sets used in our experiment are public, The Bunny, Dragon and Armadillo are available at the Stanford 3D scanning repository https://graphics.stanford.edu/data/3Dscanrep/. The Quasimoto,

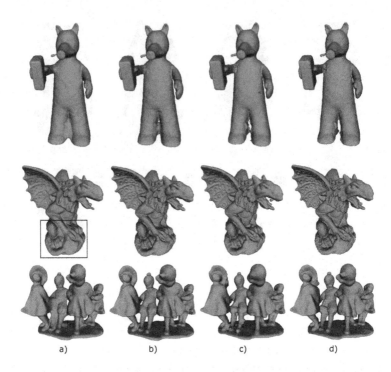

a)          b)          c)          d)

**Fig. 6.** Results obtained applying different methods to the Quasimoto (first row), Gargoyle (Second row) and Dancing Children (third row) models: a) Fourier, b) Poisson, c) MPU and d) Proposed

Gargoyle and Dancing Children are available at the AIM@SHAPE shape repository http://shapes.aim-at-shape.net.

## 6   Conclusions and Future Works

This work proposes a new implicit surface reconstruction method that combines Gaussian process regression with the Multi-level partition of unity reconstruction algorithm. Our method is able to reconstruct efficiently surfaces from point clouds with complex topology and varying sampling densities. The proposed algorithm allows to obtain good surface fitting by handling the reconstruction of regions with lack of samples, as well as surfaces with fine details and oscillations. The proposed technique obtains comparable results with respect to state of the arts algorithms, and in some point clouds it provides better results than other well established methods.

Although the performance of the proposed algorithm considerably improves over the straightforward Gaussian process regression technique, its performance can be enhanced. As future promising lines of research we plan to incorporate in our algorithm the sparse Gaussian process regression in order to reconstruct

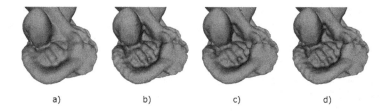

a)        b)        c)        d)

**Fig. 7.** Zoom of the region delimited by the black square in Figure 6 for each method:
a) Fourier, b) Poisson, c) MPU and d) Proposed

**Table 2.** Comparison results with the mean angle distance $d_N(\mathcal{I}, M)$

|  | Fourier | Poisson | MPU | Proposed |
|---|---|---|---|---|
| Quasimoto | 3.1553744 | 4.0908161 | 3.6098870 | 5.1690453 |
| Gargoyle | 6.5167079 | 6.7571828 | 6.5892170 | 6.3601625 |
| Dancing children | 4.7449945 | 5.0911412 | 5.9065290 | 4.0602553 |

surfaces from a small subset of the point cloud. Another direction of research is
the study of other kernel functions with the purpose of improving the preservation of fine details. Finally, we will develop a study to improve the robustness of
our algorithm so that it can handle noisy point clouds.

**Acknowledgments.** The first author was partially supported by the National
Council of Science and Technology (CONACYT). The second author wants to
thank the PROMEP Project that supported this work.

# References

1. Amenta, N., Bern, M.: Surface reconstruction by voronoi filtering. Discrete and
   Computational Geometry 22, 481–504 (1999)
2. Amenta, N., Choi, S., Kollury, R.: The power crust, unions of balls, and the medial
   axis transform. Computational Geometry 19, 103–108 (2000)
3. Boissonat, J.D., Cazals, F.: Smooth surface reconstruction via natural neighbour
   interpolation of distance functions. Computational Geometry 22, 185–203 (2002)
4. Dey, T.K.: Curve and Surface Reconstruction: Algorithms with Mathematical
   Analysis (2007)
5. Mederos, B., Amenta, N., Velho, L., de Figueredo, L.H.: Surface reconstruction for
   noisy point clouds. In: Symposium on Geometry Processing, pp. 53–62 (2005)
6. Carr, J.C., Beatson, R.K., Cherrie, J.B., Mitchell, J.T., Right, W.R., McCallum,
   C.B., Evans, R.T.: Reconstruction and representation of 3D objects with radial
   basis functions. In: ACM SIGGRAPH 2001, pp. 67–76. ACM Press (2001)
7. Turk, G., O'brien, J.F.: Modelling with implicit surfaces that interpolate. ACM
   Transactions on Graphics 21, 855–873 (2002)
8. Levin, D.: Mesh-independent surface interpolation (2003)
9. Adamson, A., Alexa, M.: Approximating and intersecting surfaces from points. In:
   Symposium on Geometry Processing, pp. 230–239 (2003)

10. Kollury, R.K.: Provably good moving least squares. ACM Transactions on Algorithms 4, 106–112 (2008)
11. Guennebaud, S., Gross, M.: Algebraic point set surfaces. ACM Transaction on Graphics 26, 1–23 (2010)
12. Kazhdan, M.M., Bolitho, M., Hoppe, H.: Poisson surface reconstruction. In: Symposium on Geometry Processing, pp. 61–70 (2006)
13. Kazdan, M.M.: Reconstruction of solid models from oriented point sets. In: Symposium on Geometry Processing, pp. 73–82 (2005)
14. Manson, P.G., Schaeffer, S.: Streaming surface reconstruction using wavelets. Computer Graphics Forum 27, 1411–1420 (2008)
15. Ohtake, Y., Belyaev, A., Alexa, M., Turk, G., Seidel, H.P.: Multi-level partition of unity implicits. In: ACM SIGGRAPH, pp. 27–31. ACM Press (2003)
16. Ohtake, Y., Belyaev, A., Seidel, H.P.: Sparse surface reconstruction with adaptive partition of unity and radial basis function. In: Graphical Models, pp. 150–165 (2005)
17. Rasmussen, C.E., Williams, C.: Gaussian Processes for Machine Learning. MIT Press (2006)
18. Smith, M., Posner, I., Newman, P.: Efficient non-parametric surface representations using active sampling for push broom laser data. In: Robotics: Science and Systems Conference (2010)
19. Gerardo-Castro, M.P., Peynot, T., Ramos, F.: Laser-radar data fusion with gaussian process implicit surfaces. In: The 9th International Conference on Field and Service Robotics, vol. 105, pp. 289–302 (2015)
20. Dragiev, S., Toussaint, M., Gienger, M.: Gaussian process implicit surfaces for shape estimation and grasping. In: IEEE International Conference on Robotics and Automation, ICRA 2011, pp. 9–13 (2011)
21. Williams, O., Fitzgibbon, A.: Gaussian process implicit surfaces. In: Gaussian Process in Practice (2007)
22. Taylor, J.S., Cristianini, N.: Kernel Methods for Pattern Analysis. Cambridge University Press (2004)
23. Lewiner, T., Lopes, H., Vieira, A.W., Tavares, G.: Efficient implementation of marching cubes' cases with topological guarantees. Journal of Graphics Tools 8, 1–15 (2003)
24. Berger, M., Levine, J.A., Nonato, L.G., Taubin, G., Silva, C.T.: A benchmark for surface reconstruction. ACM Transactions on Graphics (2013)

# Monocular Visual Odometry Based Navigation for a Differential Mobile Robot with Android OS

Carla Villanueva-Escudero, Juan Villegas-Cortez, Arturo Zúñiga-López, and Carlos Avilés-Cruz

Universidad Autónoma Metropolitana, Azcapotzalco. Departamento de Electrónica, San Pablo Xalpa No.180, Col. Reynosa Tamaulipas, CP 02200, México, D.F. cavies98@gmail.com, {juanvc,azl,caviles}@correo.azc.uam.mx

**Abstract.** In this work, a real time Monocular Visual Odometry system to estimate camera position and orientation based solely on image measurements is proposed. The system is built on the basis of the fundamentals of Structure from Motion theory, and requires only a single camera to estimate positional information. Experiments were conducted on flat ground, under controlled light conditions environment, in which and an Android mobile device camera was employed as the processor and the system sensor due to ease of acquisition and low price. The proposed system resulted in absolute navigation error rates ranging from 0.14% to 0.4% of the travelled distance at processing rates of up to 5Hz.

## 1 Introduction

Visual odometry (VO) is the process of estimating the egomotion of an agent (e.g., vehicle, human, or robot) using only the input of a single or multiple cameras attached to it. Application domains include robotics, wearable computing, augmented reality, and automotive [1]. The term VO was coined in 2004 by Nister in his landmark paper [2]. The term was chosen for its similarity to wheel odometry, which incrementally estimates the motion of a vehicle by integrating the number of turns of its wheels over time. Likewise, VO operates by incrementally estimating the pose of the vehicle through the examination of the changes that motion induces on the images of its onboard cameras. VO operates effectively, if there is sufficient illumination in the environment and the scene is static and with enough texture to allow the extraction of apparent motion. Also, consecutive frames should be captured to ensure that they have sufficient scene overlap.

The advantage of VO with respect to wheel odometry is that VO is not affected by wheel slip in uneven terrain or other adverse conditions. It has been demonstrated that, compared to wheel odometry, VO provides more accurate trajectory estimates, with relative position error ranging from 0.1 to 2%. This capability makes VO an interesting supplement to wheel odometry and, additionally, to other navigation systems such as global positioning system (GPS), inertial measurement units (IMUs), and laser odometry (similar to VO, laser odometry estimates the egomotion of a vehicle by matching consecutive laser scans).

A. Gelbukh et al. (Eds.): MICAI 2014, Part I, LNAI 8856, pp. 281–292, 2014.

Traditionally, autonomous agents obtain positional information by fusing data from the most varied sensors such as lasers, sonars, and Inertial Measurement Units in the statistically grounded framework of Simultaneous Localization and Mapping (SLAM). SLAM systems track the robot position and also the map of the environment by propagating probability density functions over time with filtering approaches like Kalman Filters and Particle Filters. Camera based SLAM was also been proposed, in the so called Visual Simultaneous Localization and Mapping (VSLAM) [2], [3], in which visual landmarks are detected and tracked into image sequences. Nonetheless, VSLAM systems have undesirable characteristics such as limited map sizes and complicated map initialization [4].

In a different direction, Visual Odometry systems (e.g. [5], [6]) track the camera pose using algorithms that adapt Structure from Motion (SFM) techniques for real time sequential and incremental operations instead of the original batch and global optimization approaches utilized in 3-D video based reconstruction. Accordingly, at each time step features (geometric entities or points located at distinctive regions) are extracted from images and matched with those from the previous frame. The change of position and orientation between the current camera pair (relative pose) is then estimated, thus enabling both the 3-D structure of the scene and also the current camera pose to be computed. The algorithms involved in this process are modeled on the mathematical foundations of Projective Geometry [7].

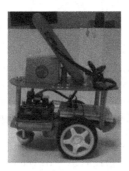 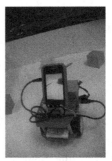

**Fig. 1.** Differential mobile robot

Based on the above, we designed and implemented a Monocular Visual Odometry system featuring a single camera as the only sensor used, Figure 1 shows our Monocular Visual Odometry Mobile Robot System. Our proposed solution has in its core a FAST [8] feature tracker capable of matching key points even with considerably large perspective distortions among images and a SFM based solution built upon the Five Point Algorithm [9] and the framework of RANSAC [10]. Once the initial reconstruction of the scene is obtained, incorrect matches are discarded and key points with already estimated 3-D position are used to assess the current camera pose. In the following sections, we elaborate the rest of this work as follows. In Section 2, approaches similar to the proposed system are presented along with their characteristics. The mathematical theory and the notation grounded on the SFM subarea are shown in Section 3. Section 4 shows the overview of our method performance. The conducted experiments are presented in Section 5, and in Section 6, conclusions drawn from this work as well as future directions are mentioned.

## 2   Related Work

Although a number of Visual SLAM solutions (e.g. [11], [12]) are currently being an active focus of research in the robotics community, we are interested in investigating visual position estimation methods with a compute and forget strategy incorporated, i.e. algorithms that do not utilize visual maps to develop long term localization. This class of localization approaches named Visual Odometry is characterized by SFM solutions processing images as they are sequentially acquired in time. These solutions constitute a constant object of study and hence originate novel black-box approaches in monocular [2], [13], [14], stereo [15] and omnidirectional [16] versions and also standalone systems relying on heavy nonlinear optimization routines [17].

The pioneering work of Nister and colleagues [2] inspired many monocular Visual Odometry systems due to its innovative Five Point Algorithm [9] used in approaches with calibrated cameras. In a different direction, the work of Campbell et al. [13] proposed a system with known and fixed camera position and orientation relative to the ground, enabling the recovery of the robots position after tracking and projecting features on the camera reference frame. Scaramuzza et al. [14] exploited the properties of nonholonomic vehicles to develop a particular motion model method to estimate the position of a vehicle when only few feature points were available; it is based on RANSAC [10]. The stereo solution following the black-box approach proposed by Andrew Howard [15] found sets of features that were mutually consistent regarding their 3-D location, which were assumed to obey a rigidity constraint. Tardif et al. [16] employed an omnidirectional camera in a vision based solution to track vehicles position in urban environments in which camera position estimates were decoupled from orientation estimates. Finally, Mouragnon et al. [17] developed a standalone vision based position estimation system similar to the one proposed by Nister et al. [2] formulating an error minimization strategy employing sliding window Bundle Adjustment techniques.

## 3   Theory

### 3.1   Monocular Visual Odometry

In the monocular VO, both relative motion and 3-D structure must be computed from 2-D bearing data. Since the absolute scale is unknown, the distance between the first two camera poses is usually set to one. As a new image arrives, the relative scale and camera pose with respect to the first two frames are determined using either the knowledge of the 3-D structure or the trifocal tensor [18].

Successful results with a single camera over long distances (up to several kilometers) have been obtained in the last decade using both perspective and omnidirectional cameras [19], [20].

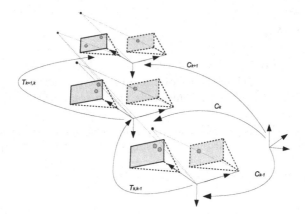

**Fig. 2.** Illustration of the visual odometry problem. Relative poses, or positions of a camera system, $(T_{k,k-1})$, are computed from visual features and concatenated to get the absolute poses $C_k$ with respect to the initial coordinate frame at $k = 0$.

### 3.2    Formulation of the VO Problem

Let us consider that an agent that is moving through an environment and takes images with a rigidly attached camera system at discrete time instants $k$. In case of a monocular system, the set of images taken at time $k$ is denoted by equation 2. Figure 2 illustrates this setting. For the sake of simplicity, the camera coordinate frame is assumed to be the agent coordinate frame. In case of a stereo system, the coordinate system of the left camera may be used as the origin.

Two camera positions at adjacent time instants $k - 1$ and $k$ are related by the rigid body transformation $T_{k,k_1}$ with 1 form:

$$T_{k,k-1} = \begin{bmatrix} R_{k,k-1} & t_{k,k-1} \\ 0 & 1 \end{bmatrix} \tag{1}$$

where $R_{k,k-1}$ is the rotation matrix, and $t_{k,k-1}$ the translation vector. The set $T_{1:n} = T_{1,0}, ...., T_{n,n-1}$ contains all subsequent motions. To simplify the notation, from now on, $T_k$ will be used instead of $T_{k,k-1}$. Finally, the set of camera poses denoted by equation 3, contains the transformations of the camera with respect to the initial coordinate frame at $k = 0$. The current pose, $C_n$, can be computed by concatenating all the transformations $T_k(k = 1...n)$, and, therefore, $C_n = C_{n-1}T_n$ , with $C_0$ being the camera pose at the instant $k = 0$, can be arbitrarily set by the user.

$$I_0 : n = I_0, ..., I_n. \tag{2}$$

$$C_0 : n = C_0, ..., C_n. \tag{3}$$

### 3.3   Camera Model

Our model assumes a pinhole projection system: the image is formed by the intersection of the light rays from the objects through the center of the lens (projection center). Let $X[x, y, z]^T$ be a scene point in the camera reference frame and $p = [u, v]^T$ its projection on the image plane measured in pixels. The mapping from the 3-D world to the 2-D image is given by the perspective projection:

$$\lambda = \begin{bmatrix} u \\ v \\ l \end{bmatrix} = KX = \begin{bmatrix} \alpha_u & 0 & u_0 \\ 0 & \alpha_v & v_0 \\ 0 & 0 & 1 \end{bmatrix} \begin{bmatrix} x \\ y \\ z \end{bmatrix} \tag{4}$$

where $\lambda$ is the depth factor, $\alpha_u$ and $\alpha_v$ the focal lengths, and $u_0, v_0$ the image coordinates of the projection center. These parameters are called *intrinsic parameters*. When the field of vision of the camera is larger than $40°$, the effects of the radial distortion become visible and can be modeled using a second- (or higher-) order polynomial. The derivation of the complete model can be found in computer vision textbooks, such as [18] and [21]. Let $\tilde{p} = [\tilde{u}, \tilde{v}, 1]^T = K^{-1}[u, v, 1]^T$ be the normalized image coordinates. Normalized coordinates will be used throughout in the following sections.

### 3.4   Motion Estimation

Motion estimation constitutes the core computation step reached at each image in a VO system. More precisely, the camera motion between the current image and the previous one is computed. Hence, the full trajectory of the camera and the agent (assuming that the camera is rigidly mounted) can be recovered. This section explains how the transformation $T_k$ between two images $I_{k-1}$ and $I_k$ can be computed from two sets of corresponding features $f_{k-1}$, and $f_k$ at time instants, $k - 1$ and $k$, respectively. Features can be either points or lines. Due to the lack of lines in unstructured scenes, point features are commonly used in VO.

**3-D-to-2-D: Motion from 3-D Structure and Image Feature Correspondences.** As pointed out by Nister et al. [2], motion estimation from 3-D-to-2-D correspondences is more accurate than the estimation from 3-D-to-3-D correspondences. Transformation $T_k$ is computed from the 3-D-to-2-D correspondences, $X_{k-1}$ and $p_k$. $X_{k-1}$ can be estimated from stereo data or, in the monocular case, from the triangulation of the image measurements, $p_{k-1}$ and $p_{k-2}$. The latter, however, requires image correspondences across three views.

In this case the overall formulation consists in finding the $T_k$ that minimizes the image reprojection error trough:

$$arg\,\frac{min}{T_k} = \sum_i ||P_k^i - \hat{P}_{k-1}^i||^2, \tag{5}$$

where $\hat{P}_{k-1}^i$ is the reprojection of the 3-D, $X_{k-1}^i$, into image $I_k$, according to the transformation $T_k$. This problem is known as *perspective from n points (PnP) (or resection)*, and there are many different solutions for it [22].

The 3-D-to-2-D motion estimation assumes that the 2-D image points come only from one camera. For the monocular case, it is necessary to triangulate 3-D points and estimate the pose from 3-D-to-2-D matches in an alternating fashion. This alternating scheme is often referred to as SFM. The VO algorithm with 3-D-to-2-D correspondences is summarized as follows:

**Algorithm 1. VO from 3-D-to-2-D Correspondences**

1. Do only once:
   (a) Capture two frames $I_{k-2}$, $I_{k-1}$
   (b) Extract and match features between them
   (c) Triangulate features from $I_{k-2}$ and $I_{k-1}$
2. Do at each iteration:
   (a) Capture a new frame $I_k$
   (b) Extract features and match them with the previous frame $I_{k-1}$
   (c) Compute camera pose (PnP) from 3-D-to-2-D matches
   (d) Triangulate all new feature matches between $I_k$ and $I_{k-1}$
   (e) Iterate from 2(a).

# 4   Monocular Visual Odometry Solution

## 4.1   Overview

A sequence of image pairs, $(I_{k-1}, I_k)$, acquired by a camera with fixed and known intrinsic parameters, indexed at time step $k$, are supplied to the Monocular Visual Odometry system, which estimates the current camera pose $[R_k|t_k]$, according to the pipeline shown in Figure 3. The computed pose is then referenced into a global coordinate system which was arbitrarily chosen as the reference frame centered in the first camera. The initial position of the robot is established always in the coordinates $(0, 0)$. The estimation of the camera pose is made with the image measurements that comply a sequential processing pipeline, as follows. A set of key points are extracted from each acquired image and matched with those extracted in the previous frame. An initial reconstruction to be used as the global reference frame, is computed using the first image pair, $(I_1, I_2)$, and the relative pose (Essential Matrix) between them. At each new image, $I_k$, the camera pose is computed using the known 3-D structure of the already initialized key points and their respective 2-D projections. Previously unseen features are then estimated, extending the initial point cloud and allowing pose estimation for subsequent image pairs, $(I_{k-1}, I_k)$. This process is detailed in the next section.

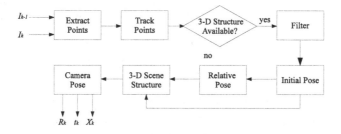

**Fig. 3.** Monocular visual odometry method

## 4.2  Feature Extraction and Matching

The system works by extracting FAST [8] features from each acquired image. This specific class of key points can be rapidly computed at the image scale-space. Likewise, the descriptor vectors allow efficient tracking across images. In doing so, key points are invariantly matched both to rotation and scale changes, and hence exhibit the desired *wide baseline matching* property, which enables distinctive points to be tracked even if the two images were very different from one another.

## 4.3  Relative Pose Estimation

The pose relating a pair of images, $I$ and $I'$, can be estimated given a set of previously matched point correspondences (6). To that end, we report to the efficient Five Point Algorithm [9], which calculates an Essential Matrix by giving at least five key point correspondences. It is important to ensure that the Essential Matrix is being estimated with sufficient robustness to any possible (and frequent) erroneous key point correspondence. Hence, the RANSAC *(RANdom SAmple Consensus)* [10] framework was employed to estimate the relative pose. RANSAC calculates on average each new robot position in 0.46 seconds.

$$\left[ x_i \; x_i' \right]_{i=1}^{i=M} \tag{6}$$

$$\left[ y_j \; y_j' \right]_{j=1}^{j=N} \tag{7}$$

## 4.4  Camera Pose Estimation

If there are sufficient available reconstructed points, given by 3-D points and the 2-D projection $(X, x)$, the pose of the camera, in which the 2-D projections were extracted, can be estimated by a type of algorithm known as *Perspective-n-Point* (PNP) [22].

### 4.5    Reconstruction in a Global Reference Frame

Each image pair, $(I_{k-1}, I_k)$, different from the first pair formed by $(I_1, I_2)$, results in a scene reconstruction, which is incorrectly referenced to the coordinate system of the image $I_{k-1}$. Consequently, a mechanism to estimate camera poses and 3-D structure, in the global reference frame (centered in the first image $I_1$), becomes necessary. On that basis, we used an effective strategy that uses previously reconstructed features to estimate the current camera pose and extend the initial reconstruction computed with the first pair $(I_1, I_2)$. Therefore, each image pair, $(I_{k-1}, I_k)$ with $k > 2$ (i.e. initial reconstruction has already been computed) proceeds as follows. Commonly, after extracting and matching key points, *the relative pose procedure is executed with the sole purpose of filtering the correct matches.* That is, given the whole set of point correspondences (6), we collect the set 7(correspondences classified by RANSAC as inliers), *which already have its 3-D coordinate initialized.*

## 5    Experiments and Results

The version of the system used in the experiments consisted of a a non-optimized C/C++ and Android 2.3 (Gingerbread) implementation, compiled on a Mac OS X 10.7.5 environment using efficient Computer Vision routines available in OpenCV 4 Android libraries. The hardware platform comprised of an Android mobile device (Motorola Photone 4G) with a Core 2 Duo 1Ghz processor and 1GB of RAM. The general system view in which we implemented our methodology is illustrated in Figure 4. All images in the experiments were captured by the mobile device camera, with resolutions of $960 \times 540$ pixels, with 236.5 kb on average. This is subject to the resolution of the camera, and the mobile device processing limitations to improve the performance of the system.

In order to evaluate our proposed Monocular Visual Odometry system, we carried out a navigation experiment performed in an indoor scenario, changing the position of the objects to be localized and the position the obstacles that had to be avoided during the navigation, see Figure 5. Thus, the image sequences used in the presented experiments comprised different situations.

Two representative experiments illustrate the performance of our proposed system. All datasets were taken from images collected in the same indoor environment. All the obstacles in the environment were type static objects with defined shapes (cubes) and 3 different colors. This selection was taken in order to facilitate decision-making. On the other hand, the position of the obstacles was arbitrary, in order to permit the system to take the correct decision; even for the case of impossible navigation.

In the first experiment, the image sequence had a total of 28 images with natural lighting. It was composed of statict objects (three cubes: one red, one blue and one yellow). The navigation of the robot consisted of a $S$ shaped trajectory of 112cm (44.4 in) long. For the second image sequence, the robot made a left turn while navigating in an artificially lit environment with three obstacles. A

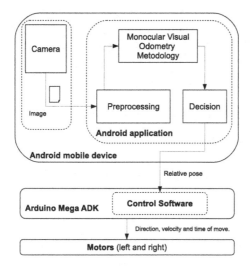

**Fig. 4.** Differential mobile robot system

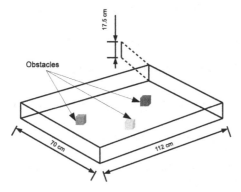

**Fig. 5.** Navigation environment

total of 28 images were used in this last experiment and the robot navigated a path of 23.45cm (9.305 in) long.

For each image, the Monocular Visual Odometry system estimates the robot position. The latter enables a direct comparison of the result given by our method against those ones estimated by other sensors. At this point, we observe that due to the fact that our method calculates the complete position in 6DOF (freedom degrees), the positions in the x, y and z axis were the only ones considered for the comparison with the actual terrain.

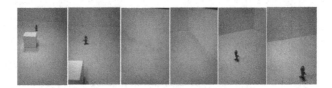

**Fig. 6.** First image sequence used in the experiments

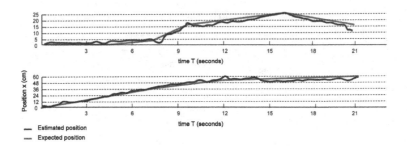

**Fig. 7.** Graphic of results first experiment

## 5.1 Monocular Visual Odometry Precision

The precision of the proposed system was assessed comparing the positional visual estimates, $V_k$, and the Ground Truth, $G_k$. For each resulting path, an instant error measure, $E_k$ was calculated with the Euclidian distance, between each position datum at each time step $k$. Moreover, a relative measure was acquired by expressing the instant error $E_k$ as a percentage of the total distance travelled, $D_{tot}$, after the trajectory traversal, as shown in 8.

$$\epsilon_k = \frac{d(V_k, G_k)}{D_{tot}} \times 100 \qquad (8)$$

Some sample frames used by the proposed Monocular Visual Odometry system are shown in Figure 9.

The same information can be visualized for the second image sequence in Figure 8. Observing the resulting path, we clearly note the similarity between the Visual Odometry trajectory and the Ground Truth. The instant error $\epsilon_k$ remained below 6%, with a final positional error of 2.19% and mean of 0.4% at all time steps for the first sequence. For the second sequence, the instantaneous error from 0.04% to 5.72%; these figures were at the final reached. The average was equal to 0.14%. Actually, we emphasize that for the second experiment, the Monocular Visual Odometry system computed position estimates with more precision than the encoder based odometry, which resulted in positions with a mean error of 3.36% (resulting in 6.54% of error at the final position).

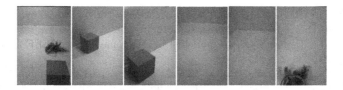

**Fig. 8.** Second image sequence used in the experiments

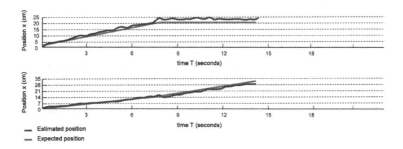

**Fig. 9.** Graphic of results second experiment

## 6   Conclusions

This work presented a Monocular Visual Odometry system built on the fundamentals of Structure from Motion theory. Only purely visual measurements were used to estimate the camera position and orientation on the challenging monocular configuration, offering thereby a black-box solution ready to be deployed on standalone operations for position estimation or to be integrated in multiple sensor localizing frameworks. The proposed Monocular Visual Odometry achieved average error rates ranging from 0.14% to 0.4% (compared to the Ground Truth) processing frames at a maximum rate of  5Hz. Future works will focus on testing our method in outdoor environments. To that end it is necessary to solution for the problem posed by the illumination.

## References

1. Scaramuzza, D., Fraundorfer, F.: Visual odometry, part i: The first 30 years and fundamentals. IEEE Robotics and Automation, 80–91 (2011)
2. Nister, D., Naroditsky, O., Bergen, J.: Visual odometry. In: IEEE Computer Society Conference on Computer Vision and Pattern Recognition (2004)
3. Longuet-Higgins, H.: A computer algorithm for reconstructing a scene from two projections. Nature 293(10), 133–135 (1981)
4. Harris, C., Pike, J.: 3d positional integration from image sequences. In: Proc. Alvey Vision Conf., pp. 87–90 (1988)
5. Frahm, J.M., Georgel, P., Gallup, D., Johnson, T., Raguram, R., Wu, C., Jen, Y.H., Dunn, E., Clipp, B., Lazebnik, S., Pollefeys, M.: Building rome on a cloudless day. In: Conf. Computer Vision, pp. 368–381 (2010)

6. Moravec, H.: Obstacle avoidance and navigation in the real world by a seeing robot rover. PhD thesis, Stanford University (1980)
7. Matthies, L., Shafer, S.: Error modeling in stereo navigation. IEEE J. Robot. Automat. 3(3), 239–248 (1987)
8. Fraundorfer, F., Scaramuzza, D.: Visual odometry, part ii: Matching, robustness, optimization, and applications. IEEE Robotics and Automation, 78–90 (2012)
9. Nister, D.: An efficient solution to the five point relative pose problem. IEEE Transactions on Pattern Analysis and Machine Intelligence 26(6), 756–777 (2004)
10. Fischler, M.A., Bolles, R.C.: Random sample consensus: A paradigm for model fitting with applications to image analysis and automated cartography. Artificial Intelligence Center, SRI International (1981)
11. Davison, A.J.: Real time simultaneous localisation and mapping with a single camera. In: IEEE International Conference on Computer Vision (2003)
12. Lategahn, H., Geiger, A., Kitt, B.: Visual slam for autonomous ground vehicles. In: IEEE International Conference on Robotics and Automation (2011)
13. Campbell, J., Sukthankar, R., Nourbakhsh, I.R., Pahwa, A.: A robust visual odometry and precipice detection system using consumer grade monocular vision. In: IEEE International Conference on Robotics and Automation (2005)
14. Scaramuzza, D., Fraundorfer, F., Siegwart, R.: Real time monocular visual odometry for on road vehicles with 1 point ransac. In: IEEE International Conference on Robotics and Automation (2009)
15. Howard, A.: Real time stereo visual odometry for autonomous ground vehicles. In: IEEE/RSJ International Conference on Intelligent Robots and Systems (2008)
16. Tardif, J.P., Pavlidis, Y., Daniilidis, K.: Monocular visual odometry in urban environments using an omnidirectional camera. In: IEEE/RSJ International Conference on Intelligent Robots and Systems (2008)
17. Mouragnon, E., Lhuillier, M., Dhome, M., Dekeyser, F., Sayd, P.: Real time localization and 3d reconstruction. In: IEEE Computer Society Conference on Computer Vision and Pattern Recognition (2006)
18. Hartley, R., Zisserman, A.: Multiple View Geometry in Computer Vision. 2nd edn. Cambridge U.K. (2004)
19. Nister, D., Naroditsky, O., Bergen, J.: Visual odometry for ground vehicle applications. J. Field Robot 23, 3–20 (2006)
20. Scaramuzza, D., Siegwart, R.: Appearance guided monocular omnidirectional visual odometry for outdoor ground vehicles. IEEE Trans. Robot. (Special Issue on Visual SLAM) 24(5), 1015–1026 (2008)
21. Ma, Y., Soatto, S., Kosecka, J., Sastry, S.: An invitation to 3d vision from images to models. Springer (2003)
22. Moreno-Noguer, F., Lepetit, V., Fua, P.: Accurate non-iterative o(n) solution to the pnp problem. In: IEEE International Conference on Computer Vision, pp. 1–8 (2007)

# Comparison and Analysis of Models to Predict the Motion of Segmented Regions by Optical Flow

Angel Juan Sanchez Garcia[1], Maria de Lourdes Velasco Vazquez[1],
Homero Vladimir Rios Figueroa[2], Antonio Marin Hernandez[2],
and Gerardo Contreras Vega[1]

[1] Faculty of Statistics and Informatics, University of Veracruz, Xalapa,
Veracruz, Mexico
[2] Department of Artificial Intelligence, University of Veracruz, Xalapa,
Veracruz Mexico
{angesanchez,lovelasco,hrios,anmarin,gcontreras}@uv.mx

**Abstract.** Computer vision systems can predict the motion of objects if the movement behavior is analyzed over time, ie, it is possible to find out future values based on previously observed values. In this paper we present an statistical analysis which is aimed to compare two models to predict the position of moving objects in next frames. The models presented are the Kalman filter and an analysis of time series using an ARIMA model. Scenarios with different characteristics are presented as test cases. Segmentation of moving objects is done through the clustering of optical flow vectors for similarity, which are obtained by Pyramid Lucas and Kanade algorithm.

**Keywords:** prediction, motion, optical flow, ARIMA model, Kalman filter.

## 1 Introduction

Computer vision tries to describe the world that we can see in one or more two-dimensional images and to reconstruct its properties [1], such as shape, illumination, color, motion and spatial order of objects, but also the behavior of the elements that are in the images. Computer vision provides us the information for "smart" interaction with the environment without being physically in contact with it [2].

In monocular vision, an important goal is to recover from multiple images over time, the relative motion between an observer and the environment. The structure of the environment obtained is used to generate relative distances between points on a surface in the scene and the observer [3]. For that reason, many applications that incorporate computer vision are used to track moving objects. So, not only we would like that a computer can identify and track any object which is in motion, but we would like that the movement could be predicted to perform some specific task, such as, to focus the camera.

A. Gelbukh et al. (Eds.): MICAI 2014, Part I, LNAI 8856, pp. 293–303, 2014.

To analyze the motion of objects, is necessary to find the objects of interest in a set of frames from a video stream. The optical flow is often used to identify object that have moved from one scene to another, being that it arises from relative motion between the object and the observer [4] [5]. With the analysis of motion over time, we can create a model that allows us to predict, with some confidence, the position of the object in the following frames.

So that, we propose a comparison to evaluate the behavior of two models in prediction of moving objects. Three scenarios were used as test cases. In the scenario 1 is shown the prediction of person moving from right to left, in the second scenario is shown a vehicle moving to the camera passing for a side from it and in the third scenario an arm with a chess board moving randomly.

This paper is organized as follow. In section 2, related work about tracking and prediction motion are presented. the process to get the points to track is shown in section 3. The description of models to analyze is provided in Section 4. In Section 5 the description of analysis used to compare both models is explained. In Section 6 the details of the experiments and the results are shown. Finally section 7 draws some conclusions.

## 2   Related Work

For decades, it has attempted to identify moving objects, track them, and to anticipate their movement. In recent years, optical flow has been used for segmenting moving objects. In [6] the authors show results of an application to segment moving cars from points of interest formed by optical flow vectors obtained by the method of pyramid Lukas - Kanade. Since in this application is only for cars, it only detect moving objects from a priori information on the object type. Moving objects are detected from the image regions with nonzero optical flow vectors and grouped according to the moving speed and Euclidean distance. The Segmentation of the detected objects is performed using a priori information of the same shape, so that we look to identify objects without any particular shape.

Once defined the regions that are in motion in an image sequence, we could predict the motion of regions in consecutive frames. A common technique for tracking and motion prediction is the Kalman Filter. This method has been used in several areas when it is looking to describe the motion of objects and that somehow it could be found or measured the position of these. In [7] the Kalman filter was used to generate a model that it could predict the movement of regions. However, other approaches have been used to predict the motion in sequences of images. In [8] is proposed a model for the interframe correspondences existing between pixels of an image sequence. These correspondences form the elements of a field called the motion field. In their model, spatial neighborhoods of motion elements are related based on a generalization of autoregressive(AR) modeling of time-series. Also in [9] a framework for predicting future positions and orientation of moving obstacles in a time-varying environment using autoregressive model (AR) is described. The AR model has been used in other fields, because it has a low complexity of computation [10], for example in the motion of vehicles [10][11], or in the medical field to predict the evolution of a tumor [12][13]. Even the AR model can be used to modify the model performed in Kalman filter [14]. However, using AR model does not involve to get parameters of the trend in a time series.

On the other hand, In [15] an aggregation approach is proposed for traffic flow prediction that is based on the moving average (MA), exponential smoothing (ES), autoregressive MA (ARIMA), and neural network (NN) models. However the aggregation approach assembles information only from relevant time series from the traffic flow volume that is collected 24 h/day over several years. Other approaches have been used to predict the motion as in [16], where it is presented a method for motion vector prediction from perspective motion models in random access scenarios with hierarchical group of picture structures. In [17]the authors investigate the influence of quantizing the motion vectors on the statistical properties of the prediction error signal. They also computed the power spectral density and the variance of the prediction error.

Also, in the field of prediction the motion of vehicles, the authors in [18] present algorithms for long-term vehicle motion estimation based on a vehicle motion model that incorporates the properties of the working environment and information collected by other mobile agents and fixed infrastructure collection points. However, these algorithms are prepared to predict long-term estimates of vehicle positions. They use a limited number of data collection points distributed around the field to update the estimates. Also, in the field of tracking vehicles, in [19], is proposed a two stage probabilistic prediction model that uses nonparametric Gaussian Process (GP) regression to model continuous complex actions combined with a parametric model for known system dynamics. This two stage model is applied to the case of anticipating driver behavior and vehicle motion. With theses references, it is important to note that there is a significant trend to use probability models in predicting movement.

## 3    Segmentation

The ability to detect motion is crucial for vision and guided behavior by the sense of sight [20]. To identify object that have moved from one scene to another, the optical flow is often used. For the identification and segmentation of moving objects in regions, it is used the methodology proposed in [21], which consists in to select the points of interest in the image where the optical flow can be reliable. Harris called to these points of interest *corners* [22] and they are obtained by the method of Shi and Tomassi [23]. Later the optical flow is calculated by the method of Lucas and Kanade [24] only at points of interest. In the figure 1 are shown examples of the optical flow vectors in the three scenarios.

After obtaining the optical flow vectors, they are grouped by similarity. To create each region that define each object, the clusters of vectors are made based on 3 characteristics: proximity, direction and magnitude. For each group of vectors, their convex hull is obtained to address the problem of discontinuity of optical flow regions and segment the region [21]. To determine whether two points

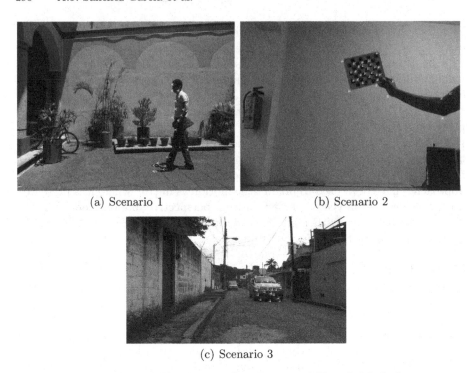

(a) Scenario 1                    (b) Scenario 2

(c) Scenario 3

**Fig. 1.** Optical Flow Vectors from Lucas and Kanade Method

belong to the convex hull from the set of points $S$. Two points $\mathbf{P}(x_1, y_1)$ and $\mathbf{Q}(x_2, y_2)$ belong to the set of the covex hull $C$ if and only if all points $\mathbf{R}(x_3, y_3)$ belonging to $S$(except $\mathbf{P}$ and $\mathbf{Q}$) when they are evaluated in the equation of the line through the points $\mathbf{P}$ and $\mathbf{Q}$, are on one side of the line (the sign must have a single value for every point $R$, either positive or negative). In other words, Equation 1 is satisfied or Equation 2 is satisfied, but not both.

$$\mathbf{P}(x_1, y_1) \in C, \mathbf{Q}(x_2, y_2) \in C \leftrightarrow \forall \mathbf{R}(x_3, y_3) \in S :$$
$$(y_2 - y_1)x_3 - (x_2 - x_1)y_3 < (y_2 - y_1)x_1 - (x_2 - x_1)y_1 \qquad (1)$$

$$\mathbf{P}(x_1, y_1) \in C, \mathbf{Q}(x_2, y_2) \in C \leftrightarrow \forall \mathbf{R}(x_3, y_3) \in S :$$
$$(y_2 - y_1)x_3 - (x_2 - x_1)y_3 > (y_2 - y_1)x_1 - (x_2 - x_1)y_1 \qquad (2)$$

Once a polygon is obtained, it is necessary to interact with a representative point of the polygon in the modeling process. Therefore, the centroid of each polygon is taken as reference for measuring the position of the object along the frames. Figure 2 shows examples of the segmentation procedure for each scenario and their centroids.

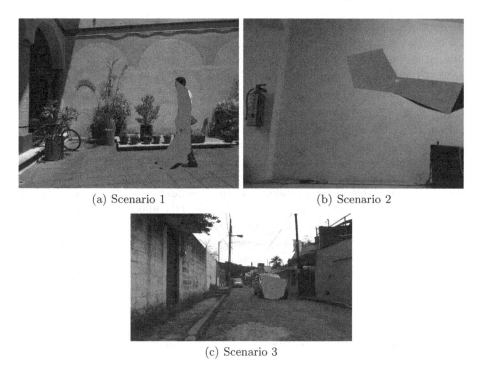

(a) Scenario 1                    (b) Scenario 2

(c) Scenario 3

**Fig. 2.** Segmentation of moving objects

# 4    Description of the Models

## 4.1    Kalman Filter

The Kalman filter has risen to great prominence in a wide variety of signal processing contexts. This model has two phases: prediction and adjustment. In this last phase, the parameters of the model are adjusted depending on the error caused in the prediction phase. The idea in the Kalman filter is that, under a strong but reasonable set of assumptions, it will be possible, given a history of measurements of a system, to build a model for the state of the system that maximizes the a posteriori probability of those previous measurements [25].

There are three important assumptions required in the theoretical construction of the Kalman filter:

1. The system being modeled is linear
2. The noise that measurements are subject to is "white", and
3. This noise is also Gaussian in nature.

The first assumption means that the state of the system at time $k$ can be modeled as some matrix multiplied by the state at time $k$-$1$. The additional assumptions that the noise is both white and Gaussian means that the noise is not correlated in time and that its amplitude can be accurately modeled using only an average and a covariance [26]. We can generalize the description of the state at time $k$ to be the following function of the state at time step $k-1$:

$$x_k = Fx_{k-1} + Bu_k + w_k \qquad (3)$$

Here $x_k$ is an n-dimensional vector of state components and F is an n-by-n matrix, sometimes called the *transfer matrix*. The vector $u_k$ allows external controls on the system, and it consists of a c-dimensional vector referred to as the control inputs; $B$ is an n-by-c matrix that relates these control inputs to the state change. The variable $w_k$ is a random variable (usually called the process noise) associated with random events or forces that directly affect the actual state of the system. We assume that the components of $w_k$ have Gaussian distribution $N(0, Q_K)$ for some n-by-n covariance matrix $Q_k$ ($Q$ is allowed to vary with time, but often it does not).

we measure the m-dimensional vector of measurements $z_k$ given by:

$$z_k = H_k x_k + v_k \qquad (4)$$

where $H_k$ is an m-by-n matrix and $v_k$ is the measurement error, which is also assumed to have Gaussian distributions $N(0, R_k)$ for some m-by-m covariance matrix $R_k$.

## 4.2    ARIMA Model

Time series forecasting is the use of a model to predict future values based on previously observed values. ARIMA *Autoregressive Integrated and Moving Average* is a probabilistic model which assumes that errors have a normal distribution with mean zero and variance $\sigma^2$. This assumption is called *White Noise*. Also, this assumes that there is no autocorrelation in the errors. The expression used to represent this assumption is:

$$\varepsilon_t \sim N(0, \sigma^2) \qquad (5)$$

*The autoregressive (AR) model* [27][28] specifies that the output variable depends linearly on its own previous values. Its set-up is based on using data observed in the past to develop the AR model coefficients.

*Moving Average* is one of widely known technical indicator used to predict the future data in time series analysis [29]. MA is a common average of the previous $n$ data points in time series data. Each point in the time series data is equally weighted.

The autoregressive and moving average process, denoted as $ARMA(p,q)$, is a combination of an autoregressive process of order $p$ and moving average process of order $q$. This combination can be written as it is shown in the equation (6):

$$X_t = c + \phi_1 X_{t-1} + \phi_2 X_{t-2} + ... + \phi_p X_{t-p} + \varepsilon_t + \theta_1 \varepsilon_{t-1} + \theta_2 \varepsilon_{t-2} + ... + \theta_q \varepsilon_{t-q} \qquad (6)$$

Where $\varepsilon_t$ errors satisfy a white noise sequence. The ARIMA model symbolized as $ARIMA(p,d,q)$, follows a similar process that $ARMA(p,q)$ processes, only now in the initial model is taken into account that the series is not stationary and it is possible that differentiations of some order are needed. Therefore $p$ denotes the number of autoregressive model parameters, $d$ denotes the order of the differentiations required to solve problems of non-stationarity and $q$ denotes the number of parameters required moving averages. This kind of model is crucial, because it helps us to engage the *trend* and *periodicity* in the time series to the model, if these elements are presented. To select the values of $p$ and $q$, several models are generated and tested to select the adjusted model with lower values of Akaike information criterion $AIC$ (which is a measure of the relative quality of a statistical model for a given set of data) and $\sigma^2$.

## 5    Description of Analysis

We intend to compare which model best fits to the real values. These analyzes are performed separately for the movement in the axis $x$ and axis $y$. Figure 3 shows an example of comparing series from Kalman Filter model, ARIMA model and the real series. In Figure 3 is presented the series for scenario 1, and since the segmented region is moving from right to left, it can be seen that series on the axis $x$ has negative trend, but the axis $y$ remains almost constant. Also, we can see that the Kalman Filter series has a lot of variability, although its behavior is similar to the original series. To eliminate variability, we base the statistical analysis on the cumulative distribution.

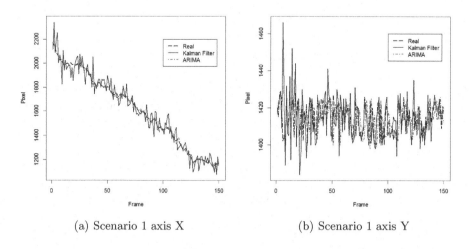

(a) Scenario 1 axis X                    (b) Scenario 1 axis Y

**Fig. 3.** Example of comparison between all original series

We used the non-parametric two-sample Kolmogorov-Smirnov test. Its objective is to test the null hypothesis that two populations have the same response distributions against the alternative that the response distribution are different. We chose Kolmogorov-Smirnov test because, unlike others test as Wilcoxon-Man-Witney test, the first is an omnibus test with good power against general alternatives in which both populations can differ in both shape and locations [30]. Figure 4 shows an example of the comparison of cumulative distributions of the series.

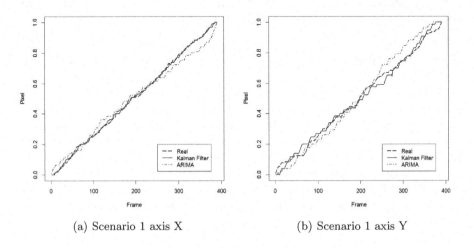

(a) Scenario 1 axis X                          (b) Scenario 1 axis Y

**Fig. 4.** Example of smoothing of the time series for scenario 1

## 6    Experiments and Results

For the experiments, in the scenarios 1 and 3 were used images of 2592 x 1944 pixels and in the scenario 2 where used images of 1920 x 1080 pixels. In all cases the images were taken from a video with a frequency of 30 images per second. The results were obtained offline. Although the images were taken in RGB format, the image processing was performed on a single channel, i.e. gray scale. To know if the time series in the ARIMA model was stationary, the Phillps-Perron test [31] was used. Table 1 shows the average of the differences between predicted values for each model and the real values.

The analysis of each scenario are shown in tables 2, 3 and 4, where the functions of cumulative distributions of the Kalman Filter and ARIMA models are compared against real values in the axis $x$ and axis $y$.

**Table 1.** Average of errors in prediction of each scenario

| Scenario | Models compared | Average difference |
|:---:|:---:|:---:|
| 1 | Kalman Filter - axis $x$ | 44.66153846 |
| 1 | Kalman Filter - axis $y$ | 13.16923077 |
| 1 | ARIMA - axis $x$ | 5.384615385 |
| 1 | ARIMA - axis $y$ | 8.561538462 |
| 2 | Kalman Filter - axis $x$ | 11.22857143 |
| 2 | Kalman Filter - axis $y$ | 4.585714286 |
| 2 | ARIMA - axis $x$ | 7.457142857 |
| 2 | ARIMA - axis $y$ | 4.328571429 |
| 3 | Kalman Filter - axis $x$ | 26.97142857 |
| 3 | Kalman Filter - axis $y$ | 9.442857143 |
| 3 | ARIMA - axis $x$ | 17.88571429 |
| 3 | ARIMA - axis $y$ | 7.228571429 |

**Table 2.** Kolmogorov Smirnov test for function of comulative distributions in scenario 1

| Model | Maximum difference | p-value |
|:---|:---:|:---:|
| KalmanFilter vs real values (axis x) | 0.0692 | 0.9144 |
| KalmanFilter vs real values (axis y) | 0.0923 | 0.6369 |
| ARIMA vs real values (axis x) | 0.0308 | 0.9999 |
| ARIMA vs real values (axis y) | 0.1308 | 0.2163 |

**Table 3.** Kolmogorov Smirnov test for function of comulative distributions in scenario 2

| Model | Maximum difference | p-value |
|:---|:---:|:---:|
| KalmanFilter vs real values (axis x) | 0.0714 | 0.9941 |
| KalmanFilter vs real values (axis y) | 0.0571 | 0.9998 |
| ARIMA vs real values (axis x) | 0.0571 | 0.9998 |
| ARIMA vs real values (axis y) | 0.0429 | 0.9999 |

**Table 4.** Kolmogorov Smirnov test for function of comulative distributions in scenario 3

| Model | Maximum difference | p-value |
|:---|:---:|:---:|
| KalmanFilter vs real values (axis x) | 0.1571 | 0.3531 |
| KalmanFilter vs real values (axis y) | 0.1429 | 0.4727 |
| ARIMA vs real values (axis x) | 0.0571 | 0.9998 |
| ARIMA vs real values (axis y) | 0.0857 | 0.9592 |

# 7   Conclusions

A comparison between two models to predict the motion of segmented regions is presented. While the Kalman filter model generates a model from the first pair of frames (although it starts with random values), the ARIMA model requires a set of frames to predict the position in the next frame. Analysis of the cumulative distributions allows us to analyze the shapes of the distributions without involving variability. In Tables 2, 3 and 4 is shown that the probability values were not significant, this means that the estimated values obtained from the Kalman Filter and ARIMA models are very close to real model, however the ARIMA model is the one with best fit.

# References

1. Szeliski, R.: Computer Vision. Algorithms and Applications. Springer, USA (2013) ISBN: 978-184882-935-0
2. Horn, P.: Robot Vision. The MIT Press, USA (1993) ISBN: 0-262-08159-8
3. Negahdaripour, S.: A direct Method for locating the Focus of Expansion, Tecnical Report. A. I. Memo No 939 (1987)
4. Gibson, J.J.: The Perception of the Visual World. Riverside Press, Cambridge (1950)
5. Gibson, J.J.: The Senses Considered as Perceptual Systems, Houghton-Mi Win, Boston (1966)
6. Mora, D., Paez, A., Quiroga, J.: Deteccion de objetos Moviles en una Escena utilizando Flujo optico. In: XIV Simposio de tratamiento de señales, imagenes y vision artificial, STSIVA 2009 (2009)
7. Sanchez, A., Rios, H., Marin, A., Acosta, H.: Tracking and Prediction of Motion of Segmented Regions Using the Kalman Filter. In: Proceedings of the CONIELE-COMP 2014, vol. 3, pp. 88–93. IEEE (2014), doi:ISBN:978-1-4799-3468-3
8. Rajagopalan, R., Orchard, M.T., Brandt, R.D.: Motion Field Modeling for Video Sequences. IEEE Transactions on Image Processing 6(11) (1997)
9. Elnagar, A., Gupta, K.: Motion Prediction of Moving Objects Based on Autoregressive Model, Systems, Man and Cybernetics. IEEE Transactions on Part A: Systems and Humans 28(6) (1998)
10. Wei, D., Ye, J., Wu, X., Liang, L.: Time Series Prediction for Generalized Heave Displacement of a Shipborne Helicopter Platform. In: SECS International Colloquium on Computing, Communication, Control, and Management (2008) (2008)
11. Jun, L., Sumei, W., Ke, P., Jun, X., Yun, W., Tao, Z.: Research on On-line Measurement and Prediction for Vehicle Motion State. In: International Conference on Digital Manufacturing and Automation (2010)
12. Ichiji, K., Sakai, M., Homma, N., Takai, Y., Yoshizawa, M.: Lung Tumor Motion Prediction Based On Multiple Time-Variant Seasonal Autoregressive Model for Tumor Following Radiotherapy. In: IEEE/SICE International Symposium System Integration, SII (2010)
13. Ichiji, K., Homma, N., Sakai, M., Takai, Y., Narita, Y., Abe, M., Sugita, N., Yoshizawa, M.: Respiratory Motion Prediction for Tumor Following Radiotherapy by using Time-variant Seasonal Autoregressive Techniques. In: 34th Annual International Conference of the IEEE EMBS (2012)

14. Huang, S.H., Tsao, J., Yang, T.C., Cheng, S.: Model-Based Signal Subspace Channel Tracking for Correlated Underwater Acoustic Communication Channels. IEEE Journal of Oceanic Engineering 39(2) (2014)
15. Man, T., Wong, S.C., Jian, X., Zhan, G.: An Aggregation Approach to Short-Term Traffic Flow Prediction. IEEE Transactions on Intelligent Transportation Systems 10(1) (2009)
16. Tok, M., Esche, M., Sikora, T.: A dynamic model buffer for parametric motion vector prediction in random-access coding scenarios. In: IEEE International Conference on Image Processing, ICIP (2013)
17. Vandendorpe, L., Cuvelier, L., Maison, B.: Statistical properties of prediction error images in motion compensated interlaced image coding. In: Proceedings of the International Conference on Image Processing, vol. 3 (1995)
18. Shan, M., Worrall, S., Masson, F., Nebot, E.: Using Delayed Observations for Long-Term Vehicle Tracking in Large Environments. IEEE Transactions on Intelligent Transportation Systems (2014)
19. Hardy, J., Havlak, F., Campbell, M.: Multiple-step prediction using a two stage Gaussian Process model. In: American Control Conference, ACC (2014)
20. Albrecht, D.G., Geisler, W.S.: Motion selectivity and the contrast-respons function of simple cells in the visual cortex. In: Vis. Neurosci., pp. 531–546 (1991)
21. Sanchez, A., Rios, H.: Segmentacion de objetos en movimiento por flujo optico y color sin informacion a priori de la escena, Research in computing science. Avances en Inteligencia Artificial 62, 151–160 (2013)
22. Harris, C., Stephens, M.: A combined corner and edge detector. In: Proceedings of the 4th Alvey Vision Conference, pp. 147–151 (1988)
23. Shi, J., Tomassi, J.: Good features to track. In: 9th IEEE Conference on Computer Vision and Pattern Recognition (1994)
24. Lucas, B.D., Kanade, T.: An iterative image registration technique with an application to stereo vision. In: Proceedings of the 1981 DARPA Imaging Understanding Workshop, pp. 121–130 (1981)
25. Kalman, R.: A new approach to linear filtering and prediction problems. Journal of Basic Engineering 82, 35–45 (1960)
26. Bradski, G., Kaebler, A.: Learning OpenCV. Computer vision with the OpenCV library, 1st edn. Oreilly (2008)
27. Haykin, S.: Nonlinear Method of Spectral Analysis. Springer (1979)
28. Kay, S.M., Marple, S.L.: Spectrum Analysis- a modern perspective. Proc. IEEE 69, 1380–1419 (1981)
29. Hansun, S.: A New Approach of Moving Average Method in Time Series Analysis, Microwave Symposium Digest. New Media Studies (CoNMedia) (2013)
30. StatXact, Statistical software for Exact Nonparametric Inference, user manual, Cytel Statistical Software (2004)
31. Phillps, P., Perron, P.: Testing fr a unit root in time series regression. Biometrika, vol 7(2), 335–346 (1988)

# Image Based Place Recognition and Lidar Validation for Vehicle Localization

Yongliang Qiao, Cindy Cappelle, and Yassine Ruichek

IRTES-SET, UTBM, 90010 Belfort Cedex, France
{yongliang.qiao,cindy.cappelle,yassine.ruichek}@utbm.fr

**Abstract.** In this paper, we propose a system for vehicle localization that combines two sensors: a camera and a lidar. An image based place recognition approach is used to determine the vehicle localization when the vehicle revisited a previously visited location. Unlike systems that only rely on visual appearance recognition for localization, we also integrate lidar measurements information in order to validate the vision based place recognition results. Effectively, false positives recognition can be detected and rejected by checking the coherency of the image based recognition results with the results of lidar measurements matching with ICP (iterative closest point) algorithm. In case of false image based recognized places, vehicle position can be computed using only lidar based ICP method. The vehicle position is effectively estimated using the last known position and the transformation between the corresponding lidar measurement and the current one obtained by applying ICP. By employing the camera and lidar sensors, the deficiencies of each individual sensor can be overcome. Experiments were conducted in two different surrounding areas. The obtained results show that the proposed method permit to avoid the well-known long-term accumulated error of dead-reckoning localization and lidar data can help to reject false positives of place recognition.

**Keywords:** Vehicle localization, Place recognition, Multi-sensor approach, ICP.

## 1 Introduction

Localization plays an essential and important role for ADAS (Advanced Driver Assistance Systems) and unmanned driving. GPS has been the most popular tool for vehicle global localization. But in some particular dense urban environments, satellite signals might be blocked or affected by buildings. The limited visibility and bad geometry of satellites or the multi-path problem will then decrease the localization accuracy and availability. Other sensors are then often added to the localization system to complete the GPS information. Among these sensors, perception sensors (as camera or lidar) are often used. One of the vision based approach for localization is SLAM (Simultaneous Localization and Mapping). Good progress has been achieved in SLAM, but is still far from being an established and reliable technology. A big problem is the lack of robustness. In this

A. Gelbukh et al. (Eds.): MICAI 2014, Part I, LNAI 8856, pp. 304–315, 2014.
© Springer International Publishing Switzerland 2014

paper, we examine the vehicle localization problem basing on place recognition by combining camera and lidar sensor data.

Most localization methods based on place recognition techniques typically adopt an image retrieval approach [1][2][3]. One of the state-of-the-art place recognition technique is Fast Appearance-Based Mapping (FAB-MAP), which employs Bag-of-Words (BOW) image retrieval systems and a Bayesian framework [4]. FAB-MAP uses Chow-Liu trees algorithm [5] to measure the co-occurring visual words to achieve robust image matching. This approach enables to recover the vehicle current position from reference key images. Visual features such as SIFT and SURF are convenient under small variations in lighting and orientation [6], but are prone to failure under complex and similar environments (ludicrous situations, such as grassy areas, multi-paned windows and occasional wall patterns). Thus, query image, taken from the current location might be matched to the content of one or more previous images stored in a large database. This would eventually lead to the fail of the mapping result. Conversely, lidar sensors are robust to variations in lighting and orientation, but rely on the presence of structures in the scene. In this work, we seek to combine the strengths of the two sensing modalities to improve the robustness of the visual place recognition system and create a system that can perform in different areas or at different times. Our approach aims at developing advanced localization method based on place recognition by combining image and lidar observations to achieve better localisation accuracy. In this study, we propose a vehicle localization using not only GPS observations but also appearance based place recognition to solve the demerits of each observation. We combine the visual and range data to improve the robustness of the place recognition system and improve the localization accuracy. The structure of this paper is organized as follows: Section 2 introduces the related works; Section 3 details the proposed vehicle localization method; and Section 4 presents some experimental results with real data acquired by our experimental vehicle. Finally, conclusions and perspectives are given in Section 5.

## 2   Related Works

Recently, one popular technique for vision based vehicle localization is image retrieval method (see [4] for a review). In [7], similarity between two images is defined as the normalized inner product of two image appearance vectors. A similarity matrix is constructed to find revisited location in a sequence. In GraphSLAM [8], the authors use a similar BOW technique but are able to update their vocabulary as each new image is processed rather than through off-line supervised learning. Compared with the original algorithm FAB-MAP 2.0 [9] uses an inverted index retrieval architecture that requires modification of the way the probabilities of revisits are computed and updated.

Place recognition can also be applied on 2D range data. In paper [10], a lidar based SLAM is proposed: a Monte Carlo Localization scheme is adopted for vehicle position estimation, based on synthetic lidar measurements and odometry information. In [11], statistical and range histogram features are used as inputs to an AdaBoost classifier. Algorithms that use multiple sensors for place recognition have also been proposed. In [12], Tipaldi et al introduce geometrical FLIRT phrases (GFPs) as a novel retrieval method for very efficient and precise place recognition. GFPs perform approximate 2D range data matching, to handle complicated partial matching patterns and are robust to noise. In [13], Bosse and Zlot evaluate several detector/descriptor-pairs of 2D range data for the task of place recognition in a graphical submap-based SLAM application.

In [14], [15] and [16], raw laser scans are used for relative pose estimation. Laser range scans are used in conjunction with EKF-SLAM in [17]. The authors introduced an algorithm where landmarks are defined by templates composed of raw sensed data which do not need to rely on geometric landmarks. In paper[18], machine learning approach is used on range sensors data for loop closure detection problems. A multi-scale interest region operator, Fast Laser Interest Region Transform is proposed in paper [19]. It can be used in conjunction with RANSAC to address the loop closing and global localization problems.

There is relatively little related works that combine visual and range data to improve the robustness of the place recognition system. Localisation algorithms based on both laser scans and vision have shown to be robust. The work presented in [12] performs loop closure detection using visual cues and laser data. Shape descriptors such as angle histograms and entropy are used to describe and match the laser scans. A loop closure is only accepted if both visual and spatial appearance comparisons credited the match. In [20], laser range scans are fused with images to form descriptors of the objects used as landmarks. The laser scans are used to detect regions of interest in the images through polynomial fitting of laser scan segments while the landmarks are represented using visual features. Jack Collier et al [21] describe a multi-sensor appearance based place recognition system suitable for robotic mapping. Bag-of-Words approach is applied on features extracted from both visual and range sensors. By applying this technique to both sensor streams simultaneously, they can overcome the deficiencies of each individual sensor. However, this approach is computationally intensive.

## 3   Proposed Vehicle Localization Approach

The system presented here is a multi-sensor extension of the FAB-MAP system described in papers [4] and [9]. The system is outlined in Figure 1. For each place, the image information and lidar data are acquired. We first conduct place recognition based on image, and then use lidar measurements for validation. If the image based place recognition result is coherent with lidar measurements then the current position is confirmed. Otherwise, the recognition result is supposed to be a false positive, the current position of the vehicle is then computed using the last known position and the transformation (computed by ICP algorithm) between the previous lidar data and the current one (refered in the rest of the paper as lidar based odometry method).

The system consists of two phases: training and testing. In the training phase, each image is associated with corresponding GPS position and lidar scan.

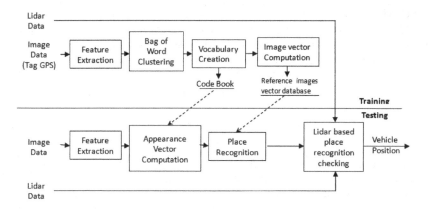

**Fig. 1.** Architecture of the proposed system

The first step of training phase is the image SURF feature extraction. Then, Bag-of-Words Kmeans clustering is performed in the feature space to group similar features and create the vocabulary.

During the testing phase, new features are extracted from real-time image, as shown in Figure 1. A probabilistic detector model converts the extracted features into an appearance vector that determines which words are present in the current scene. For a vocabulary of $n$ words, the associated appearance vector is denoted by $Z_k = Z_1, ..., Z_n$, where the binary $z$ value 1 indicates the presence of the word in the current frame. The appearance vectors are then fed to the scene recognition module where the current image is compared with training images. The corresponding images are determined using a Bayesian model. The image with the highest probability above a threshold is determined to be a tentative recognition location. If a tentative place recogniton has been found, the lidar scan corresponding to the current image and the lidar data associated to the matched reference image are compared using ICP in order to confirm (or disprove) the image based place recognition result. If the image based place recognition result is confirmed by the lidar, the image retrieval is considered as a true positive. The transformation between the current tested image and the associated reference image (from the training database) is then computed. From this transformation and the known GPS position of the associated reference image, the position corresponding to the current tested image can be calculated. In case of false positive recognition, the vehicle current position is computed using ICP method based only on lidar information.

### 3.1   Image Based Place Recognition

We use FAB-MAP as appearance based place recognition method. In this section, we describe the used place recognition system briefly. A more in depth description can be found in [6] and [8].

## a. FAB-MAP Algorithm

FAB-MAP compares the appearance of current visual scene and past locations by representing images with BW (Bag of Words) techniques. The location which has the highest probability is considered as the same as the previously visited location. The probability of matching to location $L_i$ given all observations $Z^k$, which includes the current observation $Z_k$, is calculated by recursive Bayes:

$$p(L_i|Z^k) = \frac{P(Z_k|L_i)p(L_i|Z^{k-1})}{p(Z_k|Z^{k-1})} \tag{1}$$

Here, the prior probability of a location $p(L_i|Z^{k-1})$ is estimated using a naive motion model based on image information. $P(Z_k|L_i)$ is Observation Likelihood. The probability is normalized by $p(Z_k|Z^{k-1})$.

## b. Bag-of-Words (BOW) method

In Bag-of-Words, appearance-based feature detector is used to find interest points in the image and to represent the appearance of the local region. The feature point locations are discarded and each feature is matched to a list of *a priori* generated visual words (also called "codebook"). The codebook is generated by clustering a large amount of features, extracted from a training dataset, to form a finite list (commonly thousands) of general appearances often encountered in the environment. The observation $Z_k$ corresponding to the image at time $k$ is then reduced to a binary vector indicating the codebook words that are present in the image:

$$Z_k = [z_1, z_2, \cdots, z_{|v|}] \tag{2}$$

where the individual observation of codebook word $i$ is $z_i$.

## c. Chow-Liu trees algorithm

The naive Bayes approach can significantly be improved by using Chow-Liu trees in FAB-MAP. Full distribution of observation likelihood between images is estimated using a Chow-Liu dependency tree from training data. Chow-Liu trees algorithm makes a minimum spanning tree which maximizes information entropy $I$ defined as follows:

$$I(z_i, z_j) = \sum_{z_i \in \Omega, z_j \in \Omega} p(z_i, z_j) \log \frac{p(z_i, z_j)}{p(z_i)(z_j)} \tag{3}$$

where $z_i$ are the visual words observed in the image. The high coocurring images pairs was selected by maximizing the entropy between the word $i$ and word $j$. Then the likelihood becomes high even if there are disturbances in the scene such pedestrians, cars and so on.

### 3.2    lidar Based Validation

Place recognition based on FAB-MAP approach does not consider the spatial relationship of features distribution. In addition, quantization of image descriptor vectors also loses some useful information. In order to obtain precise positions, it is necessary to validate that the place recognition results are true positives. After the image retrieval system has identified a revisited place, a validation scheme based on lidar data is applied.

By using the ICP algorithm, we compute the transformation (rotation and translation) between the current lidar data and the lidar data corresponding to the training image associated to the current image (by the FAB-MAP algorithm). The ICP algorithm estimates the optimal 2D transformation between two points sets by iterative data association of corresponding points with nearest neighbor algorithm and least square minimization.

If an image is assained to be acquired at the same place as a training image, their corresponding lidar scans should also be the same and then the transformation between the two lidar scans should be small due to the almost same surroundings structure.

So if the lidar transformation between the scans corresponding to the two matched images is minor, the image retrieval result is validated as a true positive match. As the training images are associated with GPS measurements, the position of the associated training image is known. Even if the route for the training and testing steps are the same, in real situation, the testing trajectory on this route is not exactly the same as the training trajectory. In order to get more precision position, when the test image was retrievaled and validated, the test image position is also revised by the lidar data transformation compared with the lidar data of train image .

If the lidar based test does not validate the image retrieval result, then the image matching is considered as a false positive. The vehicle current position is then computed using the previous position and the transformation between the previous lidar scan and the current lidar scan computed using ICP (lidar based odometry).

## 4   Experimental Results

The proposed method is tested with real data acquired by our experimental GEM vehicle equipped with a stereoscopic Bumblebee XB3 system (16 Hz, image size is 1280×960), a GPS receiver (10 Hz) and a horizontal SICK LMS221 laser range finder (5Hz). Only the central camera of Bumblebee XB3 system is used, the camera field of view (FOV) is 66°. Every LRF scan provides 181 data points in a 180° arc with a 1° angular resolution and a maximum range of 80m.

The experiments are conducted in two different area types: "Block area" and "Parking area". Data were acquired and stored at different times.

For the "block area" trial (AS Fig. 3 left shown), the vehicle traversed about 0.8 km in an area surrounded by buildings and factories. Data were collected the 2012/02/10 and 2011/11/29. Data collected on 2012 are used as training data. Among the 1100 acquired frames, one frame is selected as reference image each 10 frames. The training database in then composed of 110 reference images, whose corresponding GPS position and lidar data are also known.

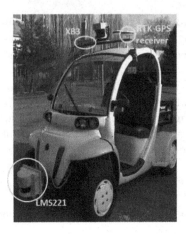

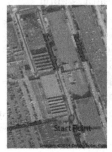

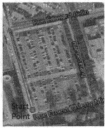

**Fig. 2.** Experimental vehicle equipped with a stereoscopic system, a LRF and a GPS receiver

**Fig. 3.** Experimental field: the left one is "block area" surrounded by factories and buildings while the right one is "parking area" which is mostly nature scene

The testing database is composed of the whole data collected in November 2011 (1600 images). As the lidar accqusition rate is slower than the camera, we have corresponding lidar scans for only 500 images.

For the "parking area"trial, the vehicle traversed about 0.6 km in an area surrounded by buildings and trees. The reference data was selected by interval of 10 frames among the 1950 frames collected in Feb.18, 2012. So there are 195 reference positions. The testing data includes the 1590 frames collected in Feb.19, 2014, and 497 images have the corresponding lidar data.

### 4.1   Place Recognition Based on FAB-MAP and lidar Validation

Feature extraction is important for place recognition. FAB-MAP expresses locations as gathering of words which are based on image features. Here, SURF features were selected to extract image feature. However, wrong recognition in bad light or in some similar scenes can occur as illustrated in Figure 4. It shows a false positive matching from image retrieval method due to lighting influence. It can be seen visually that the scale is quite different, i.e. one image is acquired closer to the building than the other one. Their corresponding lidar scans present then a huge difference. In fact, the GPS distance between these two frames is around 200 metres.

In order to make place recognition more robust, we use the classic iterative closest point (ICP) between the lidar scans corresponding to the mached training/testing images to verify the true match. The image retrieval is validated only if the translation distance between the two lidar scans is less than 3 meters.

The false positive matching result as figure 4 shows ,which can be easily confirmed is a false positive and it is correctly rejected. This scenario occurs

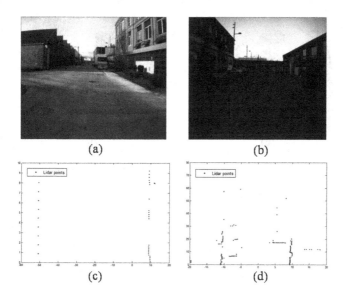

**Fig. 4.** A false image retrieval rejected by the lidar verification. The image pair false matching is shown in (a) and (b) while the corresponding lidar scans are shown in (c) and (d) respectively.

frequently in this data set due to the lighting changes or other influences in the visual imagery. It is obviously that, the matched images should have the similar lidar distance. So the lidar verification can reject the flase matching. In all cases, the lidar based verification algorithm has discarded them correctly.

Figure 5 illustrates an example of true positive. Due to space discretization and trajectories a little bit different between training and testing, it might exist several frames matched to one frame. However, when the positions between theses two frames are less than 3 meters, we still believe these matches are positive.

Using lidar based validation, a total of 137 true positives (for 500 tested images) and 246 true positives (for 497 tested images) have been detected respectively in "block area" and "parking area" (Table 1). Since our lidar based verification is very effective in discarding false positives from FAB-MAP, we obtain zero false positives in our experiment. Using the lidar verification scheme, the number of true positives decreases as expected. Effectively, it requires both image and lidar data information to recognize the scene at the same instant. But the lidar frequency is slower than camera acquisition rate. So the approach "image+lidar" is tested only on 500 images in "block area" and 497 images in "parking area" corresponding to the available lidar measurements.

## 4.2 Localization Results in "Block Area" and "Parking Area"

For testing our proposed localization method, the experiment was conducted using the two different surrounding areas. We match current test image to the train

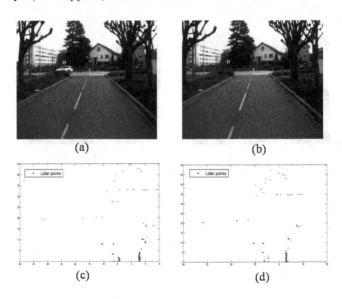

**Fig. 5.** A true positive in "parking area": the place is recognized by image retrieval and verified by lidar. The image pair is shown in (a) and (b) while the corresponding lidar scans are shown in (c) and (d) respectively.

image database. After finding a match result in the database, the corresponding lidar data will be checked to confirm the match result are true positive. If the match result is true, we can get the vehicle current position. If the match result is not true, we can use the lidar data to calculate the vehicle position basing on the last known position. Localization results by combining the image and lidar can be seen in the figure 6 and figure 7.

It shows that our localization system can do accurate estimation by combing the lidar and image data. One of the advantages is that by using lidar data and ICP method we can perform place recogniton accuratlye. For example, between the two matched points(red points), we can use the lidar data to get the vehilcle position on some unrecognition places (for some unmatched images). Therefore, we can get the minimum localization error at 0 m in some local localization, as shown in the table 2.

Table 2 shows localization error of the test route in two different areas compared with measured GPS position. It shows that the average localization error under 4 meters. We avoid the accumulative error by only using the lidar data and position error remains in a small range in our result. Considering some of the errors were caused by environment changes between experiment and reference, our system even can get more precison in some good environment. In the proposed method, we can reduce the position error in environment with less changes. Nevertheless to further refine the proposed method, we must improve the image matching perfomance and the motion estimation. From these results, the effectiveness of our proposed system is demonstrated.

**Table 1.** True Positives and False Positives from Image and from Image+Lidar in Block and Parking Area (Image* is the same images that we used in the image+ lidar approach)

|              |                 | Image | Image+Lidar | Image* |
|--------------|-----------------|-------|-------------|--------|
| Block Area   | True positives  | 358   | 137         | 102    |
|              | False Positives | 142   | 0           | 35     |
| Parking Area | True positives  | 429   | 246         | 208    |
|              | False Positives | 68    | 0           | 38     |

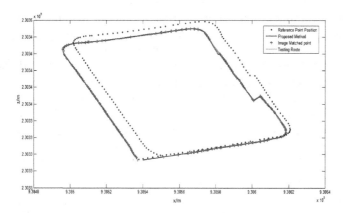

**Fig. 6.** Localization results in "Parking area"

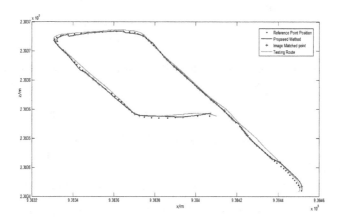

**Fig. 7.** Localization results in "Block area"

**Table 2.** Localization Error Statistics in Block Area and Parking Area

|  | Maximum Error(/m) | Minimum Error(/m) | Average Error(/m) |
|---|---|---|---|
| Block Area | 7.3930 | 0 | 3.3280 |
| Parking Area | 5.7310 | 0 | 1.2173 |

## 5  Conclusion

In this paper, we proposed a localization method by combining camera and lidar data. To reduce the false place recognition cases, lidar based ICP method was used to vertify the image matching results. It exploits the inherent strengths of both visual and lidar sensors. By this research work, we develop a place recognition system that can operate effectively for more precision in localization regardless of the different surroundings. Experimental results from different environments have shown good localization ability, and that the proposed system was capable to accurately get global position information by using small number of reference images and lidar data. For the future work, features of lidar data can also be considered to improve the place recognition accuracy.

## References

1. Ho, K., Newman, P.: Combining visual and spatial appearance for loop closure detection in slam. In: European Conference on Mobile Robots, ECMR (2005)
2. Johns, E., Yang, G.Z.: Feature co-occurrence maps: Appearance-based localisation throughout the day. In: IEEE International Conference on Robotics and Automation (ICRA), pp. 3212–3218 (2013)
3. Saito, T., Kuroda, Y.: Localization independent of location based on place recognition and gps observations. In: IEEE/SICE International Symposium on System Integration, pp. 43–48 (2012)
4. Cummins, M., Newman, P.: Fab-map: Probabilistic localization and mapping in the space of appearance. The International Journal of Robotics Research 27(6), 647–665 (2008)
5. Ho, K.L., Newman, P.: Detecting loop closure with scene sequences. International Journal of Computer Vision 74(3), 261–286 (2007)
6. Glover, A.J., Maddern, W.P., Milford, M.J., Wyeth, G.F.: Fab-map + ratslam: Appearance-based slam for multiple times of day. In: IEEE International Conference on Robotics and Automation (ICRA), pp. 3507–3512 (May 2010)
7. Glover, A., Maddern, W., Warren, M., Reid, S., Milford, M., Wyeth, G.: Open-fabmap: An open source toolbox for appearance-based loop closuredetection. In: IEEE International Conference on Robotics and Automation (ICRA), pp. 4730–4735 (2012)
8. Eade, E.D., Drummond, T.W.: Unified loop closing and recovery for real time monocular slam. In: British Machine Vision Conference (BMVC), pp. 6.1–6.10 (2008)
9. Cummins, M., Newman, P.: Appearance-only slam at large scale with fab-map 2.0. The International Journal of Robotics Research 30(9), 1100–1123 (2011)

10. Chong, Z.J., Qin, B., Bandyopadhyay, T., Ang Jr, M.H., Frazzoli, E., Rus, D.: Synthetic 2d lidar for precise vehicle localization in 3d urban environment. In: IEEE International Conference on Robotics and Automation (ICRA), pp. 1554–1559 (2013)
11. Granström, K., Schön, T., Nieto, F., Ramos, J.: Learning to close loops from range data. The International Journal of Robotics Research 30(14), 1728–1754 (2011)
12. Latecki, L.J., Lakämper, R., Wolter, D.: Shape similarity and visual parts. In: Nyström, I., Sanniti di Baja, G., Svensson, S. (eds.) DGCI 2003. LNCS, vol. 2886, pp. 34–51. Springer, Heidelberg (2003)
13. Bosse, M., Zlot, R.: Keypoint design and evaluation for place recognition in 2d lidarmaps. Robotics and Autonomous Systems 57(12), 1211–1224 (2009)
14. Hahnel, D., Burgard, W., Fox, D., Thrun, S.: An efficient fastslam algorithm for generating maps of large-scale cyclic environments from raw laser range measurements. In: IEEE/RSJ International Conference on Intelligent Robots and Systems (IROS), pp. 206–211. IEEE (2003)
15. Bosse, M., Zlot, R.: Map matching and data association for large-scale two-dimensional laser scan-based slam. The International Journal of Robotics Research 27(6), 667–691 (2008)
16. Newman, P., Cole, D., Ho, K.: Outdoor slam using visual appearance and laser ranging. In: IEEE International Conference on Robotics and Automation (ICRA), pp. 1180–1187 (2006)
17. Nieto, J., Bailey, T., Nebot, E.: Recursive scan-matching slam. Robotics and Autonomous Systems 55(1), 39–49 (2007)
18. Granstrom, K., Callmer, J., Ramos, F., Nieto, J.: Learning to detect loop closure from range data. In: IEEE International Conference on Robotics and Automation (ICRA), pp. 15–22 (2009)
19. Tipaldi, G.D., Arras, K.O.: Flirt-interest regions for 2d range data. In: IEEE International Conference on Robotics and Automation (ICRA), pp. 3616–3622 (2010)
20. Lowe, D.G.: Distinctive image features from scale-invariant keypoints. International Journal of Computer Vision 60(2), 91–110 (2004)
21. Collier, J., Se, S., Kotamraju, V.: Multi-sensor appearance-based place recognition. In: International Conference on Computer and Robot Vision, pp. 128–135 (2013)

# Frequency Filter Bank for Enhancing Carbon Nanotube Images

Jose de Jesús Guerrero Casas[1], Oscar Dalmau[2],
Teresa E. Alarcón[1], and Adalberto Zamudio[3]

[1] Centro Universitario de los Valles,
Universidad de Guadalajara,
Departamento de Ciencias Computacionales e Ingenierías,
Ameca, Jalisco, México
chuyg27@gmail.com,,
teresa.alarcon@profesores.valles.udg.mx,
[2] Centro de Investigación en Matemáticas, CIMAT AC,
Monterrey, Nuevo León, México
dalmau@cimat.mx
[3] Centro Universitario de Ciencias Exactas e Ingenierías
Universidad de Guadalajara
Guadalajara, Jalisco, México
nanozam@gmail.com

**Abstract.** Improving digital images of carbon nanotubes is an important task for characterizing nanotube structures in Nanoscience and Nanotechnology. A two-step algorithm is proposed for enhancing the information of carbon nanotube images, which are obtained by a scanning electron microscopy. In the first step it is carried out the characterization of the intensity profile of the nanotube by using the first and second derivatives along with the local variance. Then, for analyzing the intensity profile of the nanotubes, an adaptive spatial filter is designed. The first step allows to represent the intensity profile of the nanotube through a Gaussian model. In the second step, a Gaussian-matched filter Bank is designed in the frequency domain for enhancing the nanotube information, considering different values of thickness and orientation for the filter bank.

**Keywords:** Image enhancement, spatial filtering, frequency domain, thresholding, Gaussian filter, bank of filters, carbon nanotubes (CNT).

## 1 Introduction

The materials developed by nanotechnology open up a wide range of applications in medicine, electronics, chemistry, among other areas [5]. Cosmetics, tissues and accessories, special paints, food packaging, construction materials, nanoscale semiconductors, batteries durability are manufactured using nanostructures. Nanotubes made of carbon have diameters on the order of nanometers

A. Gelbukh et al. (Eds.): MICAI 2014, Part I, LNAI 8856, pp. 316–326, 2014.

and lengths of several micrometers [13] and they have physical, mechanical, electrical, optical, thermal and special chemical properties, which make it possible to improve many common materials [16,18]. Therefore the characterization of nanotube structures is a crucial step in the manufacturing process of the mentioned materials. In order to do that through a computer it is necessary to have digital images with clear information about nanotubes. This explains the use of improving algorithms in nanotube digital characterization.

On the other hand, Filter Bank is a powerful technique for signal and image processing [6,17,11]. Filter Bank has largely been used in different applications among them: texture segmentation, retina identification, image coding and image representation [9,4,14,10,15]. In particular, in [2] it is proposed an algorithm detecting blood vessels in retinal images using two-dimensional matched filters with the aim of enhancing the blood vessel information in the image. The research done in [3] combines two-dimensional matched filters with cellular automata for also detecting the blood vessels in fundus images. The main aim of this research is to enhance the carbon nanotube images. As nanotubes have a similar structure as blood vessels, in this work we propose a nanotube enhancement algorithm which is based on the design and construction of a matched filter bank [2,3]. Additionally, we provide appropriate parameters for nanotube enhancement, some of which were heuristically obtained from the study of real images. Differently from [2,3] in this work, we propose to apply the filtering in the frequency domain which brings computational improvement to the algorithm.

The structure of the paper is as follows: Section 2 describes briefly our proposal for obtaining nanotube profile and the design of the Filter Bank. Section 3 presents experimental results and discussion. In the last section we present the conclusions and future work.

## 2    The Proposal

The main objective of this work is to propose an algorithm that allows us to enhance the nanotube information in Scanning Electron Microscopy (SEM) images, Fig. 1 shows examples of this kind of images. This task is a very important for characterizing the nanotubes in SEM images because in this way one can easly detect the nanotubes in the image, and then one can measure characteristics of nanotubes, which is needed for Nanotechnologists when designing new materials and products. Although, we are interested in enhancing the nanotube information, we note that the strategy that we propose here can be used to solve a more general problem that consists in detecting large and ramified structures, for example, roads in satellite images, vessels in medical images,..., etc.

In the general case, as illustrated Fig. 1, a simple thresholding technique can not be used in order to detect the nanotubes. One finds many problems in this type of images, mainly the background of the image is not non-uniform. There also exist troubles with illumination, in some cases the background region has illumination levels similar to nanotubes which complicates the nanotube detection. Another problem with such images is the overlap of nanotubes. For the previous reasons,

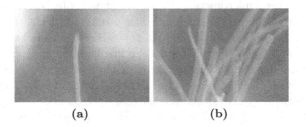

(a)                                 (b)

**Fig. 1.** Images obtained with SEM

here we propose a nanotube enhancement strategy which is composed by 2 steps. The first step consists in obtaining and studying the characteristic profile of the nanotubes. The second step consists in modeling and designing a filter bank in order to enhance the nanotube information. The filter bank is first designed in the spatial domain, as in [2,3] for retinal vessel detection, but differently from [3], we propose to apply the filtering in the frequency domain so that to obtain a better computational performance.

### 2.1   Characterization of the Intensity Nanotube Profile

As explained above, digital SEM images present background problems with locally low intensity variations. However, abrupt changes in intensity occur between the background and the region of nanotubes. Therefore, in order to find possible nanotube locations the first and second derivatives together with local variance are computed. The combination of the above criteria and a 1D box filter yields a strategy that allows the isolation, study and characterization of the nanotube profiles.

It is well-known that the first derivative provides local information about the slope and has responses close to zero in homogeneous regions, while on the edges the response gives local extreme values, i.e., maximum and minimum points, see Fig. 2 panel (a). The second derivative takes advantage of the extreme values (maximum of the absolute value) of the the first derivative and the zero-crossing

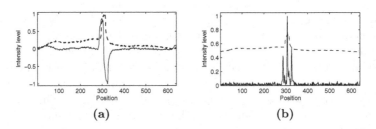

(a)                                 (b)

**Fig. 2.** Intensity profile drawn in dashed lines. (a) First derivative, (b) Second derivative.

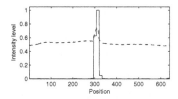

**Fig. 3.** Response to local variance in 50 blocks of the intensity profile. Intensity profile drawn in dashed lines.

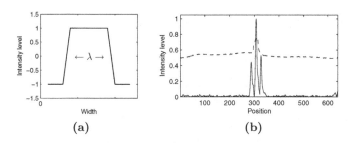

(a)                                    (b)

**Fig. 4.** (a) 1D filter box, (b) Intensity profile in dashed lines and Response to filtering with a 1D filter box in panel (a)

points that also provide information on the possible location of nanotubes, see Fig. 2 panel (b).

In order to reduce the detection uncertainty, the profile was divided in pieces or blocks of equal size and for each block it was estimated the dispersion degree of the intensity level through the variance. The highest responses can also correspond to nanotube locations, as shown in Fig. 3. Additionally, we may find possible location of nanotubes by using a 1D box filter [1], Fig. 4 (a), for this case a square pulse of width $\lambda$. Again, in this case, the response is higher at the nanotube location, Fig. 4 (b). After thresholding and combining the previous criteria, see diagram 6, one can obtain a more precise location, which means the location of the center point of the nanotube profile and also the corresponding edges, and therefore a better detection of the nanotube profile, Fig. 5.

Once the nanotube profile is detected, Fig. 5, we can study its gray level distribution. Nanotube's profile from 16 different images were averaged obtaining the curve in Fig. 5 which is similar to a Gaussian function. This justifies the modeling of the nanotube's profile as a Gaussian function. Therefore we construct a Matched Filter Bank based on a Gaussian profile for enhancing the information of nanotubes, see next Subsection, taking into consideration different orientations and thicknesses [2,3].

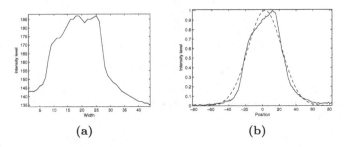

**Fig. 5.** (a) Intensity profile pertaining only to nanotube zone, (b) Average profile (curve in solid line) and the graph of a Gaussian function (curve in dashed line)

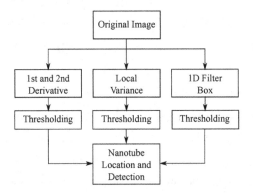

**Fig. 6.** Steps for obtaining a nanotube profile

## 2.2   Design of Matched Filter Bank

In this section we describe the Matched Filter Bank construction for nanotube enhancement. Although, the Matched Filter Bank presented here is similar to the one in [2,3], there are important details in the design of the filter bank which are different from those presented in [2,3]. So, we provide a complete description about its design and construction. As nanotubes appear in different orientations and thicknesses, one needs to design a filter bank taking into consideration the different orientations, $\theta = [\theta_1, \theta_2, \cdots, \theta_m]^T$, $\theta_j \in [0, 180)$ for $j = 1, 2, \cdots, m$, and thicknesses, $\sigma = [\sigma_1, \sigma_2, \cdots, \sigma_n]^T$, that we want to enhance, i.e., the number of filters in the bank is equal to $nm$.

The general idea is to construct a 2D convolution kernel oriented in one axis direction, Fig. 7, with a parameter $\sigma$ that controls the thickness or width of nanotubes. Afterward, the kernels are rotated according to the set of parameters $\theta$. The original convolution kernels can easily be designed by using the Gaussian function, see Subsection 2.1, as follows

$$k_{\sigma_i}(x, y) = \exp\left(-\frac{x^2}{2\sigma_i^2}\right), \quad i = 1, 2, \cdots, n, \tag{1}$$

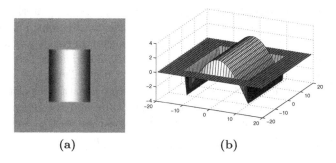

(a)                              (b)

**Fig. 7.** (a) Graphical representation of a Gaussian filter, (b) 3D view of the kernel

where $|y| < L/2$ with $L$ the length of a portion of nanotube, with thickness $2\sigma_i$, we are going to enhance. Note that the function in Eq. (1) is oriented in the $y$-axis direction and is positive, different from [2,3]. In all cases, we consider masks with size $3\sigma_i \times 3\sigma_i$, i.e., $|x| \leq 0.9\sigma_i$ and $|y| \leq 0.3\sigma_i$, and the kernel function in the $y$-direction is defined as

$$\hat{h}_{\sigma_i}(x,y) = \begin{cases} k_{\sigma_i}(x,y) \text{ if } (x,y) \in \mathcal{N}_i^{xy} \\ 0 \qquad\qquad \text{otherwise,} \end{cases} \qquad (2)$$

where $\mathcal{N}_i^{xy} = \{(x,y) \in \mathbb{R}^2 : |x| \leq 0.9\sigma_i, |y| \leq 0.3\sigma_i\}$ represents the support of the kernel in the $xy$ coordinate space. Now, the previous kernels are rotated as follows

$$\hat{h}_{\sigma_i,\theta_j}(u,v) = \hat{h}_{\sigma_i}((u,v)R_j), \forall (u,v) \in \mathcal{N}_i^{uv}, \qquad (3)$$

where $\mathcal{N}_i^{uv} = \{(u,v) \in \mathbb{Z}^2 : |u| \leq 1.5\sigma_i, |v| \leq 1.5\sigma_i\}$ and $R_j$ is a rotation matrix, i.e.,

$$R_j = \begin{pmatrix} \cos\theta_j & \sin\theta_j \\ -\sin\theta_j & \cos\theta_j \end{pmatrix}. \qquad (4)$$

Finally, the Matched Filter Bank, in the spatial domain, is obtained by centering and normalizing (3), i.e.

$$h_{\sigma_i,\theta_j}(u,v) = \begin{cases} \frac{\hat{h}_{\sigma_i}((u,v)R_j)-\mu_{ij}}{\sigma_{ij}} \text{ if } (x,y) = (u,v)R_j \in \mathcal{N}_i^{xy} \\ 0 \qquad\qquad\qquad \text{otherwise,} \end{cases} \qquad (5)$$

where

$$\mu_{ij} = \frac{1}{|\mathcal{N}_i^{uv}|} \sum_{(u,v)\in\mathcal{N}_i^{uv}} \hat{h}_{\sigma_i}((u,v)R_j), \qquad (6)$$

$$\sigma_{ij} = \sum_{(u,v)\in\mathcal{N}_i^{uv}} |\hat{h}_{\sigma_i}((u,v)R_j)|, \qquad (7)$$

and $|\mathcal{N}_i^{uv}|$ denotes the number of points $(u,v) \in \mathcal{N}_i^{uv}$ for which the point $(x,y) = (u,v)R_j$ falls in the support $\mathcal{N}_i^{xy}$, i.e., $\hat{h}_{\sigma_i,\theta_j}(u,v) \neq 0$. The centering $\mu_{ij}$ value allows to achieve responses close to zero in homogeneous regions, i.e., in smooth regions, and high responses in regions of high variation. In this way, the obtained filters have the same interpretation as those based on derivative kernels. Finally $\sigma_{ij}$ is related with amplitude and is calculated for normalizing the kernel.

The standard deviations of the Gaussians, $\sigma_i$, were heuristically obtained after observing the ratio of the thickness of the nanotube and the image size. This relation was studied and observed in many images, and it was concluded that the values of $\sigma_i$ can be obtained by the following expression:

$$\sigma_i = \kappa_i(r + c), \tag{8}$$

where $\kappa_i$ is a scale value and $r \times c$ defines the size of the image, i.e., $r$ is the number of rows and $c$ the number of columns.

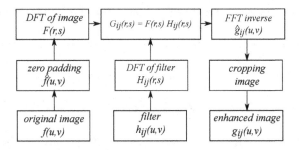

**Fig. 8.** Diagram of the filtering in the frequency domain. In this diagram $h_{ij}(u,v) = h_{\sigma_i,\theta_j}(u,v)$ and $g_{ij}(u,v)$ is the response to the filter $h_{ij}(u,v)$ when applied to the original image $f(u,v)$.

On the other hand, when working with large images, we observe that the size of convolution kernels increases due to (8). If we take also into account the number of possible rotations and the number of nanotube thicknesses that we want to enhance, i.e, the total number of filters is $nm$, then the computational time also increases. For this reason, instead of computing the filtering in the spatial domain we propose to compute the filtering in the frequency domain [12]. This is possible due to *convolution theorem* [8,7] which states that the convolution in the spatial domain equals pointwise multiplication in the frequency domain. Based on the previous property of the convolution [8,7], we present in Fig. 8 the diagram we used to filter in the frequency domain, see [7] for details. We note that the *final enhanced image* is obtained by taking the maximum response over the filter bank.

## 3   Experiments

In this section we present experiments using images obtained by Scanning Electron Microscopy. For the experiments we use real images of size $r \times c = 432 \times 640$

and $r \times c = 864 \times 1280$ pixels. The algorithms are implemented in MATLAB, and the experiments were carried out using an Intel Pentium B950 with 2 processors, 8 Gb RAM, 2.1 GHz and OS Windows 7 Home Premium. The experiments show the good quality of the proposed algorithm for nanotube enhancement and also the improvement of computational performance.

**Table 1.** Experiment with different number of rotations. Average time in seconds for the algorithms in the spatial and frequency domain. Image size $r \times c = 432 \times 640$ pixels.

| Number of rotations $m = |\theta|$ | Time in seconds Spatial domain | Time in seconds Freq. domain | Ratio Spatial/ Freq. |
|:---:|:---:|:---:|:---:|
| 4 | 3.47 | 1.54 | 2.26 |
| 8 | 9.00 | 2.75 | 3.27 |
| 12 | 14.65 | 4.01 | 3.65 |
| 16 | 20.26 | 5.32 | 3.81 |
| 20 | 25.89 | 6.63 | 3.91 |

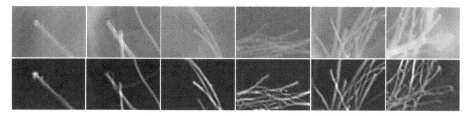

**Fig. 9.** First row: Six real images, $432 \times 640$ pixels, obtained by Scanning Electron Microscopy. Second row: Enhanced images obtained by our proposal.

In the first experiment we use 6 real images, first row in Fig. 9, and the size of the images is $r \times c = 432 \times 640$ pixels. We apply the algorithm in the spatial and the frequency domain for different number of orientations or rotations $m = |\theta|$, where $m = 4, 8, 12, 16, 20$; and the rotation angles are equally spaced, i.e., $\theta_j = \frac{180j}{m}$, $j = 0, 1, \cdots, m - 1$. The remainder parameters of the algorithms are $\kappa = \{0.01, 0.02, 0.03\}$, $\sigma = \{\sigma_i = \kappa_i(r + c)\} = \{10.72, 21.44, 32.16\}$ and the corresponding kernel sizes are $32 \times 32$, $64 \times 64$ and $96 \times 96$ respectively. In Table 1 we present the results of the first experiment. Each row of the second and third columns represents the average time (in seconds) of the algorithms, in the spatial and the frequency domain respectively, over the set images in the first row of Fig. 9. The last column represents the ratio between the average time in the spatial and the frequency domain. We note, according to Table 1, that the computational time of the algorithm in the frequency domain is less than the time in the spatial domain. It is clear that the computational time, in both cases, increases while the number of orientations increases, Table 1, but more importantly, according to the third column we note that the performance in the frequency domain also improves with respect to the algorithm in spatial domain while increasing the number of orientations in the filter bank.

The second row of Fig. 9 depicts the enhanced images using our algorithm with 12 rotations or orientations, i.e., $m = 12$. If $m = 16$ or $m = 20$ the result is very similar to the one presented in Fig. 9. As we can see, our proposal yields good nanotube enhancement for all the images, and is able to remove the background. However, in the overlapping portions of nanotubes the algorithm yields low responses.

**Table 2.** Experiment with different number of rotations. Average time in seconds for the algorithms in the spatial and frequency domain. Image size $r \times c = 864 \times 1280$ pixels.

| Number of rotations $m = \lvert\theta\rvert$ | Time in seconds Spatial domain | Time in seconds Freq. domain | Ratio Spatial/ Freq. |
|---|---|---|---|
| 4 | 60.06 | 5.87 | 10.24 |
| 8 | 165.10 | 10.91 | 15.14 |
| 12 | 266.59 | 15.71 | 16.97 |
| 16 | 373.25 | 20.79 | 17.95 |
| 20 | 480.33 | 26.32 | 18.25 |

The second experiment is similar to previous one with images of size $r \times c = 864 \times 1280$ pixels. The scale parameter is the same, i.e., $\kappa = \{0.01, 0.02, 0.03\}$ and the results of this experiment are in Table 2.

**Table 3.** Experiment for different scale values $\kappa$. Each row represents the average time in seconds for the algorithms in the spatial and frequency domain applied to images with size $r \times c = 432 \times 640$ pixels.

| Scale parameter $\kappa$ | Kernel size | Time in seconds Spatial domain | Time in seconds Freq. domain | Ratio Spatial/ Freq. |
|---|---|---|---|---|
| 0.01 | $32 \times 32$ | 1.18 | 1.07 | 1.10 |
| 0.02 | $64 \times 64$ | 3.99 | 1.28 | 3.12 |
| 0.03 | $96 \times 96$ | 10.07 | 1.88 | 5.35 |
| 0.04 | $128 \times 128$ | 17.43 | 3.10 | 5.63 |

In the third experiment we use the images with size $r \times c = 432 \times 640$ pixels in the first row of Fig. 9. In this case we fix $n = \lvert\kappa\rvert$, $m = \lvert\theta\rvert = 12$ and change the scale value $\kappa$, i.e., $0.01, 0.02, 0.03, 0.04$, therefore $\sigma$ takes de values $10.72, 21.44, 32.16, 42.88$ and the corresponding kernel sizes also change to $32 \times 32$, $64 \times 64$, $96 \times 96$ and $128 \times 128$ respectively. According to Table 3, the performance of the algorithm in the frequency domain is better than the algorithm in the spatial domain.

The last experiment is similar to the third one, and we use the same scale values $\kappa$, i.e., $0.01, 0.02, 0.03, 0.04$; but in this experiment the size of the images is $r \times c = 864 \times 1280$ pixels. Based on Table 4, we see that when the size of the kernel increases, the computational performance of the proposed algorithm in the frequency domain improves drastically with respect to the algorithm implemented in the spatial domain, see third column in Table 4.

**Table 4.** Experiment for different scale values $\kappa$. Each row represents the average time in seconds for the algorithms in the spatial and frequency domain applied to images with size $r \times c = 864 \times 1280$ pixels.

| Scale parameter $\kappa$ | Kernel size | Time in seconds Spatial domain | Time in seconds Freq. domain | Ratio Spatial/ Freq. |
|---|---|---|---|---|
| 0.01 | $64 \times 64$ | 12.99 | 3.89 | 3.34 |
| 0.02 | $128 \times 128$ | 50.64 | 4.67 | 10.85 |
| 0.03 | $193 \times 193$ | 204.60 | 7.34 | 27.89 |
| 0.04 | $257 \times 257$ | 613.78 | 13.65 | 44.96 |

# 4 Conclusions

In this paper an algorithm for detecting nanotubes profiles is presented. The proposed algorithm is based on a Matched Filter Bank which is designed and applied in both: spatial and frequency domain. In this work we provide details about the construction and parameter adjustment of the filter bank for enhancing images of carbon nanotubes obtained from SEM. The proposed algorithm gives good results for enhancement information of nanotube. The main problem of the method is the low response in overlapping portions of nanotubes. In terms of computational performance the proposed version in the frequency domain presents better results than the version in the spatial domain. In the case of large images and filters this improvement is significant. One advantage of the proposed scheme is that it can be easily adapted to enhance other nanostructures. In the last case, one just need to provide the nanostructure form and build the corresponding filter bank. As future work, we are going to extend the proposed algorithm to other nanostructures for SEM images, and also we are going to study the possibility to extend the algorithm for images obtained by Transmission Electron Microscopy (TEM).

**Acknowledgements.** This research was partially supported by the Project PROMEP/103.5/11/6834.

# References

1. Blanched, G., Charbit, M.: Digital Signal And Image Processing Using Matlab. ISTE Ltd., London (2006)
2. Chaudhuri, S., Chatterjee, S., Katz, N., Nelson, M., Goldbaum, M.: Detection of blood vessels in retinal images using two-dimensional matched filters. IEEE Transactions on Medical Imaging 8(3), 263–269 (1989)
3. Dalmau, O., Alarcon, T.: MFCA: Matched filters with cellular automata for retinal vessel detection. In: Batyrshin, I., Sidorov, G. (eds.) MICAI 2011, Part I. LNCS, vol. 7094, pp. 504–514. Springer, Heidelberg (2011)
4. Dunn, D., Higgins, W.: Optimal gabor filters for texture segmentation. IEEE Transactions on Image Processing 4(7), 847–964 (1995)
5. Euroresidentes: Principales aplicaciones actuales de la nanociencia y nanotecnología: Euroresidentes,
   http://www.euroresidentes.com/futuro/nanotecnologia/aplicaciones_nanotecnologia/nanotecnologia_aplicaciones.htm
6. Freeman, W., Adelson, E.: The design and use of steerable filters. IEEE Transactions on Pattern Analysis and Machine Intelligence 13(9), 891–906 (1991)
7. González, R., Woods, R.: Digital Image Processing. Prentice Hall Inc., New Jersey (2002)
8. González, R., Woods, R., Eddins, S.: Digital Image Processing Using Matlab. GatesMark Publishing, second edn. (2009)
9. Jain, A., Farrokhnia, F.: Unsupervised texture segmentation using gabor filters. IEEE International Conference on Systems, Man and Cybernetics 24(12), 14–19 (1991)
10. Park, C., Lee, J., Smith, M., Park, S., Park, K.: Directional filter bank-based fingerprint feature extraction and matching. IEEE Transactions on Circuits and Systems for Video Technology 14(1), 74–85 (2004)
11. Phoong, S., Kim, C., Vaidyanathan, P., Ansari, R.: A new class of two-channel biorthogonal filter banks and wavelet bases. IEEE Transactions on Signal Processing 43(3), 649–665 (March 1995)
12. Pitas, I.: Digital Image Processing Algorithms and Applications. A Wiley-Interscience Publication (2000)
13. Rivas, M., Román, J., Cosme, M.: Informe de vigilancia tecnológica madrid: Aplicaciones actuales y futuras de los nanotubos de carbono. Tech. rep., Fundación Madrid para el Conocimiento, Madrid (2007)
14. Rosiles, J.: Image and texture analysis using biorthogonal angular filter banks. Ph.D. thesis, Georgia Institute of Technology (July 2004)
15. Swamy, G., Balasubramaniam, K.: Directional filter bank-based segmentation for improved evaluation of nondestructive evaluation images. NDT and E International 40(3), 250–257 (2007)
16. Terrones, M.: Science and technology of the twenty-first century: Synthesis, properties and applications of carbon nanotubes. Annual Review of Material Research 33, 419–501 (2003)
17. Vetterli, M., Herley, C.: Wavelets and filter banks: Theory and design. IEEE Transactions on Signal Processing 40(9), 2207–2232 (1992)
18. Villalpando-Paez, F., Zamudio, A., Elias, A., Son, H., Barros, E., Chou, S., Kim, Y., Muramatsu, H., Hayashi, T., Kong, J., Terrones, H., Dresselhaus, G., Endo, M., Terrones, M., Dresselhaus, M.: Synthesis and characterization of long strands of nitrogen doped single walled carbon nanotubes. Chemical Physics Letters 424(4-6), 345–352 (2006)

# A Supervised Segmentation Algorithm for Crop Classification Based on Histograms Using Satellite Images

Francisco E. Oliva[1,*], Oscar S. Dalmau[2], and Teresa E. Alarcón[3]

[1,3]Centro Universitario de los Valles, Universidad de Guadalajara, Jalisco, México
{francisco.oliva,teresa.alarcon}@profesores.valles.udg.mx
[2]Centro de Investigación en Matemáticas, Guanajuato, México
dalmau@cimat.mx

**Abstract.** Recognizing different types of crops trough satellite imagery is an important application of Digital Image Processing in Agriculture. A supervised algorithm for identifying different types of crops is proposed. In the training stage, the studied images are preprocessed using a bilateral filter, and then the histogram of intensity levels is constructed for every crop class. The segmentation stage begins with the assignment of the likelihood of each pixel to belong to each class, which is based on the histogram information. Finally the segmentation is obtained using Gauss-Markov Measure Field. For this research Landsat-5 TM satellite images are used. The experimental work included synthetic and real images. In the case of the real image, the ground truth image was given by an expert. The results of the proposed algorithm were compared with other methods such as Maximum likelihood, Fisher linear likelihood, and Minimum Euclidean distance, among others.

**Keywords:** image segmentation, remote sensing, crop classification, histogram, likelihood estimation.

## 1 Introduction

The classification of crops in satellite imagery have been done with different techniques. The method proposed in [16] obtained a satisfying effect for the clasiffication of agricultural multispectral TM images using an Artificial Neural Networks (ANNs), in [8] was noticed that ANN is more complicated to use than statistical classifiers due to problems encountered in their design and implementation and it is always subject to adjustments in the hidden layers. In [11] Maximum Likelihood Classifier (ML) was used for the problem of crop cover mapping of a cultivated region using high resolution satellite imagery. In [4] was notice that MLC has a basic limitation that is too sensitive to the parameters values predefined by the user . In [14] was developed a method for extraction of agricultural land using information based on remote sensing imagery by combining particle swarm optimization (PSO), k-means clustering algorithm and

---

* Corresponding author.

A. Gelbukh et al. (Eds.): MICAI 2014, Part I, LNAI 8856, pp. 327–335, 2014.

Minimum Euclidean Distance (MED). In [14] the authors also noted that the performance of k-means and PSO-k-means is better than the MED method due the large number of paddy fields that were incorrectly classified as water bodies. In [9], [10] is elaborated a two step algorithm that considers spectral information together with the contextual information from neighboring pixels. The method is called ECHO (Extraction and Classification of Homogeneous Objects) spectral spatial classifier (ESS). In the proposal, firstly, the scene is segmented into statistically homogeneous regions, then the data are classified using the maximum likelihood scheme. The selection of the proper parameters in the segmentation impacts the performance of the algorithm. An improvement of this proposal is achieved in [5]. The last commented works lead to higher accuracy value of classification process respect to per- pixel approaches like ML, MED and Fisher Linear Likelihood (FLL) [7].

Inspired in the previous commented works we proposed a supervised algorithm for recognizing different types of crops on satellite imagery. In order to remove some granularities of the layers we apply a bilateral filter and then we construct a 3D histogram for each types of crops using the TM432 combination. Finally a segmentation strategy based on GMMF model is applied [6].

The rest of this paper is structured as follows: section 2 describes the steps of the proposed algorithm. In section 3 we present experiments and discussion of the results and finally in section 4 the conclusions are given.

## 2    The Proposed Algorithm

The proposed algorithm is composed of two stages: the training stage and the segmentation stage as shown in Fig. 1.

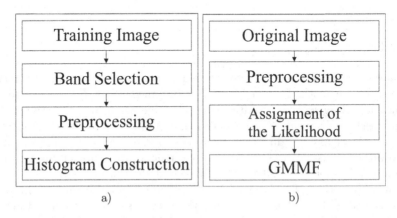

**Fig. 1.** Stages of the proposed algorithm. (a) Training stage, (b) Segmentation stage.

Next we explain each step of the elaborated algorithm.

## 2.1  Training Stage

The training step basically consists in computing a histogram which is used for the segmentation step. The main challenge here is how to select the information in order to construct the histogram. In particular we use a prior information about the classes, provided by an expert. The details of each step of the training stage are explained below.

**Band Selection:** In this research satellite images from LANSAT-5 Thematic Mapper are used (see Table 1). The information in Table 1, is taking from http://gif.berkeley.edu/. It is known that the information related to the crops are well recognized in the infrared (TM4), red (TM3) and green (TM2) bands. For that reason the color scheme TM432 is widely used for the study of vegetation as explained in http://glcfapp.glcf.umd.edu:8080/esdi/index.jsp. Therefore in this work the selected bands were TM2, TM3 y TM4.

**Table 1.** Spectral bands of the Lansat-5 Thematic Mapper (TM) Sensor

| Thematic Mapper (TM) Bands | Wavelength (µm) | Features |
|---|---|---|
| TM1 | 0.45 - 0.52 | B (Blue) |
| TM2 | 0.52 - 0.60 | G (Green) |
| TM3 | 0.63 - 0.69 | R (Red) |
| TM4 | 0.76 - 0.90 | near infrared |
| TM5 | 1.55 - 1.75 | mid-infrared |
| TM6 | 10.4 - 12.50 | thermal infrared |
| TM7 | 2.08 - 2.35 | mid-infrared |

**Preprocessing:** For enhancing the information about the crops and improving the quality of the image a bilateral filter [15] was applied on the three selected bands (TM4, TM3, TM2) independently. Bilateral filtering smooths images and preserves edges, using a non-linear combination of nearby image values. The method is noniterative and local. The filter uses a gaussian function and combines gray levels or colors based on both their spatial closeness and their gray or color similarity. Bilateral filter opts for near values considering both spatial location and gray level or color information [15].

Figure 2 shows the result of preprocessing the band TM4 using the bilateral filter with window size $3 \times 3$ and $\sigma = 1$.

**Histogram Construction:** Based on the ground truth image and considering the information of the 3 selected bands, a 3-D histogram for every class $k$ is computed, $h_k^{3D}$, $k = 1, 2, 3, \cdots, K$, where $K$ denotes the number of classes, see Equation (1).

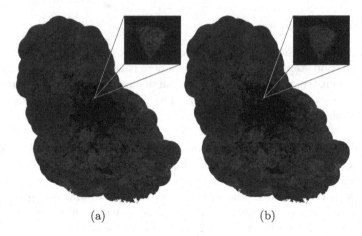

(a)                      (b)

**Fig. 2.** Preprocessing step using the TM4 band. (a) Original image, (b) Filtered image.

$$h_k^{3D}(x) = \frac{n_k(x)}{T_k}, \tag{1}$$

where the voxel $x$ is defined by the gray intensity information of the three selected bands, i.e., $x = (g_2, g_3, g_4)$, where $g_i \in \{0, 1, \cdots, 255\}$ corresponds to the TM$i$ band, with $i = \{2, 3, 4\}$. In Equation (1) $n_k(x)$ denotes the number of times the voxel $x$ was in class $k$, $T_k$ is the total number of voxels in class $k$. The constructed histograms are used for computing the likelihood of pixel of a given image to belong to each class.

The constructed histograms have information in only few voxels $x$ in the whole space, $\Omega$, which is defined by the combinations of $g_2, g_3$ and $g_4$ bands of the training image. In order to have the information in the whole space, a diffusion process is then applied according to the Equation (2):

$$h_k^{3D}(x) = \frac{\sum_{y \in \mathcal{V}_x} h_k^{3D}(y)}{|\mathcal{V}_x|}, \tag{2}$$

where $\mathcal{V}_x$ represents the neighbourhood of voxel $x$, in particular, we consider the neighboors at distance 1, i.e., $\|x - y\|_1 = 1$, $|\mathcal{V}_x|$ is the cardinality of the corresponding neighbohood. In Equation 2, $y$ denotes the neighboors of voxel $x$. As a result of the diffusion process the histogram, $h_k^{3D}$, $k = 1, 2, 3, \cdots, K$, is smoothed and for each $x \in \Omega$ one has a vector whose $k$th component is defined by $h_k^{3D}(x)$.

In order to simplify the computational cost, we can perform a further step by normalizing the histograms, so that at each voxel we have a discrete probability distribution which gives us a probabilistic interpretation, see Equation (3)

$$v_k(x) = \frac{h_k^{3D}(x)}{t(x)}, \tag{3}$$

where $v_k(x)$ is the normalized $kth$ component at voxel $x$ and $t(x) = \sum_{k=1}^{k} h_k^{3D}(x)$ the corresponding normalization factor.

## 2.2   Segmentation Step

GMMF [6] is derived from classical discrete Markov random fields, which are widely used in image processing for solving ill-posed problems. The GMMF model is an estimator of marginal distributions, see details in Ref. [6]. The functional for GMMF is the following:

$$U(p) = \sum_{r \in \mathcal{L}} \|p(r) - \hat{v}(r)\|^2 + \lambda \sum_{\langle r,s \rangle} \|p(r) - p(s)\|^2, \tag{4}$$

in the previous equation $\hat{v}(r)$ represents the normalized likelihood at pixel $r$. The value of $\hat{v}(r)$ at is derived from the Histogram construction step in the training stage, Equation (3), as follows

$$\hat{v}_k(r) = v_k(g_2(r), g_3(r), g_4(r)). \tag{5}$$

According to the GMMF model, the marginal empirical distributions $p(r)$ should be similar to the likelihood $\hat{v}(r)$ of the observations in site $r$ and they change smoothly in the lattice $\mathcal{L}$. The smoothing grade depends on the parameter $\lambda$.

The field $p(r)$ is computed through a Gauss-Saidel approach, see equation (6)

$$p_k(r) = \frac{\hat{v}_k(r) + \lambda \sum_{s \in \mathcal{N}_r} p_k(s)}{1 + \lambda |\mathcal{N}_r|}, \tag{6}$$

where $\lambda$ is the smoother parameter, $r$ indicates the pixel in the image, $s$ denotes the neighboors of pixel $r$ considering 4-connectivity. Once the vector field $p$ is estimated the optimal label field, $f(r)$ is computed as the mode of each vector $p(r)$

$$f(r) = \arg \max_{k \in \{1,2,\cdots,K\}} p_k(r). \tag{7}$$

# 3   Experiments and Discussion

In the experiment a real 7-band satellite image Lansat-5 of size $2517 \times 2800$ pixels[1] was used. This image corresponds to Guadalajara and Zapopan regions and theirs surroundings in Jalisco state, México in 2011 [13], see Fig. (3). The experimental work also included 4 synthetic images obtained from the real one. The aim in each experiment is to identify 8 types of crops Table (2).

Identification of the crops mentioned in the Table 2, has been of great interest for the statistical analysis of the growth or decrease of urban areas, because of

---

[1] Image provided by the Instituto de Información Territorial del Estado de Jalisco, México (IITEJ).

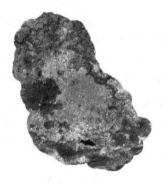

**Fig. 3.** Lansat-5 TM satellite image from Jalisco, México

**Table 2.** Types of crops studied in the proposed algorithm

| Class | Crop Name |
|-------|-----------|
| C1 | Irrigation agriculture |
| C2 | Seasonal agriculture |
| C3 | Forest |
| C4 | Scrub |
| C5 | Pastureland |
| C6 | Green area |
| C7 | Aquatic vegetation |
| C8 | Riparian vegetation |

relation between the population growth and the mentioned crops. However, the recognition task is very difficult due the similarity of the spectral characteristics for the 8 types of analyzed crops.

Below we discuss about the experimental work done in this research.

Table 3 shows a comparison of our approach with 4 reported methods: Echo spectral-spatial (ESS) [9], [10], Fisher Linear Likelihood (FLL) [7], Maximum Likelihood (ML) [11] and Minimum Euclidean Distance (MED) [12]. We used the implementation reported in https://engineering.purdue.edu/~biehl/MultiSpec/hyperspectral.html for programing the methods in the comparison.

Note that our proposal has the better overall accuracy and Kappa value. However the classes 6, 7 and 8 present a poor individual classification accuracy. The similarity of these mentioned classes with water bodies affected the classification process by our proposal. Fig. 4 shows the segmentation results obtained by our proposal and by ESS, which was the second best result according to the overall accuracy and Kappa values. The solution given by ESS presents more granularities than our solution, see Fig.4.

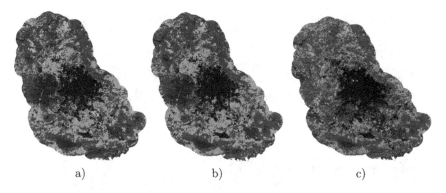

a)                        b)                        c)

**Fig. 4.** (a) Ground truth, (b) segmentation results obtained by the proposed algorithm, (c) segmentation results by ESS

**Table 3.** Numerical results of different classication methods

| Method | C1 | C2 | C3 | C4 | C5 | C6 | C7 | C8 | OverAll Accuracy | Kappa |
|---|---|---|---|---|---|---|---|---|---|---|
| ESS | 0.80 | 0.41 | 0.31 | 0.75 | 0.56 | 0.09 | 0.18 | 0.09 | 0.7773 | 0.6880 |
| FLL | 0.43 | 0.35 | 0.39 | 0.74 | 0.79 | 0.10 | 0.36 | 0.16 | 0.7770 | 0.6867 |
| ML | 0.54 | 0.40 | 0.30 | 0.73 | 0.61 | 0.11 | 0.29 | 0.29 | 0.7676 | 0.6751 |
| MED | 0.15 | 0.22 | 0.53 | 0.77 | 0.89 | 0.11 | 0.24 | 0.13 | 0.7721 | 0.6768 |
| The Proposal | 0.75 | 0.90 | 0.65 | 0.90 | 0.45 | 0.003 | 0.03 | 0.0003 | 0.8962 | 0.8499 |

Additionally, other experiments were performed using 4 synthentic images. Results of the segmentation of these synthetic images are depicted in Fig. 5.

As you can see the classification done by ESS method have a good performance, however some classes are missed. On the other hand in the segmentation obtained by our proposal, the majority of the classes are identified more accurately. Table 4 and Table 5 present numerical results about the performance of the ESS and our approach respectively. The notation I1, I2, I3, I4 in Tables 4 and 5 is related to the images represented in the first row in Fig. 5, from the left to the right.

**Table 4.** Segmentation results for synthetic images using ESS

| Image | C1 | C2 | C3 | C4 | C5 | C6 | C7 | C8 | OverAll Accuracy | Kappa |
|---|---|---|---|---|---|---|---|---|---|---|
| I1 | 0.94 | 0.97 | 0.98 | 0.97 | 0.98 | 0.90 | 0.98 | 0.49 | 0.952 | 0.942 |
| I2 | 0.87 | 0.97 | 0.98 | 0.97 | 0.98 | 0.89 | 0.96 | 0.49 | 0.934 | 0.921 |
| I3 | 0.95 | 0.98 | 0.98 | 0.96 | 0.98 | 0.97 | 0.97 | 0.01 | 0.942 | 0.927 |
| I4 | 0.95 | 0.98 | 0.98 | 0.97 | 0.98 | 0.96 | 0.98 | 0.32 | 0.951 | 0.939 |

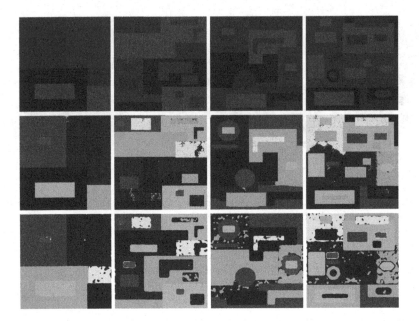

**Fig. 5.** Segmentation of synthetic images. In the first row are depicted synthetic images, the second one represents the results obtained by ESS and the last row illustrated the segmented images by our proposal.

**Table 5.** Segmentation results for synthetic images using our proposal

| Image | C1 | C2 | C3 | C4 | C5 | C6 | C7 | C8 | OverAll Accuracy | Kappa |
|-------|------|-------|-------|-------|-------|-------|-------|-------|--------------|-------|
| I1 | 0.998 | 1.000 | 0.993 | 0.998 | 0.998 | 0.021 | 0.845 | 0.884 | 0.974 | 0.967 |
| I2 | 0.977 | 1.000 | 0.995 | 0.982 | 0.989 | 0.264 | 0.806 | 0.800 | 0.947 | 0.936 |
| I3 | 0.815 | 0.998 | 0.991 | 0.989 | 0.988 | 0.833 | 0.704 | 0.919 | 0.942 | 0.928 |
| I4 | 0.913 | 0.992 | 0.987 | 0.988 | 0.991 | 0.691 | 0.856 | 0.736 | 0.928 | 0.913 |

Numerical results in Tables 4 and 5 together with the graphical representation in Fig. 5 demonstrated, in general, the good performance of the proposed segmentation strategy. In order to avoid the misclassification for the classes 6,7 and 8 we are conducting a research with other probabilistic approaches different to GMMF, like those reported in[3], [1], [2].

## 4   Conclusions

The proposed algorithm takes into account pixel information with contextual information from neighboring pixels. The proposal is based on the histogram information and the probabilistic approach called GMMF. We are addresing the current research with other probabilistic frameworks that have more computational complexity, but more accurate and robust when the features of the objects to recognize are similar.

**Acknowledgments.** The authors wish to thank IITEJ, especially to Guillermo Levine Gutiérrez, Maximiliano Bautista Andalón and Ana Teresa Ortega Minakata, for having supported with the ground truth and information needed for this research.

# References

1. Dalmau, O., Rivera, M.: A general bayesian markov random field model for probabilistic image segmentation. In: Wiederhold, P., Barneva, R.P. (eds.) IWCIA 2009. LNCS, vol. 5852, pp. 149–161. Springer, Heidelberg (2009)
2. Dalmau, O., Rivera, M.: Beta-measure for probabilistic segmentation. In: Sidorov, G., Hernández Aguirre, A., Reyes García, C.A. (eds.) MICAI 2010, Part I. LNCS, vol. 6437, pp. 312–324. Springer, Heidelberg (2010)
3. Dalmau, O., Rivera, M.: Alpha markov measure field model for probabilistic image segmentationl 412(15), 1434–1441 (2011)
4. Duda, R.O., Hart, P.E.: Pattern Classification and Scene Analysis. Wiley (1973)
5. Hastie, T., Tibshirani, R., Friedman, J.: The elements od Statiscal Learning. Data Mining, Inference, and Prediction. Springer (2001)
6. José, L., Marroquín, S.B., Calderón, F., Vemuri, B.C.: The mpm-map algorithm for image segmentation. Pattern Recognition 1, 303–308 (2000)
7. Karakahya, H., Yazgan, B., Ersoy, O.K.: A spectral-spatial classification algorithm for multispectral remote sensing data. In: ICANN, pp. 1011–1017 (2003)
8. Kavzoglu, T., Mather, P.M.: The use of backpropagating artificial neural networks in land cover classification. Int. J. Remote Sensing 24(23), 4907–4938 (2003)
9. Kettig, R.L., Landgrebe, D.A.: Computer classification of remotely sensed multispectral image data by extraction and classification of homogeneous objects. IEEE Transactions on Geoscience Electronics 14(1), 19–26 (1976)
10. Landgrebe, D.: The development of a spectral-spatial classifier for earth observational data. Pattern Recognition 12(3), 165–175 (1980)
11. Omkar, S.N., Senthilnath, J., Mudigere, D., Kumar, M.M.: Crop classification using biologically-inspired techniques with high resolution satellite image. Journal of the Indian Society of Remote Sensing 36(2), 175–182 (2008)
12. Peuquet, D.J.: An algorithm for calculating minimum euclidean distance between two geographic features. Computers& Geosciences 18(8), 989–1001 (1992)
13. Pulido, H.G., Andalón, M.B., Rubio, M.G.: Jalisco territorio y problemas de desarrollo. Iterritorial (2013)
14. Su, B., Noguchi, N.: Agricultural land use information extraction in miyajimanuma wetland area based on remote sensing imagery. Environmental Control in Biology 50(3), 277–287 (2012)
15. Tomasi, C., Manduchi, R.: Bilateral filtering for gray and color images. In: ICCV, pp. 839–846 (1998)
16. Wang, H., Zhang, J., Xiang, K., Liu, Y.: Classification of remote sensing agricultural image by using artificial neural network. In: International Workshop on Intelligent Systems and Applications, pp. 1–4 (2009)

# An Effective Visual Descriptor
# Based on Color and Shape Features for Image Retrieval

Atoany Fierro-Radilla[1], Karina Perez-Daniel[1], Mariko Nakano-Miyatakea[1],
Hector Perez-Meana[1], and Jenny Benois-Pineau[2]

[1] Postgraduate Section of ESIME Culhuacan,  Instituto Politecnico Nacional,
Av. Santa Ana No. 1000, Col. San Francisco Culhuacan
afierror@hotmail.com, mnakano@ipn.mx
[2] University of Bordeaux I, Bordeaux, France
benois-p@labri.fr

**Abstract.** In this paper we present a Content-Based Image Retrieval (CBIR) system which extracts color features using Dominant Color Correlogram Descriptor (DCCD) and shape features using Pyramid Histogram of Oriented Gradients (PHOG). The DCCD is a descriptor which extracts global and local color features, whereas the PHOG descriptor extracts spatial information of shape in the image. In order to evaluate the image retrieval effectiveness of the proposed scheme, we used some metrics commonly used in the image retrieval task such as, the Average Retrieval Precision (ARP), the Average Retrieval Rate (ARR) and the Average Normalized Modified Retrieval Rank (ANMRR) and the Average Recall (R)-Average Precision (P) curve. The performance of the proposed algorithm is compared with some other methods which combine more than one visual feature (color, texture, shape). The results show a better performance of the proposed method compared with other methods previously reported in the literature.

**Keywords:** CBIR, color descriptor, shape descriptor, dominant color, color correlogram, PHOG.

## 1   Introduction

In the last years, due to the technological advances, a large amount of devices such as: digital cameras, smart phones and tablets, have been developed in order to capture images and video data and on the other hand, a technological advance on high-speed internet connection, as well as the increasing storage capacities, leads to a growing size of databases. As a result Internet has become the largest multimedia database; a huge amount of information becomes available for a large number of users [1]. With large databases, it is a challenge to browse and retrieve efficiently the desirable information. The traditional annotation heavily relies on manual labor to label images with keywords, which unfortunately can hardly describe the diversity and ambiguity for image contents [2].

The Content-Based Image Retrieval (CBIR) system is a useful tool to resolve the above mentioned problem. The typical CBIR system performs two major tasks, the

A. Gelbukh et al. (Eds.): MICAI 2014, Part I, LNAI 8856, pp. 336–348, 2014.

first one is the feature extraction, where a set of features is extracted to describe the content of each image in the database; and the second task is the similarity measurement between the query image and each image in the database, using the extracted features [3]. Generally the CBIR is performed using some low-level visual descriptors such as color-based, texture-based and shape-based descriptors, which extract feature vectors from the images.

There are many methods which combine more than one visual descriptor [2-6], improving the image retrieval effectiveness. In [2], authors combine Linear Block Algorithm (LBA) for the global color feature extraction, Steerable Filter for the texture features extraction and Pseudo-Zernike Moments for extraction of the shape features which are rotation invariant. Authors of [3] combine color and texture features, in which the color features are extracted using the Color Layout Descriptor (CLD) and the texture features are obtained using the Gabor Filters. Another method that combines more than one visual descriptors is proposed in [6], in which the image is divided into six blocks then, the color space of each block is converted from RGB to HSV and a cumulative histogram is computed in order to obtain the color features, whereas to obtain the texture features of each block, four statistic features, such as energy, contrast, entropy and inverse difference from the Gray-Level Concurrence Matrix (GLCM), are computed.

In this paper we propose a method that combines local and global color information using the Dominant Color Correlogram Descriptor (DCCD) [7] and local shape information using the Pyramid Histogram of Oriented Gradients (PHOG) [8]. The proposed scheme is performed through three stages: In the first stage, the algorithm obtains global color features using the Dominant Color Descriptor (DCD) proposed by MPEG-7 [9, 10] as well as the shape information using the PHOG [10]. In the second stage, using color correlogram the correlation between central pixel and its neighborhood is calculated from the image represented by only dominant colors, and in the third stage, color and shape features are combined in order to obtain a new visual descriptor which improves the image retrieval performance. In order to evaluate the proposed visual descriptor, we use three metrics commonly used in the CBIR systems, such as ARP (Average Retrieval Precision), ARR (Average Retrieval Rank) and ANMRR (Average Normalized Retrieval Rank), as well as RP-curves. The performance of our proposed scheme is compared with some methods reported in the literature and the results show that the proposed visual descriptor improves the image retrieval performance.

The rest of this paper is organized as follows: In Section 2 we briefly describe some color-based descriptors commonly used in the literature. In Section 3, we briefly describe some shape-based descriptors reported in the literature. In Section 4, we present the proposed scheme. The results are shown in Section 5 and finally in Section 6 we present the conclusions of this work.

## 2    Color-Based Descriptors

Color is the basic element of image content and one of the main sensation features when a human distinguish images [9]. From the perspective of feature extraction, color-based image descriptor can be divided into two categories [12]: Global descriptor which takes into account the whole image in order to obtain the color features. In this group we have Histogram Intersection (HI) and Dominant Color Descriptor (DCD). On the other hand we have the local descriptors such as Color Correlogram (CC), Color Layout Descriptor (CLD) and Color Structure Descriptor (CSD), which obtain the color features by dividing the image into regions.

The Histogram Intersection (HI) was proposed by Swain Ballard [13]. This method is a global color descriptor and it is defined as: Given a pair of color histograms, $I$ and $M$, with $n$ bins each one, HI can be computed as:

$$HI(I, M) = \sum_{j=1}^{n} \min \left( I_j, M_j \right) \tag{1}$$

This method is robust to geometrical modification, such as rotation and scaling, as well as the variation of the image resolution [14]. The number of bins is an important factor, because the more bins are used, the image is better described but, the computational cost is increased. Another global color descriptor is the DCD, which was proposed in the MPEG-7 standard. This color descriptor replaces the whole image color information with a small number of representative colors [9]. The Dominant Color Descriptor can be defined as follows:

$$F = \{C_i, P_i\}, i = 1, 2, \ldots, N, P \in [0,1], \tag{2}$$

where $P_i$ is the percentage of the dominant color $C_i$.

The color correlogram (CC) is a local color descriptor which expresses how the spatial correlation of pairs of color changes with the distance [15] and it is defined as: For any pixel of color $c_i$ in the image, the color correlogram $(\gamma_{c_i c_j}^{(k)})$ gives the probability that a pixel at distance $k$ away from the given pixel $c_i$ has a color $c_j$. The Color Layout Descriptor (CLD) is a compact descriptor which represents the color spatial distribution of visual data [16], where the color space used in this descriptor is the YCbCr. The extraction of this descriptor consists of four stages. In the first one the image is partitioned into 64 blocks where the size of each block is W/8 and H/8 with W and H denoting the width and height of the image. In the second stage, for each block, a single dominant color is selected, then in the third stage the three components of the color space are transformed into 8x8 DCT (Discrete Cosine Transform). And finally in the fourth stage, the DCT coefficients of Y, Cb and Cr color channel are quantized and their lower coefficients are extracted to form the CLD. Another local color descriptor is the Color Structure Descriptor, which was also proposed in the MPEG-7 standard. In which an image is represented by the color distribution, and the local spatial structure of color using structuring element. It is similar to color histogram but it is semantically different. The CSD is defined as $h(m), m = 1, \ldots, M$, where the bin value $h(m)$ is the number of structuring elements containing one or more pixels with color $c_m$. Denote $I$ be the set of quantized index of an image and $S \in I$ be the set of quantized color index existing inside the sub-image region covered by the structuring element [17], the color histogram bins are accumulated according to

$$h(m) = h(m) + 1, m \in S \tag{3}$$

# 3    Shape-Based Descriptor

Shape feature is an important factor in order to identify objects as well as classification and indexing of the context semantically. In this section, three shape-based descriptors, which are Pseudo-Zernike Moments (PZM), Polar Harmonic Transform (PHT) and Pyramid Histogram of Oriented Gradients (PHOG), are described.

## 3.1    Pseudo-Zernike Moment (PZM)

The PZM consists of a set of complex polynomials that form a complete orthogonal set over the interior of the unit circle, $x^2 + y^2 \leq 1$ [2]. These polynomials are denoted as

$$V_{nm}(x, y) = V_{nm}(\rho, \theta) = R_{nm}(\rho)e^{jm\theta}, \tag{4}$$

where $\rho = \sqrt{x^2 + y^2}$ is the distance from the origin to the pixel $(x, y)$ and $\theta$ is an angle between vector $\rho$ and the $x$-axis in the clockwise direction. The radial polynomial $R_{nm}(\rho)$ is defined as:

$$R_{nm}(\rho) = \sum_{s=0}^{n-|m|} \frac{(-1)^s[(2n+1-s)!]\rho^{n-s}}{s!(n-|m|-s)!(n+|m|-s)!} \tag{5}$$

The PZM of order $n$ with repetition $m$ is defined as:

$$A_{nm} = \frac{n+1}{\pi} \iint_{x^2+y^2 \leq 1} f(x, y)V_{nm}^*(x, y)dxdy \tag{6}$$

For a digital image of size MxN, its PZM can be computed as:

$$\check{A}_{nm} = \frac{4(n+1)}{\pi MN} \sum_{i=1}^{M} \sum_{j=1}^{N} V_{nm}^*(x_i, y_j)f(x_i, y_j) \tag{7}$$

where $\Delta x = \frac{2}{M}, \Delta y = \frac{2}{N}$

The integer numbers $n$ and $m$ are defined in Table 1. A numerical instability, when high-order PZMs is required, is a serious problem of the PZM, due to the amount of factorial elements in the radial polynomial.

**Table 1.** Principal Pseudo-Zernike Moments

| Order | Moments $A_{nm}$ | No. Moments | Order | Moments $A_{nm}$ | No. Moments |
|:-----:|:----------------:|:-----------:|:-----:|:----------------:|:-----------:|
| 0 | $A_{00}$ | 1 | 4 | $A_{40}, A_{42}, A_{44}$ | 3 |
| 1 | $A_{11}$ | 1 | 5 | $A_{51}, A_{53}, A_{55}$ | 3 |
| 2 | $A_{20}, A_{22}$ | 2 | 6 | $A_{60}, A_{62}, A_{64}, A_{66}$ | 4 |
| 3 | $A_{31}, A_{33}$ | 2 | | | |

## 3.2    Polar Harmonic Transform (PHT)

The Polar Complex Exponential Transform (PCET) [18] is one of the PHT, which is defined as (8), when the order is $n$ and the repetition is $l$, $|n| = |l| = 0,1,\ldots,\infty$.

$$M_{nl} = \frac{1}{\pi}\int_0^{2\pi}\int_0^1 [H_{nl}(r,\theta)]^* f(r,\theta) r\, dr\, d\theta \tag{8}$$

where

$$H_{nl}(r,\theta) = R_n(r)e^{il\theta} \tag{9}$$

The radial kernel is a complex exponential in the radial direction, that is

$$R_n(r) = e^{i2\pi n r^2} \tag{10}$$

For a digital image of size MxN, the PCET can be computed as:

$$M_{nl} = \frac{1}{\pi}\sum_{k=0}^{M-1}\sum_{l=0}^{N-1}[H_{nl}'(x_k,y_l)]^* f'(x_k,y_l)\Delta x \Delta y \tag{11}$$

where $\Delta x = \frac{2}{M}, \Delta y = \frac{2}{N}$, we finally obtain:

$$M_{nl} = \frac{4}{\pi MN}\sum_{k=0}^{M-1}\sum_{l=0}^{N-1}[H_{nl}'(x_k,y_l)]^* f'(x_k,y_l) \tag{12}$$

## 3.3    Pyramidal Histogram of Oriented Gradients (PHOG)

The Pyramidal Histogram of Oriented Gradients (PHOG) is a spatial shape descriptor which represents the spatial distribution of edges and it is formulated as a vector representation [8]. The operation of PHOG consists of the following four steps.

1. Edge contour extraction: The contour of input image can be extracted using the Canny edge detector.
2. Cell division: The edge detected binary image is divided into cells at several pyramid levels. For example, in the first pyramid level, the edge image is divided into 2×2 cells and in the second pyramid level, each cell furthermore is divided into 2×2 sub-cells. The cell division is repeated until desirable resolution levels of pyramid.
3. HOG calculation: The Histogram of Oriented Gradients (HOG) of each cell is calculated at each pyramid resolution level. The HOG of each cell in the same pyramid level is concatenated to form a vector.
4. PHOG extraction: The final PHOG is a concatenation of all HOG vectors generates in all pyramid levels.

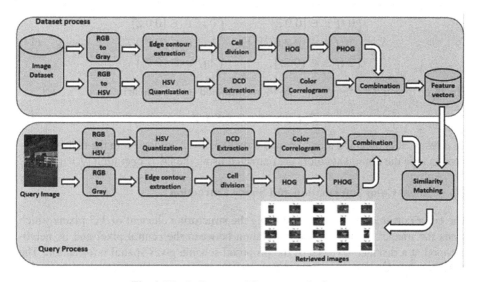

**Fig. 1.** Block diagram of the proposed scheme

# 4    Proposed Visual Descriptor

In this paper we propose a new visual descriptor which is a combination of the global and local color information based on the DCCD and the shape feature based on the PHOG. The block diagram of the proposed method is shown in fig. 1.

## 4.1    Global Color Information Extraction

In this paper we selected the HSV (Hue, Saturation, Value) color space because it is similar in the manner that human distinguish the colors [7]. In order to reduce computational cost, the quantization in the HSV color space is performed using a non-linear quantization, which is given by

$$H = \begin{cases} 0 \; if \; h & \in [316,20) \\ 1 \; if \; h & \in [20,40) \\ 2 \; if \; h & \in [40,75) \\ 3 \; if \; h & \in [75,155) \\ 4 \; if \; h & \in [155,190) \\ 5 \; if \; h & \in [190,270) \\ 6 \; if \; h & \in [270,295) \\ 7 \; if \; h & \in [295,316) \end{cases} \tag{13}$$

$$S = \begin{cases} 0 \ if \ s \ \in [0,0.2] \\ 1 \ if \ s \ \in (0.2,0.7] \\ 2 \ if \ s \ \in (0.7,] \end{cases}, V = \begin{cases} 0 \ if \ v \ \in [0,0.2] \\ 1 \ if \ v \ \in (0.2,0.7] \\ 2 \ if \ v \ \in (0.7,] \end{cases} \tag{14}$$

The three quantized components are then combined into one matrix:

$$C = 9 \times H + 3 \times S + V \tag{15}$$

As a result, it is obtained a matrix with only 8x3x3=72 colors. From the matrix calculated in (15) the dominant colors are extracted using the DCD operation [9,10].

### 4.2    Local Color Information and Shape Extraction

The color correlogram is computed using the structuring element of 3x3 pixels which scans the image, calculating the correlation between the central pixel and its neighborhood at a distance k=1. Thus, the proposed scheme gives spatial information. The color correlogram can be computed as:

$$\gamma_{c_i c_i}(I) \triangleq Pr_{p_1 \in I_{c_i}, p_2 \in I_{c_i}} [p_2 \in I_{c_i} | |p_1 - p_2| = 1] \tag{16}$$

where $c_i$ is $i$-$th$ color and $p_1$ and $p_2$ are any two pixels in the input image $I$.

In the proposed scheme, we used auto-color correlogram, in which two pixels have the same the color. As a result we obtain a color-based descriptor called the Dominant Color Correlogram Descriptor (DCCD) and is defined as:

$$DCCD = \{C_i, CC_i\} \tag{17}$$

where $CC_i$ is the color auto-correlogram of the $i$-$th$ dominant color $C_i$.

The shape feature extraction is done using the PHOG descriptor mentioned in 3.3, in which we used 3 pyramid levels and 8 bins for computing the HOG in each level.

### 4.3    Combination of Features

In the literature there are many manners to combine more than one visual feature, in this paper we used the linear combination method used in [16], which is as follows.

$$nC = \frac{C}{\max (C)}, \ nS = \frac{S}{\max (S)} \tag{18}$$

$$Q = \omega nS + (1 - \omega)nC \tag{19}$$

where $C$ and $S$ are color and shape distances between the query and dataset image, respectively. Firstly the two distances are normalized by (18) and combined lineally by (19) to obtain the similarity $Q$, where $\omega$ is the weight of a particular visual feature. If this similarity is smaller, two images are considered as more similar.

**Table 2.** Performance of color-based descriptors using dataset 1

| Method | ANMRR | ARR | | | ARP | | |
|---|---|---|---|---|---|---|---|
| | | $\alpha=2$ | $\alpha=1$ | $\alpha=1$ | $\alpha=0.5$ | $\alpha=0.25$ |
| CC [15] | 0.3126 | 0.7577 | 0.5923 | 0.5923 | 0.7846 | 0.8923 |
| HI [13] | 0.2507 | 0.8115 | 0.6269 | 0.6269 | 0.7923 | 0.9077 |
| DCD [9] | 0.2576 | 0.8154 | 0.6154 | 0.6154 | 0.7846 | 0.8615 |
| LBA [2,10] | 0.3579 | 0.6808 | 0.5642 | 0.5642 | 0.7154 | 0.8154 |
| CLD [3,16, 21] | 0.3358 | 0.7385 | 0.5731 | 0.5731 | 0.7154 | 0.8000 |
| CSD [17] | 0.3145 | 0.7538 | 0.5846 | 0.5846 | 0.7538 | 0.8769 |
| DCCD [7] | **0.2266** | **0.8231** | **0.6808** | **0.6808** | **0.8538** | **0.9231** |

**Table 3.** Performance of color-based descriptors using dataset 2

| Method | ANMRR | ARR | | | ARP | | |
|---|---|---|---|---|---|---|---|
| | | $\alpha=2$ | $\alpha=1$ | $\alpha=1$ | $\alpha=0.5$ | $\alpha=0.25$ |
| CC [15] | 0.3228 | 0.7200 | 0.5870 | 0.5870 | **0.7620** | **0.8880** |
| HI [13] | 0.3174 | 0.7610 | 0.5760 | 0.5760 | 0.7380 | 0.8640 |
| DCD [9] | 0.3384 | 0.7420 | 0.5590 | 0.5590 | 0.6920 | 0.8480 |
| LBA [2,10] | 0.3478 | 0.7320 | 0.5500 | 0.5500 | 0.7040 | 0.8000 |
| CLD [3,16, 21] | 0.3194 | **0.7620** | 0.5740 | 0.5740 | 0.7280 | 0.8360 |
| CSD [17] | 0.4431 | 0.6190 | 0.4630 | 0.4630 | 0.6200 | 0.7680 |
| DCCD [7] | **0.3086** | 0.7590 | **0.5960** | **0.5960** | 0.7560 | 0.8840 |

## 5    Experimental Results

As we mentioned before, there are many visual descriptors, such as color-based, texture-based and shape-based, also, there are many methods which combine these descriptors in order to improve the image retrieval performance. We analyzed and evaluate some algorithms using three different datasets; the dataset 1 is composed by 500 images, divided into 25 categories with 20 ground truth images per category. The dataset 2 is composed by 1000 images, divided into 20 categories with 50 ground truth images per category, and the dataset 3 is called Corel Dataset 1k [19, 20] which is composed by 1000 images, divided into 10 categories with 100 ground truth images per category. The first two datasets (dataset 1 and dataset 2) are randomly selected by authors, considering different percentage of query images respect to the dataset size and the third one is commonly used in CBIR evaluation. The color-based descriptors were evaluated using dataset 1 and dataset 2 and the results are shown in table 2 and table 3.

In the table 2 and 3, we can observe that, the results obtained by the DCCD, proposed in [7], are better than the others. The RP-curves, shown in figures 2 and 3, can describe the performance of the descriptors in the image retrieval task:

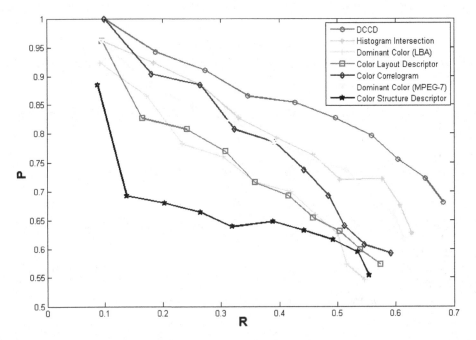

**Fig. 2.** RP-curve using dataset 1

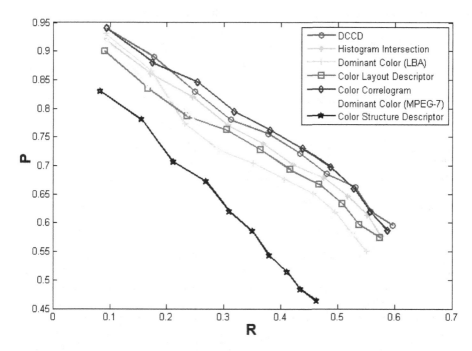

**Fig. 3.** RP-curve using dataset 2

The shape-based shape-based descriptors, PZM, PCET, PCT and PHOG, are evaluated. The evaluation was done using dataset 1, and the results are shown in the following table:

**Table 4.** Performance of shape-based descriptors using dataset 1

| Method | ANMRR | ARR | | ARP | | |
|--------|-------|-----|-----|-----|-----|-----|
| | | $\alpha=2$ | $\alpha=1$ | $\alpha=1$ | $\alpha=0.5$ | $\alpha=0.25$ |
| **PZM** [2] | 0.7177 | 0.3808 | 0.2000 | 0.2000 | 0.2308 | 0.3692 |
| **PCET** [18] | 0.7212 | 0.3642 | 0.2231 | 0.2231 | 0.2615 | 0.3692 |
| **PCT** [18] | 0.7066 | 0.3554 | 0.2423 | 0.2423 | 0.2538 | 0.3692 |
| **PHOG** [8] | **0.5825** | **0.4462** | **0.3538** | **0.3538** | **0.4692** | **0.6308** |

From tables 2, 3 and 4 and figures 2 and 3, we can observe that the DCCD and the
PHOG perform better than the other descriptors, so we decided to combine the DCCD
color-based descriptor and the PHOG shape-based descriptor in this paper. We used
the combination of two feature vectors given by (19) with three different weight ω
[16] and a simple concatenation of two feature vectors.

**Table 5.** Combination of two feature vectors with different weght ω using dataset 1

| Method | ANMRR | ARR | | ARP | | |
|--------|-------|-----|-----|-----|-----|-----|
| | | α=2 | α=1 | α=1 | α=0.5 | α=0.25 |
| Q ω=0.8 | 0.3933 | 0.6385 | 0.5077 | 0.5077 | 0.7000 | 0.8000 |
| Q ω=0.5 | 0.2364 | 0.8077 | 0.6769 | 0.6769 | 0.8154 | 0.9231 |
| Q ω=0.3 | **0.2150** | **0.8309** | **0.6846** | **0.6846** | **0.8615** | **0.9538** |
| Conca-tenation | 0.2227 | 0.8231 | 0.6808 | 0.6808 | 0.8538 | 0.9385 |

The table 5 shows that using weight $\omega = 0.3$, the performance of image retrieval task is better, which means the contribution of color feature is more important than the shape feature in the CBIR. As we mentioned before, the proposed scheme combines color and shape features based on the DCCD and the PHOG using the combination method given by (19) to obtain the similarity Q. We compared the proposed scheme with the method proposed in [2], which combines color, texture and shape features, using the dataset 1 and dataset 2. In the evaluation, we employed three metrics commonly used in the CBIR, such as Average Normalized Retrieval Rank (ANMRR), Average Retrieval Rate (ARR) and Average Retrieval Precision (ARP) [7, 14]. The number of queries must be at least 1% of the dataset size [12]. For dataset 1, we used 13 queries for evaluation equivalent to the 2.6% and for dataset 2 we used 20 queries equivalent to the 2% of the dataset size. The comparison results between the proposed scheme and [2] are shown in table 6.

**Table 6.** Comparison with the previous method [2]

| dataset 1 | | | | | | |
|-----------|-------|-----|-----|-----|-----|-----|
| Method | ANMRR | ARR | | ARP | | |
| | | α=2 | α=1 | α=1 | α=0.5 | α=0.25 |
| [2] | 0.3425 | 0.7308 | 0.5346 | 0.5346 | 0.7308 | 0.8615 |
| Proposed | **0.2150** | **0.8309** | **0.6846** | **0.6846** | **0.8615** | **0.9538** |
| dataset 2 | | | | | | |
| [2] | 0.3672 | 0.6750 | 0.5420 | 0.5420 | 0.7020 | 0.8400 |
| Proposed | **0.2698** | **0.7800** | **0.6550** | **0.6550** | **0.8120** | **0.9320** |

Using Corel Dataset 1k, we compare the proposed algorithm with the algorithms proposed in [3-6]. The evaluation method used here is the same one used in [3], in which 80 queries are used corresponding to the 8% of the dataset size. The query images are the same used in [3] and the number of retrieved images to compute the

Average Precision (AP) is the same as well. The results are shown in table 7. From the table, we can conclude the proposed method globally outperforms four previously proposed methods [3-6].

**Table 7.** Comparison with several methods [3-6]

| Class name | [3] | [4] | [5] | [6] | Proposed |
|---|---|---|---|---|---|
| Tribe | 54 % | 44.1% | 32.3% | 41% | **61%** |
| Beach | 38% | 30.6% | **61.2%** | 32% | 46.6% |
| Buildings | 40% | 38.2% | 39.2% | 37% | **41.09%** |
| Buses | 64% | **67.6%** | 39.5% | 66% | 62.93% |
| Dinosaurs | 96% | 97.2% | **99.6%** | 43% | 93.52% |
| Elephants | **62%** | 33.8% | 55.7% | 39% | 41.78% |
| Roses | 68% | 88.8% | **89.3%** | 87% | 77.51% |
| Horses | 75% | 63.2% | 65.2% | 35% | **77.35%** |
| Mountains | 45% | 31.3% | **56.8%** | 34% | 42.79% |
| Food | 53% | 34.9% | 44.1% | 31% | **68.59%** |
| Average | 59.5% | 52.97% | 58.29% | 44.5% | **61.26%** |

# 6    Conclusions

In this paper we proposed a scheme which combines color and shape features for the content-based image retrieval (CBIR) task. The proposed scheme extracts both global and local color information using the DCCD and the shape feature based on boundary information of objects using the PHOG. Two features are combined by weighted linear combination. We set a greater color-weight because the color feature provides the most distinguishable information compared with the shape features. The comparison of the proposed algorithm with four previously proposed algorithms, which combine more than one visual descriptor, shows the better performance of the proposed algorithm.

**Acknowledgements.** We thanks to the National Council of Science and Technology of Mexico (CONACyT), to ANR of France and the National Polytechnic Institute for the financial support during the realization of this research.

# References

1. Penatti, O., Valle, E., Torres, S.: Comparative study of global color and texture descriptors for web image retrieval. J. Vis. Comm. Image Representation 23, 359–380 (2012)
2. Wang, X.Y., Yu, Y.J., Yang, H.Y.: An effective image retrieval scheme using color, texture and shape features. Computer Standards & Interfaces 33, 59–68 (2011)
3. Jalab, H.A.: Image retrieval system based on color layout descriptor and global filters. In: IEEE Conf. on Open System, pp. 32–36 (2011)
4. Pujari, J., Hiremath, P.: Content-based image retrieval based on color, texture and shape features. Signal and Image Processing, 239–242 (2010)
5. Hafiane, A., Zavidovique, B.: Local relational string and mutual matching doe image retrieval. Information Processing &Manegement 44, 1201–1212 (2008)
6. Kavitha, C., Prabhakara, B., Govardhan, A.: Image retrieval based on color and texture features of the image subblocks. Int. J. Comput. Appl. 15, 33–37 (2011)
7. Fierro, A., Perez, K., Nakano, M., Benois, J.: Dominant color correlogram descriptor for content-based image retrieval. In: 3rd Int. Conf. on Image, Vision and Computing (2014)
8. Yang, B., Guo, L., Jin, L., Huang, Q.: A novel feature extraction method using pyramid histogram of orientation gradients for smile recognition. In: 16th IEEE Int. Conf. on Image Processing, pp. 3305–3308 (2009)
9. Shao, H., Wu, Y., Cui, W., Zhang, J.: Image retrieval based on MPEG-7 dominant color descriptor. In: 9th Int. Conf. for Young Scientist, pp. 753–757 (2008)
10. Yang, N., Chang, W., Kuo, C., Li, T.: A fast MPEG-7 dominant color extraction with new similarity measure for image retrieval. J. of Vis. Commum. & Image Representation 19, 92–105 (2008)
11. Johnson, G., Song, X., Montag, E., Fairchild, M.: Derivation of a color space for image color difference measurement. Color Research and Appl. 5, 387–400 (2010)
12. Talib, A., Mahmuddin, M., Husni, H., Loay, E.G.: A weighted dominant color descriptor for content-based image retrieval. J. of Vis. Commun. & Image Representation 24, 345–360 (2013)
13. Swain, M., Ballard, D.: Color indexing. Int. J. of Computer Vision 7, 11–32 (1991)
14. Fierro, A., Nakano, M., Perez, H., Cedillo, M., Garcia, F.: An efficient color descriptor based on global and local color features for image retrieval. In: Int. Conf. on Elect. Eng. Comput. Science and Automatic Control, pp. 233–238 (2013)
15. Huang, J., Kumar, S., Mitra, M., Zhu, W., Zabih, R.: Image indexing using color correlogram. In: Conf. on Computer Vision Pattern Recognition, pp. 762–768 (1997)
16. Bleschke, M., Madonski, R., Rudnicki, R.: Image retrieval system based on combined MPEG-7 texture and color descriptors. In: Int. Conf. Mixed Design of Integrated Circuit and Systems, pp. 635–639 (2009)
17. Wong, K., Po, L., Cheung, K.: Dominant color structure descriptor for image retrieval. IEEE Trans. on PAMI 32, 1259–1270 (2010)
18. Yap, P., Jiang, X., Kot, C.: Two-dimensional polar harmonic transform for invariant image representation. IEEE Trans. on PAMI 32, 1259–1270 (2010)
19. Li, J., Wang, J.: Automatic linguistic indexing of pictures by a statistical modeling approach. IEEE Trans on PAMI 25, 1075–1088 (2003)
20. Wang, J., Li, J., Wiederhold, G.: SIMPLIcity semantic-sensitive integrated matching for picture libraries. IEEE Trans. on PAMI 23, 947–964 (2001)
21. Kasutani, E., Yamada, A.: The MPEG-7 color layout descriptor: A compact image feature description for high-speed image/video segment retrieval. In: Int. Conf. on Image Processing, pp. 674–667 (2001)

# Compressive Sensing Architecture
# for Gray Scale Images

Gustavo Gonzalez-Garcia, Alfonso Fernandez-Vazquez,
and Rodolfo Romero-Herrera

School of Computer Engineering, ESCOM
National Polytechnic Institute, IPN
Unidad Profesional Adolfo Lopez Mateos
Av. Juan de Dios Batiz s/n
Esq. Miguel Othon de Mendizabal, Col. Lindavista
Mexico City, 07738, Mexico

**Abstract.** This paper proposes a compressive sensing architecture for
$128 \times 128$ pixels gray scale images. The proposed architecture is implemented in an FPGA platform. Due to speed and area advantages, the
random numbers block generator is implemented using Linear Feedback
Shift Register (LFSR) technique. The resulting random matrix is stored
in a Random Access Memory (RAM) block. In addition, a second RAM
is employed to store the sampled image. We also implement an Universal Asynchronous Receiver Transmitter (UART) to receive and transmit
data. Besides the previous blocks, we design an Arithmetic/Logic Unit
(ALU), which performs the operations in compressive sensing settings.
In this way, a Unit Control (UC) based on a Mealy type state machine
directs operations in our architecture. The purpose of the UC is three-
fold. First, the UC uses the UART to receive the sample image and store
it in the corresponding RAM block. Second, the UC directs the matrix
multiplication operation to the ALU and obtains the compressed image.
Finally, the UART transmits the compressed image to a base station.
The main characteristics of our architecture are the following: the maximum frequency of operation is 30 MHz, the power consumption is 37
mW, and the average time processing is 4.5 ms.

**Keywords:** Compressed Sensing, FPGA, Images, Reconfigurable Architecture.

## 1 Introduction

Traditional data compression relies on Nyquist theory and is composed by three
main steps, i.e., sampling, digital processing, and coding. In this setting, well
known data compression standards for audio and image compression can be jpg,
mp3, mpg, among others. The main drawbacks of this method are the following: 1) the sampling process generally includes big redundant data, which are
removed after digital processing and coding 2) in real world, the signals of interests do not possess band limited as is required by the Nyquist theory, and

A. Gelbukh et al. (Eds.): MICAI 2014, Part I, LNAI 8856, pp. 349–355, 2014.

3) a device with physical limitations imposes distortion in the reconstruction of the original signal. To overcome those disadvantages, a new data acquisition paradigm has been proposed, i.e., compressive sensing. This approach is a universal technique to compress sparse signals [2]. Sparse signals are more common in real word than band limited signals [5]. Compressive sensing allows the reconstruction of the desired signal with high accuracy, which are sampled below the Nyquist criterion [1,5].

In this way, recently, the TamaRISC-CS system has been proposed [2,3]. The proposed system is an application-specific instruction-set processor (ASSP) operating operating in the subthreshold regime. This characteristic allows to accomplish 62X speed-up and 11.6X power savings. This implies that the power consumption is 70nWat 1kHz. Another interesting approach is given in [4], where compressing sensing is applied to biosignal acquisition systems to reduce the data rate and realizes ultra-low-power performance. The proposed system achieves compression factors greater than 16X for ECG and EMG signals. Finally, in [6], the authors suggest the use of compressing sensing for MAGNETIC RESONANCE IMAGING (MRI). In addition, some hardware limitations are discussed in order to successfully apply compressive sensing in MRI applications.

The main goal of this paper is to propose a reconfigurable softcore architecture for data acquisition based on compressive sensing. In order to evaluate the proposed architecture, we implement the corresponding building block into VHDL (VHSIC (Very High Speed Integrated Circuit) Hardware Description Language). The architecture is designed such that it can handle gray scale images of size $128 \times 28$ pixels. Furthermore, we carried out the implementation of the reconfigurable softcore in an FPGA (Field Programmable Gate Arrays).

The rest of the paper is organized as follows. Section 2 reviews the basic theory of compressive sensing. Sections 3 deals with the hardware description of our architecture while Section 4 presents the main results of the proposed approach. Finally, Section 5 concludes the paper.

## 2   Basic Theory

This section reviews the theory of compressive sensing. Consider a discrete vector signal $\mathbf{x}$, which can be expressed by means of a redundant representation or frame, i.e.,

$$\mathbf{x} = \sum_{i=1}^{N} s_i \psi_i, \tag{1}$$

where $s_i$, for $i = 1, \ldots, N$, are the frame coefficients, $\psi_i$ is the frame $i$, and $N$ is the number of frames [1,5]. Alternatively, equation (1) can be rewritten as [1,5]

$$\mathbf{x} = \mathbf{\Psi s}, \tag{2}$$

where $\mathbf{\Psi}$ is the resulting frame matrix of size $N \times N$, that is, $\mathbf{\Psi} = [\psi_1 \psi_2 \cdots \psi_N]$, and $\mathbf{s}$ is a vector of coefficients $s_i$, i.e., $\mathbf{s} = [s_1 s_2 \cdots s_N]^{\mathrm{T}}$. The signal $\mathbf{x}$ is $K$-sparse if it is a linear combination of only $K$ vectors $\psi_i$ for $K < N$, that is, only $K$ of the $s_i$ coefficients in (1) are nonzero and $(N - K)$ are zero.

Consequently, in compressive sensing, the compressed signal is obtained from $K$ measurements, which are performed as

$$\mathbf{y} = \mathbf{\Phi x},\qquad(3)$$

where $\mathbf{\Phi}$ is the measurement matrix with size $K \times N$ and $\mathbf{y}$ with size $K \times 1$ is the resulting compressed vector. The compression ration is therefore $K/N$. Substituting (2) into (3), we have

$$\mathbf{y} = \mathbf{\Gamma s},\qquad(4)$$

where $\mathbf{\Gamma} = \mathbf{\Phi\Psi}$ is called random sensing matrix with size $K \times N$. Usually, each entry for the matrix is a random variable with either uniform or normal distribution and variance $2/K$.

This paper deals with the implementation of the compressive sensing based on equations (3) and (4). The proposed reconfigurable architecture is described in Section 3.

## 3   Proposed Reconfigurable Architecture

### 3.1   Building Blocks

The proposed architecture is an specific purpose softcore. The system is based on a RISC architecture of 8 bits. Additionally, an Universal Asynchronous Receiver Transmitter (UART) is implemented to receive and transmit data. The implemented control unit is based on a Mealy state machine, which perform the compressive sensing algorithm. Figure 1 shows the main building blocks of the architecture, that is, arithmetic-logic unit (ALU), image memory, frame memory, control unit, multiplier block, and UART block.

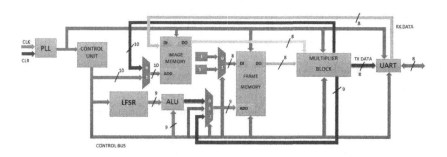

**Fig. 1.** Main building blocks of the proposed architecture

In the following we discuss in detail the main building blocks of the architecture.

## 3.2 ALU

The ALU performs basic operations like additions, subtractions, XOR, AND, NADN, OR, and NOR. The considered ALU is synthesized using look-ahead (anticipated carry) in VHDL. This characteristic improves the speed of the architecture.

## 3.3 Image Memory

The image memory is a $(16K \times 8)$ RAM (Random Access Memory). The main objective of this RAM is to store the raw gray scale image. The size of the image is $128 \times 128$ pixels. Each pixel is represented by 8 bits word.

## 3.4 Frame Memory

The image memory is a $(8K \times 8)$ RAM, which stores the measurement matrix $\Phi$. In order to simplify the computation of the matrix multiplication in equation (4), we follow the ideas in [2,3], where the entries of the random sensing matrix can be either 1 or $-1$. To do that, we first set to the value 1 the RAM memory. As a second step, we generate pseudo random numbers, which contain the positions of the RAM memory where the value 1 is substituted by 1. In this setting, the matrix multiplication operation is reduced to summations and subtractions operations.

## 3.5 Multiplication Block

In this section of the softcore, we implement a multiplication block, which consists of multiplier blocks and adders. The main task of this block is to perform the matrix multiplication $\Psi x$, i.e., each row of the matrix $\Phi$ is multiplied by the column vector $x$. Subsequently, the corresponding compressed coefficients are obtained by adding the resulting vector. The compressed vector is stored in a RAM memory and is transmitted by the UART block.

## 3.6 UART Block

We also implement an UART protocol to transmit or to receive data from a second device. The data can be the raw data or the compressed data.

## 3.7 Unit Control

This is the main building block in our softcore. This block is based on a Mealy state machine, which is composed by six states shown in Figure 2. The ASM (Algorithmic State Machine) chart for the implementation of the states is described in Section 3.9.

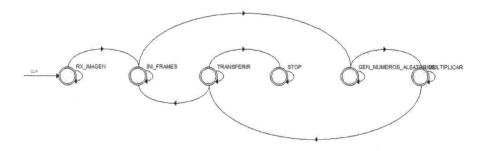

**Fig. 2.** State diagram

### 3.8 Random Number Generator

At this stage, the main idea is to maximize the performance of the proposed architecture and to implement a dedicated block to generate the random numbers. Therefore, in order to improve the speed and area consumption, the random numbers block generator is implemented using Linear Feedback Shift Register (LFSR) technique.

### 3.9 ASM Chart for Compressive Sensing

To develop an algorithm for compressive sensing, we propose an ASM chart, which is illustrated in Figure 3. In the first step, we reset registers and memories. The following step store the random matrix $\Phi$. The random numbers are generated and are stored in a $64 \times 128$ RAM memory as is shown in Figure 2. In this way, the UART block receives the gray scale image $\mathbf{x}$ from a second device using serial protocol. The compressed samples are obtained by means of the product $\Phi\mathbf{x}$ and the compressed vector $\mathbf{y}$ is stored in RAM memory. Finally, the vector $\mathbf{y}$ is transmitted to the second device. In this process, the original images with $2^{14}$ samples is reduced to 1000 samples. This means, we have a compression ratio of 0.061.

## 4   Results

We implement the proposed architecture into VHDL. The synthesis of each building block is obtained from Altera Quartus II Web Edition ver. 13.0 and the employed hardware is an FPGA Cyclone IV EEP4CE115F29C7. The simulation is carried out using the environment Altera ModelSim 10.1. Table 1 shows the main results. The first row provides the total combinational functions, which directly impacts the total area. In addition, the remaining parameters are obtained under the following conditions, the voltage source is 1200 mV and the working temperature is 85°C.

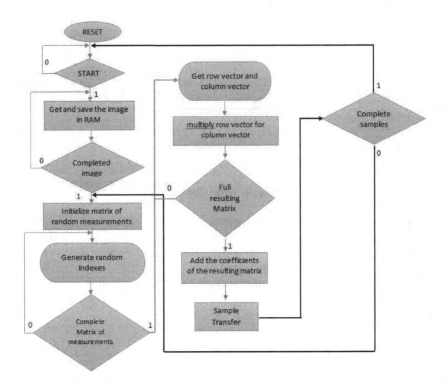

**Fig. 3.** ASM chart

**Table 1.** Synthesis results of the proposed architecture and optimization analysis

| | |
|---|---|
| Total combinational functions | 13355 |
| Dedicated logic registers | 12014 |
| Embedded Multiplier elements | 0 |
| Maximum Frequency | 30 MHz |
| Core Static Thermal Power Dissipation | 102 mW |
| Thermal Power Dissipation | 37 mw |
| Execution time of the algorithm | 4.5 ms |

## 5    Conclusions

This paper presents an specific purpose architecture for compressive sensing and its VHDL implementation. The proposed architecture is an alternative solution to the existing architectures in the literature. As a difference with that solutions, our approach is a simple solution since no silicon synthesis is necessary. We describe the main building blocks along with the proposed algorithm for compressive sensing. In this approach, the number of compressed samples is 1000 for an image of size 128 × 128 pixels. This suggests that our architecture for compressive sensing is a useful tool for data acquisition.

**Acknowledgments.** This work was supported by SIP-IPN project 20141476.

# References

1. Baraniuk, R.G.: Compressive sensing [lecture notes]. IEEE Signal Processing Magazine 24(4), 118–121 (2007)
2. Constantin, J., Dogan, A., Andersson, O., Meinerzhagen, P., Rodrigues, J., Atienza, D., Burg, A.: TamaRISC-CS: An ultra-low-power application-specific processor for compressed sensing. In: 2012 IEEE/IFIP 20th International Conference on VLSI and System-on-Chip (VLSI-SoC), pp. 159–164 (October 2012)
3. Constantin, J., Dogan, A., Andersson, O., Meinerzhagen, P., Rodrigues, J., Atienza, D., Burg, A.: An ultra-low-power application-specific processor with sub-$v_T$ memories for compressed sensing. In: Burg, A., Coşkun, A., Guthaus, M., Katkoori, S., Reis, R. (eds.) VLSI-Soc 2012. IFIP Advances in Information and Communication Technology, vol. 418, pp. 88–106. Springer, Heidelberg (2013), http://dx.doi.org/10.1007/978-3-642-45073-0_5
4. Dixon, A., Allstot, E., Gangopadhyay, D., Allstot, D.: Compressed sensing system considerations for ECG and EMG wireless biosensors. IEEE Transactions on Biomedical Circuits and Systems 6(2), 156–166 (2012)
5. Donoho, D.: Compressed sensing. IEEE Transactions on Information Theory 52(4), 1289–1306 (2006)
6. Lustig, M., Donoho, D., Santos, J., Pauly, J.: Compressed sensing MRI. IEEE Signal Processing Magazine 25(2), 72–82 (2008)

# A Novel Approach for Face Authentication
# Using Speeded Up Robust Features Algorithm

Cyntia Mendoza-Martinez*, Jesus Carlos Pedraza-Ortega,
and Juan Manuel Ramos-Arreguin

Universidad Autonoma de Queretaro, Queretaro, Mexico
isc_cmendoza@hotmail.com

**Abstract.** In this paper, we propose a modified face authentication method based on the image preprocessing (histogram equalization, HE) and with SURF algorithm (Speeded Up Robust Features) in the feature extraction step. In particular, our methodology aims at determining a person's authenticity when he/she has a few facial expressions, different backgrounds or a variance in lighting. We evaluated the performance of this method using public face databases like The Extended Cohn-Kanade Dataset (CK+) and Caltech Faces. We made some test using sixty images (thirty per database), Equal (E) or Different (D) and according to the match between images (for example Image 1 and Image 2) and a defined threshold, our method determines if a person is authenticated or not. The results showed that with the database CK+ was obtained 93% and with Caltech Faces 86% of accuracy in the authentication process, these results were compared with those obtained by some algorithms like LDA, PCA, SIFT and SURF (without preprocessing) and we can conclude that the authentication rate was improved.

**Keywords:** Biometrics, Computer vision, Face authentication, Image processing, OpenCV, Python, SURF.

## 1 Introduction

Biometrics refers to the identification of a person on the basis of their physical and behavioral characteristics. Some biometric systems include features of fingerprints, hand geometry, voice, iris, etc., and can be used for identification. Most biometric systems are based on the collection and comparison of biometric characteristics which can provide identification [1]. In the recent years, a number of recognition and authentication systems based on biometric measurements have been proposed. Algorithms and sensors have been developed to acquire and process many different biometric traits. Moreover, the biometric technology is being used in novel ways, with potential commercial and practical implications to our daily activities [2]. Today's world security issues are the most important segment among all. Therefore, a segment of authentication and face recognition plays a major role. When a person or a system checks the person's identity against another person then we are in process of authentication. That means the one who is authenticated can confirm that he/she is the person with whom is compared.

---

* Corresponding author.

A. Gelbukh et al. (Eds.): MICAI 2014, Part I, LNAI 8856, pp. 356–367, 2014.

There are two essential type of authentication: verification, this is a process of confirming identity of any person by comparing the input data with ones existing in database, this is called 1:1 authentication method and the second one is identification, in this case we are matching the input data with all samples (named N) in the database with a view to retrieving the data related for the person, this system called 1:N represents the authentication model, where $N \geq 2$ [3]. The most common algorithms used in this field are LDA and PCA [4], SIFT [5] and SURF [6]. However, the principal limitations of the systems that use these algorithms are their dependence on the lighting conditions, positions, shapes and sizes of the face.

Within this paper, we concern about face authentication based on SURF algorithm. The contribution is to add a pre-processing filter in the feature extraction step and pay attention to the problems before mentioned to improve the results in the process of authentication. The remaining of this paper is organized as follows: in Section 2 we present a description of SURF algorithm (Speeded Up Robust Features), after that in Section 3 we explain a detailed description of our proposal. Later, Section 4 provides the reader with information about the experimentation made and the experimental results obtained from it. Finally, in Section 5, our conclusions and future work are presented.

## 2 Speeded Up Robust Features

SURF is a robust local feature detector [6], first presented by Herbert Bay et al. in 2006. The SURF algorithm is composed of three consecutive steps [7], the first one is called interest point detection, the second one is build the descriptor associated with each interest points and finally the descriptor matching. In the next section we are going to explain about those three steps of the algorithm.

### 2.1 Interest Point Detection

In [6] and [8] it describes that a Hessian matrix can be used as a good detector for its high performance in computational time and accuracy. Scale selection can be achieved through the determinant of the Hessian or Hessian–Laplace detector.

Given a point $p = (x, y)$ in the image I, the Hessian matrix $H(p, \sigma)$ in p at scale $\sigma$ is defined as follows:

$$H(p, \sigma) = \begin{pmatrix} L_{xx}(p, \sigma) & L_{xy}(p, \sigma) \\ L_{xy}(p, \sigma) & L_{yy}(p, \sigma) \end{pmatrix}. \tag{1}$$

Where $L_{xx}(p, \sigma)$ is the convolution of the second-order Gaussian derivative $\frac{\partial^2}{\partial x^2} g(\sigma)$ with the image I in point p, and similarly for $L_{xy}(p, \sigma)$ and $L_{yy}(p, \sigma)$. Although Gaussian filters are optimal for scale-space analysis, it has been implemented an alternative to these filters in the SURF detector called box-filters, this is due to a series of limitations of these filters (in practice they have to be discretized and cropped).

These filters approximate the second-order Gaussian derivatives and can be evaluated at a very low computational cost using an integral image $I_\Sigma(x)$ at a location p = (x, y), it represents the sum of all pixels in the input image I within a rectangular region formed by the origin and p. Also (x, y) defines the position of the point in the integral image. Once the integral image has been computed, it takes only three additions to calculate the sum of the intensities over any rectangular area. After that, the scale-space is analyzed by the elevation of filter size, instead of reducing the image size as in the SIFT detector, this difference can be seen in Fig. 1.

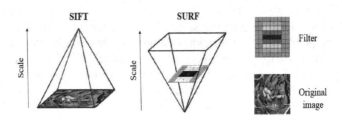

**Fig. 1.** Instead of iteratively reducing the image size (left, SIFT), the use of integral images allows the up-scaling of the filter at constant cost (right, SURF)

The advantage of using box filters and integral image principles is the high computational efficiency for the SURF approach compared to the SIFT approach since we only change the box filter size in the SURF approach while changing the image size and applying the filter to each image size in the image pyramid in the SIFT approach.

In the SURF approach, the box filter (Fig. 2) starts with a 9×9 size filter as the initial scale layer where it is referred as scale s = 1.2 (the approximated Gaussian derivative with the value σ = 1.2) and instead of having image pyramids, the original image will be filtered by bigger masks, denoted them by $D_{xx}$, $D_{yy}$ and $D_{xy}$.

The weights applied to the rectangular regions are kept simple for computational efficiency, and it is expressed as follows:

$$\det(H_{aprox}) = D_{xx}D_{yy} - (wD_{xy})^2 . \tag{2}$$

The relative weight w of the filter responses is used to balance the expression for the Hessian's determinant. This is needed for the energy conservation between the Gaussian kernels and the approximated Gaussian kernels, in this case $|x|_F$ is the Frobenius norm, w is given by the following equation:

$$w = \frac{|L_{xy}(1.2)|_F \; |D_{yy}(9)|_F}{|L_{yy}(1.2)|_F \; |D_{xy}(9)|_F} = 0.912 \dots \cong 0.9 . \tag{3}$$

In practice, the w factor is constant, as this did not have a significant impact on the results in the experiments [6].

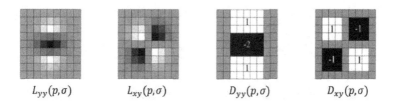

$$L_{yy}(p,\sigma) \qquad L_{xy}(p,\sigma) \qquad D_{yy}(p,\sigma) \qquad D_{xy}(p,\sigma)$$

**Fig. 2.** Left to right: The (discretized and cropped) second-order Gaussian partial derivative in y ($L_{yy}$) and xy-direction ($L_{xy}$), respectively; after the approximation for the second-order Gaussian partial derivative in y ($D_{yy}$) and xy-direction ($D_{xy}$). The grey regions are equal to zero.

## 2.2 Building the Descriptor Associated with Each Interest Points

In order to be invariant to rotation, in [6] is identified a reproducible orientation for the interest points. For that purpose, first are calculated the Haar-wavelet responses in x and y direction, the used filters to compute the responses are shown in Fig. 3 where the black color have the weight -1 and the white color have the weight +1. For the extraction of the descriptor, the first step consists of construct a square region centered on the interest point and oriented along the direction determined by the orientation selection method described in [8]. The region is split up regularly into smaller 4x4 square sub-regions.

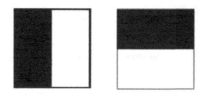

**Fig. 3.** Haar wavelet filters to compute the responses in x (left) and y direction (right)

This preserves important spatial information, as shown to the left of Fig. 4. For each sub-region, we compute Haar wavelet responses at 5x5 regularly spaced sample points samples (for illustrative purposes, we show only 2x2 sub-divisions here). For each field, we collect the sums $d_x$, $|d_x|$, $d_y$, $|d_y|$, computed relatively to the orientation of the grid, as shown to the right of Fig. 4. For reasons of simplicity, we call $d_x$ the Haar wavelet response in horizontal direction and $d_y$ the Haar wavelet response in vertical direction.

To increase the robustness towards geometric deformations and localization errors, the responses $d_x$ and $d_y$ are first weighted with a Gaussian (with value $\sigma = 3.3s$) centered at the interest point. Concatenating the sums for all 4x4 sub-regions, gives as result a descriptor vector of length 64 for each interest point. The wavelet responses are invariant to a bias in illumination (offset). Invariance to contrast (a scale factor) is achieved by turning the descriptor into a unit vector.

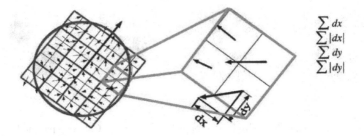

**Fig. 4.** Building the descriptor associated with an interest point

### 2.3 Descriptor Matching

In matching step, the descriptor vectors are matched between different images. The matching is based on a distance between the vectors, e.g. the Mahalanobis or Euclidean distance [6]. In conclusion, descriptor matching is a representation of the correspondence between each interest point identified in two images, only features are compared if they have the same type of contrast as can be appreciated in Fig. 5:

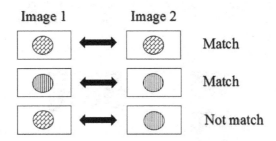

**Fig. 5.** Match between interest points of two images (Image 1 vs. Image 2)

## 3     Proposed Approach

We have developed this methodology using Python 2.7 as programming language, Eclipse as development environment and some libraries of OpenCV, however, all the information is presented in a clear and easy way. As can be observed in Fig. 6, the authentication process can be divided into five steps: Face image, Face detection, Feature detection, Feature match and Decision.

The whole methodology is described in Fig. 7. Before implementing SURF algorithm, we proposed to apply an image preprocessing (which one belongs to the feature extraction step, as can be seen in the blue box from Fig. 7) to improve the second and third step within authentication process, this will be described later on.

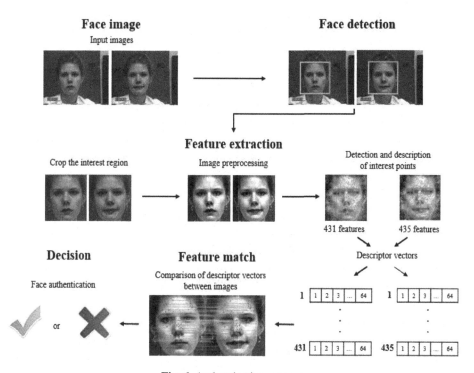

**Fig. 6.** Authentication process

In the face image step we used some images taken from two public face databases. The first image set was obtained from The Extended Cohn-Kanade Dataset (CK+) which one was proposed by Lucey et al. [9], this is a complete expression database for action unit and emotion-specified expression that is used for testing purposes.

This database contains 100 university students. They ranged in age from 18 to 30 years. Sixty-five percent were female, 15 percent were African-American, and three percent were Asian or Latino. Subjects were instructed by an experimenter to perform a series of 23 facial displays that included single action units and combinations of action units. Image sequences from neutral to target display were digitized into 640 by 480 or 490 pixels and with PNG format.

The second image set was obtained from Caltech Faces, this is a frontal face dataset collected by Markus Weber at California Institute of Technology [10]. The database contains 450 face images which ones were digitized into 896 by 592 pixels with JPEG format, 27 or so unique people under with different lighting/expressions/backgrounds.

In Fig. 8 some examples of these databases can be observed, they include men and woman, different lighting conditions and backgrounds, color images and grayscale.

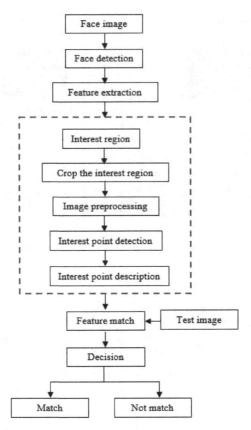

**Fig. 7.** Proposed methodology: Face image, Face detection, Feature extraction, Feature match and Decision

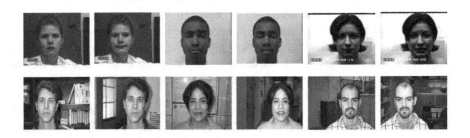

**Fig. 8.** Examples of databases CK+ (upper) and Caltech Faces (lower)

In the face detection step, we apply Haar like feature detection algorithm which can be used for object detection, e.g. in the upper right from Fig. 6. More information about this step can be consulted in [11]. In the feature extraction step we apply our improved phase of preprocessing, the goal is to obtain the faces samples ready for the forthcoming steps, an advantage of this process is that we only select an interest region to detection and description of features. More information can be consulted in [12].

Next, we select an interest region taking as reference the green box marked from the previous step and this region is cropped, as can be observed in middle left from Fig. 6. After that, we realize the histogram equalization (HE) in the image (in middle from Fig. 6), this is one on the most widely used methods of enhancing contrast effectively and simply [13] and modifies the pixel values in such a way that the intensity histogram of the resulting image becomes uniform. The output image then makes use of all the possible brightness values, thus, resulting in enhanced contrast [14]. The next step is to apply the SURF algorithm to features extraction on an image, the purpose is to obtain detectors and descriptors of interest points, as can be seen in middle right from Fig. 6.

We continue with feature match step where an input image (Face image, first step) and a test image (this image could be similar or different from the input image), both images are compared according to the features detected before for each image, this step can be observed on Fig. 6. In this case, each image has X features (descriptors, where $X \geq 1$) of dimension 64. So, we match each feature between images to find features with lowest Euclidean distance.

Then, we take all the features that were found in both images, after that we compared both features to identify how many matches have between two images. Finally, we have the decision step, it means that according to the number of matches between images we determine if the input image correspond to the test image. This is known such as Match or Not match as can be observed at the end of Fig. 7.

In our case and according to the matching method described in [15], to make sure that an input image (Image 1) corresponds with test image (Image 2), does not matter their expressions e.g. if Image 1 is neutral and Image 2 is angry, sad with surprised, fear with happy, etc., we defined a threshold of 20 (also based on our previous experiments) it means if with our approach it detects at least 20 matches between images, the process is considered as valid authentication, otherwise the authentication process will be considered as failed. In order to validate our proposal, we tested 60 face images (30 face images per database) and the results are shown in the next section.

## 4    Experimental Results

First, Table 1 shows the software and hardware that we used in our tests.

**Table 1.** Software and Hardware used for our approach

| Software and Hardware | |
|---|---|
| Eclipse | Version: Kepler (integrated development environment) |
| Python | Version: 2.7 (programming language). |
| OpenCV libraries | Version: 2.4 |
| Computer model | Notebook HP ENVY 15. |
| Operative System | Windows 8, 64 bits. |
| Processor | Intel® Core™ i7 CPU 2.4 GHz. |
| Memory (RAM) | 16.0 GB. |

In this study we made a series of experiments to verify: data acquisition with different image formats (PNG and JPEG), face detector step, feature extraction step, feature match (threshold of acceptation: at least 20 matches between images) and decision step. In data acquisition step, we used two different face databases: The Extended Cohn-Kanade Dataset (CK+) and Caltech Faces, each database contains different characteristics that helped us to validate our approach. In face detector step, we have used Haar like feature detection algorithm, it is important to mention that we have tested with different images dimensions, backgrounds and illumination conditions. In feature extraction step (The results are shown in Table 2 and an example is given in Fig. 9), we also need to evaluate the performance of the experiments according to:

- True positive (TP): When Image 1 matches with Image 2 (both are Equal "E") and the decision is: match between images.
- False positive (FP): When Image 1 do not match with Image 2 (Image 1 is Different "D" to Image 2) and the decision is: match between images, but the decision is false because Image 1 is different to Image 2.
- True negative (TN): When Image 1 do not match with Image 2 (both are D) and the decision is: no match between images.
- False negative (FN): When Image 1 matches with Image 2 (both are E) and the decision is: no match between images, but the decision is false because Image 1 is equal to Image 2.

**Table 2.** True and False positives, and True and False negatives

| Database | TP | FP | TN | FN | Authenticity rate |
|----------|-----|-----|-----|-----|-------------------|
| CK+ | 60% | 0% | 33% | 7% | 93% |
| Caltech Faces | 53% | 0% | 33% | 13% | 86% |

In order to validate our approach, in some cases both images are similar e.g. Image 1 could be with a neutral facial expression and Image 2 could be with a surprised facial expression and both images correspond to the same person. In other cases Image 1 could be with a happy facial expression and also Image 2 but correspond to different people. Table 3 contains the results about the number of feature extraction in each database, where Test is the number of experiment, St correspond to status of images (Equal, E or Different, D), Cp is the comparison between images (Female, F or Male, M), e.g. F - M is a comparison between images of a woman and a man, and finally Img is the number of image (Image 1 and Image 2).

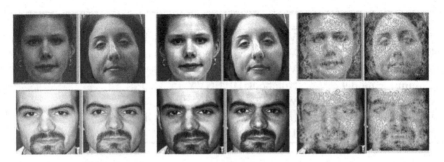

**Fig. 9.** Left to right: interest region, equalized image and feature extraction

**Table 3.** Feature extraction results

| | CK+ | | | | Caltech Faces | | | |
|---|---|---|---|---|---|---|---|---|
| Test | St | Cp | Img 1 | Img 2 | St | Cp | Img 1 | Img 2 |
| 1 | E | F-F | 431 | 435 | D | M-M | 833 | 998 |
| 2 | D | F-F | 288 | 435 | E | M-M | 666 | 1064 |
| 3 | E | F-F | 693 | 679 | E | M-M | 667 | 801 |
| 4 | D | F-M | 467 | 774 | E | M-M | 746 | 1112 |
| 5 | E | M-M | 450 | 510 | D | F-F | 1064 | 506 |
| 6 | E | M-M | 945 | 959 | E | M-M | 749 | 658 |
| 7 | D | M-M | 494 | 768 | E | F-F | 604 | 776 |
| 8 | E | M-M | 767 | 873 | E | F-F | 725 | 853 |
| 9 | E | F-F | 621 | 453 | D | M-M | 984 | 816 |
| 10 | E | F-F | 401 | 312 | E | F-F | 506 | 735 |
| 11 | E | F-F | 383 | 362 | D | F-M | 1141 | 687 |
| 12 | D | F-M | 383 | 391 | E | M-M | 891 | 915 |
| 13 | E | M-M | 428 | 497 | E | M-M | 1172 | 886 |
| 14 | E | M-M | 484 | 535 | D | F-M | 839 | 587 |
| 15 | D | F-M | 440 | 547 | E | M-M | 629 | 1124 |

In feature match step and according to the results obtained in feature extraction step, Table 4 shows the total number of matching between images. Finally, the decision step is given by the range of acceptance (in our case the threshold of acceptation was at least 20 matches between images). Fig. 10 is an example of match between images.

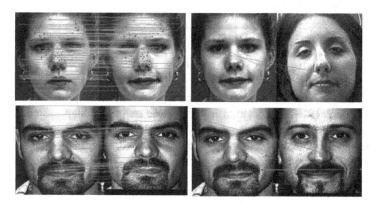

**Fig. 10.** In the upper left corner we have match between similar images of women and in the upper right corner with different images. The same case in the lower left and right corners but with men.

Finally, we evaluated the performance of the proposed methodology against the most common algorithms used in this field like LDA and PCA [16], SIFT and SURF (without preprocessing) [17]. Table 5 shows the results obtained in the tests.

**Table 4.** Match between images

| Test | CK+ | Caltech Faces |
|------|-----|---------------|
| 1    | 104 | 4             |
| 2    | 5   | 20            |
| 3    | 56  | 51            |
| 4    | 4   | 32            |
| 5    | 78  | 5             |
| 6    | 101 | 51            |
| 7    | 4   | 47            |
| 8    | 35  | 24            |
| 9    | 30  | 4             |
| 10   | 13  | 18            |
| 11   | 42  | 7             |
| 12   | 5   | 42            |
| 13   | 106 | 36            |
| 14   | 102 | 5             |
| 15   | 5   | 15            |

**Table 5.** Comparison between LDA, PCA, SIFT and SURF

| Algorithm | Authenticity rate |
|-----------|-------------------|
| LDA | 88.75% |
| PCA | 83.57% |
| SIFT | 81.00% |
| SURF (without preprocessing) | 81.47% |
| SURF (with preprocessing) | 86-93% |

# 5    Conclusions and Future Work

In this paper, we proposed a novel approach for face authentication using Speeded Up Robust Features (SURF) algorithm in the feature extraction step. This methodology was tested on the databases The Extended Cohn-Kanade Dataset (CK+) and Caltech Faces, which include pose, lighting, facial expressions and different background. Experimental results showed that compared with methods like LDA, PCA, SIFT and SURF (without preprocessing), our methodology improved the authentication rate. In future work, we need to perform a deep analysis of image preprocessing, at the same time, the facial expression effect in the authentication of faces.

**Acknowledgments.** This research was supported by CONACYT through the project 302491 and also we would like to thank Universidad Autonoma de Queretaro and Fondo para el Fortalecimiento de la Investigacion (FOFI) UAQ-2013, for the support in this work.

# References

1. Brumnik, R., Podbregar, I., Ivanuša, T.: Reliability of Fingerprint Biometry (Weibull Approach). In: Riaz, Z. (ed.) Biometric Systems, Design and Applications, pp. 3–4. InTech (2011) ISBN: 978-953-307-542-6

2. Yang, J., Poh, N.: Recent Application in Biometrics. InTech (2011) ISBN 978-953-307-488-7

3. Kremić, E., Subaşi, A.: The Implementation of Face Security for Authentication Implemented on Mobile Phone. The International Arab Journal of Information Technology (2011)

4. Lu, X.: Image Analysis for Face Recognition. Michigan State University, East Lansing, Míchigan, United States, Personal notes (2003)

5. Lowe, D.G.: Distinctive image features from scale-invariant keypoints. International Journal of Computer Vision 60(2), 91–110 (2004)

6. Bay, H., Tuytelaars, T., Van Gool, L.: SURF: Speeded up robust features. In: Leonardis, A., Bischof, H., Pinz, A. (eds.) ECCV 2006, Part I. LNCS, vol. 3951, pp. 404–417. Springer, Heidelberg (2006)

7. Oyallon, E., Rabin, J.: An analysis and implementation of the SURF method, and its comparison to SIFT. Image Processing on Line (2013)

8. Boullosa, O.: Estudio comparativo de descriptores visuales para la detección de escenas cuasi-duplicadas (Comparativestudy of visual descriptorsfordetectingnearduplicatescenes), Madrid, Spain (2011)

9. Lucey, P., Cohn, J.F., Kanade, T., Saragih, J., Ambadar, Z., Matthews, I.: The Extended Cohn-Kanade Dataset (CK+): A complete expression dataset for action unit and emotion-specified expression. In: Proceedings of the Third International Workshop on CVPR for Human Communicative Behavior Analysis (CVPR4HB 2010), San Francisco, USA, pp. 94–101 (2010)

10. Weber, M.: Unsupervised Learning of Models for Object Recognition. PhD. Thesis, California Institute of Technology, Pasadena, California (2000)

11. Park, K.Y., Hwang, S.Y.: An improved Haar-like feature for efficient object detection. Pattern Recognition Letters 42, 148–153 (2014)

12. Travieso, C.M., Del Pozo, M., Alonso, J.B.: Facial Identification Based on Transform Domains for Images and Videos. In: Riaz, Z. (ed.) Biometric Systems, Design and Applications, pp. 978–953. InTech (2011) ISBN: 978-953-307-542-6

13. Paik, J.K.: Image processing method and system using gain controllable clipped histogram equalization. U.S. Patent No 7,885,462 (2011)

14. Han, J.H., Yang, S., Lee, B.U.: A novel 3-D color histogram equalization method with uniform 1-D gray scale histogram. IEEE Transactions on Image Processing 20(2), 506–512 (2011)

15. Cao, Z., Yin, Q., Tang, X., Sun, J.: Face recognition with learning-based descriptor. In: 2010 IEEE Conference on Computer Vision and Pattern Recognition (CVPR), pp. 2707–2714. IEEE (2010)

16. Zainudin, M., Radi, H., Abdullah, S., Rahim, R.A., Ismail, M.: Face Recognition using Principle Component Analysis (PCA) and Linear Discriminant Analysis (LDA). IJECS-IJENS 12, 50–55 (2012)

17. Gou, G., Huang, D., Wang, Y.: A hybrid local feature for face recognition. In: Anthony, P., Ishizuka, M., Lukose, D. (eds.) PRICAI 2012. LNCS, vol. 7458, pp. 64–75. Springer, Heidelberg (2012)

# On-Line Dense Point Cloud Generation from Monocular Images with Scale Estimation

Ander Larranaga-Cepeda, Jose Gabriel Ramirez-Torres,
and Carlos Alberto Motta-Avila

LTI-CINVESTAV
Km. 5.5 Carr. a Soto la Marina
Cd.Victoria, TAMPS
Mexico
{alarranaga,grtorres}@tamps.cinvestav.mx

**Abstract.** This paper introduces an approach for on-line marker-based three dimensional modeling with scale estimation and heightmap construction from monocular images. The presented system is also capable of an off-line marker-less 3D reconstruction from monocular images with increased detail. This method is designed for the flexible use with an Unmaned Aerial Vehicle (UAV); this means that, despite being tested with a Parrot AR.Drone 1.0, it is easily portable to other more capable UAV models. The followed approach was an adaptation of the patch-based Multiview Stereo (PMVS) algorithm for on line point cloud generation. The system achieved 1.05 processed images per second on average, slightly surpassing the planed objective of 1 processed image per second. The height estimation error ranges between 1-1.5% with a manual marker detection and 4-5% with automatic marker detection, which seems accurate enough for autonomous navigation and path planning. As future work, tests with a better UAV, processing time reduction, marker-less height map construction, autonomous indoor navigation and collaborative on-line 3D modeling are planned.

## 1 Introduction

An unmanned aerial vehicle (UAV) is defined as a powered, aerial vehicle that does not carry a human operator, uses aerodynamic forces to provide vehicle lift and can fly autonomously or be piloted remotely [1]. UAVs are classified according to the type of wing (fixed/rotary wing) and to its taking off capabilities (vertical take-off or short take off and landing) [2]. Good performance, low cost, vertical take off and landing capabilities allowing access to hazardous areas for humans, low weight and low noise figure among the main advantages of using UAVs. Non remote control UAVs are able to perform just automatic tasks such as marker-based navigation, take off or land [3]. In order to expand UAVs range of possibilities we must assure a safe and autonomous navigation through unknown environments. Being able to explore an unknown environment leads to many

A. Gelbukh et al. (Eds.): MICAI 2014, Part I, LNAI 8856, pp. 368–379, 2014.

non trivial problems such as knowing the UAV position in a GPS denied area or avoiding obstacles when navigating through them. To solve many of these problems, a metric representation of the environment can be constructed based on the received data from a sensor, that is, a map containing distance, height and angle data of the flown area.

The surface elevations, the orography, are a key aspect in autonomous navigation of robotic aerial vehicles. The most common way to describe a terrain's orography is through a colored map known as heightmap where every color represents a certain height range. Its generation is a computerized process involving the digital representation of the Earth's surface and it is known as a Digital Elevation Model (DEM), Digital Terrain Model (DTM) or Digital Surface Model (DSM) [4][5]. The digital terrain models are used for extracting terrestrial parameters, generating a three dimensional map with relief data, correcting aerial photography, analyzing GPS data and flight planning among others.

There are several UAV-based digital terrain model generation proposals [6][7][3], however, the purpose of this paper is to provide a new solution using a low cost UAV equipped with a single camera. The addition of more sophisticated equipment increases significatively the UAV's prize and it precludes the access to particulars and organizations with low budget. A solution based on a commercial UAV equipped with a monocular camera would provide an easy and affordable way for the generation of digital terrain models without making a significant investment, being useful for academic and civilian purposes. The selected UAV model is an AR.Drone 1.0 launched by the French company Parrot, however and due to the constrains of its camera, the presented work has been designed to fit most of the available low cost UAVs and the imagery acquisition was performed with a Canon Powershot digital camera.

This work proposes a framework for both on line and off line generation of a point cloud based on a three dimensional model with scale estimation and heightmap construction allowing the navigation of a UAV through it. The paper is organized as follows: Section 2 describes the previous work in three dimensional modeling, heightmap generation and odometry and navigation algorithms for the AR.Drone UAV, Section 3 describes the structure of the proposed framework, Section 4 provides the experimental results, Section 5 presents a data analysis and interpretation and finally, Section 6 summarizes and presents some final conclusions.

## 2  Previous Work

### 2.1  AR.Drone

The selected UAV for accomplishing our purpose is the Parrot AR.Drone 1.0. Nevertheless, the framework has been designed for being easily portable to a more capable UAV. Every so often new models are available in the market with better specifications so portability was a requirement during the development of this system. Many algorithms and frameworks have been presented by other authors for the AR.Drone but three dimensional modeling has not been addressed yet due to resolution and quality constrains. For this reason, although the AR.Drone 1.0 was used to design a marker based control, images were taken with a digital camera as mentioned earlier. Better image quality will only generate a better 3D model. The proposed algorithm has focused mainly on indoor navigation [8], odometry and path estimation [9][10].

## 2.2   Image-Based 3D Reconstruction

A few approaches addressing the three dimensional reconstruction from monocular images have been published. Due to the complexity of this task, many authors suggest the possibility of employing additional sensors for this purpose [11] or a stereoscopic camera [12] to get depth data from the images and discard monocular cameras for not being suitable for 3D modeling [11]. Other approaches are focused on Visual SLAM based on an Extended Kalman Filter (EKF) and a three dimensional facade reconstruction with scale uncertainty [13][14]. To this date, a published paper addressing the problem of on line heightmap construction from monocular images has not been found due to the unknown scale factor. In structure-from-motion (SfM) with a single camera the scene can be only recovered up to a scale, but no absolute dimensions can be computed [15]. To solve the scale uncertainty, we must assure the presence of a known reference in the scene so the absolute scale can be recovered from the relative dimensions of the reference in it. This procedure entails another particularity that must be solved and that is the fact that the location of the plane XY of the point cloud coordinate system has to be also known and parallel to the actual ground of the scene. The easiest way to avoid this problem is to employ a marker that could be easily detected by an algorithm for marker detection such as the method proposed by Garrido-Jurato *el al.* [16] and also providing the camera pose $[R|t]$ matrix centered on the marker.

Off-line 3D reconstruction from images has been successfully addressed with algorithms like Patch-based Multiview Stereo (PMVS) [17] and SfM approaches such as A Contrario Structure from Motion (ACSfM) [18] that are able to provide a dense and highly detailed point cloud. However, the required processing time for image matching and camera pose computing is too high for on-line three dimensional reconstruction system and on the other hand, the scale factor is also unknown.

## 2.3   Scale Estimation for Heightmap

Published works with the same purpose and infrastructure were not found. There are several proposals when it comes to heightmap generation via aerial images, but most of them are based on GPS [19][20] and stereoscopic cameras [7] to get depth data. Weiss's *et al.* [20] approach creates a three dimensional model in real time after manually measuring the scale factor, however, GPS denied environments are not considered. The approach is similar to Davison's [21] where they add an A4 sheet to the scene for automatically computing the absolute

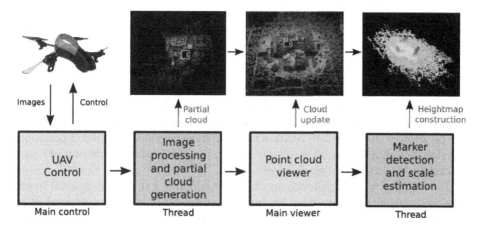

Images ↓  Control ↑     ↑ Partial cloud     ↑ Cloud update     ↑ Heightmap construction

| UAV Control | Image processing and partial cloud generation | Point cloud viewer | Marker detection and scale estimation |

Main control        Thread        Main viewer        Thread

**Fig. 1.** Framework's on-line 3D modeling and heightmap reconstruction schema

scale. Researchers have come out with several robust descriptors for defining an object in a three dimensional space [22][23][24] but most of them do not consider occlusions and cannot deal properly with several instances of the same object in a scene. That's the case of the classic geometric hashing algorithm which, despite being commonly used for detection of 3D objects [25], is somehow sensitive to the presence of occlusions and clutter [26][27].

## 3    Framework Proposal

The UAV must be able to overfly a indoor area or a terrain, build a point cloud and construct a heightmap from it. The simplest way of determining a path to follow is by means of markers. The Garrido-Jurato *el al.* [16] marker method was used for establishing checkpoints on the terrain. For example, if the UAV detects the marker number two that means that it should turn around 90 degrees and keep going straight until another marker is found. The marker provides three additional and useful advantages: the first one is the real time camera pose matrix estimation without having to perform image matching whose computational cost would make impossible the on line approach. The second one is that the *a priori* knowledge of the size of the marker will allow to find out the point cloud's scale factor and the third one is that it defines the ground level of the scene, that is, the parallel to the XY plane of the coordinate system which is necessary for height estimation.

Parallel to the navigation and photography taking, a point cloud should be generating and updating in the graphical viewer. A patch-based PMVS algorithm [17] was adapted to work in the system. Corners and edges are detected with Harris [28] and difference of gaussians (DoG) [29] respectively. Each point of interest is known as a patch and every patch could appear in more than one image. Each patch keeps growing by finding epipolar consistency in the nearest neighbor of the same patch in another image and they merge according to a photometric consistency criteria measured with cross-correlation. The process works as follows: for every three images a temporary point cloud is generated and it is added to a general cloud which will be updated in the viewer with every addition. Despite the fact that the algorithm does not have an on line nature, it was observed that the processing time of sets of three images of 640x480 pixels adjusted to the time boundary established at the beginning of the research, i.e. one frame per second. In this way, the point cloud increases its number of points as the UAV advances through the environment. The camera pose matrix based on the position of the camera in relation to the marker provides the needed precision for the correct addition of every auxiliary point cloud and avoids outliers and deformations on the modeled objects.

Tombari's *et al.* [30] approach for object detection in a three dimensional space was the implemented algorithm for the marker detection in the point cloud. It is based in a Hough Transform variant [31], formerly used for edge detection in 2D images, adapted for 3D spaces. There are two point clouds: one that will be called *scene*, which is the environment to model itself, and another one called *model* which is a template of the object being searched. The total number of points in both clouds are counted and their normal vectors are computed according to Khoshelman *et al.* [32]. Then, a uniform sampling is performed in order to reduce the number of points dividing the cloud into small squares and approximating all the points within every square to its centroid. This procedure is also useful to reduce computational cost. SHOT descriptors are computed for the remaining points [33] and corresponding points are looked for based on Euclidean distance. If any are found, BOARD algorithm [34] assigns a local reference frame (LRF) to each one in order to make them rotation and translation invariant. Finally, Hough voting is performed to create a histogram of local reference frame orientations. A variable threshold defines the number of point correspondences found and then it can be concluded whether the reference object is present at the scene or not. If the marker has been found, a search for its corners is performed to measure it. The relative size in the point cloud and the absolute size of the marker allow to solve the scale uncertainly. The last step is to modify the RGB values of every point in the cloud according to the real height of it after computing a range based on the extremes in the Z axis. For viewing purposes, an open source and freely available library called Point Cloud Library (PCL) was used for the viewer implementation.

The whole system was programmed in C/C++ and structured in two parts, one for the control of the UAV and for processing the image stream, which also orders to a thread though a pipe to start generating an temporary cloud whenever three images are available, and a second one for adding the temporary cloud to the global one, updating the viewer and start in a thread the search of the marker. The system schema is represented in Fig.1.

A marker based control will not always be possible in big environments or in hazardous areas. For this matter, a way of generating an off-line three dimensional model from images was designed for the system. In this case, we should know the exact $[R|t]$ transformation matrix based on the point cloud's baseline to

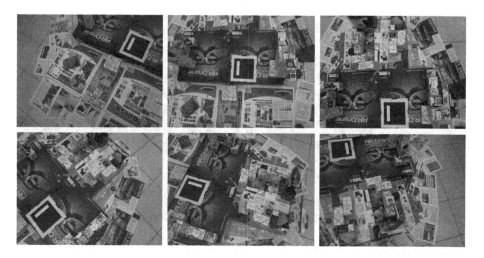

**Fig. 2.** Example of the images used for the presented results

adjust the model floor or zero level to the actual XY plane. Due to its difficulty, this functionality has been limited to the generation of a 3D model regardless a scale factor. This task was accomplished with the ACSfM algorithm [18] which performs image matching with SIFT [35] to compute the camera pose matrices. Finally, the whole set of images is processed with PMVS and the point cloud is generated.

## 4   Results

Two scenarios with different marker sizes where used to validate our proposal. The 3D model and heightmap are shown for both of the scenarios and for one of them an off-line reconstruction was performed with the whole image set to compare the quality between the on line and off line approach.

### 4.1   On-line 3D Modeling

72 images of 640x480 pixels were processed for the generation of the model shown in Fig. 2. Due to camera constrains and because of the need to validate our proposal, images were taken with a Canon Powershot digital camera and sent to the algorithm via simulation. The growing process of the global cloud is shown in Fig.3 and Fig.4 shows the model's 3D profile.

### 4.2   Marker Detection and Heightmap Generation

The heightmap was generated for both scenarios in Fig. 5 and the results are shown in Fig. 6. The dimensions of four known heights $A$, $B$, $C$ and $D$ were used to measure the error. Scenario one is equipped with a 14 by 14 centimeter

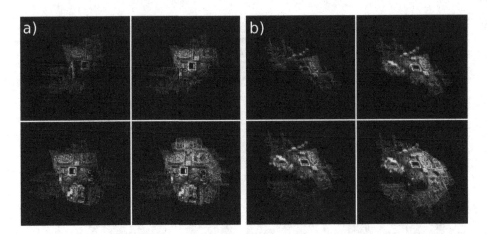

**Fig. 3.** Point cloud on-line growing a) plan view and b) profile view

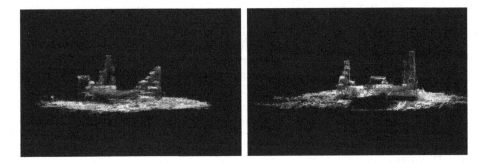

**Fig. 4.** 3D profile of the generated model

**Table 1.** The selected height's real dimensions in scenario one and two

| Scenario | Height A [m] | Height B [m] | Height C [m] | Height D [m] |
|---|---|---|---|---|
| 1 | 0.235 | 0.39 | 0.16 | -0.14 |
| 2 | 0.39 | 0.395 | 0.55 | 0.24 |

maker and scenario two with a 21 by 21 centimeter marker to evaluate the error for equal resolution images with different marker sizes. Measured dimensions of $A,B,C$ and $D$ in both scenarios are shown in Table 1. Table 2 and Table 3 show the estimated height and the error for each scenario respectively.

### 4.3   Off-line 3D Modeling

The presented 3D model was generated from the same 72 640x480 images used in the previous section. The model from different perspectives is shown in Fig.7.

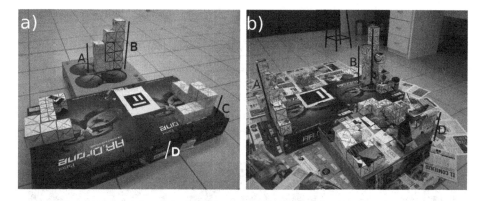

**Fig. 5.** a) Validation scenario one and b) Validation scenario two

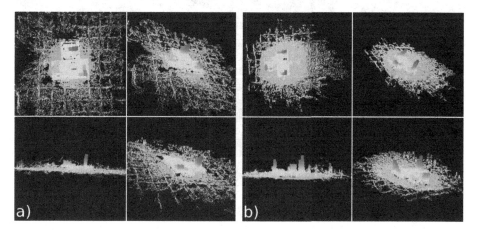

**Fig. 6.** a) Generated heightmap for the scenario one and b) heightmap for the scenario two

**Table 2.** Height estimation results for 14 centimeter marker side in scenario one

| A [m] | B [m] | C [m] | D [m] | Average error [%] | Threshold |
|-------|-------|-------|-------|-------------------|-----------|
| 0.2308 | 0.4046 | 0.1719 | -0.1369 | 3.79 | 0.01 |
| 0.2645 | 0.4477 | 0.1952 | -0.1523 | 14.53 | 0.015 |
| 0.3176 | 0.5474 | 0.2310 | -0.1962 | 40.01 | 0.020 |
| - | - | - | - | - | 0.030 |
| - | - | - | - | - | 0.1 |

## 5   Discussion

The results reported in Table 2 and Table 3 were obtained with 14 centimeter and 21 centimeter markers sides. They are slightly different because not only the marker side and the threshold in Hough voting affect in the scale estimation

**Table 3.** Height estimation results for 21 centimeter marker side in scenario two

| A [m] | B [m] | C [m] | D [m] | Average error [%] | Threshold |
|---|---|---|---|---|---|
| 0.4195 | 0.4098 | 0.5645 | 0.2471 | 4.22 | 0.01 |
| 0.4261 | 0.4039 | 0.5707 | 0.2457 | 4.41 | 0.015 |
| 0.4329 | 0.4143 | 0.5814 | 0.2525 | 6.70 | 0.020 |
| 0.4398 | 0.4181 | 0.5777 | 0.2513 | 7.09 | 0.030 |
| 0.5171 | 0.4985 | 0.7001 | 0.3071 | 28.51 | 0.1 |

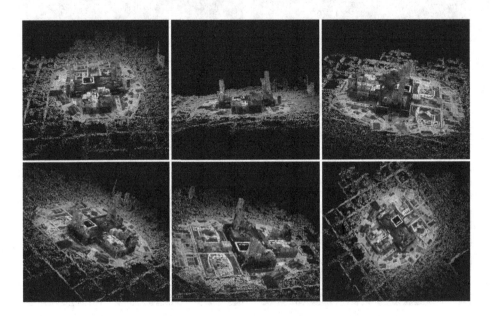

**Fig. 7.** Different perspectives of the off-line 3D generated model

process. The image quality and resolution have a significant influence on the camera pose computing and on the marker detection in the point cloud. The proposed framework also allows to manually select the marker corners, case where the error ranges between 1-1.5%. This lead us to conclude that scale estimation relies on an accurate marker side detection and at the same time, camera pose matrix precision relies on the visual quality of the marker. That is, the higher the image quality and resolution the better results and faster processing time. For autonomous navigation, 640x480 images provide a heightmap in an adequate processing time, enough to accurate fulfill the established requirements of the present work. The aim was at least 1 frame per second and 1.05 frames per second on average were reached in our test. Due to the UAV's constrains, we cannot assert a reliable performance of the proposed framework in outdoor environments with high altitude aerial images. The combination of a SfM algorithm for computing camera poses and a patch-based point cloud generation algorithm provided an accurate, dense and highly detailed 3D model in the off-line approach. This case supposed that the UAV overflew the environment for image acquisition and the system started processing when the UAV landed. As it has been commented before, the point cloud in Fig.7 is up to scale but no absolute scale was recovered. It was achieved a heightmap reconstruction with a manual reference and after applying a transformation matrix to the point cloud in a performed test, however, the rotation angle in each axis and the values of the translation vector were obtained after several trial and error attempts.

## 6    Conclusion

Based on the results it can be concluded that the generated three dimensional model is comparable and even better in terms of visual quality and processing time when compared to the previous work presented in Section 2 in both the on-line and off-line approaches. Also, the height estimation error for the 21 centimeter side marker was smaller than for the 14 centimeter one but suitable and accurate enough in both cases for a safe autonomous navigation through the scenario. It is planned as future work to test the presented framework with real aerial images to study how the area of the environment and the altitude of the UAV affects to the height estimation and height map generation. Processing time reduction, marker-less height map construction, autonomous indoor navigation and collaborative on-line 3D modeling are also planned in the future.

**Acknowledgment.** The authors would like to acknowledge the support of CONACyT for the Master of Science scholarship fund for Ander Larranaga and Carlos Alberto Motta and the support of the CINVESTAV-LTI for the facilities to perform this work. We would also like to acknowledge the authors of the following libraries: OpenMVG, OpenCV, PMVS2 and Point Cloud Library.

## References

1. Gertler, J.: Us unmanned aerial systems. Congressional Research Service (2012)
2. Cetinsoy, E., Dikyar, S., Hancer, C., Oner, K., Sirimoglu, E., Unel, M., Aksit, M.: Design and construction of a novel quad tilt-wing UAV. Mechatronics 22, 723–745 (2012)
3. Sanfourche, M., Delaune, J., Besnerais, G.L.: Perception for UAV: Vision-based navigation and environment modeling. Journal AerospaceLab 4, 1–19 (2012)
4. Sirmacek, B., d'Angelo, P., Krauss, T., Reinartz, P.: Enhancing urban digital elevation models using automated computer vision techniques. In: International Conference on Pattern Recognition (2010)
5. Weibel, R., Heller, M.: Digital Terrain Modelling (1993)
6. Call, B.: Obstacle avoidance for unmanned air vehicles. Master's thesis, Brigham Young University (2006)
7. Besnerais, G., Sanfourche, M., Champagnat, F.: Dense height map estimation from oblique aerial image sequences. Computer Vision and Image Understanding 109, 204–225 (2008)

8. Bills, C., Chen, J., Saxena, A.: Autonomous MAV flight in indoor environments using single image perspective cues. In: International Conference on Robotics and Automation, ICRA (2011)
9. Jimenez-Lugo, J., Zell, A.: Framework for autonomous onboard navigation with the AR.Drone. In: International Conference on Unmanned Aircraft Systems, pp. 575–583 (2013)
10. Engel, J., Sturmand, J., Cremers, D.: Camera-based navigation of a low-cost quadrocopter. In: 2012 IEEE/RSJ International Intelligent Robots and Systems (IROS), vol. 320 (2012)
11. Pollefeys, M., Nistér, D., et al.: Detailed real-time urban 3d reconstruction from video. International Journal of Computer Vision 78, 143–167 (2008)
12. Wen-Chung, C., Shu-An, L.: Real-time feature-based 3d map reconstruction for stereo visual guidance and control of mobile robots in indoor environments. In: 2004 IEEE International Conference on Systems, Man and Cybernetics, vol. 6, pp. 5386–5391 (2008)
13. Diskin, Y., Asari, V.: Dense point-cloud creation using superresolution for a monocular 3d reconstruction system. In: Proc. SPIE 8399, Visual Information Processing XXI, pp. 83990–N–83990N–9 (2012)
14. Motta, C.: Reconstrucc in tridimensional de fachadas de edificios empleando imgenes monoculares obtenidas por un veculo areo no tripulado autnomo. Master's thesis, Centro de Investigacin y de Estudios Avanzados del Instituto Politcnico Nacional (February 2014)
15. Scaramuzza, D., Fraundorfer, F., Pollefeys, M., Siegwart, R.: Absolute scale in structure from motion from a single vehicle mounted camera by exploiting nonholonomic constraints. In: 2009 IEEE 12th International Conference on Computer Vision, pp. 1413–1419 (2009)
16. Garrido-Jurado, S., Muñoz-Salinas, R., Madrid-Cuevas, F., Marín-Jiménez, M.: Automatic generation and detection of highly reliable fiducial markers under occlusion. Pattern Recognition 47(6), 2280–2292 (2014)
17. Furukawa, Y., Ponce, J.: Accurate, dense, and robust multi-view stereopsis. Pattern Analysis and Machine Intelligence 32(8), 1362–1376 (2010)
18. Moulon, P., Monasse, P., Marlet, R.: Adaptive structure from motion with a contrario model estimation. In: Lee, K.M., Matsushita, Y., Rehg, J.M., Hu, Z. (eds.) ACCV 2012, Part IV. LNCS, vol. 7727, pp. 257–270. Springer, Heidelberg (2013)
19. Barazzetti, L., Scaioni, M.: Orientation and 3D modelling from markerless terrestrial images: Combining accuracy with automation. The Photogrammetric Record, vol. 25, p. 2010 (2013)
20. Weiss, S., Achtelik, M., Kneip, L., Scaramuzza, D., Siegwart, R.: Intuitive 3D maps for MAV terrain exploration and obstacle avoidance. Journal of Intelligent and Robotics Systems 61(1-4), 473–493 (2011)
21. Davison, A.: Real-time simultaneous localisation and mapping with a single camera. In: 2003 Proceedings of the Ninth IEEE International Conference on Computer Vision, vol. 2, pp. 1403–1141 (2003)
22. Mian, A., Bennamoun, M., Owens, R.: On the repeatability and quality of keypoints for local feature-based 3d object retrieval from cluttered scenes. International Journal of Computer Vision 89, 348–361 (2010)
23. Chen, H., Bhanu, B.: 3d free-form object recognition in range images using local surface patches. Pattern Recognition Letters 28, 1252–1262 (2007)
24. Zhong, Y.: Intrinsic shape signatures: A shape descriptor for 3d object recognition. In: Proc. 3DRR Workshop (in conj. with ICCV), pp. 689–696 (2009)

25. Lamdan, Y., Wolfson, H.: Geometric hasing: A general and efficient model-based recognition scheme. In: Proc. Int. Conf. on Computer Vision, pp. 238–249 (1988)
26. Gwimson, W., Huttenlocker, D.: On the sensitivity of geometric hashing. In: Proc. Int. Conf. on Computer Vision, pp. 334–338 (1990)
27. Lamdan, Y., Wolfson, H.: On the error analysis of geometric hashing. In: Proc. IEEE Conf. on Computer Vision, pp. 22–27 (1991)
28. Harris, C., Stephens, M.: A combined corner and edge detector. In: Proceedings of the 4th Alvey Vision Conference, pp. 147–151 (1988)
29. Marr, D., Hildreth, E.: Theory of edge detection. In: Proceedings of the Royal Society of London, pp. 215–217 (1980)
30. Tombari, F., Stefano, L.D.: Object recognition in 3d scenes with occlusions and clutter by hough voting. In: 4th Pacific-Rim Symposium on Image and Video Technology, pp. 349–355 (2010)
31. Hough, P.: Method and means for recognizing complex patterns (1962)
32. Khoshelham, K.: Extending generalized hough transform to detect 3d objects in laser range data. In: Proc. ISPRS Workshop on Laser Scanning, pp. 206–210 (2007)
33. Tombari, F., Salti, S., DiStefano, L.: Unique signatures of histograms for local surface description. In: ECCV 2013 Proceedings of the 11th European Conference on Computer Vision Conference on Computer vision, pp. 356–369 (2010)
34. Petrelli, A., Stefano, L.D.: On the repeatability of the local reference frame for partial shape matching. In: 13th International Conference on Computer Vision (ICCV), pp. 2244–2251 (2011)
35. Lowe, D.: Distinctive image features from scale-invariant key points. International Journal of Computer Vision 60(2), 91–110 (2004)

# An Improved Colorimetric Invariants and RGB-Depth-Based Codebook Model for Background Subtraction Using Kinect

Julian Murgia[1], Cyril Meurie[2], and Yassine Ruichek[1]

[1] IRTES-SeT, UTBM, 90010 Belfort Cedex, France
{julian.murgia,yassine.ruichek}@utbm.fr
[2] Univ Lille Nord de France, F-59000 Lille,
IFSTTAR, LEOST, F59650, Villeneuve d'Ascq
cyril.meurie@ifsttar.fr

**Abstract.** In this paper we propose to join the benefits of multiple invariant information into the well-know background subtraction method "Codebook". Indeed, this method mainly repose on a color model allowing a separate process of color and intensity distortion. In order to manage hard situations involving high illumination changes, we propose to enhance this model with the use of two supplementary steps: 1/ transforming the input color image using a colorimetric invariant in order to obtain a color-invariant image whatever the illumination conditions; 2/ using depth information as a new data inside the Codebook model, thus performing an RGB-D fusion during the segmentation process.

**Keywords:** Image color analysis, subtraction techniques, segmentation, object detection, colorimetric invariants, RGB-D, fusion.

## 1 Introduction

Objects detection is a very common step in severals applications of Intelligent Transportation Systems. Its use is integrated into many applications in various domains, such as videosurveillance, pedestrian and/or vehicle detection, detection of hazardous situations in public transports[7][19][18].

Multiple methods have been proposed to address this issue [3][2][15], from simplest techniques to more sophisticated. Basically, background subtraction consists in modeling the background from a sequence of images, then compare this background model to every new frame obtained from the camera to finally obtain a foreground segmentation. Depending on each method, the model computation can be made at pixel level of image, or at region-level after a simplification of image. The representation of every part of the model is independant.

Among the most known representations, multimodal distribution methods are known to provide the better results, such as the very common method Generalized Mixture Of Gaussians (MOG) [21][22]. In this case, each pixel is modeled by a mixture of $n$ gaussian distributions depending on the pixel value. Then, a

A. Gelbukh et al. (Eds.): MICAI 2014, Part I, LNAI 8856, pp. 380–392, 2014.
© Springer International Publishing Switzerland 2014

match is being searched between each pixel of the new frame and the model. If a match is found, then the pixel is background, else it is foreground. This kind of representation allows a modeling of more complex backgrounds but the method depends on a learning parameter.

Kim et al. propose the Codebook algorithm [13] that doesn't make use of a learning rate parameter and provides generally good detection results. Recent results shows that even if the Codebook can adapt to little illumination changes, it is very sensible to strong changes which can occur in the scene when the model is not yet adapted. This paper is an attempt to tackle this kind of problems.

In the past few years, great use was made of RGB-D cameras such as Kinect distributed by Microsoft®, or Xtion Pro Live distributed by Asus®. These sensors provide high-resolution depth maps in real time at a very low cost. Depth information is estimated by the combination of an infra-red emitter and a standard CMOS sensor. The camera determines the quantity of infra-red light reflected by the scene. The closer the object, the greater the quantity of light reflected.

The use of a fourth component in BGS method can be tackled in different ways: considering it as a separate information, thus performing a background subtraction on RGB components in one hand and the new information in the other hand, and only after fuse the results using a simple boolean condition [14], or include the new information into the background model [8]. In most of cases, noise can be observed in resulting segmentations.

The use of colorimetric invariants proposed previously helped the algorithm to provide usable segmentations even when the background model is desynchronized from the current scene [16]. But, as color information is highly dependant of observation conditions (dark, lit, fog, rain, snow...), colorimetric invariance is not necessarily sufficient to provide strong results. To improve further in this direction, additional invariant data can then be used by the algorithm to perform an ever better segmentation. The Codebook representation method is flexible enough to make use of color and brightness information but also any kind of supplementary data for the model can be provided. We then propose in this paper to merge the use colorimetric invariants with RGB-D fusion inside the Codebook algorithm.

In this paper, we will first describe the main components involved in our contribution. That is, a recap of the Codebook method and its improvement for the use of depth information will be done in Part 2. A brief recall of the concept of colorimetric invariants will be made in Part 3, as well as a short presentation of those which turned out to be the most interesting in our cases. Finally, results and observations will be given in Part 4.

## 2 Codebook

Background modelisation is made by the Codebook method proposed by Kim et al [13]. This method has become a reference in many fields of research such as detection and tracking of moving objects. It is robust and efficient in a wide number of use cases, including dynamic backgrounds (tree foliages, foutains, sea shores, flags...) and little illumination changes.

This algorithm was driven by the following observation: false detections are generally situated in dark zones of the image. Therefore, as the color of pixels define their darkness or brightness, color should be used as an important factor in the comparison of two pixels. This reflection led to the creation of a new color model used inside the algorithm to evaluate separately color and brightness of pixels.

## 2.1   Learning

Codebook algorithm consists in a clustering of the image to build a background model from a learning period. This model is represented by a list of Codebooks (1 per pixel) each containing a certain number of codewords. A codeword is created (or updated if the observed pixel's representation is similar to an existing codeword) for each pixel of every frame of the learning sequence. A codeword contains two vectors, respectively R,G and B values of the pixel, and other data such minimum and maximum observed brightness, temporal data and frequency of occurrence. During this phase, a new codeword obtained for a given pixel is integrated in the background model if it satisfies two conditions:

1. brightness constraint: the intensity must lie in the interval $[L_{low}; L_{high}]$ determined from all the minimum $L_{min}$ and maximum $L_{max}$ brightness observed for this pixel. This range of brightness delimits the range under which a codeword is considered as shadow, and above which it is considered as highlight. For each codeword, we have :

$$L_{low} = \alpha L_{min},$$
$$L_{high} = min(\beta L_{max}, \frac{L_{min}}{\alpha}) \tag{1}$$

where $\alpha < 1$ and $\beta > 1$ are fixed parameters of the algorithm.

2. color distorsion constraint: the color distorsion $\delta$ of the pixel and the codeword must lie under a given threshold $\epsilon$. This $\delta$ value is calculated from input pixel RGB values and the tested codeword.

After the background model construction, the algorithm optimizes its size by determining Codewords corresponding to pixels erroneously integrated as background pixels. A Codeword $m$ is defined by a pair of vectors $V_m = [\bar{R}, \bar{G}, \bar{B}]$ and $Aux_m = [I^m_{min}, I^m_{max}, f_m, \lambda_m, t, l]$. $V_m$ defines the average value of each component. $I^m_{min}$ and $I^m_{max}$ define minimum and maximum brightness respectively, of all observations that match to codeword $m$. $\lambda_m$ denoted as Maximum Negative Run-Length (MNRL) is defined as the longest interval of time during which the codeword $m$ has not been updated. $p$ and $q$ define first and last times of update of codeword $m$, respectively.

## 2.2  Foreground/Background Detection

The final background model represents the parts of an image that does not move. It is then possible to compare each Codebook to determine whether an observed pixel belongs to background or not. More simply, the existence of a similar Codeword in the model for this pixel's Codebook is tesed, using the same constraints quoted before. If a Codeword matches this pixel, then it belongs to background (black in segmentations). If no match is found, this pixel is marked as foreground (white in segmentations). After foreground detection phase is executed for each pixel, the algorithm updates the background codebooks model.

## 2.3  Codebook RGB-D

Disparity information can be used into the Codebook algorithm by incorporating a new data obtained from the disparity map. As disparity is a 1D information, it can be treated the same way as brightness. The modification made to the algorithm is the addition of a new value in the first vector of Codewords, containing the disparity of the corresponding pixel, that is: $V_m = [\bar{R}, \bar{G}, \bar{B}, \bar{D}]$. Also, new values are added into the second vector of Codeword: low disparity $D_{low}$ and high disparity $D_{hi}$ values, representing the disparity range allowed for input values, as defined in Equation 2.

$$D_{low} = \alpha_D D_{max}$$
$$D_{hi} = min\{\beta_D D_{max}, \tfrac{D_{min}}{\alpha_D}\} \tag{2}$$

having $D_{min}$ and $D_{max}$ respectively the minimum and maximum disparities observed for this pixel. $\alpha_D$ and $\beta_D$ are thresholds in the depths distortion, defined the same way as for brightness distortion. $\alpha_D$ value is typically between 0.4 and 0.7, $\beta_D$ between 1.1 and 1.5. Then, the new disparity distortion function described in Equation 3 is used during both learning and process phase:

$$disparityDist(D, \langle D_{min}, D_{max}\rangle) = \begin{cases} true & isInvalid(D) \vee (D_{hi} \leq D \leq D_{low}) \\ false & otherwise \end{cases}$$

$$\tag{3}$$

$D$ is the tested disparity, and $isInvalid()$ function determines whether $D$ is erroneous. Typically, a disparity value of 0 denotes an invalid disparity. A matching between the observed pixel and an existing codeword means it satisfies those three conditions: color, brightness and disparity distorsions. The decision function determining whether a pixel $x$ matches a codeword $c_m$ is described in Equation 4. If a pixel matches a codeword in the background model, it is also considered as background (BG), else as foreground (FG).

$$decision(x) = \begin{cases} BG & if\ (colorDist(x) \leq \epsilon_1 \vee \\ & (\epsilon_1 < colorDist(x, c_m) \leq \epsilon_2 \\ & \wedge disparityDist(D, \langle D_{min}, D_{max}\rangle)))\wedge \\ & brightnessDist(I, \langle I_{min}, I_{max}\rangle)\wedge \\ & disparityDist(D, \langle D_{min}, D_{max}\rangle) \\ FG & otherwise \end{cases} \tag{4}$$

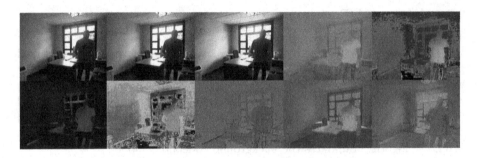

**Fig. 1.** Color invariants and color models used. From left to right and top to bottom: original RGB, Greyworld, RGB-Rank, L*a*b*, HSL, Opposite Colorspace, l1l2l3, c1c2c3, YIQ, YCbCr.

Equation 4 describes the pixel classification decision. If the disparity attached to this pixel is valid and comprised between acceptable thresholds, the decision function takes it into account. Otherwise,only color and brightness distorsions are considered. If a matching occurs, the pixel is set as background. Otherwise, it is classified as foreground.

After the segmentation process is done, we applied a chain of morphological operators in order to remove false positives remaining in the background, and holes filling to get plain silhouettes when possible.

## 3   Color Invariance

Prior to any Codebook-related action, we propose to apply a colorimetric invariant to modify the color aspect of the image to give it the aspect it would have under a canonical illuminant. This concept assumes that one can perceive the color of an object, whichever the color of the illuminant. To perform this task, it is necessary to estimate this illuminant color. Multiple methods can achieve this, which can be sorted into 3 categories:

1. Use of low-level characteristics: these methods are based on low-level statistics or a dichromatic reflection model, physics-based
2. Use of a learning phase: the illuminant is determined using a model obtained from a learning dataset
3. A combination of these two methods.

Every colorimetric invariance method does not produce identic images. They often need to create a new model, adapted to the characteritics they make use of. Therefore, no method can be considered as "universal". Some works also consist in a combination of multiple strategies: Gijsenij et al. [12] showed that different colorimetric invariance algorithms perform better on different types of images; Bianco et al. [1] proposed a CART-based algorithm to choose the best colorimetric invariant for a given image, using a decision forest technique. In this paper, we prefer testing several colorimetric invariants: Greyworld [4],

Affine Normalization [17], Chromaticity Space, Comprehensive Normalization [10], Opposite Colorspace, Reduced Coordinates, m1m2m3, l1l2l3 and c1c2c3 [11], YIQ [5], YCh1Ch2 [6], YCbCr, RGB-Rank [9], CIE L*a*b*, HSL color models [20].

Figure 1 shows some invariant images tested from one RGB image and used as input images in the Codebook algorithm.

# 4    Results and Observations

## 4.1    Dataset, Tests and Metrics

Images acquisitions have been made in a room six times at different moments of day, implying different lighting conditions. The scenario for all bases is the same: a person enters the room, walk before his desk, then after, sits down on a chair, stays for a while, then stands up and walks out. Figure 2 shows six images taken from each database. In certain cases, the curtains are closed and light can be turned off, in order to simulate a very difficult case when the room is very dark.

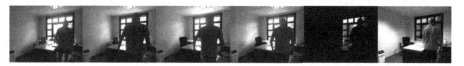

**Fig. 2.** Original color images from images L1 to L6

These six cases provide different tests to determine the benefits of the RGB-D fusion inside the Codebook when applied to different bases and not up-to-date learning bases, because illuminations and colors are very different from one base to another. That is, learnings are applied on 50 frames (RGB and disparity maps obtained from the Kinect) from each learning base, with every tested colorimetric invariant or color model. From each of these learnings, we compute segmentations for all six processing bases, using corresponding colorimetric invariant / color model as well. Thus, a naming convention was created for each test performed: we call $Lx$ the learning bases and $Px$ the processing bases, where $x$ is the number of the corresponding base as enumerated before. Consequently, a test named L1_P3 defines a test where the learning was done with base 1 and the process was done with base 3. Of course, a colorimetric invariant name (or color model) is attached to every test.

The use of color-invariant images is supposed to increase the robustness of the Codebook model. As a consequence, the codebook algorithm was also modified to avoid the model update occurring after the detection phase of the Codebook process. This way, we were able to obserse the effects of colorimetric invariants on adaptative as well as fixed RGB and RGB-D codebook model. Non-adaptative codebooks correspond to algorithms which do not update their background model while adaptative codebooks do update their model. This detail is critical in the way to compare results, since these two modes do not correspond to the same algorithm anymore. Therefore, adaptive Codebooks results can be compared only with each other, as non-adaptive Codebooks can be compared only amongst them.

To evaluate our method and be able to perform a quantitative analysis, hand-segmented ground truths were produced. Relatives measures Recall and Precision were then calculated using true/false positives and true/false negatives (TP, FP, TN, FN) for *both* foreground and background classes. This choice is motivated by the fact that considering the effectiveness of the Codebook (RGB) algorithm, the improvements the new method including disparity will mostly be situated in the background zones of the images. These measures are then combined into an accuracy metric, F-Measure *FM* to evaluate the quality of the segmentions. Recall, Precision and F-Measure are defined as follows:

$$Recall_{fg} = \frac{TP}{TP+FN}, \qquad Recall_{bg} = \frac{TN}{TN+FP},$$
$$Precision_{fg} = \frac{TP}{TP+FP}, \qquad Precision_{bg} = \frac{TN}{TN+FN}, \qquad (5)$$
$$FM_c = \frac{2.(Recall_c.Precision_c)}{Recall_c+Precision_c}$$

Tests were performed with a learning base image L1 constituted of 50 images. Codebook values used are: $\alpha_c = 0.4, \beta_c = 1.7, \alpha_D = 0.75, \beta_D = 1.25, \epsilon_1 = 10, \epsilon_2 = 16$. These values were determined empirically to allow the algorithm to produce interesting enough results with every tested database.

## 4.2    Results and Analysis

Tables 1 and 3 display mean F-measures corresponding to Codebook RGB algorithms, non-adaptative and adaptative respectively. Positive (bold values) and negative values describe respectively improvement and deterioration, refering to values obtained without any use of colorimetric invariants or color spaces. More precisely, Chromaticity Space, RGB-Rank, c1c2c3, L*a*b* and HSL provided the best results amongst all tested colorimetric invariants and color models. Red and green values indicate for each line the maximum and minimum value, respectively. In the case of non-adaptative Codebook RGB, gains appear important. Chromaticity Space especially provide the best results improvements, between +22% and +77% for background regions and between 0% and +46% for foreground regions, even though improvements are brought by every colorimetric invariant displayed in Table 1.

Depth information usage in non-adaptative Codebook RGB-D to improve these results showed interesting results as well, as showed in Table 2. In this table, F-Measures appear a little lower than in Table 1, even though improvements still remain situated between +33% and +70% in background, and between +13% and 42% in foreground. Again, Chromatictiy Space showed the best results in this case.

Figures 3, 4 and 5 show segmentations obtained when the learning was performed on L1 (first database, corresponding to the top-left corner image) with three algorithm versions presented, respectively adaptative Codebook RGB, non-adaptative Codebook RGB-D and adaptative Codebook RGB-D. Tests were

**Table 1.** F-Measures gains and deteriorations for non-adaptative Codebook RGB

|  | cs | | rgb-r | | c1c2c3 | | hsl | | yiq | | ych1ch2 | | lab | |
|---|---|---|---|---|---|---|---|---|---|---|---|---|---|---|
|  | bg | fg | bg | fg | bg | fg | bg | fg | bg | fg | bg | fg | bg | fg |
| L1_P1 | 45,5% | 45,7% | 31,8% | 20,2% | 43,5% | 39,6% | 31,2% | 15,3% | 26,7% | 22,6% | 8,2% | 9,2% | 41,1% | 45,0% |
| L1_P2 | 57,3% | 43,6% | 40,7% | 12,5% | 52,4% | 32,3% | 31,0% | 6,3% | 40,9% | 15,3% | 10,2% | 1,0% | 51,2% | 37,0% |
| L1_P3 | 60,2% | 39,6% | 43,5% | 11,9% | 45,0% | 23,8% | 20,4% | 4,9% | 12,9% | 38,4% | 6,4% | 0,4% | 39,4% | 22,2% |
| L1_P4 | 34,7% | 31,6% | 23,3% | 16,8% | 33,0% | 25,7% | 21,1% | 8,3% | 19,6% | 10,7% | -10,8% | -1,6% | 36,2% | 41,9% |
| L1_P5 | 22,9% | 0,4% | 2,9% | 0,2% | 21,1% | 0,3% | 14,5% | 0,5% | 22,7% | 0,2% | 12,3% | 0,4% | 6,2% | 0,3% |
| L1_P6 | 76,8% | 14,8% | 43,6% | 4,2% | 57,2% | 8,0% | 23,9% | 2,0% | 9,4% | 1,1% | 19,0% | 1,4% | 8,4% | 1,2% |
| Average | 49,6% | 29,3% | 31,0% | 11,0% | 42,0% | 21,6% | 23,7% | 6,2% | 22,0% | 8,9% | 7,5% | 1,8% | 30,4% | 24,6% |

**Table 2.** F-Measures gains and deteriorations for non-adaptative Codebook RGB-D

|  | cs | | rgb-r | | c1c2c3 | | hsl | | yiq | | ych1ch2 | | lab | |
|---|---|---|---|---|---|---|---|---|---|---|---|---|---|---|
|  | bg | fg | bg | fg | bg | fg | bg | fg | bg | fg | bg | fg | bg | fg |
| L1_P1 | 34,9% | 38,1% | 26,4% | 33,8% | 33,9% | 31,8% | 22,1% | 6,9% | 13,5% | 6,7% | -2,7% | -4,2% | 28,2% | 31,9% |
| L1_P2 | 51,9% | 41,3% | 43,2% | 25,6% | 48,5% | 30,8% | 11,5% | 1,1% | 15,8% | 4,1% | -4,5% | -1,1% | 40,3% | 31,5% |
| L1_P3 | 50,1% | 41,5% | 41,9% | 23,7% | 45,8% | 29,8% | 15,4% | 4,5% | -4,9% | 2,3% | -4,7% | -0,8% | 25,6% | 20,0% |
| L1_P4 | 18,7% | 22,2% | 13,0% | 19,5% | 16,7% | 15,3% | 7,2% | 0,4% | -9,7% | -5,7% | -31,3% | -12,1% | 29,1% | 21,0% |
| L1_P5 | 14,4% | 0,6% | -1,6% | 0,0% | 13,8% | 0,6% | 9,1% | 0,4% | 33,6% | 3,0% | 5,5% | 0,1% | 3,6% | 0,3% |
| L1_P6 | 70,3% | 13,5% | 51,7% | 6,1% | 56,0% | 8,5% | 24,7% | 2,2% | 2,0% | 0,6% | 19,0% | 1,4% | 3,4% | 0,6% |
| Average | 40,0% | 26,2% | 29,1% | 18,1% | 35,8% | 19,4% | 15,0% | 2,6% | 8,4% | 1,8% | -3,1% | -2,8% | 20,1% | 18,9% |

**Table 3.** F-Measures gains and deteriorations for adaptative Codebook RGB

|  | cs | | rgb-r | | c1c2c3 | | hsl | | yiq | | ych1ch2 | | lab | |
|---|---|---|---|---|---|---|---|---|---|---|---|---|---|---|
|  | bg | fg | bg | fg | bg | fg | bg | fg | bg | fg | bg | fg | bg | fg |
| L1_P1 | 3,0% | -19,2% | 1,8% | 0,3% | 2,6% | -16,8% | 3,3% | 10,3% | 3,2% | 0,2% | 1,5% | 3,5% | 3,0% | -15,5% |
| L1_P2 | -0,1% | 0,0% | 0,6% | 0,0% | 0,0% | 0,0% | -0,2% | 0,0% | -0,4% | 0,0% | -0,8% | 0,0% | 0,3% | 0,0% |
| L1_P3 | -0,2% | 5,7% | 0,6% | 3,7% | -0,1% | -4,7% | 0,8% | 14,7% | -0,5% | -0,3% | -3,1% | -2,5% | 0,3% | -2,3% |
| L1_P4 | 0,4% | 7,0% | 0,3% | 4,7% | -0,2% | -2,0% | 0,4% | 8,9% | 0,6% | 1,0% | 0,8% | 7,7% | -0,1% | -1,7% |
| L1_P5 | -1,9% | -11,3% | -7,8% | 16,2% | -3,3% | -16,5% | -0,5% | -2,1% | -5,2% | -13,0% | 1,5% | -6,7% | -1,5% | -6,9% |
| L1_P6 | -1,2% | -52,1% | -0,7% | -11,5% | -1,6% | -50,9% | 0,8% | -19,5% | -0,5% | -8,4% | -1,4% | -10,5% | -0,8% | -37,3% |
| Average | 0,0% | -11,7% | -0,8% | 2,2% | -0,4% | -15,2% | 0,5% | 2,1% | -0,5% | -3,4% | -0,2% | -0,8% | 0,2% | -10,6% |

**Table 4.** F-Measures gains and deteriorations for adaptative Codebook RGB-D

|  | cs | | rgb-r | | c1c2c3 | | hsl | | yiq | | ych1ch2 | | lab | |
|---|---|---|---|---|---|---|---|---|---|---|---|---|---|---|
|  | bg | fg | bg | fg | bg | fg | bg | fg | bg | fg | bg | fg | bg | fg |
| L1_P1 | 1,4% | 10,6% | -0,2% | 0,2% | 1,4% | 13,3% | 0,3% | 12,1% | -1,3% | 1,8% | -0,9% | 4,9% | -0,4% | 0,6% |
| L1_P2 | -1,4% | 12,0% | 0,5% | 4,4% | 0,7% | 17,5% | -0,3% | 15,8% | -0,7% | 6,5% | -0,4% | 6,9% | 0,2% | 5,3% |
| L1_P3 | -0,1% | 8,6% | 0,6% | 4,9% | 0,4% | 14,1% | 0,5% | 12,7% | -0,8% | 3,1% | -1,4% | 4,8% | 0,1% | 1,1% |
| L1_P4 | -0,8% | 11,5% | 0,3% | 4,2% | 0,7% | 14,1% | 0,6% | 13,4% | 0,9% | 6,2% | 0,8% | 10,3% | 0,1% | 2,5% |
| L1_P5 | -1,6% | 17,9% | -5,8% | 24,3% | -4,3% | 8,5% | 0,2% | 14,0% | -5,3% | -9,6% | 0,4% | -3,8% | -2,0% | -3,9% |
| L1_P6 | -0,4% | -29,9% | -0,1% | -4,6% | -0,4% | -23,1% | 0,2% | 4,7% | -0,6% | -6,5% | -0,8% | -0,9% | 0,1% | -12,2% |
| Average | -0,2% | 5,1% | -0,8% | 5,6% | -0,2% | 7,4% | 0,2% | 12,1% | -1,3% | 0,2% | -0,4% | 3,7% | -0,3% | -1,1% |

processed on all databases, from L1 to L6 in the following order, with every colorimetric invariant and color model separately. Learning and process phases were done using the same colorimetric invariant or color model for both phases.

The quality of segmentations obtained with adaptative Codebook RGB (Figure 3) is low as no average F-Measure came upper than 2.2% and 0.5% improvement in foreground and background classes respectively. This did not allow a post-processing operation to provide better results. Noise is observed in the background parts of images and foreground silhouettes were not homogen enough to allow a proper reconstruction.

Figures 4 and 5, in another hand, display results making use of depth information. In these two cases, a post-processing was applied consisting in performing morphological operations (closing, opening, holes filling) in order to remove noise and false positives in the background as well as to improve silhouettes shapes.

Figure 5 shows results with the adaptative Codebook as it provided the best results (with post-processing). These segmentations lead to some first qualitative

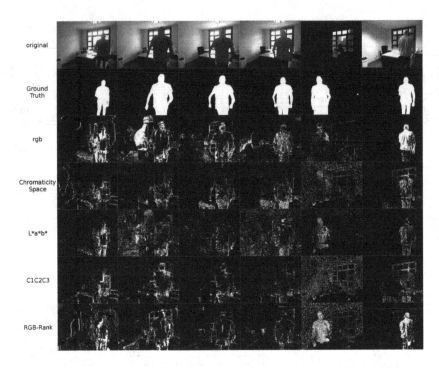

**Fig. 3.** Segmentations obtained with algorithm adaptative Codebook RGB with a learning on L1. From left to right: P1 to P6 processes. Bottom lines display most interesting colorimetric invariants and color models according to our results.

observations: when processing original images (line 3) depending on the moment of day, hollowed foreground appear and noised background remain in results. Tests driven with the use of colorimetric invariants helped the filling of foreground silhouettes, especially in L1_P5 case: at the price of a higher background noise (-0.2%), c1c2c3 increased the foreground F-Measure by 7.4%. In certain test cases though (L1_P4), the improvement is less visible.

Certain colorimetric invariants such as YCbCr, YCh1Ch1 or m1m2m3 do not converge towards one similar image. Depending on the moments of the day, two images which look originally similar can look very different when using one colorimetric invariant on both. Moreover, certain colorimetric invariants (ie: l1l2l3, Opposite colorspace, HSL...) do not output "real world color" images. This state of fact explains some results less interesting than others, depending on databases.

Previous qualitative observations are confirmed by F-Measure values. Results obtained in [16] with Codebook RGB are very similar, as we obtain slightly better results with certain colorimetric invariants increasing F-Measures. Non-adaptative Codebooks (RGB and RGB-D) effectively improve more importantly the F-Measure values for both foreground and background classes than adaptative Codebooks do. Table 1 demontrates these improvements as F-Measure increase up to 78% for background and 45% foreground (with Codebook RGB

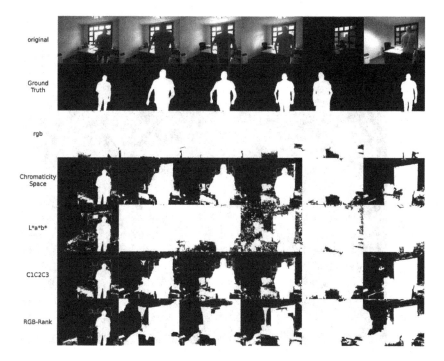

**Fig. 4.** Segmentations obtained with algorithm non-adaptative Codebook RGB-D with a learning on L1. From left to right: P1 to P6 processes. Bottom lines display most interesting colorimetric invariants and color models according to our results. Segmentations are filtered with morphological operators.

and Chromaticity space color invariant). Table 2 also shows improvements as F-Measure increase up to 70% for background and more than 40% in foreground (with Codebook RGB-D and Chromaticity space color invariant). More globally, these results confirm the interest of the use of colorimetric invariant to improve the segmentation of moving objects.

As statued previously, depth inclusion into the codebook algorithm globally improves segmentations quality by $+7\%$ for foreground class and $+5\%$ for background class when using original RGB images jointly with depth values in $L_x\_P_x$ cases (learning and processing bases are the same).

When learning and process times are different $(L_x\_P_y)$ cases, of course F-Measure decrease since these cases are more difficult. When no colorimetric invariant is used, foreground F-Measures decrease below 22% and 50%. But even then, colorimetric invariants such as c1c2c3, Chromaticity space, RGB-Rank, HSL and YCh1Ch2 improve foreground F-Measure in certain cases by more than 40%. One can also notice that these average values are widely reduced by L1_P6 average F-Measures. This denotes a limit of the method: very time-shifted databases are diffult for the algorithm to manage, and colorimetric invariants are not sufficient enough to limit this effect, which denote the need of a proper learning update even if it can be shifted. When no improvement is brought,

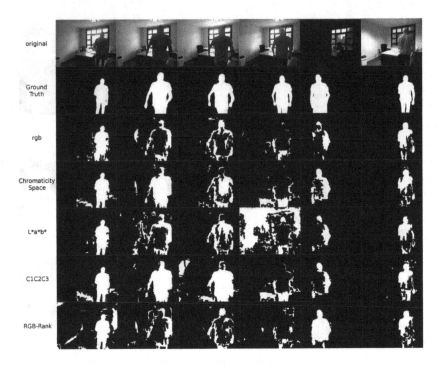

**Fig. 5.** Segmentations obtained with algorithm adaptative Codebook RGB-D with a learning on L1. Bottom lines display most interesting colorimetric invariants and color models according to our results. Post-processing is applied after segmentation.

no noticeable deterioration exists either. This means that for best colorimetric invariants, results are at least very close to results obtained when using original images, at best they are better. Little deteriorations are observed in background class while this method interestingly improves detection quality of foreground class. These results confirm the benefits of the joint use of depth in a background subtraction technique as well as the use of modified images with colorimetric invariants or different color spaces.

## 5    Conclusion

In this paper, we have proposed a new solution for foreground detection methods involving colorimetric invariance and RGB-D fusion. Depth information collected from active sensors were used together with different colorimetric invariant modified images, thus occasionally providing better segmentation results. This method opens a door for future works dealing with difficult, indoor and outdoor environments which often cause detection problems because of important lighting changes. Future works should propose a different way to manage the color constancy inside the background model, and determine the best colorimetric invariance method according to each situation.

# References

1. Bianco, S., Ciocca, G., Cusano, C., Schettini, R.: Automatic color constancy algorithm selection and combination. Pattern Recognition 43(3), 695–705 (2010)
2. Bouwmans, T., Baf, F.E.: Statistical background modeling for foreground detection: A survey. In: Handbook of Pattern Recognition and Computer (2010)
3. Bouwmans, T., Baf, F.E., Vachon, B., et al.: Background modeling using mixture of gaussians for foreground detection-a survey (2008)
4. Buchsbaum, G.: A spatial processor model for object colour perception. Journal of the Franklin Institute (1980)
5. Buchsbaum, W.H.: Color TV Servicing, third edition. Prentice Hall, Englewood Cliffs (1975)
6. Carron, T.: Segmentation d'images couleur dans la base Teinte Luminance Saturation: approche numerique et symbolique. PhD thesis, Universite de Stanford (1995)
7. Truong Cong, D.-N., Khoudour, L., Achard, C., Meurie, C., Lezoray, O.: People re-identification by spectral classification of silhouettes. Signal Processing 90(8), 2362–2374 (2010), Special Section on Processing and Analysis of High-Dimensional Masses of Image and Signal Data
8. Fernandez-Sanchez, E.J., Diaz, J., Ros, E.: Background subtraction based on color and depth using active sensors. Sensors 13(7), 8895–8915 (2013)
9. Finlayson, G.D., Hordley, S.D., Schaefer, G., Tian, G.Y.: Illuminant and device invariant colour using histogram equalisation. In: Pattern Recognition (2005)
10. Finlayson, G.D., Schiele, B., Crowley, J.L.: Comprehensive colour image normalization (1998)
11. Gevers, T.: Arnold W.M. Smeulders. Color-based object recognition. Pattern Recognition (1999)
12. Gijsenij, A., Gevers, T.: Color constancy using natural image statistics and scene semantics. IEEE Transactions on Pattern Analysis and Machine Intelligence (2010)
13. Kim, K., Chalidabhongse, T.H., Hanuood, D., Davis, L.: Background modeling and substraction by codebook construction (2004)
14. Leykin, A.: Robust multi-pedestrian tracking in thermal-visible surveillance videos. In: In and Beyond the Visible Spectrum Workshop at the International Conference on Computer Vision and Pattern Recognition, vol. 136, pp. 0–136 (2006)
15. Mcivor, A.M.: Background Subtraction Techniques (2000)
16. Murgia, J., Meurie, C., Ruichek, Y.: Improvement of moving objects detection in continued all-day illumination conditions using color invariants and color spaces (2013)
17. Obdrzalek, S., Matas, J., Chum, O.: On the interaction between object recognition and colour constancy. In: Proc. International Workshop on Color and Photometric Methods in Computer Vision (2003)
18. Salmane, H., Ruichek, Y., Khoudour, L.: Gaussian Propagation Model Based Dense Optical Flow for Objects Tracking. In: Campilho, A., Kamel, M. (eds.) ICIAR 2012, Part I. LNCS, vol. 7324, pp. 234–244. Springer, Heidelberg (2012)
19. Salmane, H., Ruichek, Y., Khoudour, L.: Using Hidden Markov Model and Dempster-Shafer Theory for Evaluating and Detecting Dangerous Situations in Level Crossing Environments. In: Batyrshin, I., González Mendoza, M. (eds.) MICAI 2012, Part I. LNCS, vol. 7629, pp. 131–145. Springer, Heidelberg (2013)
20. Smith, A.R.: Color gamut transform pairs. In: SIGGRAPH Comput. Graph (1978)

21. Stauffer, C., Grimson, W.E.L.: Adaptive background mixture models for real-time tracking. In: IEEE Computer Society Conference on Computer Vision and Pattern Recognition, vol. 2, p. 2246 (1999)
22. Zivkovic, Z., van der Heijden, F.: Recursive unsupervised learning of finite mixture models. IEEE Transactions on Pattern Analysis and Machine Intelligence 26(5), 651–656 (2004)

# Novel Binarization Method for Enhancing Ancient and Historical Manuscript Images

Saad M. Ismail and Siti Norul Huda Sheikh Abdullah

Center for Artificial Intelligence Technology,
Faculty of Information Science and Technology,
Universiti Kebangsaan Malaysia, 43600 UKM Bangi, Selangor, Malaysia
Ababnah2002@yahoo.com, mimi@ftsm.ukm.my

**Abstract.** Ancient documents are often subject to background damage. Examples of background damage containing various quality are uneven background, ink bleed, or ink bleed and expansion of spots. Image processing provides a variety of approaches for dealing with this deterioration in the quality of manuscripts to make them readable. Unlike DIBCO dataset, Jawi- Malay manuscripts are among the ancient manuscripts that have undergone varying degrees of complex damage and distortions. State of the art methods unable to improve their image and readability. To deal with these challenges, this paper proposes a new adaptive binarization method which consists of several steps beginning with global enhancement and local adaptive thresholding, and ending with post-processing. For the purpose of evaluation, the method was compared with state of the art methods using the Relative Foreground Area Error (RAE) measurement and the ANOVA analysis of variance tool. The results showed that the proposed method gave the smallest RAE with differ significantly with respect to RAE value compared with other methods, which means that it produced better image results and readability.

**Keywords:** Ancient Jawi-Malay Manuscript, Degraded Image Enhancement, Global Thresholding, Adaptive Thresholding.

## 1 Introduction

A manuscript is any document written by hand, as opposed to being printed or reproduced in some other way. Ancient and historical manuscripts often have degraded or damaged backgrounds due to the process of aging over several decades. Some of the degraded conditions or factors are due to environmental influences, and worn out and ancient ink quality. The ancient Malay manuscripts, which are normally written in Jawi script, are among the famous manuscripts for which little research can be found in the literature, and research is now being carried out to improve them and to make them readable. These documents still exist until today but the quality has been degraded [17], and the increased complexity of the images has resulted in different levels of quality within the single image itself. Examples of ancient Malay manuscripts are given in Fig. 1.

A. Gelbukh et al. (Eds.): MICAI 2014, Part I, LNAI 8856, pp. 393–406, 2014.
© Springer International Publishing Switzerland 2014

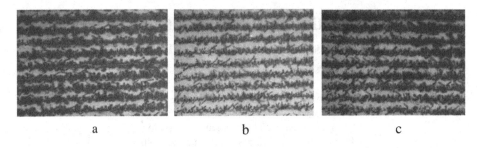

a                              b                              c

**Fig. 1.** Several examples of images of ancient Jawi-Malay manuscripts [10] that have different qualities were used in this experiment. From the left: (a) ink bleed-expands spots  (b) uneven background, and (c) ink bleeds images.

As a result of mounting interest in the analysis of historical photographs, documents and manuscripts, researchers are faced with many challenges. The degraded conditions of historical documents (e.g., images have different qualities due to the uneven background, ink bleed, or ink bleed and expansion of spots, etc.) have motivated researchers to develop suitable methods for improving and processing such images [16] [17]. Binarization and enhancement algorithms are suitable for dealing with these challenges [19] [20] [21]. Several binarization and enhancement techniques have been proposed over the last few years for dealing with problems concerning the images, especially the degraded images of documents [22] [23]. Binarization methods consist of simple thresholding methods and compound methods. The simple thresholding methods are used to determine the thresholding value, where the pixels are separated into black and white. They are easy to implement and provide high performance in most cases, but in some cases they fail and require some factors to be manually determined [12]. The compound algorithms consist of several steps. Some compound algorithms are based on document features and recognition stages [5, 8], while others are based on adding preparatory steps to an existing simple thresholding method [4, 13], and still others are based on filters, segmentation, text extraction, pre-processing and post-processing [1, 3].

The aim of this paper is to propose a new binarization method to solve most of the challenges, such as uneven background, ink bleed, or ink bleed and expansion of spots, etc., by producing better binarization results in the degraded and ancient historical images. This paper is organized as follows: Section 2 presents the background and literature on the methods which are the basis for this new, proposed method; Section 3 presents the details of the proposed method; Section 4 gives the experimental results and the comparison with other methods; and finally, the conclusion is presented in Section 5.

## 2    Review of Related Methods

Many techniques have been proposed in the literature aimed at solving problems with document images and their enhancement [16]. Some of them are simple thresholding methods or compound methods consisting of several steps. This paper focuses on the most widely used methods and those methods that are aimed at the enhancement of ancient Malay manuscript images, namely the Bataineh [2], Niblack [11], NICK [6] and Sauvola[18] methods. These methods were chosen as they are applied on many databases like the DIBCO dataset [13] series, which contain images with problems concerning ink bleed around the textual information and low contrast between the background and the object. These problems have been found to be a major issue in the preservation of ancient Jawi-Malay handwritten manuscripts in the Malaysian National Library. Fig.1 shows some examples of Jawi-Malay manuscript images with different quality levels that are suffering extra degraded.

**Niblack Method [11]:** The Niblack binarization method was proposed by Niblack [11] and it is one of the most commonly used methods. The thresholding values of each window over the image are calculated separately by the following formula:

$$T = m + k \quad , \tag{1}$$

where the window size is determined by the user; m is the mean value,    is the standard deviation value of the pixels inside the window, and k is a constant ($0 \leq k \leq 1$) [13]. However, the disadvantage of this method is that it produces a large amount of black noise in the empty windows, as shown in Fig.2 (b).

**NICK Method [6]:** The NICK method, developed by Khurshid et al., is an improvement over the Niblack binarization method [11]. It aims to solve the problem of black noise in the Niblack binarization method and low contrast by shifting the thresholding value downward. The thresholding formula is as given below:

$$T = m + k \sqrt{\frac{(\Sigma p^2 - m^2)}{NP}} \tag{2}$$

where k is a factor in the range of [−0.1, −0.2]; $p_i$ is the pixel value of the greyscale levels in the image; NP is the total number of pixels in the image; and m is the mean value. The method solves most of problems but it still fails when the contrast is too small or the text is in thin pen strokes, as shown in Fig.2(c).

**Bataineh's Method [2]:** This method suggests an adaptive threshold for low contrast images and thin pen stroke problems using the adaptive window generation and adaptive thresholding value based on global and local image information. The thresholding formula is as given below:

$$T_W = m_g - \frac{m_w^2 - \sigma_w}{(m_g + \sigma_w)(\sigma_{adaptive} + \sigma_w)} \tag{3}$$

$$\sigma_{adaptive} = \frac{\sigma_w - \sigma_{min}}{m_{max} - \sigma_{min}} Max_{level} \tag{4}$$

Where $Tw$ is the grey-level value of the thresholding value of the binarization window, $m_W$ is the grey-level of the mean value of the pixels in the binarization window, $m_g$ is the grey-level of the mean value of the global image pixels; $\sigma_{Adaptive}$ is the grey-level of the adaptive standard deviation of the binarization window as defined in the equation(4), $\sigma_W$ is the standard deviation of the target window, $\sigma_{min}$ is the minimum standard deviation value of all the windows, $\sigma_{max}$ is the maximum standard deviation value of all the windows and $max_{Level}$ is the maximum grey-level value.

$$I_{binary}(x,y) = \begin{cases} Black, & i(x,y) < T_w \\ White, & i(x,y) \geq T_w \end{cases}, \qquad (5)$$

where I (x, y) is the binary image and $i(x, y)$ is the input pixel value of the image. This method gives relatively better results for solving problems. However, NICK method fails to cater low contrast images and thin pen strokes, as can be seen in Fig.2(d).

**Sauvola algorithm [14]:** It is a modification of that of Niblack, performs better in the documents with a background containing a light texture or too variation and uneven illumination. In the Sauvola modification, the binarization is given by:

$$T = m.\left(1 - k.\left(1 - \frac{\sigma}{R}\right)\right), \qquad (6)$$

where $R$ is the dynamic carried of the standard deviation $\sigma$, and the parameter $k$ takes positive values in the interval [0.2, 0.5]. In [14] study, Sauvola used $R=128$ and $k=0.5$ values.

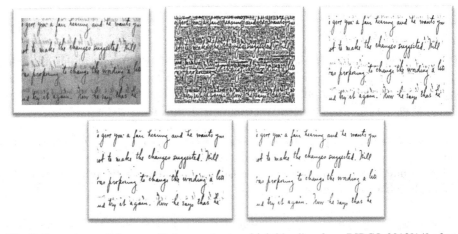

**Fig. 2.** Example result image with low contrast and ink bleeding from DIBCO 2012[14] after applying the Niblack(b)[11], NICK(c)[6] and bataineh(d)[2] methods, the original image(a)

## 3     Proposed Binarization Method

In the proposed method, we compromise problems and weaknesses of the simple methods. Therefore, we develop a capable method for dealing with most challenges with high performance particularly effective in solving low contrast problem between the foreground and background and   text information loss. The diagram of the proposed binarization method is illustrated in Fig. 3. This method consists of image enhancement, proposed local thresholding for binarization and smoothing filter as post-processing for binary image. The details of each stage are described in this section.

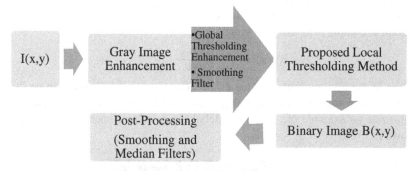

**Fig. 3.** The proposed Image Binarization Flowcharts

### 3.1    Gray Image Enhancements

The presence of noise in images, especially in historical documents, is unavoidable. This noise is introduced by image scanning, recording or transmission and may cause errors in the processing of these documents. In order to allow better quality of the input image, the application of noise reduction algorithms seems to be necessary. Several techniques [24] were proposed for reducing the noise sensitivity, such as special filters or noise and shadow removal. The better the noise removal methods, the better the binarized image will return. For this purpose the global threshold with average filter are proposed and applied.

In the first part of the global thresholding technique, the average intensity value of the grey-level image is calculated as shown in Eq.(6) and then subtracted from the intensity value of the image as shown in Eq.(7), while in the second part, histogram stretching is performed. Thus, the remaining pixels will expand and take up all the grey-levels. The input for the method is assumed to be grey-level images. A more details of the global thresholding enhancement technique are given in the following steps. The calculation of the threshold average pixel ($T_{AVP}$) used as a threshold for an M×N document image I (x, y), is given by the formula:

$$T_{AVP} = \frac{\sum_x \sum_y I(x,y)}{M \times N} \tag{7}$$

he next step is to subtract the image I (x, y) from the background ($T_{AVP}$). Note that "1" stands for the background and "0" for the foreground. The formula that is used for image subtraction, $I_s(x,y)$ is as below:

$$I_s(x,y) = I(x,y) - T_{\text{AVP}} + 1 \qquad (8)$$

After the subtraction process, many pixels are moved to the side of the background, while the rest of the pixels fade away. After the subtraction step, the intensity of the image is adjusted by a histogram stretching technique and extending the values to the whole greyscale range from 0 to 1. The background pixels retain their values, while the rest of the pixel values should extend from 0 to 1. The relation used for the histogram stretching is as the following:

$$I(x,y) = 1 - \frac{1 - I_s(x,y)}{1 - i} \ , \qquad (9)$$

where $i$ = the minimum pixel value in the $I_s(x,y)$ image which given in eq.(8). The previous section used global thresholding and average filter to reduce image noise. We illustrate an example of proposed global image enhancement with average filter as shown in Fig.3.

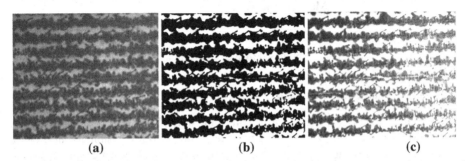

**(a)**                          **(b)**                          **(c)**

**Fig. 3.** Example of Global Thresholding Enhancement (a) original image (b) after subtracts image using Eq (8), and (c) histogram stretching image using Eq (9).

### 3.2    The Proposed Local Binarization

Achieving the best local threshold value extraction, we have exploited the positivity of the global thresholding and the local information of image as the following steps:

### 3.2.1    Global Threshold Value

Image thresholding based on gray level histogram information is a simple and important technique for segmentation, the purpose of which is to identify the regions of image objects correctly. At present there exist many threshold selection methods based on the histogram of the image. Minimum error thresholding originated by Kittler and Illingworth (1986) [7] is one popular method. The proposed method used this method to extract the global threshold value as a first step in proposed adaptive thresholding. This process to extract the global threshold value by Kittler method has been formulated as follow:

Let the pixels of a given image be represented in L gray levels [1, 2... L]. The number of pixels at level (i) is denoted by Ni and the total number of pixels by N = n1 + n2 +...+ nl. In order to simplify the discussion, the gray-level histogram is normalized and regarded as a probability distribution as shown in (Eq.10):

$$P_i = \frac{ni}{N} \quad , \quad Pi \geq 0, \sum_{i=1}^{L} P(i) = 1 \tag{10}$$

Now suppose that we divide the pixels into two classes C0 and C1 (background and objects) by a threshold at threshold T; C0 denotes pixels with levels [1... T], and C1 denotes pixels with levels [T + 1... L]. Then the probabilities of class occurrence (P), the class mean levels (M), and standard deviation ( ) respectively, are given by:

$$P_0 = P(c_0) = \sum_{i=1}^{T} P_i \tag{11}$$

$$P_1 = P(c_1) = \sum_{i=T+1}^{L} P_i \tag{12}$$

$$M_0 = \sum_{i=1}^{T} \frac{iP_i}{P_0} \tag{13}$$

$$M_1 = \sum_{i=T+1}^{L} \frac{iP_i}{P_1} \tag{14}$$

$$\sigma_0 = \left( \frac{\sum_{j=1}^{T}(iP_i - M_0)^2}{P_0} \right)^2 \tag{15}$$

$$\sigma_1 = \left( \frac{\sum_{i=T+1}^{L}(iP_i - M_1)^2}{P_1} \right)^2 \tag{16}$$

For a threshold $T \in \{0, 1 \ldots L\}$, Kittler and Illingworth [7] derives the minimum error criterion function as given in Eq.14:

$$J(T) = 1 + 2[P_0(T) \log_0(T)] + P_1(T) \log_1(T)] - 2[P_0(T) \log P_0(T)) + P_1(T) \log P_1(T)] \tag{17}$$

For optimal global threshold value we minimize the J (T) then the threshold value calculated as shown in (eq.18):

$$T = \text{argmin } J(T) - 0.5 \tag{18}$$

### 3.2.2 Local Threshold and Binarization

Global binarization methods are very fast and produce good result for less degraded image, but for more complex degraded image, global binarization is less significant in most cases.    On the other hand, local binarization overcomes this problem by computing threshold values individually by using a local neighborhood pixels. We compute the proposed local threshold value by taking into account of local mean ($M_L$) for each window size in I(x,y) image    (Eq.19):

$$M_L = \frac{I(x,y)}{W_{size}} \quad , \tag{19}$$

where $M_L$ is mean value for all pixels, I(x,y) is the gray image and $W_{size}$ is the window size. Then we propose the local thresholding value namely $TH_W$ by combining the equations (18, 19) with critical constant factor (K) used for determining the number of edge pixels considered as object pixels. This relation is shown as in Eq.17:

$$TH_W = M_L\left(\frac{(1-T)}{K}\right) \tag{20}$$

where THW is the local threshold value, $M_L$ is the local mean value for I(x,y) image pixels based on $W_{size}$, k is a constant value (we sugges k=100 for obtaining the best result). Based on this $TH_W$ values, the binarization process is defined in (Eq.18). If the value of the current pixel is I(x,y) less than $TH_W$ then it is set to black, otherwise it is set to white.

$$binaryI(x,y) = \begin{cases} black, & I(x,y) < TH_W \\ white, & otherwise \end{cases} \tag{21}$$

where binary I(x,y) is the binary image, $TH_W$ is the locale threshold value and I(x,y) is the gray image.

### 3.3    Post-processing

After performing the adaptive binarization, we use the median and average smoothing filter  to remove some small noises. **The median and average filters:** median filter is a nonlinear digital filtering technique, is normally used to reduce noise in an image, for every pixel, a 3×3 neighborhood with the pixel as center is considered (Fig 4c). Then, a smoothing filter is use to reduce the amount of intensity variation between one pixel and the next (Fig.4e).

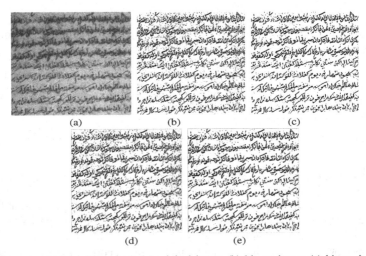

**Fig. 4.** Example of binarization result (a) original image (b) binary image (c) binary image with median filter (d) binary image with smoothing filter (e) binary image with median and smoothing filter.

## 4    Experimental Results and Discussion

We carried out a comparative study to evaluate the performance of our algorithm on eleven ancient Hang Tuah Malay manuscript which consists of extra ordinary degraded images taken from the Malaysian National Library [16]. As mentioned previously, there are several levels of image quality, so the image were divided into three levels of quality, namely uneven background, ink bleed, and ink bleed-expansion of spots images. For evaluation purposes, the proposed method was compared with other common methods recommended in the literature which are considered as efficient and simple, like the Bataineh [2], Niblack [11], NICK [6] and Sauvola[18] methods. Fig.6, presents some of the image results produced by Bataineh [2], Niblack [11], NICK [6], Sauvola[18] and proposed methods. For analytical experiment, we measure our experiment was using Relative Foreground Area Error (RAE) criterion. Then we perform ANOVA analysis to check their significance test.

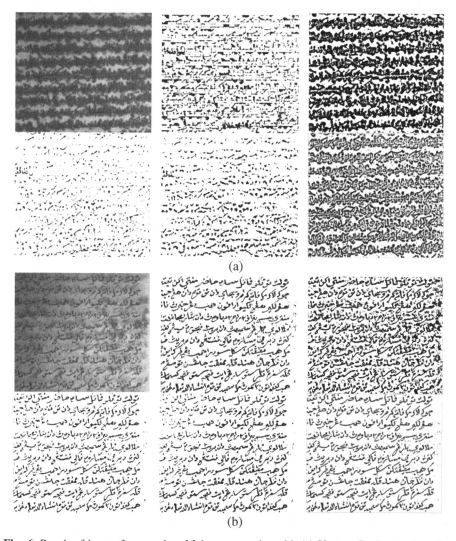

(a)

(b)

**Fig. 6.** Result of image from ancient Malay manuscript with (a) Uneven Background quality level (b) Ink-Bleed quality level (c) Ink-Bleed and Expansion Spot quality level. From the left to Right: Original, Bataineh [2], Niblack [11], NICK [6], Sauvola[18] and proposed methods.

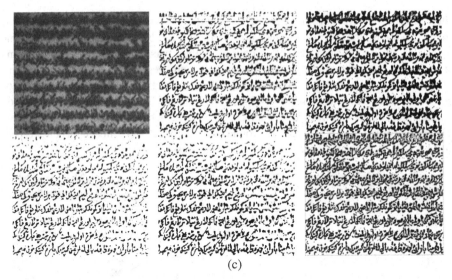

(c)

**Fig. 6.** (*Continued*)

## - RAE Value Criterion

RAE criterion was first proposed and modified later by Sezgin and Sankur [16]. It is a comparison of object properties, more specifically the area of the detected and expected foreground. It calculates the expected values within [0, 1], and the measure which is the earliest or closest to zero gives the best binarization results. The RAE value is defined by the following formula:

$$I_{binary}(x, y) = \begin{cases} \frac{A_0 - A_k}{A_0}, & A_k < A_0 \\ \frac{A_k - A_0}{A_k}, & \text{otherwise} \end{cases} \quad (19)$$

where $A_0$ is the area of reference image and $A_k$ is the area of the binarization or foreground image. The score values for three types of degraded document images after processed by the Bataineh [2], Niblack [11], NICK [6], Sauvola[18] and proposed binarization methods are shown in Table 1 and fig.7.

As mentioned earlier, the RAE is one of the most widely used measures for the comparison of object properties, such as area and shape, as obtained from the segmented image with respect to the reference image where, for a perfect match of the segmented region, the RAE must be closest to zero, which means there are few error pixels in the object area. In this research, five methods were applied to eleven images chosen from ancient Malay manuscript images, which included varying degrees of quality. The results, as shown in the above table, indicate that the proposed method got the best RAE result of 0.0442 compared to the Bataineh [2], Niblack [11], NICK [6],

**Table 1.** The RAE values and their averages for ancient Malay Manuscript images with different quality levels for the Bataineh [2], Niblack [11], NICK [6], Sauvola[18] and proposed methods.

| Quality image | Image | Proposed method | Sauvola[18] | Bataineh method [2] | Niblack method [11] | NICK method [6] |
|---|---|---|---|---|---|---|
| | | | RAE value | | | |
| Uneven Background Images | Im63 | 0.0390 | 0.0619 | 0.3258 | 0.1600 | 0.1311 |
| | Im65 | 0.0271 | 0.0531 | 0.3377 | 0.1748 | 0.1347 |
| | Im67 | 0.0150 | 0.0462 | 0.2965 | 0.1497 | 0.1360 |
| | Im69 | 0.0276 | 0.0662 | 0.1931 | 0.1570 | 0.1428 |
| | Im77 | 0.0212 | 0.0744 | 0.1356 | 0.1480 | 0.1331 |
| Ink-Bleed Images | Im99 | 0.0420 | 0.0721 | 0.3429 | 0.1855 | 0.1620 |
| | Im101 | 0.0662 | 0.0717 | 0.3905 | 0.1712 | 0.1766 |
| | Im107 | 0.0624 | 0.0544 | 0.3812 | 0.1553 | 0.1421 |
| Ink-Bleed and Expansion Spot Images | Im61 | 0.0525 | 0.0841 | 0.4025 | 0.1294 | 0.1177 |
| | Im109 | 0.0675 | 0.0733 | 0.4509 | 0.1432 | 0.1122 |
| | Im111 | 0.0658 | 0.0522 | 0.4117 | 0.1412 | 0.1224 |
| Average | | **0.0442** | **0.0645** | **0.3335** | **0.1559** | **0.1373** |

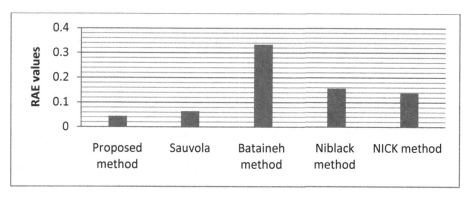

**Fig. 7.** The averages RAE values for ancient Malay Manuscript images for the proposed, Sauvola[18] Bataineh [2], Niblack [11] and NICK [6] methods. Where the small value is the best result.

and Sauvola[18] methods, which achieved 0.3335, 0.1559, 0.1373 and 0.0645, respectively. It can be said that the proposed method has achieved the expected results in improving the images, which include different types of degradation such as ink bleed-expansion spots, uneven background, and ink bleed images, thus making them as readable as possible.

-    **Statistical Analysis of Variance RAE Value**

The ANOVA tool performs a simple analysis of variance on data RAE for 5 methods (Bataineh [2], Niblack [11], NICK [6], Sauvola[18] and proposed). The analysis provides a test of the hypothesis that each of the 5 methods used do not differ significantly with respect to RAE generated by them against the alternative hypothesis that 5 methods used differ significantly with respect to RAE generated by them. The following tables show the summary of ANOVA single factor i.e. Table2.

**Table 2.** Anova: Single Factor for RAE value

| Methods | Count images | m-rank | Average | Variance |
|---|---|---|---|---|
| Proposed method | 11 | 12 | 0.044209 | 0.000388 |
| Sauvola method | 11 | 21 | 0.064509 | 0.00014 |
| Bataineh method | 11 | 54 | 0.333491 | 0.009059 |
| Niblack method | 11 | 44 | 0.155936 | 0.000267 |
| NICK method | 11 | 34 | 0.137336 | 0.000351 |

| Source of Variation | SS | DF | MS | F | P-value | F crit |
|---|---|---|---|---|---|---|
| Between Groups | 0.575551 | 4 | 0.143888 | 70.50475 | 6.2E-20 | 2.557179 |
| Within Groups | 0.102041 | 50 | 0.002041 | | | |
| Total | 0.677592 | 54 | | | | |

Based on the p-value of (Table2) above it can be concluded that the 5 methods used differ significantly with respect to RAE value generated by them.

# 5    Conclusion

The ancient and historical Malay manuscripts dating from hundreds to thousands of years old often have bad or damaged backgrounds. The great interest in ancient manuscripts coupled with the lack of attention especially among image processing researchers, inspires us to explore new methods for handling our extra ordinary degraded images. The proposed method provides a simple and efficient way of improving the degraded images of ancient Malay manuscripts, which have different levels of quality. Furthermore, our proposed method achieves smaller average RAE to other state-of-the-art methods, namely the Bataineh [2], Niblack [11], NICK [6] and Sauvola[18] methods. In the future work, we opt to improve our proposed method by focusing on the pre-processing part  and complimenting other state of the art methods. Thus, it may increase better accuracy and more readable image results.

**Acknowledgement.** The authors would like to thank the Ministry of Education, Malaysia and Universiti Kebangsaan Malaysia for providing facilities and financial support under Fundamental Research Grant Scheme No. FRGS/1/2014/ICT07/UKM/02/5 entitled "Overlapped Irregular Shape Descriptor Based On Non-Linear Approach".

# References

1. Armanfard, N., Valizadeh, M., Komeili, M., Kabir, E.: Document image binarization by using texture-edge descriptor. In: IEEE 14th International CSI Computer Conference, CSICC 2009 (2009)
2. Bataineh, B., Abdullah, S.N.H.S., Omar, K.: An adaptive local binarization method for document images based on a novel thresholding method and dynamic windows. Journal of Pattern Recognition Letters 32, 1805–1813 (2011)
3. Cecotti, H., Belad, A.: Dynamic filters selection for textual document image binarization. In: IEEE 19th International Conference on Pattern Recognition, ICPR 2008 (2008)
4. Chong-Yang, Z., Jing-Yu, Y.: Binarization of document images with complex background. In: IEEE 2010 6th International Conference on Wireless Communications Networking and Mobile Computing, WiCOM (2010)
5. Chou, H., Lin, H., Chang, F.: A Binarisation Method With Learning-Built Rules for Document Images Produced By Cameras. Pattern Recognition 43(4), 1518–1530 (2010)
6. Khurshid, K., Siddiqi, I., Faure, C., Vincent, N.: Comparison of Niblack Inspired Binarization Methods for Ancient Documents. In: 16th International Conference on Document Recognition and Retrieval, SPIE, USA (2010)
7. Kittler, J., Illingworth, J.: Minimum error thresholding. Pattern Recognition 19(1), 41–47 (1986)
8. Lelore, T., Bouchara, F.: Document image binarisation using markov field model. In: IEEE 10th International Conference on Document Analysis and Recognition, ICDAR 2009 (2009)
9. Li-Jing, T., Kan, C., Yan, Z., Xiao-Ling, F., Jian-Yong, D.: Document image binarization based on NFCM. In: IEEE 2nd International Congress on Image and Signal Processing, CISP 2009 (2009)
10. Manuscripts, National Library of Malaysia (Perpustakaan Negara Malaysia, PNM) (April 27, 2009), http://www.pnm.gov.my/pnmv3/index.php?id=84
11. Niblack, W.: An introduction to digital image processing. Strandberg Publishing Company (1985)
12. Ntogas, N., Veintzas, D.: A binarization algorithm for historical manuscripts. WSEAS International Conference. In: Proceedings. Mathematics and Computers in Science and Engineering, World Scientific and Engineering Academy and Society (2008)
13. Pratikakis, I., Gatos, B., Ntirogiannis, K.: ICFHR 2012 competition on handwritten document image binarization (H-DIBCO 2012). In: 2012 International Conference on Frontiers in Handwriting Recognition (ICFHR). IEEE (2012)
14. Sezgin, M., Sankur, B.: Survey Over Image Thresholding Techniques and Quantitative Performance Evaluation. J. Electron Imaging 13(1), 146–165 (2004)
15. Tong, L., Chen, K., Zhang, Y., Fu, L., Duan, Y.: Document Image Binarisation Based on NFCM. In: 2nd International Congress on Image and Signal Processing 2009, CISP 2009, Zarzis, Tunisia, October 17-19, pp. 1–5 (2009)

16. Venkata Rao, N., Srinivasa Rao, A.V., Balaji, S., Reddy, L.P.: Cleaning of Ancient Document Images Using Modified Iterative Global Threshold. International Journal of Computer Science Issues (IJCSI) 8(6) (2011)
17. Yahya, S.R., Sheikh Abdullah, S.N.H., Omar, K., Liong, C.-Y.: Adaptive binarization method for enhancing ancient malay manuscript images. In: Wang, D., Reynolds, M. (eds.) AI 2011. LNCS, vol. 7106, pp. 619–627. Springer, Heidelberg (2011)
18. Sauvola, J., PietikaKinen, M.: Adaptive document binarization. In: Proceedings of the Fourth International Conference on Document Analysis and Recognition. IEEE (2000)
19. Mukherjee, A., Kanrar, S.: Image Enhancement with Statistical Estimation. arXiv preprint arXiv:1205.1365 (2012)
20. Wolf, C.: Document ink bleed-through removal with two hidden Markov random fields and a single observation field. IEEE Transactions on Pattern Analysis and Machine Intelligence 32(3), 431–447 (2010)
21. Tonazzini, A., Salerno, E., Bedini, L.: Fast correction of bleed-through distortion in grayscale documents by a blind source separation technique. International Journal of Document Analysis and Recognition (IJDAR) 10(1), 17–25 (2007)
22. Okamoto, A., Yoshida, H., Tanaka, N.: A Binarization Method for Degraded Document Images with Morphological Operations. In: International Conference on Machine Vision Applications, Kyoto, Japan (2013)
23. Chaki, N., Shaikh, H.S., Saeed, K.: Exploring Image Binarization Techniques. In: Biswas, S., Nori, K.V. (eds.) FSTTCS 1991. LNCS, vol. 560, Springer, Heidelberg (1991)
24. Ben Messaoud, I., Amiri, H., El Abed, H., Margner, V.: New binarization approach based on text block extraction. In: 2011 International Conference on Document Analysis and Recognition (ICDAR). IEEE(2011)

# Preferences for Argumentation Semantics

Mauricio Osorio[1], Claudia Zepeda[2], and José Luis Carballido[2]

[1] Universidad de las Américas Puebla
osoriomauri@gmail.com
[2] Benemérita Universidad Atónoma de Puebla
{czepedac,jlcarballido7}@gmail.com

**Abstract.** We propose an engineering approach for assembling argumentation theory with a preference approach, which allows us to give as input an argumentation problem with preferences and return the stable argumentation extensions that fulfill the preferences.

**Keywords:** Preferences, ordered disjunction, argumentation semantics.

## 1  Introduction

In this paper, we propose an engineering approach for assembling argumentation theory with a preference approach, which allows us to give as input an argumentation problem with preferences and obtain the stable argumentation extensions that fulfill the preferences. Specifically, what we propose here is to use graphs to represent argumentation problems, since graphs are useful to represent the meaning of data including its relations according to humans' view. Given an argumentation framework we define a directed graph where the nodes represent the arguments and each arrow represents an attack of one argument to other, thus providing a visual and convenient representation of the argumentation framework. At the same time, we enrich the search for solutions of an argumentation problem, by implementing a way to choose one solution over others. Here, inspired in the semantics of logic programs with ordered disjuntion (LPOD) defined by Brewka in [2], we propose to define a partial order on the stable extensions of an argumentation framework according to the preferences, however, unlike the Brewka's method our approach does not generate stable extensions, our approach obtains just the stable extensions corresponding to the argumentation framework and sorts these extensions according to a partial order defined by the preferences. Argumentation theory has become an interesting research line in Artificial Intelligence and includes developing theoretical models, prototype implementations, and application studies [1,6].The objective of argumentation theory is to analyze the fundamental mechanism that persons use in argumentation, and to explore ways to implement this mechanism as computer systems. Several approaches have been proposed for capturing representative patterns of inference in argumentation theory, but Dung's approach (presented in [4]) is a unifying framework which has played an influential role in argumentation research and Artificial Intelligence. Dung's approach is regarded as an

A. Gelbukh et al. (Eds.): MICAI 2014, Part I, LNAI 8856, pp. 407–418, 2014.

abstract model where the main concern is to find the set of arguments which are considered as acceptable i.e., to find sets of arguments which represent coherent points of view. The strategy for analyzing the attack relationships, and then inferring the sets of acceptable arguments, is based on extension based semantics. Dung defines four extension based semantics: grounded semantics, stable semantics, preferred semantics, and complete semantics. Although each abstract argumentation semantics represents a different pattern of inference in argumentation theory, all of them have as common point the concept of admissible set[1]. When Dung introduced his abstract argumentation approach, he proved that his approach can be regarded as a special form of logic programming with negation as failure. He defined a logic programming codification in order to map an argumentation framework $AF$ into a logic program $P_{AF}$. In particular Dung showed that the stable model semantics [5] is a convenient logic programming semantics to capture the stable semantics of an argumentation framework, i.e., the stable models of a logic program correspond to the stable extensions of an argumentation framework.

However, to the best of our knowledge, currently there is no approach that chooses some stable extensions of an argumentation framework over others according to a criterion of preferences following Brewka's approach. Our point of view combines answer set programming and Brewkas approach for preferences, taking advantage of the fact that Brewkas method is well known and has already a prototype of software on which we can do tests. Our approach can be represented by figure A.

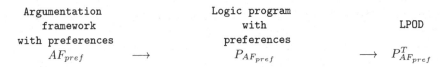

**Fig. A.** Diagram of our proposal

In order to give a better idea of our proposal, we present an example of an argumentation problem with preferences about tourism. We illustrate its graph representation, the representation of the preferences and the stable argumentation extensions that fulfill the preferences. Subsequently, throughout this paper we present the technical details which lead to the results of this example.

*Example 1.* A tourist, with limited cash to spend, is planning on visiting Mexico. She is looking for 4-star or 3-star hotel deals in the areas of Puebla and Acapulco, the two places she would like to visit. She likes activities in colonial cities but, in Puebla she will not be able to find cheap seafood, which she loves. On the other hand, she loves a variety of activities in the water, something she can not enjoy in Puebla, however she is aware of the possibilities of a tropical storm in the area of Acapulco during the time of her trip. Moreover, we can assume that the tourist

---

[1] An admissible set represents a coherent point of view in a conflict of arguments.

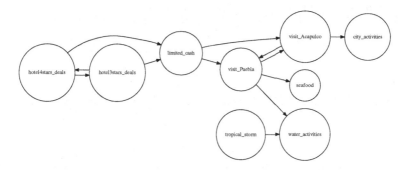

**Fig. 1.** Graph representation of $AF := \langle AR, Attacks \rangle$ with $Pref = \{(city\_activities, seafood), (hotel4stars\_deals, hotel3stars\_deals)\}$

prefers city activities over seafood and 4-stars hotels over 3-stars hotels. How can she deicide where to go on her vacation given that she can not afford visiting both cities?

This argumentation problem can be regarded as a directed graph, as shown in Figure 1.

The directed graph in Figure 1 can also be represented by the following argumentation framework with preferences.

$AF_{pref} := (\langle AR, attacks \rangle, Pref)$ where
$AR = \{limited\_cash, hotel4stars\_deals, hotel3stars\_deals, visit\_Puebla,$
$\quad\quad visit\_Acapulco, water\_activities, city\_activities, seafood, tropical\_storm\}$
$Attacks = \{(hotel4stars\_deals, limited\_cash), (hotel3stars\_deals, limited\_cash),$
$\quad\quad (visit\_Acapulco, visit\_Puebla), (limited\_cash, visit\_Puebla),$
$\quad\quad (limited\_cash, visit\_Acapulco), (visit\_Puebla, visit\_Acapulco),$
$\quad\quad (visit\_Puebla, water\_activities), (tropical\_storm, water\_activities),$
$\quad\quad (visit\_Acapulco, city\_activities), (visit\_Puebla, seafood)\}$
$Pref = \{(city\_activities, seafood), (hotel4stars\_deals, hotel3stars\_deals)\}.$

We can see that each preference is represented as a finite ordered sequence of accepted arguments like $(a_1, \ldots, a_n)$ which intuitively indicates that the accepted argument $a_1$ is preferred to the accepted argument $a_2$, and the accepted argument $a_2$ is preferred to the accepted argument $a_3$, and so on. Hence in our example, the tourist's preference for city activities over seafood is represented as $(city\_activities, seafood)$ which intuitively indicates that the accepted argument $city\_activities$ is preferred to the accepted argument $seafood$. We will see that the stable argumentation semantics of $AF$ indicates that there are four stable extensions where preferences will be applied to obtain the stable extensions that fulfill better the preferences. These stable extensions are:

| | Arguments accepted | Arguments defeated |
|---|---|---|
| 1 | $visit\_Puebla, hotel4stars\_deals,$ $city\_activities, tropical\_storm$ | $visit\_Acapulco, hotel3stars\_deals,$ $water\_activities, seafood, limited\_cash$ |
| 2 | $visit\_Acapulco, hotel4stars\_deals,$ $seafood, tropical\_storm$ | $visit\_Puebla, hotel3stars\_deals,$ $city\_activities, water\_activities, limited\_cash$ |
| 3 | $visit\_Puebla, hotel3stars\_deals,$ $city\_activities, tropical\_storm$ | $visit\_Acapulco, hotel4stars\_deals,$ $water\_activities, seafood, limited\_cash$ |
| 4 | $visit\_Acapulco, hotel3stars\_deals,$ $seafood, tropical\_storm$ | $visit\_Puebla, hotel4stars\_deals,$ $city\_activities, water\_activities, limited\_cash$ |

In an intuitive way, we can see that two of the stable extensions indicate that the tourist visits Puebla, where she finds a hotel with the right prices and enjoys the activities proper of the city. In the other one, two of the stable extensions indicate that she visits Acapulco where she finds a hotel with the right prices and will be able to practice sea activities as well as enjoy sea food, although she will be at risk of facing a storm that could ruin her vacation. Now, considering that the tourist prefers city activities over seafood and 4-stars hotels over 3-stars hotels represented as the following set of preferences $\{(city\_activities, seafood), (hotel4stars\_deals, hotel3stars\_deals)\}$ we can verify that the stable extension that fulfills better the preferences is $\{visit\_Puebla, city\_activities, hotel4stars\_deals, tropical\_storm\}$. This stable extension coincides with what our intuition expected.

In section 2, we review some basic concepts about the stable argumentation semantics and logic programs with ordered disjunction. In section 3, we describe our approach. Finally, in section 5, we present our conclusions.

## 2    Background

In this section, we review the theoretical concepts of argumentation proposed by Dung in [4], we review also the definition of LPODs introduced by Brewka in [2]. From now on, we assume that the reader is familiar with the notion of propositional logic, an *interpretation*, *validity* and normal logic programs (see [9] for details of these notions). In this paper, a logic programming semantics $S$ is a mapping defined on the family of all programs which associates to a given program a subset of its 2-valued (classical) models. We say that $M$ is a *minimal model* of $P$ if and only if there does not exist a model $M'$ of $P$ such that $M' \subset M$, $M' \neq M$ [9].

**Argumentation Semantics.** The basic structure of Dung's argumentation approach is an argumentation framework which captures the relationships between the arguments.

**Definition 1.** *[4] An argumentation framework is a pair* $AF := \langle AR, attacks \rangle$, *where AR is a finite set of arguments, and attacks is a binary relation on AR, i.e., attacks* $\subseteq AR \times AR$.

For instance, if $AF := \langle \{a, b, c, d\}, \{(a, a), (a, c), (b, c), (c, d)\} \rangle$, then we say that $a$ *attacks* $c$ (or $c$ is attacked by $a$) if $attacks(a, c)$ holds. Similarly, we say that a set $S$ of arguments attacks $c$ (or $c$ is attacked by $S$) if $c$ is attacked by an argument in $S$. Any argumentation framework can be regarded as a directed graph. Dung defined his argumentation semantics based on the basic concept of *admissible set*.

**Definition 2.** *[4] Let $AF := \langle AR, attacks \rangle$ be an argumentation framework. A set $S$ of arguments is said to be conflict-free if there are no arguments $a$, $b$ in $S$ such that $a$ attacks $b$. An argument $a \in AR$ is acceptable with respect to a set $S$ of arguments if and only if for each argument $b \in AR$: If $b$ attacks $a$ then $b$ is attacked by $S$. A conflict-free set of arguments $S$ is admissible if and only if each argument in $S$ is acceptable w.r.t. $S$. We say that $E \subseteq AR$ is an stable extension of $AF$ if $E$ is an admissible set of $AF$ that attacks every argument in $AR \setminus E$. The set of stable extensions of $AF$, denoted by* stable_extensions($AF$), *will be referred to as the stable semantics of $AF$.*

Now, we review the relationship between argumentation semantics and logic programming semantics. In particular between the stable argumentation semantics and the *stable* logic programming semantics. This relationship is based on the proposal [8] of regarding an argumentation framework as a logic program. Hence, we describe a mapping from an argumentation framework $AF$ into a logic program $P_{AF}$. In this mapping we use the predicate $def(x)$ to represent that "the argument $x$ is defeated". This mapping also includes clauses such as $def(x) \leftarrow \neg def(y)$ to capture the idea that argument $x$ is defeated when anyone of its adversaries $y$ is not defeated.

**Definition 3.** *[8] Let $AF = \langle AR, attacks \rangle$ be an argumentation framework,*
$$P_{AF}^{d_1} = \bigcup_{x \in AR} \{def(x) \leftarrow \neg def(y) \mid (y, x) \in attacks\}, \text{ and}$$
$$P_{AF}^{d_2} = \bigcup_{x \in AR} \{\bigcup_{y:(y,x) \in attacks} \{def(x) \leftarrow \wedge_{z:(z,y) \in attacks} def(z)\}\}.$$

For a given atom $x$ in the definition of $P_{AF}^{d_2}$ there may not be a $z$ as described, in that case the corresponding conjunction $\wedge_{z:(z,y) \in attacks} def(z)$ is empty leaving the fact $def(x) \leftarrow$ in $P_{AF}^{d_2}$. The reader familiar with argumentation theory can observe that essentially, $P_{AF}^{d_1}$ captures the basic principle of *conflict-freeness* [8]. We can see that $P_{AF}^{d_1} \cup P_{AF}^{d_2}$ only identifies the defeated arguments. In order to identify the accepted arguments, we define $P_{AF}$ as follows.

**Definition 4.** *[8] $P_{AF} = P_{AF}^{d_1} \cup P_{AF}^{d_2} \cup \bigcup_{x \in AR} \{acc(x) \leftarrow \neg def(x)\}$.*

Finally, we know that the stable argumentation semantics can be characterized by a logic programming semantics [3]. In order to introduce this characterization, we introduce the following definition. Let $E$ be a set of arguments: $tr(E) = \{acc(a) \mid a \in E\} \cup \{def(b) \mid b$ is an argument and $b \notin E\}$.

**Theorem 1.** *[3] Let $AF = \langle AR, attacks \rangle$ be an argumentation framework, $E \subseteq AR$. Then $E$ is a stable extension of $AF$ iff $tr(E)$ is a stable model of $P_{AF}$.*

Up to this point we can obtain the stable extensions but we have not said anything about preferences.

**Logic Programs with Ordered Disjuntion.** Now we review Logic Programs with Ordered Disjunction, abbreviated as LPODs, introduced by Brewka in [2]. We present the formal definition of an LPOD and its semantics. We see that an LPOD can include rules with disjunctions of literals where the order in which these literals are written in each disjunction represents an order of preferences. We also see how the semantics of LPODs first proposes to generate the answer sets of an LPODs and then defines a partial order over these answer sets to select the preferred ones. In order to define LPOD's, the connective ordered disjunction × is added to the set of connectives of propositional formulas. The intuition behind LPODs is to express knowledge about preferences in a simple way. A (propositional) LPOD consists of rules of the form[2]: $C_1 \times \ldots \times C_n \leftarrow A_1, \ldots, A_m, \neg B_1, \ldots, \neg B_k$ where the $C_i$, $A_j$ and $B_l$ are ground literals. The rule head can be interpreted as: if possible $C_1$, if $C_1$ is not possible then $C_2$, ..., if all of $C_1, \ldots, C_{n-1}$ are not possible then $C_n$. The literals $C_i$ are called choices of the rule. As usual we omit $\leftarrow$ whenever $m = 0$ and $k = 0$, that is, if the rule is a fact. Moreover, we write $\leftarrow body$ whenever $n = 0$, that is, if the rule is a constraint. Now we define the semantics of LPODs.

**Definition 5.** *Let $r = C_1 \times \ldots \times C_n \leftarrow body$ be a rule. For $k \leq n$ we define the kth option of $r$ as $r^k = C_k \leftarrow body, \neg C_1, \ldots, \neg C_{k-1}$. Let $P$ be an LPOD. $P$ is a split program of $P$ if it is obtained from $P$ by replacing each rule in $P$ by one of its options. A set of literals $S$ is an answer set of $P$ if it is a consistent answer set of a split program $P$ of $P$. Let $S$ be an answer set of an LPOD $P$. We say taht $S$ satisfies the rule $C_1 \times \ldots \times C_n \leftarrow A_1, \ldots, A_m, \neg B_1, \ldots, \neg B_k$*

- *to degree 1 if $A_j \notin S$, for some $j$, or $B_i \in S$, for some $i$,*
- *to degree $j$ ($1 \leq j \leq n$) if all $A_j \in S$, no $B_i \in S$, and $j = \min\{r | C_r \in S\}$.*

**Definition 6.** *For a set of literals $S$, let $S_i(P)$ denote the set of rules in $P$ satisfied by $S$ to degree $i$. Let $S_1$ and $S_2$ be answer sets of an LPOD $P$. $S_1$ is preferred to $S_2$ ($S1 > S2$) iff there is $i$ such that $S_2^i(P) \subset S_1^i(P)$, and for all $j < i$, $S_1^j(P) = S_2^j(P)$. A set of literals $S$ is a preferred answer set of an LPOD $P$ iff $S$ is an answer set of $P$ and there is no answer set $S_1$ of $P$ such that $S_1 > S$.*

*Example 2.* Let $P$ be the following LPOD:

$$1) \ a \times c \times d.$$
$$2) \ b \leftarrow \neg a.$$
$$3) \ c \leftarrow \neg d.$$
$$4) \ d \leftarrow \neg c.$$

The three split programs of $P$ are:

| $P_1$ : | $P_2$ : | $P_3$ : |
|---|---|---|
| $a.$ | $c \leftarrow \neg a.$ | $d \leftarrow \neg a, \neg c.$ |
| $b \leftarrow \neg a.$ | $b \leftarrow \neg a.$ | $b \leftarrow \neg a.$ |
| $c \leftarrow \neg d.$ | $c \leftarrow \neg d.$ | $c \leftarrow \neg d.$ |
| $d \leftarrow \neg c.$ | $d \leftarrow \neg c.$ | $d \leftarrow \neg c.$ |

---

[2] In this work we consider only default negation, but this does not contradict the results as given in [2].

We obtain four answer sets: $M_1 = \{a, c\}$, $M_2 = \{a, d\}$, $M_3 = \{b, c\}$ and $M_4 = \{b, d\}$. $M_1$ and $M_2$ satisfy all rules of $P$ to degree 1, $M_3$ satisfies 1) to degree 2 but the rest of rules to degree 1, $M_4$ satisfies 1) to degree 3 but the rest of rules to degree 1. The preferred answer sets are thus $M_1$ and $M_2$.

Note that the ordered disjunction rules contribute to generate the answer sets and not just to choose them, and our interest in Brewka's method is only in the way of choosing but without generating. Currently, there is a modification of SMODELS[3] that can be used to compute preferred answer sets under the ordered disjunction semantics called PSMODELS[4].

## 3 Preferences for Argumentation Semantics

Once the background is showed, we will illustrate the use of semantics for LPOD's to select stable extensions that fulfill better the preferences, namely we extend the stable argumentation semantics to *stable argumentation semantics with preferences*. Our approach is inspired on the semantics of ordered disjunction logic programs (LPOD's) proposed by Brewka [2]. We adapt Brewka's approach to one approach with preferences but without disjunctions. Let us illustrate what we mean considering again the LPOD $P$ of example 2:

$$1) \ a \times c \times d.$$
$$2) \ b \leftarrow \neg a.$$
$$3) \ c \leftarrow \neg d.$$
$$4) \ d \leftarrow \neg c.$$

Brewka's approach generates four answer sets, $M_1 = \{a, c\}$, $M_2 = \{a, d\}$, $M_3 = \{c, b\}$ and $M_4 = \{d, b\}$, due to the disjunction (rule 1), subsequently these answer sets are partially ordered, thus the preferred answer sets are $M_1$ and $M_2$. However, we are interested in adapting Brewka's approach such that 1) acts like a preference specification that does not contribute to generate answer sets and only indicates the order to select the answer sets generated by rules that do not include the ordered disjunction operator. Thus in our proposed approach, program $P$ is rewritten as the following logic program with preferences:

$$1) \ a \rhd c \rhd d.$$
$$2) \ b \leftarrow \neg a.$$
$$3) \ c \leftarrow \neg d.$$
$$4) \ d \leftarrow \neg c.$$

Rule 1) indicates the preference, which intuitively indicates that the accepted argument $a$ is preferred to the accepted argument $c$, and the accepted argument $c$ is preferred to the accepted argument $d$. We can verify that with our proposal this new program generates only two answer sets $\{c, b\}$ and $\{d, b\}$ due to rules 2), 3) and 4), and according to the preference (rule 1) $\{c, b\}$ is the preferred.

---

[3] http://www.tcs.hut.fi/Software/smodels/
[4] http://www.tcs.hut.fi/Software/smodels/priority/

Thus, our approach will provide an order for the stable extensions in terms of the preferences but, in opposition to Brewka's approach, which generate answer sets based on the ordered disjunction, our method does not generate stable extensions but only keeps those of the original program $P_{AF}$. Briefly, we propose to obtain the semantics of an argumentation framework with preferences as follows: First, we extend the definition of an argumentation framework by adding a list of preferences to it. Then, we transform the argumentation framework with preferences into a logic program with preferences; the rules that represent the preferences use the connective $\triangleright$. See the first transformation shown in the diagram of Figure A. Finally, we transform the logic program with preferences into a particular and special LPOD whose preferred answer sets will be mapped to the stable extensions that fulfill better the preferences. See the second transformation shown in the diagram of Figure A. Let us extend the definition of an argumentation framework by adding a lists of preferences to it. First, we define a preference as a finite ordered sequence of accepted arguments like $(a_1, \ldots, a_n)$, which intuitively indicates that the accepted argument $a_1$ is preferred to the accepted argument $a_2$, and the accepted argument $a_2$ is preferred to the accepted argument $a_3$, and so on.

**Definition 7.** *An argumentation framework with preferences (AFP) is pair* $AF_{pref} := (AF, Pref)$, *where* $AF = \langle AR, attacks \rangle$ *is an argumentation framework and* $Pref := \{(a_1^1, \ldots, a_{n_1}^1), \ldots, (a_1^m, \ldots, a_{n_m}^m)\}$, *is a finite set of preferences.*

In order to obtain the semantics of an AFP, we define a logic program with preferences associated to it and denoted as $P_{AF_{pref}}$. This associated logic program, corresponds to the union of the logic program $P_{AF}$ (see section 2) with a particular set of rules of preference, denoted as $R_{pref}$. The set $R_{pref}$ is defined as $\{a_1^1 \triangleright \ldots \triangleright a_{n_1}^1, \ldots, a_1^m \triangleright \ldots \triangleright a_{n_m}^m\}$, where $a_1^i \triangleright \ldots \triangleright a_{n_i}^i$ is called a rule of preference and represents the i-th sequence in the set $Pref$.

**Definition 8.** *Let* $AF_{pref} := (AF, Pref)$ *be an AFP. We define the logic program with preferences associated to* $AF_{pref}$ *as follows:* $P_{AF_{pref}} = P_{AF} \cup R_{pref}$.

*Example 3.* If we consider the AFP of example 1 then, its logic program with preferences $P_{AF_{pref}}$ is $P_{AF} \cup R_{pref}$, with $R_{pref} = \{acc(city\_activities) \triangleright acc(seafood), acc(hotel4stars\_deals) \triangleright acc(hotel3stars\_deals)\}$.

### 3.1   Computing the Stable or Preferred Extensions of an AFP

In what follows, we explain how to represent our approach in terms of LPODs. We will show how this can be done in answer set programming. In this way, we address the problem of computing stable extensions of an argumentation framework according to a set of preferences. We achieve this by encoding each rule of preference in $R_{pref}$ as an ordered disjunction rule that will be part of the set $R_{od}$ and developing a set of rules $T_{a_i}$ for each accepted argument $a_i$ in a preference of $Pref$ of the given AFP. The intuitive idea of each of these sets

$T_{a_i}$ is explained below. Thus, given an APF we obtain its stable extensions that fulfill better the set of preferences, by means of the preferred answer sets of a particular LPOD defined by the union of logic programs $P_{AF}$, $R_{od}$ and the sets $T_{a_i}$. Since $P_{AF}$ has already been discussed in Section 2, we will begin by defining the set $R_{od}$.

**Definition 9.** *Given a logic program* $P_{AF_{pref}} = P_{AF} \cup R_{pref}$, *of an AFP, we define the set* $R_{od} = \{a_1^{\bullet} \times \ldots \times a_n^{\bullet} | a_1 \rhd \ldots \rhd a_n$ *is a rule of preference in* $R_{pref}\}$ *where each* $a_i^{\bullet}$ *in each ordered disjunction rule of* $R_{od}$ *is a new atom that does not appear in* $P_{AF_{pref}}$ *and appears in only one rule of* $R_{od}$.

*Example 4.* Let us consider the $P_{AF_{pref}}$ of example 3. We can see that $R_{od}$ is the following set of two ordered disjuntion rules:

$r_1$: $acc(city\_activities)^{\bullet} \times acc(seafood)^{\bullet}$
$r_2$: $acc(hotel4stars\_deals)^{\bullet} \times acc(hotel3stars\_deals)^{\bullet}$

Now, we define the set of rules $T_{a_i}$ for each accepted argument $a_i$ in a preference of $Pref$ of the given AFP.

**Definition 10.** *Let* $AF_{pref} := (AF, Pref)$ *be an AFP, where* $AF = \langle AR, attacks \rangle$ *and* $Pref := \{(a_1, \ldots, a_n), (b_1, \ldots, b_m), \ldots\}$. *We define* $T_{a_i}$ *as the following set of rules for each* $a_i$ *in each preference of the set* $Pref$:

$$a) \leftarrow \neg a_i, a_i^{\bullet},$$
$$b)\ a_i^{\bullet} \leftarrow \neg a_i^{\circ},$$
$$c)\ a_i^{\circ} \leftarrow \neg a_i,$$
$$d) \leftarrow a_i, a_i^{\circ}\},$$

*where* $a_i^{\circ}$ *is a new atom defined for each* $a_i^{\bullet}$. *We call* $T$ *the union of all* $T_{a_i}$, *i.e.,* $T = \bigcup_{a_i} T_{a_i}$.

The intuition behind the set of rules $T_{a_i}$ is as follows: rule c) indicates that $a_i^{\circ}$ is defined as $\neg a_i$; rule b) indicates that $a_i^{\bullet}$ is defined as $\neg a_i^{\circ}$, i.e., $a_i^{\bullet}$ is defined as $\neg\neg a_i$. Here we should notice that double negation of $a_i$ has a weaker meaning than $a_i$, that is "one does not want that $a_i$ is not in the model is not equivalent to $a_i$ must be in the model". Rules a) and d) precludes a literal and its negation to be in a model. This interpretation of double negation is implicitly built in the semantics of answer sets. The set of rules $T_{a_i}$ do not allow the introduction of models (in this case stable extensions) besides those of the original $P_{AF}$.

*Example 5.* If we consider the AFP of example 1 then, the set $T_{city\_activities}$ is:

$\leftarrow \neg acc(city\_activities), acc(city\_activities)^{\bullet},$
$acc(city\_activities)^{\bullet} \leftarrow \neg acc(city\_activities)^{\circ},$
$acc(city\_activities)^{\circ} \leftarrow \neg acc(city\_activities),$
$\leftarrow acc(city\_activities), acc(city\_activities)^{\circ}$

In a similar way we can define a set of four rules for $T_{seafood}$, $T_{hotel4stars\_deals}$, and $T_{hotel3stars\_deals}$. Thus, $T = T_{city\_activities} \cup T_{seafood} \cup T_{hotel4stars\_deals} \cup T_{hotel3stars\_deals}$.

Now, given an AFP, we define its logic program with ordered disjunction $P_{AF_{pref}}^{T}$ as the union of logic programs $P_{AF}$, $R_{od}$ and the set $T$.

**Definition 11.** *Given an AFP, we define its LPOD as the program $P^T_{AF_{pref}}$ as* $P_{AF} \cup R_{od} \cup T$.

The preferred answer sets of this LPOD give the desired stable extensions that fulfill better the preferences when intersecting them with the original language of the AFP.

**Theorem 2.** *Let $AF_{pref} := (AF, Pref)$ with $AF = \langle AR, attacks \rangle$ be an AFP and $P^T_{AF_{pref}}$ be its LPOD. Let S be a preferred answer set of $P^T_{AF_{pref}}$ then, $S \cap AR$ is a stable extension of $AF_{pref}$ that fulfills better the set of preferences Pref.*

*Example 6.* Let us consider again the AFP of example 1. Recall that $R_{od}$ is the following set of rules (see example 4): $r_1 : acc(city\_activities)^\bullet \times acc(seafood)^\bullet$, $r_2 : acc(hotel4stars\_deals)^\bullet \times acc(hotel3stars\_deals)^\bullet$.
According to examples 3, 4 and 5, we can see that the LPOD of this AFP is

$$P^T_{AF_{pref}} = P_{AF} \cup R_{od} \cup T$$

Now we obtain the preferred answer sets of this LPOD according to the definition of Brewka (see section 2) as follows. First, we define the split programs of $P^T_{AF_{pref}}$:

$P_1 = P_{AF} \cup \{acc(city\_activities)^\bullet, \; acc(hotel4stars\_deals)^\bullet\} \cup T$.

$P_2 = P_{AF} \cup \{acc(city\_activities)^\bullet,$
$\qquad acc(hotel3stars\_deals)^\bullet \leftarrow \neg acc(hotel4stars\_deals^\bullet\} \cup T$.

$P_3 = P_{AF} \cup \{acc(seafood)^\bullet \leftarrow \neg acc(city\_activities)^\bullet,$
$\qquad acc(hotel4stars\_deals)^\bullet\} \cup T$.

$P_4 = P_{AF} \cup \{acc(seafood)^\bullet \leftarrow \neg acc(city\_activities)^\bullet,$
$\qquad acc(hotel3stars\_deals)^\bullet \leftarrow \neg acc(hotel4stars\_deals)^\bullet\} \cup T$.

Let us continue obtaining the models of $P^T_{AF_{pref}}$ that correspond to the models of the four split programs:

| Answer | Arguments accepted | Arguments defeated |
|--------|--------------------|--------------------|
| $M_1$ | $visit\_Puebla, hotel4stars\_deals,$ $city\_activities, tropical\_storm$ $city\_activities^\bullet, hotel4stars\_deals^\bullet$ $seafood^\circ, hotel3stars\_deals^\circ$ | $visit\_Acapulco, hotel3stars\_deals,$ $water\_activities, seafood,$ $limited\_cash$ |
| $M_2$ | $visit\_Acapulco, hotel4stars\_deals,$ $seafood, tropical\_storm$ $seafood^\bullet, hotel4stars\_deals^\bullet,$ $city\_activities^\circ, hotel3stars\_deals^\circ$ | $visit\_Puebla, hotel3stars\_deals,$ $city\_activities, water\_activities,$ $limited\_cash$ |
| $M_3$ | $visit\_Puebla, hotel3stars\_deals,$ $city\_activities, tropical\_storm$ $city\_activities^\bullet, hotel3stars\_deals^\bullet$ $seafood^\circ, hotel4stars\_deals^\circ$ | $visit\_Acapulco, hotel4stars\_deals,$ $water\_activities, seafood,$ $limited\_cash$ |
| $M_4$ | $visit\_Acapulco, hotel3stars\_deals,$ $seafood, tropical\_storm$ $seafood^\bullet, hotel3stars\_deals^\bullet,$ $city_a ctivities^\circ, hotel4stars_d eals^\circ,$ | $visit\_Puebla, hotel4stars\_deals,$ $city\_activities, water\_activities,$ $limited\_cash$ |

Now, to distinguish between more intended and less intended answer set, we obtain the degree of satisfaction of rules $r_1$ and $r_2$ for each answer set. The degree of $r_1$ w.r.t. $M_1$, denoted as $degree(r_1)_{M_1}$ is 1, since $acc(city\_activities)^\bullet$ is in $M_1$ and it occupies position 1 in the finite ordered sequence of accepted arguments $Pref$. The degree of $r_1$ w.r.t. $M_2$, denoted as $degree(r_1)_{M_2}$ is 2, since $acc(seafood)^\bullet$ is in $M_2$ and it occupies position 2 in the finite ordered sequence of accepted arguments $Pref$. In a similar way we can verify that $degree(r_1)_{M_3} = 1$, $degree(r_1)_{M_4} = 2$, $degree(r_2)_{M_1} = 1$, $degree(r_2)_{M_2} = 1$, $degree(r_2)_{M_3} = 2$, $degree(r_2)_{M_4} = 2$.

We use the degrees of satisfaction of rules to define a preference relation on answer sets. The preference relation is based on set inclusion of the rules satisfied to certain degrees. For each stable model $M$, we obtain the set of extended ordered disjunction rules in $P^T_{AF_{pref}}$ satisfied by $M$ to degree $i$, denoted by $M^i(P^T_{AF_{pref}})$. Then,

$$M^1_1(P^T_{AF_{pref}}) = \{r_1, r_2\}, M^1_2(P^T_{AF_{pref}}) = \{r_1\}, M^1_3(P^T_{AF_{pref}}) = \{r_1\}, M^1_4(P^T_{AF_{pref}}) = \{\}$$
$$M^2_1(P^T_{AF_{pref}}) = \{\ \}, \qquad M^2_2(P^T_{AF_{pref}}) = \{r_2\}, M^2_3(P^T_{AF_{pref}}) = \{r_2\}, M^2_4(P^T_{AF_{pref}}) = \{r_1, r_2\}$$

We can see that $M_1$ is preferred to $M_2$, denoted as $M_1 > M_2$, since $M^1_2(P^T_{AF_{pref}}) \subset M^1_1(P^T_{AF_{pref}})$. In a similar way, we can verify that $M_1 > M_3$, and $M_1 > M_4$. The preferred answer set of $P^T_{AF_{pref}}$ is $M_1$. According to Theorem 2, the stable extension of $AF_{pref}$ that fulfills better the set of preferences $Pref$ is:

$$M_1 \cap AR = \{acc(visit\_Puebla), acc(hotel4stars\_deals), acc(city\_activities),$$
$$acc(tropical\_storm), def(visit\_Acapulco), def(hotel3stars\_deals),$$
$$def(water\_activities), def(seafood), def(limited\_cash),$$
$$def(hotel3stars\_deals)\}$$

As we mention at the end of Introduction Section, this stable extension coincides with what our intuition expected.

## 4  Preferences for the Preferred Argumentation Semantics

Here, we consider other interesting argumentation semantics defined by Dung in [4], the *preferred argumentation semantics*. We should note that the name of this semantics is not because this semantics is selecting the preferred extensions of an argumentation framework according to some preference criterion, that is, the word *preferred* is just the identifier of this semantics and this name was given by the author of this semantics. We can verify very straightforward that our approach works to select the preferred extensions that fulfill better a set of preferences, we only should replace the definition of stable argumentation semantics by the definition of preferred argumentation semantics. If we take into account the background of argumentation given in section 2 then, the definition of the preferred argumentation semantics given by Dung is as follows.

**Definition 12.** *[4] A preferred extension of an argumentation framework AF is a maximal (w.r.t. inclusion) admissible set of AF. The set of preferred extensions of AF, denoted by* preferred_extensions(AF), *will be referred to as the preferred semantics of AF.*

It is important to say that the preferred argumentation semantics can be characterized by a disjunctive logic program [7]. Thus, in order to obtain the preferred extensions of an argumentation framework we can use a mapping function that constructs a disjunctive logic program, such that the stable models of it correspond to the preferred extensions of the argumentation framework. The mapping is very similar to the mapping given in definitions 3 and 4, we only should replace in this mapping the rules $def(x) \leftarrow \neg def(y)$ by $def(x) \vee def(y)$. For instance, the rule $def(hotel4stars\_deals) \leftarrow \neg def(hotel3stars\_deals)$ in program $P_{AF}$ of example 1 is replaced with the rule $def(hotel4stars\_deals) \vee def(hotel3stars\_deals)$. Formally, given an argumentation framework $AF = \langle AR, attacks \rangle$, we define $P_{AF}^{d_1^\vee} = \bigcup_{x \in AR}\{def(x) \vee def(y) \mid (y,x) \in attacks\}$ and we replace $P_{AF}^{d_1}$ with $P_{AF}^{d_1^\vee}$ in definition 4, i.e., we define $P_{AF}^\vee = P_{AF}^{d_1^\vee} \cup P_{AF}^{d_2} \cup \bigcup_{x \in AR}\{acc(x) \leftarrow \neg def(x)\}$. Thus, $E \subseteq AR$ is a preferred extension of $AF$ iff $tr(E)$ is a stable model of $P_{AF}^\vee$. In this way, the preferred extensions and the stable extensions of an argumentation framework correspond to the stable models of particular logic programs.

## 5   Conclusions

This paper describes a proposal to enrich the search for solutions of an argumentation problem, by implementing a way to choose one solution over others.

## References

1. Bench-Capon, T.J.M., Dunne, P.E.: Argumentation in artificial intelligence. Artificial Intelligence 171(10-15), 619–641 (2007)
2. Brewka, G.: Logic Programming with Ordered Disjunction. In: Proceedings AAAI-2002(2002)
3. Carballido, J.L., Nieves, J.C., Osorio, M.: Inferring Preferred Extensions by Pstable Semantics. Revista Iberomericana de Inteligencia Artificial 13(41), 38–53 (2009)
4. Dung, P.M.: On the acceptability of arguments and its fundamental role in nonmonotonic reasoning, logic programming and n-person games. Artificial Intelligence 77(2), 321–358 (1995)
5. Gelfond, M., Lifschitz, V.: The Stable Model Semantics for Logic Programming. In: Kowalski, R., Bowen, K. (eds.) 5th Conference on Logic Programming, pp. 1070–1080. MIT Press (1988)
6. Nevar, C.I.C., Maguitman, A.G., Loui, R.P.: Logical models of argument. ACM Comput. Surv. 32(4), 337–383 (2000)
7. Nieves, J.C., Osorio, M., Cortés, U.: Preferred extensions as stable models. Theory and Practice of Logic Programming (TPLP) 8(4), 527–543 (2008)
8. Nieves, J.C., Osorio, M., Zepeda, C.: A schema for generating relevant logic programming semantics and its applications in argumentation theory. Fundamenta Informaticae 106(2-4), 295–319 (2011)
9. van Dalen, D.: Logic and structure, 3rd Augmented edn. Springer, Berlin (1994)

# Computing Preferred Semantics: Comparing Two ASP Approaches vs an Approach Based on 0-1 Integer Programming

Mauricio Osorio, Juan Díaz, and Alejandro Santoyo

Universidad de las Americas en Puebla,
Sta. Catarina Martir, Cholula, Puebla, 72820 Mexico
{osoriomauri,alejandro1.santoyo}@gmail.com, juana.diaz@udlap.mx
http://www.udlap.mx

**Abstract.** Dung's abstract argumentation frameworks has been object of intense study not just for its relationship with logical reasoning but also for its uses within artificial intelligence. One research branch in abstract argumentation has focused on finding new methods for computing its different semantics. We present a novel method, to the best of our knowledge, for computing preferred semantics using 0-1 integer programming, and also experimentally compare it with two answer set programming approaches. Our results indicate that this new method performed well.

**Keywords:** Argumentation Frameworks, Binary Programming, Answer Set Programming, Preferred Semantics.

## 1 Introduction

Argumentation theory has become an increasingly important and exciting research topic in Artificial Intelligence (AI), with research activities ranging from developing theoretical models, prototype implementations, and application studies [1], [2]. The main purpose of argumentation theory is to study the fundamental mechanism humans use in argumentation and to explore ways to implement this mechanism on computers.

Currently formal argumentation research has been strongly influenced by abstract argumentation theory of Dung [3]. This approach is mainly orientated to manage the interaction of arguments by introducing a single structure called Argumentation Framework (AF). An argumentation framework is basically a pair of sets: a set of arguments and a set of disagreements between arguments called attacks. Indeed an argumentation framework can be regarded as a directed graph in which the arguments are represented by nodes and the attack relations are represented by arcs. In Figure 1, one can see an example of an argumentation framework and its graph representation.

In [3], four argumentation semantics were introduced: stable semantics, preferred semantics, grounded semantics, and complete semantics. The central notion of Dung's semantics is the acceptability of the arguments. Even though

A. Gelbukh et al. (Eds.): MICAI 2014, Part I, LNAI 8856, pp. 419–430, 2014.

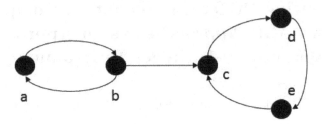

**Fig. 1.** Graph Represetation of $AF := \langle\{a, b, c, d, e\}, \{(a, b), (b, a), (b, c), (c, d), (d, e),$ $(e, c)\}\rangle$

each of these argumentation semantics represents different patterns of selection of arguments, all of them are based on the basic concept of admissible set. Informally speaking, an admissible set presents a coherent and defendable point of view in a conflict between arguments. For instance, by considering the argumentation framework of Figure 1, one can find the following admissible sets: $\emptyset, \{a\}, \{b\}, \{b, d\}$.

One research branch in abstract argumentation has been to find new methods for computing its different semantics, *i.e.* the search for acceptable (*w.r.t.* certain criteria) sets of arguments. Charwat *et al.* [4] surveys the approaches that has been used so far for computing argumentation frameworks semantics, and divided them into reduction and direct approaches. The direct approach consists in developing new algorithms for computing argumentation frameworks semantics, but our interest is in the reduction approach.

The reduction approach consists in using the software that was originally developed for other formalisms [4]. Thus, a given argumentation framework has to be formalized in the targeted formalism, like: constraint-satisfaction [5], propositional logic [6], and answer-set programming [7], [8].

To the best of our knowledge, there is just a previous work [9] where authors indirectly used 0-1 integer programming for computing preferred semantics, since their approach was based on a mapping from an argumentation framework $AF$ into a logic program with negation as failure $\Pi_{AF}$ to Clark's completion $Comp(\Pi_{AF})$ [10] to 0-1 integer program $lc(\Pi_{AF})$ [11], which then was solved by a mathematical programming solver.

In this work, we present a novel method, to the best of our knowledge, for directly computing preferred semantics using 0-1 integer programming with no mapping. Additionally, we experimentally compare it with two ASP approaches: the ASPARTIX approach[12] using its general encoding for preferred semantics[1], and the approach presented by Osorio *et al.* [10], where authors showed that preferred extensions can be characterized by the stable model semantics of a logic program. Our results indicate that this new method performed well, and even outperforms the ASP approaches for other semantics [13].

The paper is organized as follows. Section 2 gives some background on argumentation. Section 3 presents a procedure based on solving a series of 0-1

---

[1] http://www.dbai.tuwien.ac.at/research/project/argumentation/systempage/

integer programming problems for computing preferred extensions. Section 4 presents the experiment results as well as the used methodology. Finally, Section 5 presents some conclusions and future work.

## 2   Background

For space reasons, we assume that readers are familiar with the basic notions of 0-1 integer programming and answer set programming, otherwise readers can find good introductions in [14] for 0-1 integer programming, and in [7] for answer set programming. Additionally in [8] readers can find a survey of answer set programming approaches for computing argumentations semantics.

In this section we define some basic concepts of Dung's argumentation approach. The first one is the argumentation framework. An argumentation framework captures the relationships between arguments.

**Definition 1.** *[3] An argumentation framework is a pair $AF := \langle AR, attacks \rangle$, where AR is a finite set of arguments, and attacks is a binary relation on AR, i.e. attacks $\subseteq AR \times AR$.*

Any argumentation framework can be regarded as a directed graph. For instance, if $AF := \langle \{a, b, c, d, e\}, \{(a, b), (b, a), (b, c), (c, d), (d, e), (e, b)\} \rangle$, then $AF$ is represented as it is shown in Figure 1. We say that $a$ *attacks* $b$ (or $b$ is attacked by $a$) if $attacks(a, b)$ holds. Similarly, we say that a set $S$ of arguments attacks $b$ (or $b$ is attacked by $S$) if $b$ is attacked by an argument in $S$.

Dung defined his argumentation semantics based on the basic concept of *admissible set*, which can be understood in terms of *defense* of arguments and in terms of *conflict-free* sets, as follows:

**Definition 2.** *[15] Let $AF := \langle AR, attacks \rangle$ be an argumentation framework, $A \in AR$ and $S \subseteq AR$, then:*

1. *$A^+$ as $\{B \in AR \mid A$ attacks $B\}$ and*
2. *$S^+$ as $\{B \in AR \mid A$ attacks $B$ for some $A \in S\}$.*
3. *$A^-$ as $\{B \in AR \mid B$ attacks $A\}$ and*
4. *$S^-$ as $\{B \in AR \mid B$ attacks $A$ for some $A \in S\}$.*
5. *$S$ is conflict-free iff $S \cap S^+ = \emptyset$.*
6. *$S$ defends an argument $A$ iff $A^- \subseteq S^+$.*
7. *$F : 2^{AR} \to 2^{AR}$ as $F(S) = \{A \in AR \mid A$ is defended by $S\}$.*

Now it is possible to define the semantics (extensions) in terms of admissible sets as follows:

**Definition 3.** *[15] Let $AF := \langle AR, attacks \rangle$ be an argumentation framework and $S \subseteq AR$ be a conflict-free set of arguments, then:*

1. *$S$ is admissible iff $S \subseteq F(S)$.*
2. *$S$ is a complete extension iff $S = F(S)$.*

3. *S is a preferred extension iff S is a maximal (w.r.t. set inclusion) complete extension.*

The preferred semantics as defined in [3] can also be defined in terms of *admissible sets* as it was shown in [15]. Thus we have the following equivalent definitions for preferred semantics:

**Proposition 1.** *[15] Let $AF := \langle AR, attacks \rangle$ be an argumentation framework and let $S \subseteq AR$. The following statements are equivalent: 1).- S is a maximal complete extension (Definition 3 item 3), and 2).- S is a maximal admissible set (Definition 7 in [3]).*

## 3   Computing Preferred Semantics by 0-1 Integer Programming

In this section we show the 0-1 integer programming model, its encoding in FICO Xpress Mosel[2] language and its operation for computing the preferred semantics of a given argumentation framework.

### 3.1   Preliminary Definitions

A 0-1 integer program works with decision variables to find the solution to a given problem formulation. Therefore, the first step is to define the required binary decision variables, which will be related to the reference set $S$ mentioned in definitions 2, 3 and Proposition 1, as follows:

$$S_i = \begin{cases} 0 & \text{if } i \notin Optimal\ Solution \\ 1 & \text{if } i \in Optimal\ Solution \end{cases} \quad \forall\ i \in AR \quad (1)$$

This decision variables definition is part of the preferred semantics problem formulation presented in Subsection 3.2. Now, consider that it is required to have a mechanism to work with attacks more suitable than working with the adjacency matrix of a given argumentation framework, then we define:

**Definition 4.** *Let $AF := \langle AR, attacks \rangle$ be an argumentation framework, then: $R_i^- = \{j \in AR : (j, i) \in attacks\}\ \forall i \in AR$, is the set of nodes attacking node i, and $R^- = \{R_i^- : i \in AR\}$.*

Considering Definitions 2, 3, and 4 we restate the admissible set definition in order to be able to derive the linear constraint that assures admissibility.

**Definition 5.** *Let $AF := \langle AR, attacks \rangle$ be an argumentation framework, and set $S \subseteq AR$, then S is admissible iff $\forall i \in S, \forall j \in R_i^-, \exists k \in S, ((k, j) \in attacks))$.*

This definition becomes constraint (4) in the problem formulation. In the next Subsection we present the preferred semantics problem formulation and explain the objective function and constraints, as well as the iterative process for computing all the extensions.

---

[2] http://www.fico.com/en/wp-content/secure_upload/
Xpress-Mosel-User-Guide.pdf

## 3.2   Preferred Semantics Problem Formulation

Consider that a mathematical solver searches in the solution space for one optimal solution for a given problem formulation. Therefore, if we want all the extensions of a given argumentation framework, it is required to solve a series of binary programming models, one for each extension.

The 0-1 integer problem formulation to compute the $t^{th}$ preferred extension of a given argumentation framework is the following, including (1):

$$max \; f(S) = \sum_{i \in AR} S_i \tag{2}$$

$$S_i + S_j \leq 1 \qquad\qquad \forall i \in AR, \forall j \in R_i^- \tag{3}$$

$$\sum_{k \in R_j^-} S_k \geq S_i \qquad\qquad \forall i \in AR, \forall j \in R_i^- \tag{4}$$

$$\sum_{i \in C^r} S_i \geq 1 \qquad\qquad \forall r = 1, \ldots, t-1 \tag{5}$$

$$S_i \in \{0, 1\} \qquad\qquad i = 1, ..., |AR| \tag{6}$$

In (1) we have the decision variables definition and constraint (6) defines the problem's domain. Now, if it the 0-1 program formulation with a given argumentation framework has an optimal solution then we define:

**Definition 6.** *The set* $M = \{i \in AR : S_i = 1\}$ *is the optimal solution to the 0-1 problem formulation, and* $C = \{i \in AR : S_i = 0\}$ *the solution's complement.*

We can think of the preferred semantics in terms of a serie of solutions that this model finds in each iteration, as follows:

$$\{M^1, M^2, ..., M^q\} : |M^1| \geq |M^2| \geq ... \geq |M^q|$$

Since an argumentation framework semantics is made up of several sets, we use $M^t$ to denote the solution of the binary subproblem in iteration $t$ and $q$ to denote the amount of preferred extensions that a given argumentation framework has, such that $q \geq 1$ and $q \in \mathbb{N}$. The expression states also that the $M^1$ has the largest possible cardinality, and that $|M^1| \geq |M^2| \geq ... \geq |M^q|$ such that $|M^q|$ has the smallest possible cardinality.

The following paragraphs explain each constraint of the preferred semantics problem formulation in terms of the properties that preferred extensions must fulfill, namely: conflic-freeness, admissibility, and maximality *w.r.t.* set inclusion.

*Conflict-Freeness.* Note that the definition of a conflict-free set in Definition 2 item 5 is not stated in terms of attacks's directions but just in terms of attacks between arguments, without considering the directions of them. In this way, such a definition is considering an arc just as an edge, and therefore the whole argumentation framework can be regarded as an undirected graph, at least with regard to the conflict-free set problem.

In graph theory [16], a *stable set* is a set of vertices no two of which are adjacent, and it is also commonly known as an *independent set*. Thus, the typical stable set problem of an undirected graph in graph theory can be seen as the conflict-free set problem of an argumentation framework in abstract argumentation. This is important because the stable set problem has been widely studied within the mathematical programming community.

A stable set in a graph is *maximum* if the graph contains no larger stable set and *maximal* if the set cannot be extended to a larger stable set; a maximum stable set is necessarily maximal, but not conversely [16]. Thus, we also can think of the problem of finding the maximum independent set problem as the *maximum conflict-free set* problem.

There is a well-known 0-1 integer programming formulation for the maximum independent set problem. Given a graph $G = (V, E)$ ($AF := \langle AR, attacks \rangle$), where $V(G)$ is the set of vertices ($AR$), and $E(G)$ is the set of edges (*attacks*), and considering Definition 4 instead the adjacency matrix $x$ for graph $G$, the problem formulation [17] for computing a *maximum conflict-free set* (or *maximum independent set*) is made up of (1), (2), (3), and (6):

Note that the expression $S_i + S_j \leq 1$, in constraint (3), will be just fulfilled when $S_i = 1$ or $S_j = 1$ but not both and when $S_i = 0$ and $S_j = 0$, therefore at most one arguments will be selected which guarantees us that solution will be a *conflict-free set*.

**Maximality with Regard to Set Inclusion.** The model's objective function (2) guarantees us that we will find a *maximum cardinality set* which will be the solution $M^t$, and constraint (5) will avoid that $M^{t+1}$ be any subset of $M^t$, thus (2) and (5) guarantee us *maximality with regard to set inclusion*.

**Admissibility.** The intuition of Definitions 1, 2 and 3 is that an *admissible set S* should defend each of its arguments, and Definition 5 just restates it in terms of Definition 4. Note that in Definition 5 the existential quantifier suggests that constraint (4) should be $\sum_{k \in R_j^-} S_k \geq 1$, but we use $\sum_{k \in R_j^-} S_k \geq S_i$ since the constraint must be fulfilled $\forall i \in AR^3$. This way, the translation from this definition to constraint (4) is a straightforward task.

Thus, constraint (4) guarantees that the set $M^t$ is admissible, and we know that $M^t$ is a *maximum cardinality set*, and from Proposition 1 we know that then it is also a *preferred extension*.

---

[3] There are two special cases: $S_i = 0$ and $S_i = 1$. In the first one, it does not matter the total of $\sum_{k \in R_j^-} S_k$ because $S_i \notin Solution$, thus in the second case we will have $\sum_{k \in R_j^-} S_k \geq 1$ which means that there will be at least one argument defending argument $i$ since $S_i \in Solution$.

## 3.3   Preferred Extension Program

Notice that the problem formulation made up of (2), (3), (4) and (6) already can be used for computing the first preferred extension of a given argumentation framework. To this end, this program should be coded using a mathematical programming language like *mosel*[4], which is a straightforward task, since the mathematical language was developed for expressing mathematical formulas, and even though we can not show the complete code for space reasons, the following code stands for the whole mathematical model:

```
! Objective Function
  z:= sum(i in nodos) S(i)
! Constraints
  forall(i in nodos, j in R(i)) S(i) + S(j) <= 1
  forall(i in nodos, j in R(i)) sum(k in R(j)) S(k) >= S(i)
  forall(i in nodos) S(i) is_binary
  maximize(z)
```

We will denote this program as $BIP$ in order to make reference to it.

## 3.4   Preferred Semantics

Note that once the model is implemented in a mathematical programming language, the program just compute one preferred extension, the one with the largest cardinality. In order to compute an additional extension it is required to solve the model again, but adding an additional constraint to avoid getting previous solution and any subset of it, which will force to get another different extension with at most the same cardinality. In this setting, it is required to iterate to find all the extensions of a given argumentation framework until there is no optimal solution.

Then, in order to find the constraint that we have to add, consider Definitions 6, and let $P$ be the solution in iteration $t + 1$, and $M$ the solution in iteration $t$, thus:

$$P \subseteq M \leftrightarrow \forall x(x \in P \to x \in M) \leftrightarrow \forall x(x \notin P \vee x \in M)$$
$$P \nsubseteq M \leftrightarrow \exists x(x \in P \wedge x \notin M) \leftrightarrow \exists x(x \in P \wedge x \in C)$$

The intuition of this result is that it is required that solution in iteration $t+1$ has at least one element from solution's complement in iteration $t$. Constraint (5) is defined from this intuition. Note that the mosel code must take care of the special case where $|M| = |AR|$.

Now, considering that $PE$ should contain all the preferred extensions of a given argumentation framework, and $MC$ a set of additional (5) constraints, then the algorithm for computing the $q$ extensions of a given argumentation framework is the following:

---

[4] http://www.fico.com/en/products/fico-xpress-optimization-suite/

1  Set $PE = \emptyset$, $MC = \emptyset$;
2  Solve $BIP \cup MC$;
3  **while** *optimal solution found* **do**
4  |    Let M be the optimal solution, and C its complement;
5  |    Add M to PE;
6  |    Add $\sum_{i \in C} S_i \geq 1$ to $MC$;
7  |    Solve $BIP \cup MC$;
8  **end**

**Algorithm 1.** For Computing all Preferred Extensions of a Given AF

Now it is possible to state the following theorem:

**Theorem 1.** *Let AF be an argumentation framework, $R^-$ as in Definition 4, M is a solution of BIP, and PE is computed as described in Algorithm No. 1, then PE is the set of all preferred extensions of AF.*

*Proof. Sketch: Consider the following items:*

1. *The Objective function (2), and constraints (3) and (4) guarantee us that M is a conflict-free set of maximum cardinality which also is admissible.*
2. *By items 1 and by Proposition 1 we know that a maximal admissible set is also a maximal complete extension, and by Definition 3 we know that a maximal complete extension is also a preferred extension. Therefore M is a preferred extension.*
3. *Now, notice that in each iteration, due to the constraint added to MC in step 6 in iteration t, the solution M (if exists), obtained in step 4 must not be a superset or subset of any previous solutions already in PE, and must be of maximum cardinality among the solutions that satisfy $BIP \cup MC$, therefore M is maximal w.r.t. set inclusion.*

## 4    Experimental Evaluation

In order to measure the performance of the 0-1 integer program, it was compared with two answer set programming approaches: the ASPARTIX[18] which we will call just ASP1, and the Osorio's approach [10] which we will call ASP2. Additionally, the approach based on 0-1 integer programming will be called BIP (Binary Integer Programming).

### 4.1    Experiment Description

The ASP1 code was originally developed in DLV and is capable to compute several extensions, among them the preferred extensions. For space reasons we can not present the code used to compute the preferred extensions, however the program is available at ASPARTIX's web page[5].

---

[5] http://www.dbai.tuwien.ac.at/research/project/argumentation/systempage/

The ASP2 code should be created from the argumentation framework code that describes each instance. For space reasons we can not present the method for mapping from an argumentation framework into a answer set program, however the method is described in [10].

The solver used for both answer set programming approaches was Clingo[6] due to its great performance in several answer set programming competitions [19], while, the 0-1 integer programming approach used the *ad-hoc* Xpress[7] solver. Both solver were used without any special configuration parameter. The computers used in the experiment had the following configuration: An AMD Phenom II X3 2.80 Ghz processor, 4GB of RAM, and 32-bit Windows 7 professional operating system.

The given time for solving each instance was 1000 seconds. In order to compute the global time when a solver fails solving a given instances, the time assigned is 1000 seconds.

The instances that were used during all the experiments were taken from the ASPARTIX web page[8], though it seems that they are currently not available. The name of each instance gives us some information about its inherent difficulty to be solved and it has the form: inst_G_n_p1_p2_i, that should be interpreted as follows:

**G: Generator Used:** 2: arbitrary AFs (does not use p2); 4: 4-grid AFs; 8: 8-grid AFs. Readers can find a complete description in [20]. **n:** number of arguments. **p1:** Probability for each pair of arguments (a,b) that the attack (a,b) is present for the arbitrary graphs. For the grid graphs this parameter indicates one dimension of the grid. The other is calculated with n. **p2:** Present only for grid AFs. Indicates the probability that a given attack is a mutual attack. **i:** Index for AFs with the same parameters, i.e. AFs generated with the same parameters are distinguished with this index.

### 4.2    Performance Results

A total of 1320 instances were used, the instances ranged from 20 arguments to 110 arguments with increments of 10 arguments. There were 132 instances of 20 arguments, 44 of each kind of instances, and so on for the rest of the instances.

In Figure No. 2 we show average computation times for each approach and for each kind of instances (arbitrary, 4-grid and 8-grid). It shows also that ASP2 had the best performance (near cero) for 4-grid and 8-grid instances, while the Binary Integer Program (BIP) approach had the worst one. However, ASP2 has the worst performance with arbitrary instances, while ASP1 had the best one.

In the same Figure No. 2, notice that the performance solving 4-grid instances were quite similar until 40-arguments instances, where the BIP approach started to have difficult to solve them. The ASP1 approach started to have problems

---

[6] http://potassco.sourceforge.net

[7] http://www.fico.com/en/Products/DMTools/Pages/FICO-Xpress-Optimization-Suite.aspx

[8] http://www.dbai.tuwien.ac.at/research/project/argumentation/systempage

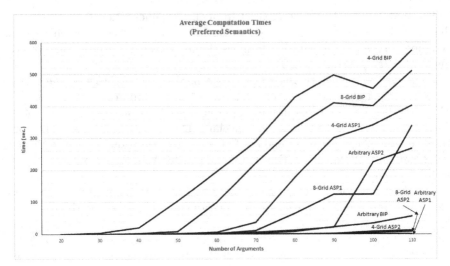

**Fig. 2.** Average Computation Times per Approach and per Kind of AF

until the 70-arguments instances. The ASP2 approach had no difficulties even with the 110-arguments instances.

The performance solving 8-grid instances were quite similar until 50-arguments instances, where the BIP approach started to have difficulties to solve them. The ASP1 approach started to have problems until the 70-arguments instances. The ASP2 approach had no difficulties even with the 110-arguments instances.

The performance solving arbitrary instances were quite similar until 90-arguments instances, where the ASP2 approach started to have difficult to solve them. The BIP approach performed quit well even for 110-arguments instances. The ASP1 approach had no difficulties even with the 110-arguments instances.

In Figure No. 3 we show the timeouts percentages for each approach and for each kind of instance. Each time that the approach could not compute a given instance within the time limit of 1000 seconds, it was computed as a timeout. It is not surprising that the graph behaviour is very similar to the behaviour of Figure No. 2, since the timeouts are directly related to the approach difficult to solve certain kind of instances. Note that several lines are not visible since all of them were always cero.

### 4.3   Interpretation and Discussion

In Figures No. 2 and 3 we see that ASP2 was better in 4-grid and 8-grid instances, while ASP1 was better in Arbitrary instances. On the other hand, even though that BIP was 2nd place in just Arbitrary instances, there are some issues that we should point out:

BIP's performance in Arbitrary instances was close to 1st place (ASP1), in 8-grid instances BIP's performance was close to ASP1 and ASP2 until after 50 nodes instances, and until after 40 nodes instances in 4-grid instances.

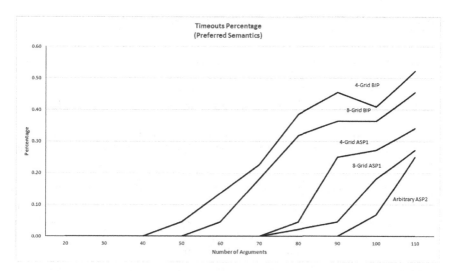

**Fig. 3.** Timeout per Approach and per kind of AF

Additionally, we can say that ASP1 and BIP are similar in the sense that both were created to compute the preferred semantics of any argumentation framework, while ASP2 requires a mapping from a given argumentation framework into a logic program, which can just be used to compute the preferred semantics of that specific argumentation framework.

## 5    Conclusions

We have presented a novel method for computing preferred semantics using binary integer programming, and we found that the performance is comparable with answer set programming approaches.

Additionally, it is well known that binary integer programs can be improved, in order to compute more efficiently its objective function, by using mathematical programming techniques. It means that it is possible to improve the performance of this novel approach for computing preferred semantics.

This new approach constitutes an alternative for computing argumentation frameworks semantics using mathematical programming techniques, and even though we used an state of the art mathematical programming solver, there exists several mathematical programming libraries for java, C++ and other general purpose languages. As future work we will analize the possible connection with the work of Gabbay [21].

## References

1. Bench-Capon, T., Dunne, P.E.: Argumentation in artificial intelligence. Artificial Intelligence 171(10-15), 619–641 (2007),
   http://www.sciencedirect.com/science/article/pii/S0004370207000793

2. Rahwan, I., Simari, G.R. (eds.): Argumentation in Artificial Intelligence. Springer (2009)
3. Dung, P.M.: On the acceptability of arguments and its fundamental role in non-monotonic reasoning, logic programming and n-person games. Artificial Intelligence 77(2), 321–358 (1995)
4. Gaggl, S.A., Wallner, J.P., Wolfran, S., Charwat, G., Dvorak, W.: Implementing abstract argumentation: A survey. Institut Fur Information Systeme, Tech. Rep. (2013)
5. Dechter, R.: Constraint Processing. Morgan Kaufmann Publishers Inc. (2003)
6. Biere, A., Heule, M., van Maaren, H., Walsh, T. (eds.): Handbook of Satisfiability. Frontiers in Artificial Intelligence and Applications, vol. 185. IOS Press (2009)
7. Brewka, G., Eiter, T., Truszczyński, M.: Answer set programming at a glance. Commun. ACM 54(12), 92–103 (2011)
8. Toni, F., Sergot, M.: Argumentation and answer set programming. In: Balduccini, M., Son, T.C. (eds.) Logic Programming, Knowledge Representation, and Nonmonotonic Reasoning. LNCS, vol. 6565, pp. 164–180. Springer, Heidelberg (2011)
9. Preferred Extensions as Minimal Models of Clark's Completion Semantics, vol. 68 (2013)
10. Nieves, J.C., Osorio, M., Cortés, U.: Preferred Extensions as Stable Models. Theory and Practice of Logic Programming 8(4), 527–543 (2008)
11. Bell, C., Nerode, A., Ng, R.T., Subrahmanian, V.S.: Mixed integer programming methods for computing nonmonotonic deductive databases. Journal of the ACM 41(6), 1178–1215 (1994)
12. Egly, U., Alice Gaggl, S., Woltran, S.: Answer-set programming encodings for argumentation frameworks. Argument & Computation 1(2), 147–177 (2010), http://www.tandfonline.com/doi/abs/10.1080/19462166.2010.486479
13. Osorio, M., Santoyo, A., Diaz, J.: Computing semi-stable semantics of af by 0-1 integer programming. Submitted to LANMR 2014 (2014)
14. Wolsey, L.A.: Integer Programming. Discrte Mathematics and Optimization. John Wiley & Sons, Inc. (1998)
15. Caminada, M.W.A., Carnielli, W.A., Dunne, P.E.: Semi-stable semantics. J. Log. Comput. 22(5), 1207–1254 (2012)
16. Bondy, J.A., Murty, U.S.R.: Graph Theory. Graduate Texts in Mathematics. Springer (2008); Axler, S. (ed.)
17. Butenko, S.: Maximum independent set and related problems, with aapplications. Ph.D. dissertation, University of Florida (2003)
18. Egly, U., Gaggl, S.A., Woltran, S.: ASPARTIX: Implementing argumentation frameworks using answer-set programming. In: Garcia de la Banda, M., Pontelli, E. (eds.) ICLP 2008. LNCS, vol. 5366, pp. 734–738. Springer, Heidelberg (2008)
19. Calimeri, F., Ianni, G., Ricca, F.: The third open Answer Set Programming competition. CoRR, vol. abs/1206.3 (2012), http://dblp.uni-trier.de/db/journals/corr/corr1206.html#abs-1206-3111
20. Dvorák, W., Gaggl, S.A., Wallner, J.P., Woltran, S.: Making use of advances in answer-set programming for abstract argumentation systems. CoRR, vol. abs/1108.4942 (2011)
21. Gabbay, D.M.: Equational approach to argumentation networks. Argument and Computation 3(2-3), 87–142 (2012)

# Experimenting with SAT Solvers in Vampire*

Armin Biere[1], Ioan Dragan[2], Laura Kovács[2,3], and Andrei Voronkov[4]

[1] Johannes Kepler University, Linz, Austria
[2] Vienna University of Technology, Vienna, Austria
[3] Chalmers University of Technology, Gothenburg, Sweden
[4] The University of Manchester, Manchester, UK

**Abstract.** Recently, a new reasoning framework, called AVATAR, integrating first-order theorem proving with SAT solving has been proposed. In this paper, we experimentally analyze the behavior of various SAT solvers within first-order proving. For doing so, we first integrate the Lingeling SAT solver within the first-order theorem prover Vampire and compare the behavior of such an integration with Vampire using a less efficient SAT solver. Interestingly, our experiments on first-order problems show that using the best SAT solvers within AVATAR does not always give best performance. There are some problems that could be solved only by using a less efficient SAT solver than Lingeling. However, the integration of Lingeling with Vampire turned out to be the best when it came to solving most of the hard problems.

## 1 Introduction

This paper aims to experimentally analyze and improve the performance of the first-order theorem prover Vampire [8] on dealing with problems that contain propositional variables and also other clauses that can be splitted. The recently introduced AVATAR framework [15], proposes a way of integrating a SAT solver in the framework of an automatic theorem prover. The main task that a SAT solver has in this framework is to help the theorem prover in splitting clauses. Although initial results obtained by using this framework in Vampire proved to be really efficient, it is unclear whether efficiency of AVATAR depends on the efficiency of the used SAT solver. In this paper we address this problem using various SAT solvers and experimentally evaluate AVATAR as follows. We first integrate the Lingeling [3] SAT solver inside Vampire and compare its behavior against a less efficient SAT solver already implemented in Vampire. Our experiments on a large number of problems show significantly different results when using Lingeling and/or the default SAT solver of Vampire for splitting clauses in AVATAR.

Splitting clauses is a well studied problem in the community of automated theorem provers. First, the method introduced in the SPASS [16] theorem prover tries to do splitting and uses backtracking to recover from a bad split. Another way of dealing with splittable clauses was introduced in Vampire [10] and takes care of splitting without backtracking. Both ways of splitting on a clause are highly optimized for these theorem

---

* This work was partially supported by Swedish VR grant D0497701 and the Austrian research projects FWF S11410-N23, FWF S11408-N23 and WWTF ICT C-050.

A. Gelbukh et al. (Eds.): MICAI 2014, Part I, LNAI 8856, pp. 431–442, 2014.

provers. Implementation of these splitting techniques is not trivial and can highly influence the overall performance of the prover. Therefore, in [6] the authors are performing an extensive evaluation of different ways of doing splitting and evaluate other methods using BDDs and SAT solvers for clause splitting. Although the use of splitting improves performance these splitting techniques cannot compete against the methods used in SAT solvers on propositional problems or even in SMT solver on ground instances [15].

The problem of dealing with splitting clauses in AVATAR is motivated by the way first-order theorem provers usually work. In general first-order provers make use of three types of inferences: *generating, deleting* and *simplifying* inferences. In practice, using these inferences one can notice a couple of problems. Usually the complexity for implementing different algorithms for the inference rules are dependent in the size (length) of the clauses they operate on. As an example of simplifying inference, subsumption resolution is known to be NP-complete and the algorithms that implement it are exponential in the number of literals in a clause. Another issue arises when we want to use generating inferences. In this case assuming we have two clauses containing $l_1$ and $l_2$ literals and we apply resolution on them then the resulting clause will have $l_1 + l_2 - 2$ literals. Now if these clauses are long it means we generate even longer clauses. This also raises the question of storage for these clauses for example by indexing [9] .They are a couple of methods that deal with large clauses, for example limited resource strategy [11] which is also implemented in Vampire. This method will start throwing away clauses that slow down the prover. An alternative would be to use splitting in order to make the clauses shorter and easy to be manipulated by the prover.

In this paper we study the use of splitting in the new AVATAR framework (see Section 2) for first-order theorem proving, by integrating different SAT solvers into the Vampire automated theorem prover (see Section 3). We evaluate the new approach (see Section 4) on a large set of problems in order to better understand how does the use of an state of the art SAT solver influences the AVATAR framework.

## 2   Preliminaries

This section overviews the main notions used in the paper, for more details we refer to [8,15]. In the framework of first-order logic, a *first-order clause* is a disjunction of *literals* of the following form $L_1 \lor \ldots \lor L_n$, where a literal is an atomic formula or the negation of an atomic formula. Usually when we speak about splitting we speak about clauses as being sets of literals. Due to this description of a clause we can safely assume that we do not have duplicate literals. We also assume that predicates, functions are uninterpreted and the language might contain the equality predicate (=).

In a nutshell splitting of clauses starts from the following remark. Suppose that we have a set $S$ of first-order clauses and $C_1 \lor C_2$ a clause such that the variables of $C_1$ and $C_2$ are disjoint. Then $\forall(C_1 \lor C_2)$ is equivalent to $\forall(C_1) \lor \forall(C_2)$. This transformation implies that the set $S \cup \{C_1 \lor C_2\}$ is unsatisfiable if and only if both $S \cup \{C_1\}$ and $S \cup \{C_2\}$ are unsatisfiable. In practice one can notice the fact that splittable clause usually appear when theorem provers are used in software verification applications.

Let $C_1, \ldots, C_n$ be clauses such that $n \geq 2$ and all the $C_i$'s have pairwise disjoint sets of variables. We can safely say that $SP \stackrel{\text{def}}{=} C_1 \lor \ldots \lor C_n$ is splittable into components $C_1, \ldots, C_n$. We will also say that the set $C_1, \ldots, C_n$ is a splitting of $SP$. An example of such a splittable clause can be considered any ground clause that contains multiple literals. One problem that arises in splitting is the fact that there are multiple ways of splitting a clause. But this is not a major issue since we know that there is always a unique splitting such that each component cannot be splitted more. We call this splitting of a clause maximal. Computation of such a splitting proves to always give the maximal number of components of a clause, see [10] for details.

Let us first discuss how the mapping between the first-order problem and the propositional problem is done. In the propositional problem that is sent to the SAT solver we basically keep track of clause components. In order to do that we have to use a mapping $[.]$ from components to propositional literals. The mapping has to satisfy the following properties: 1. $[C]$ is a positive literal if and only if $C$ is either a positive ground literal or a non-ground component; 2. for a negative ground component $\neg C$ we have $[\neg C] = \neg[C]$; 3. $[C_1] = [C_2]$ if and only if $C_1$ and $C_2$ are equal up to variable renaming and symmetry of equality. In order to implement this mapping Vampire uses a component index, which maps every component that satisfies the previous conditions into a propositional variable $[C]$. And for each such component $C$ the index checks whether there is already a stored component $C'$ that are equal than it returns $[C']$ as propositional variable. Doing so we ensure that we do not have multiple propositional variables that are mappings of equal components. In case there is no such component stored in the index, than a new propositional variable $[C]$ is introduced and we store the association between $C$ and $[C]$. A model provided by the SAT solver for the propositional problem is considered a component interpretation. Such a model contains only variables of the form $[C]$ or their negations and does not contain in the same time both a variable and its negation. The truth definition of a propositional variable in such an interpretation is standard. With the small difference that in case for a component $C$ neither $[C]$ not $\neg[C]$ belongs to the interpretation, than $[C]$ is considered *undefined*, meaning it is neither true nor false.

In a nutshell AVATAR works as follows. The first-order reasoning part works as usual, using a saturation algorithm [8]. The main difference with respect to a classical approach is the way it treats splittable clauses. In the case that a clause $C_1 \vee C_2 \ldots \vee C_n$ is splittable in $C_1, C_2, \ldots, C_n$ components and the clause passes the retention test it is not added to the set of *passive* clauses. Instead we add a clause $[C_1] \vee [C_2] \vee \ldots \vee [C_n]$ to the SAT solver and check if the problem added to the solver is satisfiable. If the SAT solver returns unsatisfiable, it means that we are done and report it to the first-order reasoning part. In case the problem is satisfiable, we ask the SAT solver to produce a model. This model acts as a component interpretation $I$. If in the interpretation a literal has the form $[C]$ for some component C then we pass to the first-order reasoner the component, where C is used as an assertion. Exception from this rule are those literals of the form $\neg[C]$, where C is a non-ground component. This is due to the fact that such a literal does not correspond to any component.

In our context a SAT solver has to expose an incremental behavior. By incremental we mean that the solver receives from time to time new clauses that have to be added at the propositional problem and checks whether the problem is satisfiable upon request from the first-order reasoner. If the problem is satisfiable than all it has to do is to pass back to the first-order reasoner a model (component interpretation) for all the propositional variables. Otherwise it simply has to return unsatisfiable and communicate the unsatisfiability result to the first-order reasoning part as well.

## 3  Integration

We now describe how we integrated the Lingeling SAT solver in the framework of Vampire. We also overview the options implemented in order to control the behavior of Lingeling in Vampire. Although Lingeling is used in commercial applications, the source code is publicly available. Also the default license allows Lingeling to be used in non-commercial and academic context. Our main goal after integrating the new solver in Vampire framework was to obtain better performance in the process of solving first-order problems.

In general any SAT solver is designed to accept as its input problems described in the DIMACS format [2]. We have decided to implement an interface that allows us to directly control Lingeling via its API. By using the API one can also control the options for the background SAT solver at run time depending on the strategy being deployed.

In the case when the SAT solver establishes satisfiability of a given problem, we are interested in obtaining a model for the problem. This behavior matches the intended use for the majority of SAT solver and in particular Lingeling. In the case of satisfiability though there are some situations when we would be interested in obtaining similar models. By similar models we mean that in the incremental case, if the current problem is proved to be satisfiable, we add new clauses to the solver and the solver decides that the problem is still satisfiable, we would like to obtain a model that has as few different assignments from the previous model as possible.

For the purpose of our work, we use Lingeling in an incremental manner, but there is still the question of how should we add the clauses to the solver. Incrementality in the context of SAT solving refers to the fact that a SAT solver is expected to be invoked multiple times. Each time it is asked to check satisfiability status of all the available clauses under assumptions that hold only at that specific invocation. The problem to be solved thus grows upon each call to add new clauses to the solver, for details see [5]. In the context of Vampire at some particular point the first-order reasoner can add a set of clauses to the existing problem. In order to add these clauses to the underlying SAT solver we implemented two versions of using Lingeling in the AVATAR architecture of Vampire. The first version, given in Algorithm 1, iterates over the clauses that appear in the original problem and adds them one by one to Lingeling. After we have added the entire set of clauses to the SAT solver we call for satisfiability check. We call this method of adding clauses "almost incremental" since it does not call for satisfiability check after each clause is added. Algorithm 1 is very similar to non-incremental SAT solving at each step when the first-order reasoning part asks for satisfiability check, since the call for satisfiability is done only after all the new clauses are added to the solver (line 6). Overall, the approach is still based on incrementality of the underlying SAT solver, since we keep adding clauses to the initial problem.

Another way of using the underlying solver would be to simulate the pure incremental approach, as presented in Algorithm 2. This approach is similar to the previous one with the difference that now as soon as a new clause is added to Lingeling we are also calling for a satisfiability check (line 4).

In order to be able to use any of the previous ways of integrating Lingeling in Vampire one has to be careful when adding clauses to Lingeling. Internally Lingeling tries to apply preprocessing on the problem and during preprocessing a subset of variables could be eliminated. This can lead to some problems since we eliminate a subset variables during the preprocessing and in some future step we might add some of them back to the solver. The issue that arises here is the fact that performing these operations can lead to unsoundness of the splitting solution generated by the first-order reasoner. In order to avoid the issue of not allowing the solver to eliminate variables while performing the preprocessing steps, Lingeling relies on the notion of *frozen* literals [3]. One can see a frozen literal as a literal that is marked as being important and not allowing the preprocessor to eliminate it during preprocessing steps. Using freezing of literals we are ensured that although preprocessing steps are done, it will inhibit the elimination of marked variables. In our case it actually means that one has to freeze all the literals that appear in the initial problem and also all the literals that are due to be added. The process of freezing literals is done on the fly when new clauses are added to the solver. In order to do be efficient and not freeze multiple times the same literal we keep a list of previously added and frozen literals.

| | |
|---|---|
| 1: **Input:** a set of clauses to be added | 1: **Input:** a set of clauses to be added |
| 2: **while** not all clauses added **do** | 2: **while** not all clauses added **do** |
| 3:     **Add** clause to Lingeling | 3:     **Add** clause to Lingeling |
| 4:     **Keep track** of the added clause | 4:     **Call** SAT procedure |
| 5: **end while** | 5:     **Keep track** of the added clause |
| 6: **Call** SAT procedure | 6:     **if** UNSATISFIABLE found **then** |
| 7: **if** UNSATISFIABLE found **then** | 7:         **Report** Unsatisfiability |
| 8:     **Report** Unsatisfiability | 8:     **else** |
| 9: **else** | 9:         **Return** a model |
| 10:     **Return** a model | 10:     **end if** |
| 11: **end if** | 11: **end while** |

**Fig. 1.** *"Almost" incremental* version of Lingeling in Vampire

**Fig. 2.** *Incremental* version of Lingeling in Vampire

Although the freezing of all literals proves to be a suitable solution of enforcing Lingeling not to eliminate some variables during the preprocessing steps, this also limits the power of the preprocessing implemented in the solver. One improvement could be to develop a methodology that would allow "predicting" which literals are not going to be used later on and allow the SAT solver to eliminate them if necessary.

### 3.1   Integrating and Using Lingeling in Vampire

In order to run Vampire[1] with Lingeling as a background SAT solver one has to use from command line the following option:

$$- -\text{sat\_solver lingeling}$$

---

[1] Vampire with all the features presented in this paper can be downloaded from vprover.org

By default when one enables the use of Lingeling as a background SAT solver, the solver is used as presented in Algorithm 1. This means that we add first all the clauses to the SAT solver and only then call for satisfiability check.

In case one wants to use Lingeling in Vampire as presented in Algorithm 2 the following option needs to be used

$$- - \mathtt{sat\_lingeling\_incremental}\ [\mathrm{on/off}]$$

This enables the incremental use of Lingeling as presented in the algorithm. By default this option is set to **off**.

We are also interested in generating similar models when we use incrementally the underlying solver. In order to control this behavior, one should use the option:

$$- - \mathtt{sat\_similar\_models}\ [\mathrm{on/off}]$$

By default this option is set to **off**. As for the previous options activating similar model generation has effect only in the case where Lingeling is used as background solver. In the following we present the results obtained by running Vampire with combinations of these options.

## 4  SAT Experiments in Vampire

Currently, there are all together 5 different combinations of values for the new options controlling the use of SAT solvers in Vampire. In order to benchmark these strategies we used problems coming from the TPTP [13] library. The experiments where run on the InfraGrid infrastructure of West University of Timisoara [1]. The infrastructure contains 100 Intel Quad Core processors, each one with dedicated 10GB of RAM. All the experiments presented in this paper are run with a time limit of 60 seconds and with memory limit of 2GB.

### 4.1  Benchmarks and Experiments

As a first set of problems we have considered the 300 problems from the first-order division of the CASC 2013 competition see [14]. Besides these problems we also used 6637 problems from the TPTP library. These 6637 problems are a subset of the TPTP library that have ranking greater than 0.2 and less than 1. Ranking 0.2 means that 80% of the state of the art automatic theorem provers can solve this problem, while ranking 1 means that no state of the art automated theorem prover can solve the problem.

Generally using a cocktail of strategies on a single problem proves to behave always better in first-order automated theorem proving. For this purpose we have decided to evaluate our approaches of using SAT solving in the AVATAR framework of Vampire both using a mixture of options and also using the default options implemented in Vampire.

**CASC Competition Problems.** We evaluated Vampire using all the new SAT features and kept all other options with their default values, from now on we will call this version of Vampire *default mode*. Also we evaluated the mode where we launch a cocktail of options (strategies) with small time limits and try to solve the problem, called the *casc mode*. A summary of the results obtained by running these strategies can be found in Table 1 and Table 2. All tables presented in this paper follow the same structure: the first row presents the abbreviations for all the used strategies, the second row presents the average time used by each of the strategies in order for solving the problems. Here we take into account only the time spent on the problems that can be solved using a particular strategy. The third row presents the total number of problems solved by each strategy. The last row presents the number of different problems. By different problems we mean problems that could be solved either by Vampire with the default SAT solver and not solved by any of the strategies involving Lingeling and the problems that can be solved only by at least one strategy that involves Lingeling but cannot be solved by Vampire using the default SAT solver. The abbreviations that appear in the header of each table stand for the following: *vamp* stands for Vampire using the default SAT solver, *L* stands for Vampire using Lingeling as background SAT solver, in an "almost" incremental way, *L S* similar to *L* but turning the generation of similar models on the SAT solver side on, *L I* stands for Vampire using Lingeling as background SAT solver in pure incremental way and *L I S* is similar to *L I* but with the change that it turns similar model generation on the SAT solver side.

**Table 1.** Results of running Vampire with default values for parameters on the 300 CASC problems

| Strategy | Vamp | L | L S | L I | L I S |
|---|---|---|---|---|---|
| Average Time | 3.4747 | 3.0483 | 4.2159 | 2.6728 | 3.8490 |
| # of solved instances | 142 | 146 | 156 | 143 | 144 |
| # different | 2 | 12 | 16 | 10 | 11 |

**Table 2.** Results of running Vampire using a cocktail of strategies on the 300 CASC problems

| Strategy | Vamp | L | L S | L I | L I S |
|---|---|---|---|---|---|
| Average Time | 3.4679 | 3.0615 | 4.2701 | 2.8139 | 3.7852 |
| # of solved instances | 230 | 233 | 240 | 232 | 232 |
| # different | 1 | 8 | 13 | 8 | 7 |

Table 1 reports on our experiments using the default mode of Vampire on the 300 CASC problems. Among these 300 problems, 23 problems can be solved only by either Vampire using some variations of Lingeling as background SAT solver or by Vampire using the default SAT solver. Table 2 shows our results obtained by running Vampire in casc mode on the 300 CASC problems. Among these 300 problems there are 18 problems that can be solved only by either Vampire using some variation of Lingeling as background SAT solver or by Vampire using the default SAT solver.

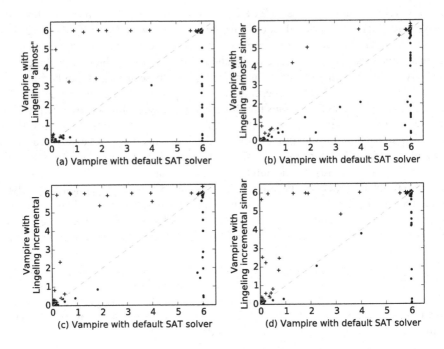

**Fig. 3.** Comparison of performance between Vampire with the default SAT solver and different Lingeling strategies run in *default* mode. Default SAT solver is compared against: (a) Lingeling "almost" incremental, (b) Lingeling "almost" incremental and similar models, (c) Lingeling incremental and (d) Lingeling incremental and similar models.

Figure 3 presents a comparison between Vampire using the default SAT solver and each of the new strategies. The scatter plots present on the x-axis the time spent by Vampire in trying to solve an instance, while on the y-axis the time spent by different strategies on the same instance. In order to have more concise figures we have decided to normalize the time spent in solving by a factor of 10. Doing so one can compare time-wise the performance of each of the strategies. A point appearing on the diagonal of the plot represents the fact that both strategies terminated in the same amount of time. A point appearing on top of the main diagonal represents the fact that Vampire using the default strategy managed to solve that instance faster than Vampire using Lingeling variations. Similar a point below the diagonal represents the fact that Vampire using the new strategy solved the problem faster than Vampire using the default SAT solver.

The plot presents one to one comparison between the strategies and the default strategy. In Figure 3 we present the results obtained by running Vampire in "default" mode but varying the SAT solver as described above. From this figure one can notice the fact that more points appear above the diagonal, meaning that the default values of Vampire are better. We can notice however that there are some problems on which Vampire with default SAT solver time out while using Lingeling they can be solved in very short time. From these plots one could conclude that taken individually these strategies and compared to the default one, they seem to be have similar behavior as the default one.

Nevertheless, if we take them together and compare them to the default strategy we notice the fact that indeed they behave better.

Table 2 and Figure 4 present a similar comparison on the same problems, using the same variations of the underlying SAT solver and the same limits as for the *default* mode.

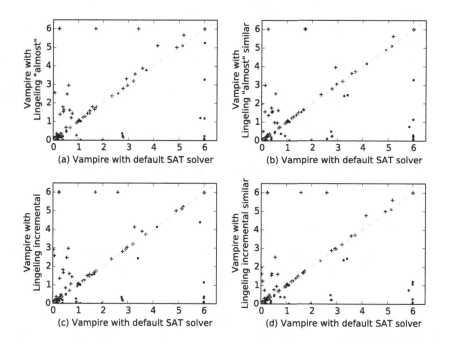

**Fig. 4.** Comparison of performance between Vampire with the Default SAT solver and different Lingeling strategies run in *casc* mode. Default SAT solver is compared against: (a) Lingeling "almost" incremental, (b) Lingeling "almost" incremental and similar models, (c) Lingeling incremental and (d) Lingeling incremental and similar models.

**Other TPTP Problems.** In a similar manner as for the 300 CASC problems we have evaluated our newly added features on a big subset of TPTP problems. The problems that have been selected for test have ranking in the interval [0.2, 1), having the status of either: *Unsatisfiable, Open, Theorem* or *Unknown*.

In Table 3 we present the summary of obtained results from running Vampire with all the variations on the set of problems in *default* mode. Table 4 presents the summary of our results obtained by running Vampire in *casc* mode on the same set of problems using the same variations as above described.

From our experiments we noticed that using Lingeling as a background SAT solver in the "almost" incremental and with the similar model generation turned on proves to perform the best among the newly implemented strategies. This sort of behavior can be due to multiple reasons. First it could be due to the fact that the solver tries to keep the model for as long as possible, due to similar model generation option. Another

**Table 3.** Results of running Vampire using default values for parameters on the 6.5K problems

| Strategy | Vamp | L | L S | L I | L I S |
|---|---|---|---|---|---|
| Average Time | 6.0440 | 5.9982 | 6.5992 | 5.6805 | 6.5025 |
| # of solved instances | 2672 | 2810 | 2925 | 2750 | 2788 |
| # different | 104 | 350 | 422 | 328 | 334 |

explanation for best performance can be the fact that using this options we do not call the SAT solver after each clause is added, but rather only after we add all the clauses generated by the first-order reasoning part, hence decreasing the time spent by the SAT solver in solving.

**Table 4.** Results of running Vampire using a cocktail of strategies on the 6.5K problems

| Strategy | Vamp | L | L S | L I | L I S |
|---|---|---|---|---|---|
| Average Time | 6.1019 | 6.0895 | 6.1139 | 6.3069 | 6.0638 |
| # of solved instances | 4788 | 4822 | 4881 | 4809 | 4792 |
| # different | 81 | 212 | 245 | 207 | 194 |

### 4.2  Analysis of Experimental Results

While integrating the new SAT solver inside Vampire and during the experiments we observed some issues that might increase the performance of future SAT solvers inside the Vampire's AVATAR architecture. **(i)** It is not necessary that a state of the art SAT solver, as Lingeling, behaves better inside the AVATAR framework. **(ii)** Integration of new solvers is less complicated than fine tuning the newly integrated solvers in order to match the performance of the default SAT solver, which is hard. **(iii)** Using an external SAT solver just in case the SAT problems are hard enough could be a good trade-off. We discuss these issues below.

**(i)** First, let us discuss the performance issue. At least in the case of Lingeling upon integration we have noticed that it behaves really nice on some of the problems while on some others it seems to fail. There are a couple of factors that could influence the behavior of such a performant tool. (1) Calling the solver many times decreases its performance. Although the solver is designed to be incremental upon adding new clauses to the problem and call for satisfiability check, it restarts. Now the problem appears when we call many times the solver. For example in the case of "pure" incremental way, we call the solver after each clause is added. Although the speed with which the check is done is incredibly fast, calling it n times makes it n times slower. (2) Due to this behavior in the worst case we have n restarts on the SAT solver side, where n is the number of clauses added to the solver. Both these points showed up in the statistics from the experiments we have performed. It is not uncommon that the first-order reasoning part will create a problem containing 10K or even 100K clauses. Now even if for one call the SAT solver spends 0.01 seconds it results in a timeout.

**(ii)** The default SAT solver implemented in Vampire follows the general structure of the MiniSAT [5] SAT solver. This architecture is an instantiation of the Conflict-Driven

Clause Learning (CDCL) [12] architecture. Although it is incremental, it deals with incrementality in a different manner. Assuming that we add a clause to the solver, first we check whether we can extend the current model so that we can satisfy also the newly added clause if the clause gets satisfied by the current model we keep the model and add the clause to the database. In case the clause is not directly satisfied by the model but does not contain any variable that is used in the model we try to satisfy the clause by extending the model. If we cannot do that, we do not restart, but rather backtrack to the point where the conflict comes from. A conflict can appear only if variables that are used in the model appear also in the newly added clause. If that is the case we take the lowest decision level among the conflict variables and backtrack to it. From there on we continue the classical SAT procedure and try to find a new model.

Using this approach, the SAT solver brings a couple of advantages for the first-order reasoning part. Due to the fact that we try to keep the model with minimal changes, we do not have to modify the indexing structures so often in the first-order part and also from our experiments we have noted that the actual SAT solving procedure gets called less often than in the case of calling for satisfiability check on an plugged-in solver.

(iii) Adding a new external SAT solver inside the framework of Vampire is not complicated. One has to take care about how the first-order reasoning part and the SAT solver communicate and do some book keeping. The issue arises when one has to fine-tune the SAT solver so that it performs well in it's new environment. Usually state of the art SAT solvers are highly optimized in order to behave well on big problems coming from industry but sometimes seem to get stuck in small problems. Also one important component of a state of the art solver is preprocessing [4], which for our purpose has to be turned off in order to ensure that we do not eliminate variables that might be used for splitting in the first-order reasoner. Due to the fact that we do not use all the power of a SAT solver we have to answer the question whether it is the case that state of the art, or commercial, solvers behave better in this context. In the case of the AVATAR architecture for an automated theorem prover producing different models for the SAT problems means that a clause gets splitted in different ways. That also translates into the fact that in some cases the use of an "handcrafted" SAT solver might produce the right model, but it also means that in other cases the state of the art solver produces the right model at the right time. This results in either solving the problem really fast or not at all. Some interesting fact that we have noticed during the experiments is the fact that the AVATAR architecture is really sensitive towards the models produced by the SAT solver.

## 5   Conclusion and Future Work

Starting from the initial results of the newly introduced AVATAR framework for an automatic theorem prover, we investigate how does a state of the art SAT solver behave in this framework. We describe the process of integrating a new SAT solver in the framework of Vampire using the AVATAR architecture. We also present a couple of decisions that have been made in order to better integrate the first-order proving part of Vampire with SAT solving. From our experiments we noticed that using a state of the art SAT solver like Lingeling inside the framework of an automated theorem prover based on AVATAR is useful and behaves well on TPTP problems. However there are also cases where using Lingeling as background solver Vampire does not perform as good as using a less efficient SAT solver.

We believe that further refinements on the SAT solver part and better fine tuning of the solver will produce even better results. We are investigating different ways of combining the Vampire built-in SAT solver with the external SAT solver such that we do not restart upon every newly added clause. Besides splitting, Vampire uses SAT solving also for instance generation [7] and indexing. We are therefore also interested in finding out whether the use of a state of the art SAT solver improves the performance of Vampire.

# References

1. HPC Center - West University of Timisoara,
   http://hpc.uvt.ro/infrastructure/infragrid/
2. Biere, A.: Picosat essentials. JSAT 4(2-4), 75–97 (2008)
3. Biere, A.: Lingeling, plingeling and treengeling entering sat competition 2013. In: SAT Competition 2013, pp. 51–52 (2013)
4. Eén, N., Biere, A.: Effective preprocessing in SAT through variable and clause elimination. In: Bacchus, F., Walsh, T. (eds.) SAT 2005. LNCS, vol. 3569, pp. 61–75. Springer, Heidelberg (2005)
5. Eén, N., Sörensson, N.: An extensible SAT-solver. In: Giunchiglia, E., Tacchella, A. (eds.) SAT 2003. LNCS, vol. 2919, pp. 502–518. Springer, Heidelberg (2004)
6. Hoder, K., Voronkov, A.: The 481 ways to split a clause and deal with propositional variables. In: Bonacina, M.P. (ed.) CADE 2013. LNCS, vol. 7898, pp. 450–464. Springer, Heidelberg (2013)
7. Korovin, K.: Inst-gen – A modular approach to instantiation-based automated reasoning. In: Voronkov, A., Weidenbach, C. (eds.) Programming Logics. LNCS, vol. 7797, pp. 239–270. Springer, Heidelberg (2013)
8. Kovács, L., Voronkov, A.: First-Order Theorem Proving and VAMPIRE. In: Sharygina, N., Veith, H. (eds.) CAV 2013. LNCS, vol. 8044, pp. 1–35. Springer, Heidelberg (2013)
9. Nieuwenhuis, R., Hillenbrand, T., Riazanov, A., Voronkov, A.: On the evaluation of indexing techniques for theorem proving. In: IJCAR, pp. 257–271 (2001)
10. Riazanov, A., Voronkov, A.: Splitting without backtracking. In: IJCAI, pp. 611–617 (2001)
11. Riazanov, A., Voronkov, A.: Limited resource strategy in resolution theorem proving. J. Symb. Comput. 36(1-2), 101–115 (2003)
12. Silva, J.P.M., Lynce, I., Malik, S.: Conflict-driven clause learning sat solvers. In: Handbook of Satisfiability, pp. 131–153 (2009)
13. Sutcliffe, G.: The TPTP Problem Library and Associated Infrastructure. J. Autom. Reasoning 43(4), 337–362 (2009)
14. Sutcliffe, G.: TPTP, TSTP, CASC, etc. In: Diekert, V., Volkov, M.V., Voronkov, A. (eds.) CSR 2007. LNCS, vol. 4649, pp. 6–22. Springer, Heidelberg (2007)
15. Voronkov, A.: AVATAR: The architecture for first-order theorem provers. In: Biere, A., Bloem, R. (eds.) CAV 2014. LNCS, vol. 8559, pp. 696–710. Springer, Heidelberg (2014)
16. Weidenbach, C.: Combining superposition, sorts and splitting. In: Handbook of Automated Reasoning, pp. 1965–2013 (2001)

# Onto Design Graphics (ODG):
# A Graphical Notation to Standardize Ontology Design

Rafaela Blanca Silva-López, Mónica Silva-López, Iris Iddaly Méndez-Gurrola,
and Maricela Bravo

Systems Department, Metropolitan Autonomous University (UAM)
Av. San Pablo No. 180, Col. Reynosa Tamaulipas, Delegación Azcapotzalco
CP. 02200, Distrito Federal, México
{rbsl,misl,iimg,mcbc}@correo.azc.uam.mx

**Abstract.** Ontology design is a complex task that requires the use of some graphical tools to assist the ontology developer. Although there have been great advances in ontology engineering research, a standard graphical notation has not been adopted yet. In this paper we propose a graphical notation for ontology design aiming at facilitating to share and reuse ontology designs between ontology users. Some authors propose the mapping of ontology elements with Unified Modeling Language (UML) components. However, a direct association between UML elements and ontology design issues does not exist. OntoDesign Graphics is an easy to learn graphical notation that it is used for displaying visually the elements of the ontology design, facilitating the design and integration of other designs clearly and efficiently.

**Keywords:** ontology design, ontology graphical notation, knowledge reuse.

## 1    Introduction

According with Gruber [1] the goals for developing ontologies is to share and understand the structure of information across people or software agents. In order to achieve these goals effectively, a graphical notation for the representation of ontology design is required.

In the last decade, a large number of ontologies covering multiple disciplinary domains have been published, from the medical field to education; majority of ontologies are public and searchable on the Internet. Each ontology has a particular purpose; however, it does not offer the necessary documentation to reuse it efficiently, in most cases, there is only a file with an Web Ontology Language (OWL) extension. When there is a documentation, it is very difficult to integrate it due to the diversity of graphical representations used by authors.

Graphical representations of ontological designs do not follow a standard as each ontology author uses different symbols to represent the elements of the ontology. The lack of a common set of symbols that help to represent the design of ontologies is an opportunity area to be covered to meet the objective of sharing the knowledge generated and to reuse not only the eXtensible Markup Language (XML) of an

A. Gelbukh et al. (Eds.): MICAI 2014, Part I, LNAI 8856, pp. 443–452, 2014.

ontology, but the documentation using a graphical representation of the ontology to understand and extend.

Since documentation is one of the pillars for the reuse of ontologies, in this paper we propose a graphical notation or symbolism for the design of ontologies, each of the elements was designed to facilitate easy learning and use, in a way that is simple to diagram and interpret. In order to evaluate the proposed OntoDesign Graphics notation, an application scenario is presented, showing the applicability of the notation.

The rest of the paper is organized as follows. In section two the state of the art is described briefly, some works of graphical modeling ontologies using Unified Modeling Language (UML) and other notations are included. In section three OntoDesign Graphics notation for the design of ontologies is described. In section four an application case developed under the proposed notation is shown. Finally conclusions are presented in section five.

## 2     State of the Art

Modeling is an essential part of large software projects and is helpful for medium and small projects as well. The work most closely related to modeling ontologies and that use some standards like UML and other notations for graphical representation, are listed below.

There are several studies that use the UML standard for ontology development, among them are the Kogut et al, in that article discusses the convergence of UML and ontologies and suggests some possible future directions [2].

Cranefield and Purvies examines the potential for object-oriented standards to be used for ontology modeling, and in particular presents an ontology representation language based on a subset of the UML together with its associated Object Constraint Language [3].

Wang and Chan in [4] investigated UML as an ontology modeling tool to facilitate the mapping from knowledge model to software model.

Baclawski et al [5] have been building tools for ontology development based on UML. This allows the many mature UML tools, models and expertise to be applied to knowledge representation systems, not only for visualizing complex ontologies but also for managing the ontology development process. Ontology languages have some features that UML does not support. That paper identifies the similarities and differences between UML and the ontology languages RDF and DAML+OIL.

Palmer et al [6] proposes a particular method which utilize UML as a design visualization tool for modeling ontologies based on the Common Logic knowledge representation language. The use of that method will enable Common Logic ontological concepts to be more readily accessible to general engineers and provide a valuable ontology design aid.

Mappings between OWL elements and UML class diagrams are precisely defined in the Ontology Definition Metamodel (ODM) published by Object Management Group (OMG) [7]. The ODM defines a set of UML metamodels and profiles for development of RDF and OWL. Kendall et al in [8] describes some of the revised approaches, and presents potential extensions to the UML profile to address requirements of OWL 2.

Also there are exists some tools and editors that help to ontology modeling. Ceccaroni and Kendall present a research on a semantically rich, graphical representation of ontologies and its utility for collaborative construction based on requirements outlined by the Agentcities initiative. A new tool, called the Visual Ontology Modeler, is described and evaluated in the context of Agentcities [9,10].

Benevides and Guizzardi [11] present a Model-Based graphical editor for supporting the creation of conceptual models and domain ontologies in a philosophically and cognitively well-founded modeling language named OntoUML.

Gomes and de Almeida in [12] described ODEd, an ontology editor that supports the definition of concepts, relations and properties, using graphic representations, besides promoting automatic inclusion of some classes of axioms and derivation of object infrastructures from ontologies.

Ontology visualization and their content and structure is important. In the past few years a number of visualization approaches were developed with the focus either on the representation of the relationships between classes or on the hierarchical structure and instances. A survey of ontology visualization methods is presented in [13] the purpose of that article is to present these techniques and categorize their characteristics and features in order to assist method selection and promote future research in the area of ontology visualization. Other developments in this area can be found in [14,15] like Knoocks (Knowledge Blocks), which is a visualization approach with focus on both the interconnections within the ontology and the instances in conjunction with their hierarchical structure.

Lohmann et al in [16] developed VOWL, a comprehensive and well-specified visual language for the user-oriented visualization of ontologies, and conducted a comparative study on an initial version of VOWL, and in others works of Lohmann et al in [17] presents ProtégéVOWL, a first implementation of VOWL realized as a plugin for the ontology editor Protégé. It accesses the internal ontology representation provided by the OWL API and defines graphical mappings according to the VOWL specification.

Finally, to move towards a unified visual notation for OWL ontologies Negru, Lohmann and Haag in [18] have made a comparative study of the user. They compare two different notations for OWL ontologies in the paper: the UML profile of the Ontology Definition Metamodel (ODM) and the Visual Notation for OWL Ontologies (VOWL).They report on a comparative user study of these notations and discuss benefits and limitations raised by the study participants. Based on these findings, they draw some general conclusions regarding the development of a unified visual notation for OWL ontologies.

Based on the works consulted, we can realizing that there are some clues about a unified visual notation for ontologies, however, there is still much research to be done, so in this work the didactic graphical notation for the ontologies design is proposed, which covers some concepts that are not supported in UML and neither other notations, the notation proposed has not yet been tested, this will be part of future work.

## 3    OntoDesign Graphics

There are several investigations related to modeling ontologies using UML. However UML focuses primarily on software development and lacks some elements to model an ontology in an easy to learn and use way. OntoDesign Graphics is a didactic graphical notation, whose goal is to have a means of representation graphic for ontologies. The core graphical elements of the proposed notation of OntoDesign Graphics and their descriptions are shown in Table 1.

**Table 1.** Symbols used to represent the graphic design of ontology in OntoDesignGraphics notation

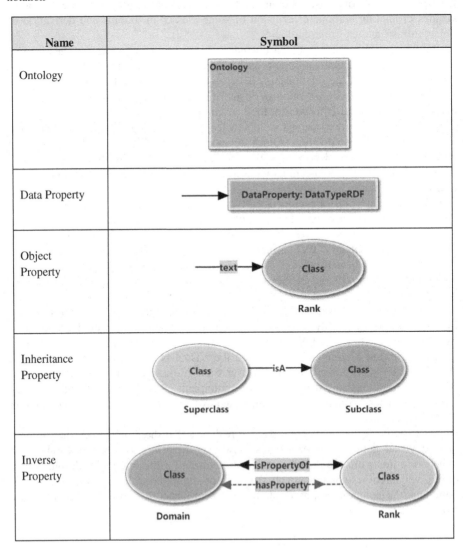

| Name | Symbol |
|------|--------|
| Ontology | |
| Data Property | |
| Object Property | |
| Inheritance Property | |
| Inverse Property | |

**Table 1.** (*continued*)

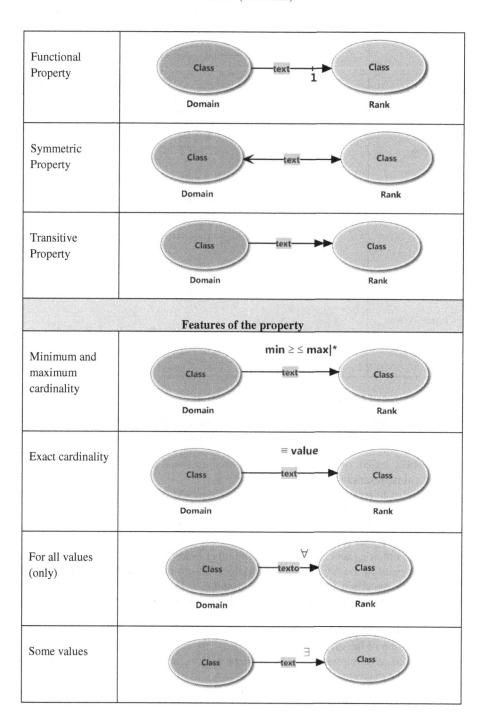

**Table 1.** (*continued*)

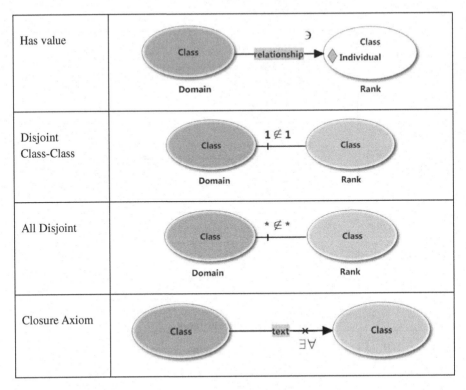

### 3.1   Features of OntoDesign Graphics Notation

A set of characteristics of OntoDesign Graphics are described below. These characteristics allow it to be a didactic notation for the graphical representation of ontologies:

- Use labels based on mathematical expressions, this gives more clarity in the graphical representation of the ontology design.
- Use ellipses to represent classes, adjust its size in width and length which improves the visual representation of the ontology design.
- Facilitates integration of multiple ontologies and the relationship between them through colors and rectangles.
- The main ontology and relationships with other ontologies were visually identified.
- Each property or axiom used in the ontology design has a graphical representation that can be specified in a single arrow joining. It is possible represent more than one feature associated with the property. For example: if it is reversed, cardinality and if it use closure axiom.
- Use colors to represent different types of relations, which supports the interpretation of the diagram.
- No need to have knowledge of XML tags used in the ontologies representation to interpret the diagram.
- Its symbolism is based on the axioms allowed by the Protégé editor for the ontology design and represent diagrams of real ontologies.

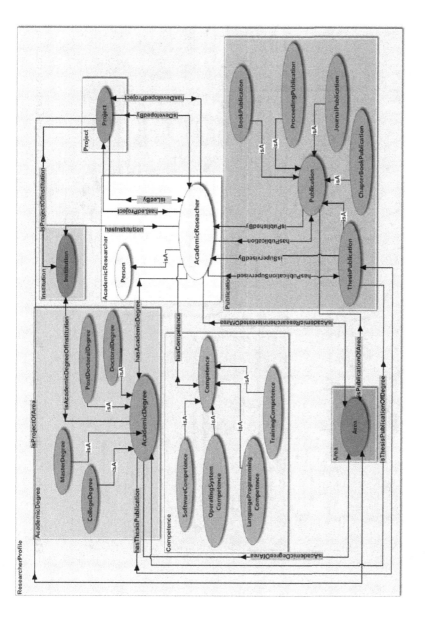

**Fig. 1.** General relationship ontologies representing research profiles in OntoDesign Graphics notation.

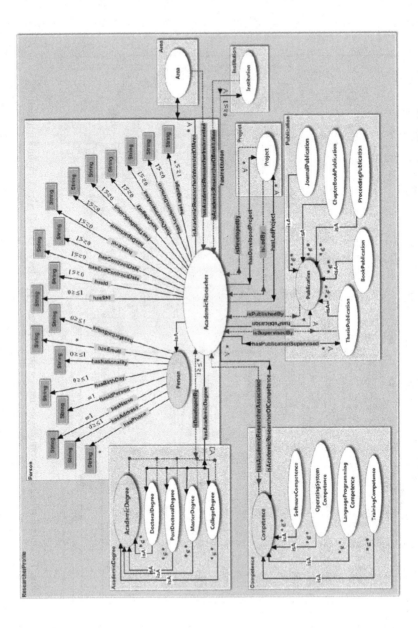

**Fig. 2.** Diagram of relationships between classes of the ontology Person using OntoDesign Graphics notation

# 4    Application Scenario

OntoDesign Graphics was used for the design of a multi-ontology for the representation research profiles. The general relations between different kinds of ontologies in graphical notation OntoDesign Graphics are shown in Figure 1.

The function of each of the ontologies representing research profiles is as follows:

— Area: Ontology representing knowledge areas of science.
— AcademicDegree: Ontology representing academic degrees granted by an institution of higher education or graduate studies.
— Institution: Ontology representing institutions such as universities, research centers, and so on.
— Competence: Ontology representing disciplinary skills associated to researchers.
— Project: Ontology representing research projects.
— Publication: Ontology representing publications by a researcher, references to journal articles, conferences, theses, book publishing, etc.
— Person: Ontology representing people within the system, focusing on researchers.

Hierarchies of classes of the ontology Person is described in Figure 2 using the OntoDesign Graphics notation.

# 5    Conclusions

There are several investigations in which proposals for defining the graphical representation of the design of an ontology are presented. They mostly focus on a mapping of the elements of an ontology with the notation defined in UML components. However, UML notation is a grammatical representation proposed for developing software for process modeling, and others. There are not elements of UML to allow a proper, clear and direct all the elements of the design of an ontology mapping.

There are many published ontologies on the Internet; however, they are not adequately documented, making very difficult their reutilization and extension for knowledge sharing and question answering.

OntoDesign Graphics is a novel proposal for a notation that allows graphical representation for the design of an ontology, visually in a single diagram all the elements of the ontology can be identified, such as classes, class hierarchy, properties, relations between classes, property restrictions, among others. Enriching documentation and facilitating the understanding of the design to other users, while promoting the generation of shared knowledge.

As a future work, we will continue with the development of a tool to support the mapping notation of OntoDesign Graphics with OWL format and vice versa. Suggest a notation for the design of ontologies and integrated into the UML notation to formalize and standardize the notation.

# References

1. Gruber, T.R.: A Translation Approach to Portable Ontology Specification. Knowledge Acquisition 5, 199–220 (1993)
2. Kogut, P., Cranefield, S., Hart, L., Dutra, M., Backawski, K., Kokar, M., Smith, J.: UML for ontology development. The Knowledge Engineering Review 17(1), 61–64 (2002)
3. Cranefield, S., Purvis, M.: UML as an Ontology Modelling Language. In: The Proceedings of the IJCAI 1999 Workshop on Intelligent Information Integration, Germany (1999)
4. Wang, X., Chan, C.W.: Ontology Modeling Using UML. In: 7th International Conference on Object Oriented Information Systems (OOIS), Calgary, Canada, pp. 59–68 (2001)
5. Baclawski, K., Kokar, M., Kogut, P., Hart, L., Smith, J., Letkowski, J., Emery, P.: Extending the Unified Modeling Language for ontology development. Software and Systems Modeling 1(2), 142–156 (2002)
6. Palmer, C., Chungoora, N., Young, R., Gunendran, A., Usman, Z., Case, K., Harding, J.: Exploiting unified modelling language (UML) as a preliminary design tool for Common Logic-based ontologies in manufacturing. International Journal of Computer Integrated Manufacturing 26(3), 267–283 (2013)
7. Ontology Definition Metamodel, http://www.omg.org/spec/ODM/1.1/
8. Kendall, E., Bell, R., Burkhart, R., Dutra, M., Wallace, E.: Towards a Graphical Notation for OWL 2. OWLED. CEUR Workshop Proceedings, vol. 529. CEUR-WS.org (2008)
9. Ceccaroni, L., Kendall, E.: A graphical environment for ontology development. In: Proceedings of the Second International Joint Conference on Autonomous Agents and Multiagent Systems, pp. 958–959. ACM (2003)
10. Ceccaroni, L., Kendall, E.: A Semantically-Rich, Graphical Environment for Collaborative Ontology Development in Agentcities. iD3, Barcelona, Spain (2003)
11. Benevides, A.B., Guizzardi, G.: A Model-Based Tool for Conceptual Modeling and Domain Ontology Engineering in OntoUML. In: Filipe, J., Cordeiro, J. (eds.) Enterprise Information Systems. LNBIP, vol. 24, pp. 528–538. Springer, Heidelberg (2009)
12. Gomes Mian, P., de Almeida Falbo, R.: Supporting ontology development with ODEd. Journal of the Brazilian Computer Society 9(2), 57–76 (2003)
13. Katifori, A., Halatsis, C., Lepouras, G., Vassilakis, C., Giannopoulou, E.: Ontology visualization methods—a survey. ACM Comput. Surv. 39(4), Article 10 (2007)
14. Kriglstein, S., Wallner, G.: Knoocks - A Visualization Approach for OWL Lite Ontologies. In: 2010 International Conference on Complex, Intelligent and Software Intensive Systems, pp. 950–955 (2010)
15. Kriglstein, S.: OWL Ontology Visualization: Graphical Representations of Properties on the Instance Level. In: 2010 14th International Conference on Information Visualisation (IV), pp. 92–97 (2010)
16. Lohmann, S., Negru, S., Haag, F., Ertl, T.: VOWL 2: User-Oriented Visualization of Ontologies. In: Lambrix, P., Hyvönen, E., Janowicz, K., Schlobach, S. (eds.) EKAW 2014. LNCS, vol. 8876. Springer, Heidelberg (2014)
17. Lohmann, S., Negru, S., Bold, D.: The ProtégéVOWL plugin: Ontology visualization for everyone. To appear in Proceedings of ESWC 2014 Satellite Events. Springer (2014)
18. Negru, S., Haag, F., Lohmann, S.: Towards a unified visual notation for OWL ontologies: insights from a comparative user study. In: Sabou, M., Blomqvist, E., Di Noia, T., Sack, H., Pellegrini, T. (eds.) Proceedings of the 9th International Conference on Semantic Systems (I-SEMANTICS 2013), pp. 73–80. ACM, New York (2013)

# A Logic for Context-Aware Non-monotonic Reasoning Agents

Abdur Rakib and Hafiz Mahfooz Ul Haque

School of Computer Science
The University of Nottingham, Malaysia Campus
{Abdur.Rakib,khyx2hma}@nottingham.edu.my

**Abstract.** We develop a logical model for resource-bounded context-aware multi-agent systems which handles inconsistent context information using non-monotonic reasoning. We extend the temporal logic $CTL^*$ with belief and communication modalities, and the resulting logic $\mathcal{L}_{DROCS}$ allows us to describe a set of rule-based non-monotonic context-aware agents with bounds on computational (time and space) and communication resources. We use OWL 2 RL ontologies and Semantic Web Rule Language (SWRL) for context-modelling and rules that enables the construction of a formal system. We provide an axiomatization of the logic and prove it is sound and complete. We illustrate the use of the logical model on a simple example.

**Keywords:** Context-aware, Rule-based reasoning, Defeasible reasoning, Multi-agent systems, Ontology.

## 1 Introduction

The term context-awareness in pervasive computing has been used relatively long ago, e.g., by Schilit and colleagues [24]. It describes the ability of a device to realise a situation and act accordingly. Thus a system is said to be context-aware if it can extract, interpret, and is able to adapt its behaviour to the current context of use [6]. In the literature, several definitions of *context* have been proposed including those presented by [25,8]. We view context is any information that can be used to identify the status of an entity. An entity can be a person, a place, a physical or a computing object. This context is relevant to a user and application, and reflects the relationship among themselves [8]. A context can be formally defined as a $\langle subject, predicate, object \rangle$ triple that states a fact about the subject where — the subject is an entity in the environment, the object is a value or another entity, and the predicate is a relationship between the subject and object. According to [8], *"if a piece of information can be used to characterize the situation of a participant in an interaction, then that information is context"*. For example, we can represent contexts *"Mary has fever categorized as High"* as $\langle Mary, hasFever, High \rangle$ and *"Mary has a carer named Fiona"* as $\langle Mary, hasCarer, Fiona \rangle$. Here, the caregiver of a patient is dynamically identified based on the care status of the caregiver. These contexts can be written using

A. Gelbukh et al. (Eds.): MICAI 2014, Part I, LNAI 8856, pp. 453–471, 2014.

first order predicates as *hasFever('Mary, 'High)* and *hasCarer('Mary, 'Fiona)* respectively.

In the literature, various techniques have been proposed to develop context-aware systems, including rule-based techniques [7,12]. In rule-based techniques a context-aware system composed of a set of rule-based agents, and firing of rules that infer new facts may determine context changes and representing overall behaviour of the system. An agent is called a rule-based agent if its behaviour and/or its knowledge is expressed by means of rules. In the setting of this paper, we call a *rule-based agent* as *context-aware agent* since it enables the system to understand and process context information expressed using first order rules. While active context-aware computing leads to a new paradigm that leverages interaction among system users and their environments, many challenges might arise on the basis of computational (time:measured in number of computational steps and space: amount of memory) and communication (number of messages need to be exchanged between devices) resources. This is due to the fact that many context-aware systems often run on tiny resource-bounded devices and in highly dynamic environments. The state of the art context-aware capable devices including PDAs, mobile phones, smart phones, GPS system, and wireless sensor nodes usually operate under strict resource constraints, e.g., battery energy level, memory, processor, and quality of wireless connection [26]. Therefore, for a given set of context-aware reasoning agents with some inferential abilities and computational (time and space) and communication resource bounds, it may not be clear whether a desired context can be inferred and if it can what computational and communication resources must be devoted by each agent. Furthermore, reasoning tasks may involve complex processing and resolve conflicting context information. Although research advances have been made in building context-aware systems for many applications, however well developed theoretical foundations considering their resource-boundedness features are still lacking. In this work, we present a logical framework for resource-bounded context-aware non-monotonic reasoning agents which is intended to be theoretically well motivated and technically well defined. We develop a logic $\mathcal{L}_{DROCS}$ which extends the temporal logic $CTL^*$ with belief and communication modalities and incorporates defeasible reasoning [19] technique (one of most prominent member of the non-monotonic reasoning techniques). The logic $\mathcal{L}_{DROCS}$ allows us to describe a set of context-aware non-monotonic reasoning agents with bounds on computational and communication resources. We provide an axiomatization of the logic and prove it is sound and complete, and using a simple example we show how we can express some interesting resource-bounded properties of a desired system.

The rest of the paper is organised as follows. In section 2, we briefly review description logics, ontologies and defeasible reasoning. In section 3, we describe our model of context-aware systems. In section 4, we develop the logic $\mathcal{L}_{DROCS}$ and show an illustrative example system, in section 5 we present related work, and conclude in section 6.

# 2 Preliminaries

## 2.1 Description Logics and Ontology

Description logics (DLs) are a well-known family of knowledge representation formalisms that can be used to represent knowledge of a domain in a structured and organized manner [3]. A DL is based on the notion of concepts (classes) and roles (binary relations), and is mainly characterized by the constructors that let complex concepts and roles to be constructed from atomic ones. A DL knowledge base ($\mathcal{KB}$) has two components: the Terminology Box (*TBox*) and the Assertion Box (*ABox*). The *TBox* introduces the terminology of a domain, while the *ABox* contains assertions about individuals in terms of this vocabulary. The *TBox* is a finite set of general concept inclusions (*GCI*) and role inclusions. A *GCI* is of the form $C \sqsubseteq D$ where $C$, $D$ are *DL*-concepts and a role inclusion is of the form $R \sqsubseteq S$ where $R$, $S$ are *DL*-roles. We may use $C \equiv D$ (concept equivalence) as an abbreviation for the two *GCIs* $C \sqsubseteq D$ and $D \sqsubseteq C$ and $R \equiv S$ (role equivalence) as an abbreviation for $R \sqsubseteq S$ and $S \sqsubseteq R$. The *ABox* is a finite set of concept assertions in the form of $a : C$ (or $C(a)$ which states that the individual $a$ is an instance of the class $C$) and role assertions in the form of $\langle a, b \rangle : R$ (or $R(a, b)$ which states that the individual $a$ is related to the individual $b$ through the relation $R$). The ability to model a domain and the decidable computational characteristics make DLs the basis for the widely accepted ontology languages such as Web Ontology Language (OWL). The Web Ontology Language version 2, OWL 2, has three sub-languages: OWL 2 EL, OWL 2 QL, and OWL 2 RL [17]. OWL 2 RL is suitable for rule-based applications, it enables additional rules such as SWRL to be added to ontologies for more expressive descriptions of an application domain.

There have been various approaches proposed for context modelling, however, ontology-based approach has been advocated as being the most promising one [4]. For example, if we are interested in modelling a smart space health care monitoring system we may use OWL concept names to capture terms that are relevant to this domain and ultimately represent the desired scenario using a set of logical statements [12]. We model context-aware systems using OWL 2 RL ontologies (and SWRL) and extract rules from an ontology following a similar approach proposed by [13] to design our rule-based non-monotonic context-aware agents. We developed a translator that takes as input an OWL 2 RL ontology in the OWL/XML format (an output file of the Protégé [20] editor) and translates it to a set of plain text rules. We use the OWL API [15] to parse the ontology and extract the set of axioms and facts. The design of the OWL API is directly based on the OWL 2 Structural Specification and it treats an ontology as a set of axioms and facts which are read using the visitor design pattern. We also extract the set of SWRL rules using the OWL API which are already in the Horn clause rule format. First, atoms with corresponding arguments associated with the head and the body of a rule are identified and we then generate a plain text Horn clause rule for each SWRL rule using these atoms. Abox axioms are already in Horn clause formats as well and they are simply rules with empty bodies.

## 2.2   Defeasible Reasoning

Defeasible reasoning is a simple rule-based reasoning technique that has been used to reason with incomplete and inconsistent information [2]. A defeasible logic theory consists of a collection of rules that reason over a set of facts to reach a set of defeasible conclusions. It also supports priorities among rules to resolve conflicts. More formally, a defeasible theory $\mathcal{D}$ is a triple $(\Re, \mathcal{F}, \succ)$ where $\Re$ is a finite set of rules, $\mathcal{F}$ is a finite set of facts, and $\succ$ is a superiority relation on $\Re$. The superiority relation $\succ$ is often defined on rules with complementary heads and its transitive closure is irreflexive, i.e., the relation $\succ$ is acyclic. Rules are defined over literals, where a literal is either a first-order atomic formula $P$ or its negation $\neg P$. For example, given a literal $l$, the complement $\sim l$ of $l$ is defined to be $P$ if $l$ is of the form $\neg P$, and $\neg P$ if $l$ is of the form $P$. In the rules, we assume variables are preceded by a question mark and constants are preceded by a single quote. In $\mathcal{D}$, there are three kinds of rules those are often represented using three different arrows.

***Strict rules*** are of the form: $P_1, P_2, \ldots, P_n \to P$ where the conclusion $P$ is valid whenever its antecedents $P_1, P_2, \ldots P_n$ are true. An example of a strict rule can be *"A person who has a patient identification number is a patient"* which can be written as **r1:** *Person(?p), PatientID(?pid), hasPatientID(?p, ?pid) → Patient(?p)*.

***Defeasible rules*** are of the form: $P_1, P_2, \ldots, P_n \Rightarrow P$ and they can be defeated by contrary evidence. An example rule can be **r2:** *Patient(?p), hasFever(?p, 'High) ⇒ hasSituation(?p, 'Emergency)*. This rule states that if the patient has a high fever then there are provable reasons to declare an emergency situation for her, unless there is other evidence that provides reasons to believe the contrary. For example, a defeasible rule **r3:** *Patient(?p), hasFever(?p, 'High), hasConsciousness(?p, 'Yes) ⇒ ∼ hasSituation(?p, 'Emergency)*. We can observe that the defeasible rule **r3** is more specific (we assume that **r3** is superior to **r2** i.e., **r3** ≻ **r2**) and it could override the rule **r2**. That is a defeasible rule is used to represent tentative information that may be used if nothing could be placed against it.

***Defeater rules*** are of the form: $P_1, P_2, \ldots, P_n \rightsquigarrow P$ and they don't support inferences directly, however, they can be used to block the derivation of inconsistent conclusions. Their only use is to prevent conclusions. For example, **r4:** *Patient(?p), hasFever(?p, 'High), hasDBCategory(?p, 'EstablishedDiabetes ⇝ hasSituation(?p, 'Emergency)*.

A rule can have multiple (ground) instances. For example, *Person('Mary), PatientID('P001), hasPatientID('Mary, 'P001) → Patient('Mary)* could be one possible instance of the rule **r1**. In the above rules, suppose the superiority relation $\succ$ among the rules are defined as follows **r1** ≻ **r4**, **r4** ≻ **r3**, **r3** ≻ **r2** and the current set of facts (contexts) are *Person('Mary), PatientID('P001), hasPatientID('Mary, 'P001), hasFever('Mary, 'High), hasConsciousness('Mary, 'Yes)* then by matching and firing those rules a defeasible conclusion ∼ *hasSituation('Mary, 'Emergency)* can be inferred.

# 3 Context-Aware Systems as Multi-agent Defeasible Reasoning Systems

We model a context-aware system as a multi-agent defeasible reasoning system which consists of $n_{Ag}(\geq 1)$ individual agents $A_g = \{1, 2, ...., n_{Ag}\}$. Each agent $i \in A_g$ is represented by a triple $(\Re, \mathcal{F}, \succ)$, where $\mathcal{F}$ is a finite set of facts contained in the working memory, $\Re = (\Re^s, \Re^d)$ is a finite set of strict and defeasible rules representing the knowledge base, and $\succ$ is a superiority relation on $\Re$. As we have mentioned in the preceding section, rules are of the form $P_1, P_2, \ldots, P_n \hookrightarrow P$ (derived from OWL 2 RL and SWRL with possible user annotation), and a working memory contains ground atomic facts (contexts) taken from ABox representing the initial state of the system. Without loss of generality, in the rest of this paper we assume $\hookrightarrow$ as either $\rightarrow$ or $\Rightarrow$. In a rule instance, the antecedents $P_1, P_2, \ldots, P_n$ and the consequent $P$ are context information. The antecedents of a rule instance form a complex context which is a conjunction of $n$ contexts. We say that two contexts are contradictory iff they are complementary with respect to $\sim$, for example, hasSituation('Mary, 'Emergency) and $\sim$hasSituation('Mary,'Emergency) are contradictory contexts. Note that in our model the set of facts translated from the ABox needs to be consistent, i.e., if it contains pair of contradictory contexts then they can be detected and removed. We assume that the set $\Re^s$ of strict rules is non-contradictory which is used to represent non-defeasible contextual information, however, the set $\Re^d$ of defeasible rules is contradictory and hence the set $\Re$ which is $\Re^s \cup \Re^d$ may also be contradictory. Conflicting contexts may be resolved using the superiority relation $\succ$ among rules. An agent $i$ can fire instances of strict rules to infer new non-contradictory contexts, while a defeasible context $P$ can be inferred if there is a rule instance whose consequence is $P$ and there does not exist a stronger rule instance whose consequence is $\sim P$. Since the translated rules from an ontology are not prioritized, we assume that the rule priorities are provided by the system designers, depending on the intended applications. We further assume that the priorities are static, i.e., the rule firing constraint does not change during the reasoning process. In our model, agents share a common ontology and communication mechanism. To model communication between agents, we assume that agents have two special communication primitives $Ask(i, j, P)$ and $Tell(i, j, P)$ in their language, where $i$ and $j$ are agents and $P$ is an atomic context not containing an $Ask$ or a $Tell$. $Ask(i, j, P)$ means '$i$ asks $j$ whether the context $P$ is the case' and $Tell(i, j, P)$ means '$i$ tells $j$ that context $P$' ($i \neq j$). The positions in which the $Ask$ and $Tell$ primitives may appear in a rule depends on which agent's program the rule belongs to. Agent $i$ may have an $Ask$ or a $Tell$ with arguments $(i, j, P)$ in the consequent of a rule; e.g., $P_1, P_2, \ldots, P_n \rightarrow Ask(i, j, P)$. Whereas agent $j$ may have an $Ask$ or a $Tell$ with arguments $(i, j, P)$ in the antecedent of the rule; e.g., $Tell(i, j, P) \rightarrow P$ is a well-formed rule (we call it trust rule) for agent $j$ that causes it to believe $i$ when $i$ informs it that context $P$ is the case. No other occurrences of $Ask$ or $Tell$ are allowed. When a rule has either an $Ask$ or a $Tell$ as its consequent, we call it a communication rule. All other rules are known as deduction rules. These include rules with $Ask$s and $Tell$s in the antecedent as well as rules containing neither an *Ask* nor a *Tell*. Note that OWL 2 is limited to unary and binary predicates and it is function-free. Therefore, in the Protégé [20] editor all the arguments of *Ask* and *Tell* are represented using constant symbols.

```
Rule    ::= Atoms '↪' Atom | ~ Atom
Atoms   ::= Atom {, Atom}*
Atom    ::= standardAtom | commmunicationAtom
standardAtom ::= description'('i-object ')'
             | individualvaluedProperty'('i-object ',' i-object ')'
             | datavaluedProperty'('i-object ',' d-object ')'
             | sameIndividuals'('i-object ',' i-object ')'
             | differentIndividuals'('i-object ',' i-object ')'
             | dataRange'(' d-object ')'
             | builtIn'(' builtinId ',' {d-object}* ')'
communicationAtom ::= 'Ask(' i ',' j ',' standardAtom ')'
             | 'Tell(' i ',' j ',' standardAtom ')'
i ::= 1 | 2 | ... | n_Ag
j ::= 1 | 2 | ... | n_Ag
builtinID ::= URIreference
i-object ::= i-variable | individualID
d-object ::= d-variable | dataLiteral
i-variable ::= 'I-variable('URIreference')'
d-variable ::= 'D-variable('URIreference')'
```

**Listing 1.1.** Abstract syntax of rules

## 4    The Logic $\mathcal{L}_{DROCS}$

We now introduce the logic $\mathcal{L}_{DROCS}$ based on [1] (which has been developed on propositional language and monotonic reasoning). Our proposed approach is based on the work of [13] who show that a subset of *DL* languages can be effectively mapped into a set of strict and defeasible rules. Intuitively, the set of translated rules corresponds to the *ABox* joined with *TBox* axioms of an OWL 2 RL ontology and SWRL rules. Let us define the internal language of each agent in the system. Let the set of agents be $A_g = \{1, 2, ...., n_{Ag}\}$, $\mathcal{C} = \{C_1, C_2, ... C_l\}$ be a finite set of concepts, $\mathcal{R} = \{R_1, R_2, ..., R_m\}$ be a finite set of roles. We also define a set $\mathcal{Q} = \{Ask(i, j, P), Tell(i, j, P)\}$, where $i, j \in A_g$ and $P \in \mathcal{C} \cup \mathcal{R}$. Let $\Re^s$ be a finite set of strict rules and $\Re^d$ be a finite set of defeasible rules. Let $\Re = \Re^s \cup \Re^d = \{r_1, r_2, ..., r_n\}$ be a finite set of rules of the form $P_1, P_2, ..., P_t \hookrightarrow P$ , where $t \geq 0$, $P_i, P \in \mathcal{C} \cup \mathcal{R} \cup \mathcal{Q}$ for all $i \in \{1, 2, ..., t\}$, $P_i \neq P_j$ for all $i \neq j$, and $\hookrightarrow$ as either $\rightarrow$ or $\Rightarrow$. More specifically, $P_i$ and $P$ are OWL atoms of the following form: $C_i(x)$ and $R_j(y, z)$. Where $C_i \in \mathcal{C}$, and $x$ is either a variable, an individual or a data value. $R_j \in \mathcal{R}$, when it is an Object property $y, z$ are either variables, individuals or data values, however, $y$ is variable or individual and $z$ is a data value when $R_j$ is a Datatype property. In Listing 1.1, we specify the abstract syntax of rules using a BNF. In this notation, the terminals are quoted, the non-terminals are not quoted, alternatives are separated by vertical bars, and components that can occur zero or more times are enclosed braces followed by a superscript asterisk symbol ($\{\ldots\}^*$). A class atom represented by `description(i-object)` in the BNF consists of an OWL 2-named class and a single argument representing an OWL 2 individual, for example an atom `Person(a)` holds if `a` is an instance of the class description `Person`. Similarly, an individual property atom represented by `individualvaluedProperty(i-object,i-object)` consists of an OWL 2 object property and two arguments representing OWL 2 individuals, for example an atom `hasCarer(a,b)` holds if `a` is related to `b` by property `hasCarer` and so on.

For convenience, we use the notation $ant(r)$ for the set of antecedents of $r$ and $cons(r)$ for the consequent of $r$, where $r \in \Re$. We fix a finite set of variables $X$ and a finite set of constants $D$ and assume $\delta$ is some substitution function from the set of variables of a rule into $D$. We denote by $\mathcal{G}(\Re)$ the set of all the ground instances of the rules occurring in $\Re$, which is obtained using $\delta$ (a more formal definition is given in Definition 2). Thus $\mathcal{G}(\Re)$ is finite. Let $\bar{r} \in \mathcal{G}(\Re)$ be one of the possible instances of a rule $r \in \Re$. $C(a)$, $R(a,b)$, $Ask(i,j,C(a))$, $Ask(i,j,R(a,b))$, $Tell(i,j,C(a))$, and $Tell(i,j,R(a,b))$ are ground atoms, for all $C \in \mathcal{C}, R \in \mathcal{R}$. The internal language $\mathcal{L}$ includes all the ground atoms and rules. Let us denote the set of all formulas (rules and ground atoms) by $\Omega$ which is finite. In the language of $\mathcal{L}$ we have a belief operator $B_i$ for all $i \in A_g$. We assume that there is a bound on communication for each agent $i$ which limits agent $i$ to at most $n_C(i) \in \mathbb{Z}^*$ messages. Each agent has a communication counter, $cp_i^{=n}$, which starts at 0 ($cp_i^{=0}$) and is not allowed to exceed the value $n_C(i)$. We divide agent's memory into two parts as rule memory (knowledge base) and working memory. Rule memory holds set of rules, whereas the facts are stored in the agent's working memory. Working memory is divided into static memory ($S_M(i)$) and dynamic memory ($D_M(i)$). The $D_M(i)$ of each agent $i \in A_g$ is bounded in size by $n_M(i) \in \mathbb{Z}^*$, where one unit of memory corresponds to the ability to store an arbitrary ground atom. The static part contains initial information to start up the systems, e.g., initial working memory facts, thus it's size is determined by the number of initial facts. The dynamic part contains newly derived facts as the system moves. Only facts stored in $D_M(i)$ may get overwritten, and this happens if an agent's memory is full or a contradictory context arrives in the memory (even if the memory is not full). Whenever newly derived context arrives in the memory, it is compared with the existing contexts to see if any conflict arises. If so then the corresponding contradictory context will be replaced with the newly derived context, otherwise an arbitrary context will be removed if the memory is full. Note that unless otherwise stated, in the rest of the paper we shall assume that memory means $D_M(i)$.

The syntax of $\mathcal{L}_{\mathcal{DROCS}}$ includes the temporal operators of $CTL^*$ and is defined inductively as follows:

- $\top$ (tautology) and *start* (a propositional variable which is only true at the initial moment of time) are well-formed formulas (wffs) of $\mathcal{L}_{\mathcal{DROCS}}$;
- $cp_i^{=n}$ (which states that the value of agent $i$'s communication counter is $n$) is a wff of $\mathcal{L}_{\mathcal{DROCS}}$ for all $n \in \{0, \ldots, n_C(i)\}$ and $i \in A_g$;

- $B_iC(a)$ (agent $i$ believes $C(a)$), $B_iR(a,b)$ (agent $i$ believes $R(a,b)$), and $B_ir$ (agent $i$ believes $r$) are wffs of $\mathcal{L}_{\mathcal{DROCS}}$ for any $C \in \mathcal{C}, R \in \mathcal{R}, r \in \Re$ and $i \in A_g$;
- $B_k Ask(i,j,C(a))$,  $B_k Ask(i,j,R(a,b))$,  $B_k Tell(i,j,C(\ a))$,  and $B_k Tell(i,j,R(\ a,b))$ are wffs of $\mathcal{L}_{\mathcal{DROCS}}$ for any $C \in \mathcal{C}, R \in \mathcal{R}, i,j \in A_g$, $k \in \{i,j\}$, and $i \neq j$;
- If $\varphi$ and $\psi$ are wffs of $\mathcal{L}_{\mathcal{DROCS}}$, then so are $\neg\varphi$ and $\varphi \wedge \psi$;
- If $\varphi$ and $\psi$ are wffs of $\mathcal{L}_{\mathcal{DROCS}}$, then so are $X\varphi$ (in the next state $\varphi$), $\varphi U\psi$ ($\varphi$ holds until $\psi$), $A\varphi$ (on all paths $\varphi$).

Other classical abbreviations for $\bot$, $\vee$, $\rightarrow$ and $\leftrightarrow$, and temporal operations: $F\varphi \equiv \top U\varphi$ (at some point in the future $\varphi$) and $G\varphi \equiv \neg F\neg\varphi$ (at all points in the future $\varphi$), and $E\varphi \equiv \neg A\neg\varphi$ (on some path $\varphi$) are defined as usual.

For convenience, we define the following sets: $CP_i = \{cp_i^{=n} \mid n = \{0, \ldots, n_C(i)\}\}$, $CP = \bigcup_{i \in A_g} CP_i$. Now we define priority relation between rules as follows.

**Definition 1 (Rule priority).** Let $pri : \Re \rightarrow N_{\geq 0}$ be a function that assigns each rule a non-negative integer. We define a partial order $\succ$ on $\Re$ such that for any two rules $r, r' \in \Re$ we say that $r \succ r'$ (rule $r$ has priority over $r'$) iff $pri(r) \geq pri(r')$, where $\geq$ is the standard greater-than-or-equal relation on the set of non-negative integers $N_{\geq 0}$.

The semantics of $\mathcal{L}_{\mathcal{DROCS}}$ is defined by $\mathcal{L}_{\mathcal{DROCS}}$ transition systems which are based on $\omega$-tree structures. Let $(S,T)$ be a pair where $S$ is a set and $T$ is a binary relation on $S$ that is total, i.e., $\forall s \in S \cdot \exists s' \in S \cdot sTs'$. $(S,T)$ is a $\omega$-tree frame iff the following conditions are satisfied.

1. $S$ is a non-empty set and $T$ is total;
2. Let $<$ be the strict transitive closure of $T$, namely $\{(s,s') \in S \times S \mid \exists n \geq 0, s_0 = s, \ldots, s_n = s' \in S$ such that $s_i T s_{i+1} \forall i = 0, \ldots, n-1\}$;
3. For all $s' \in S$, the past $\{s \in S \mid s < s'\}$ is linearly ordered by $<$;
4. There is a smallest element called the root, which is denoted by $s_0$;
5. Each maximal linearly $<$- ordered subset of $S$ is order-isomorphic to the natural numbers.

A branch of $(S,T)$ is an $\omega$-sequence $(s_0, s_1, \ldots)$ such that $s_0$ is the root and $s_i T s_{i+1}$ for all $i \geq 0$. We denote $B(S,T)$ to be the set of all branches of $(S,T)$. For a branch $\pi \in B(S,T)$, $\pi_i$ denotes the element $s_i$ of $\pi$ and $\pi_{\leq i}$ is the prefix $(s_0, s_1, \ldots, s_i)$ of $\pi$. A $\mathcal{L}_{\mathcal{DROCS}}$ transition system $\mathbb{M}$ is defined as $\mathbb{M} = (S,T,V)$ where

- $(S,T)$ is a $\omega$-tree frame
- $V : S \times A_g \rightarrow \wp(\Omega \cup CP)$; we define the belief part of the assignment $V^B(s,i) = V(s,i) \setminus CP$ and the communication counter part $V^C(s,i) = V(s,i) \cap CP$. We further define $V^M(s,i) = \{\alpha \mid \alpha \in V^B(s,i) \cap D_M(i)\}$ which represents the set of facts stored in the dynamic memory of agent $i$ at state $s$. $V$ satisfies the following conditions:

1. $|V^C(s,i)| = 1$ for all $s \in S$ and $i \in A_g$.
2. If $sTs'$ and $cp_i^{=n} \in V(s,i)$ and $cp_i^{=m} \in V(s',i)$ then $n \leq m$.

- we say that a rule $r : P_1, P_2, \ldots, P_n \hookrightarrow P$ is applicable in a state $s$ of an agent $i$ if $ant(\bar{r}) \in V(s,i)$ and $cons(\bar{r}) \notin V(s,i)$. The following conditions on the assignments $V(s,i)$, for all $i \in A_g$, and transition relation $T$ hold in all models:

  1. for all $i \in A_g$, $s, s' \in S$, and $r \in \Re$, $r \in V(s,i)$ iff $r \in V(s',i)$. This describes that agent's program does not change.

  2. for all $s, s' \in S$, $sTs'$ holds iff for all $i \in A_g$, $V(s',i) = V(s,i) \setminus \{\beta\} \cup \{cons(\bar{r})\} \cup \{Ask(j,i,C(a))\} \cup \{Tell(j, i, C(a))\} \cup \{Ask(j,i,R(a,b))\} \cup \{Tell(j, i, R(a,b))\}$. This describes that each agent $i$ fires a single applicable rule instance of a rule $r$, or updates its state by interacting with other agents, otherwise its state does not change. Where $\beta$ may be an arbitrary context or a contradictory context which can be replaced depending on the status of the memory and the newly derived or communicated context.

The truth of a $\mathcal{L_{DROCS}}$ formula at a point $n$ of a path $\pi \in B(S,T)$ is defined inductively as follows:

- $\mathbb{M}, \pi, n \models \top$,
- $\mathbb{M}, \pi, n \models start$ iff $n = 0$,
- $\mathbb{M}, \pi, n \models B_i\alpha$ iff $\alpha \in V(\pi_n, i)$,
- $\mathbb{M}, \pi, n \models cp_i^{=m}$ iff $cp_i^{=m} \in V(\pi_n, i)$,
- $\mathbb{M}, \pi, n \models \neg\varphi$ iff $\mathbb{M}, \pi, n \not\models \varphi$,
- $\mathbb{M}, \pi, n \models \varphi \wedge \psi$ iff $\mathbb{M}, \pi, n \models \varphi$ and $\mathbb{M}, \pi, n \models \psi$,
- $\mathbb{M}, \pi, n \models X\varphi$ iff $\mathbb{M}, \pi, n + 1 \models \varphi$,
- $\mathbb{M}, \pi, n \models \varphi U\psi$ iff $\exists m \geq n$ s.t. $\forall k \in [n,m)$ $\mathbb{M}, \pi, k \models \varphi$ and $\mathbb{M}, \pi, m \models \psi$,
- $\mathbb{M}, \pi, n \models A\varphi$ iff $\forall \pi' \in B(S,T)$ s.t. $\pi'_{\leq n} = \pi_{\leq n}$, $\mathbb{M}, \pi', n \models \varphi$.

We now describe conditions on the models. The transition relation $T$ corresponds to the agent's executing actions $\langle act_1, act_2, \ldots, act_{n_{A_g}} \rangle$ where $act_i$ is a possible action of an agent $i$ in a given state $s$. The set of actions that each agent $i$ can perform are: $Rule_{i,r,\beta}$ (agent $i$ firing a selected matching rule instance $\bar{r}$ of $r$ and adding $cons(\bar{r})$ to its working memory and removing $\beta$), $Copy_{i,\alpha,\beta}$ (agent $i$ copying $\alpha$ from other agent's memory and removing $\beta$, where $\alpha$ is of the form $Ask(j,i,P)$ or $Tell(j,i,P)$), and $Idle_i$ (agent $i$ does nothing but moves to the next state). Intuitively, $\beta$ may be an arbitrary context which gets overwritten if it is in the agent's dynamic memory $D_M(i)$ or it is a specific context that contradicts with the newly derived context. If agent's memory is full $|V^M(s,i)| = n_M(i)$ then we require that $\beta$ has to be in $V^M(s,i)$. When the counter value reaches to $n_C(i)$, $i$ cannot perform copy action any more. Furthermore, not all actions are possible in a given state. For example, there may not be any matching rule instance. Note also that only selected matching rule instances can be fired. That is one rule instance may be selected from the conflict set that has the highest priority. If there are multiple rule instances with the same priority, the rule instance to be executed is selected non-deterministically. More formally, we define rule selection strategy as follows:

**Definition 2 (Rule selection strategy).** *For every state $s$, agent $i$, and $r \in V(s,i)$, we say that the rule $r$ matches at state $s$ iff $ant(\bar{r}) \subseteq V(s,i)$ and $cons(\bar{r}) \notin V(s,i)$. Let $\delta : S \times A_g \to \mathcal{G}(\Re)$ be a function that generates matching rule instances of the agent $i$ at state $s$ and $\Re_{mat} \subseteq \mathcal{G}(\Re)$ denote the set of all matching rule instances of the agent $i$ at state $s$. A set $\Re_{sel}$ is said to be selected rule instances if (i) $\Re_{sel} \subseteq \Re_{mat}$; and (ii) $\forall \bar{r} \in \Re_{sel} \nexists \bar{r'} \in \Re_{sel}$ such that $pri(r') \succ pri(r)$.*

Now let us denote the set of all possible actions by agent $i$ in a given state $s$ by $T_i(s)$ and its definition is given below:

**Definition 3 (Available actions).** *For every state $s$ and agent $i$,*

1. *$Rule_{i,r,\beta} \in T_i(s)$ iff $\bar{r} \in \Re_{sel}$, $\beta$ is a contradictory context (with respect to $cons(\bar{r})$ i.e., if $\beta$ is $\alpha$ then $cons(\bar{r})$ is $\sim \alpha$ and vice versa) or $\beta \in \Omega$ or if $|V^M(s,i)| = n_M(i)$ then $\beta \in V^M(s,i)$;*
2. *$Copy_{i,\alpha,\beta} \in T_i(s)$ iff there exists $j \neq i$ such that $\alpha \in V(s,j)$, $\alpha \notin V(s,i)$, $cp_i^{=m} \in V(s,i)$ for some $m < n_C(i)$, $\alpha$ is of the form $Ask(j,i,P)$ or $Tell(j,i,P)$, and $\beta$ as before;*
3. *$Idle_i$ is always in $T_i(s)$.*

**Definition 4 (Effect of actions).** *For each $i \in A_g$, the result of performing an action $act_i$ in a state $s \in S$ is defined if $act_i \in T_i(s)$ and has the following effect on the assignment of formulas to $i$ in the successor state $s' \in S$:*

1. *if $act_i$ is $Rule_{i,r,\beta}$: $V(s',i) = V(s,i) \setminus \{\beta\} \cup \{cons(\bar{r})\}$;*
2. *if $act_i$ is $Copy_{i,\alpha,\beta}, cp_i^{=m} \in V(s,i)$ for some $m \leq n_C(i)$: $V(s',i) = V(s,i) \setminus \{\beta, cp_i^{=m}\} \cup \{\alpha, cp_i^{=m+1}\}$;*
3. *if $act_i$ is $Idle_i$: $V(s',i) = V(s,i)$.*

Now, the definition of the set of models corresponding to a system of rule-based context-aware reasoners is given below:

**Definition 5.** *$\mathbb{M}(n_M, n_C)$ is the set of models $(S,T,V)$ which satisfies the following conditions:*

1. *$cp_i^{=0} \in V(s_0, i)$ where $s_0 \in S$ is the root of $(S,T)$, $\forall i \in A_g$;*
2. *$\forall s \in S$ and a tuple of actions $\langle act_1, act_2, \ldots, act_{n_{A_g}} \rangle$, if $act_i \in T_i(s), \forall i \in A_g$, then $\exists s' \in S$ s.t. $sTs'$ and $s'$ satisfies the effects of $act_i, \forall i \in A_g$;*
3. *$\forall s, s' \in S$, $sTs'$ iff for some tuple of actions $\langle act_1, act_2, \ldots, act_{n_{A_g}} \rangle$, $act_i \in T_i(s)$ and the assignment in $s'$ satisfies the effects of $act_i, \forall i \in A_g$;*
4. *The bound on each agent's memory is set by the following constraint on the mapping $V$: $|V^M(s,i)| \leq n_M(i), \forall s \in S, i \in A_g$.*

Note that the bound $n_C(i)$ on each agent $i$'s communication ability (no branch contains more than $n_C(i)$ *Copy* actions by agent $i$) follows from the fact that $Copy_i$ is only enabled if $i$ has performed fewer than $n_C(i)$ copy actions in the past. Below are some abbreviations which will be used in the axiomatization:

- $ByRule_i(P, m) = \neg B_i P \wedge cp_i^{=m} \wedge \bigvee_{\bar{r} \in \Re_{sel} \wedge cons(\bar{r})) = P}(B_i r \wedge \bigwedge_{Q \in ant(\bar{r})} B_i Q)$.
  This formula describes a state $s$ where it may make a *Rule* transition and believe context $P$ in the next state, $m$ is the value of $i$'s communication counter, $P$ and $Q$ are ground atomic formulas.
- $ByCopy_i(\alpha, m) = \neg B_i \alpha \wedge B_j \alpha \wedge cp_i^{=m-1}$, where $\alpha$ is of the form $Ask(j, i, P)$ or $Tell(j, i, P)$, $i, j \in A_g$ and $i \neq j$.

Now we introduce the axiomatization system.

A1 All axioms and inference rules of $CTL^*$ [22].

A2 $\bigwedge_{\alpha \in D_M(i)} B_i \alpha \rightarrow \neg B_i \beta$ for all $D_M(i) \subseteq \Omega$ such that $|D_M(i)| = n_M(i)$ and $\beta \notin D_M(i)$. This axiom describes that, in a given state, each agent can store maximally at most $n_M(i)$ formulas in its memory,

A3 $\bigvee_{n=0,...,n_C(i)} cp_i^{=n}$, $n$ is value of the communication counter of an agent $i$ corresponding to its *Copy* actions.

A4 $cp_i^{=n} \rightarrow \neg cp_i^{=m}$ for any $m \neq n$, which states that at any given time the value of the copy counter of agent $i$ is unique

A5 $B_i \alpha \rightarrow \neg B_i \sim \alpha$ for any $\alpha \in S_M(i) \cup D_M(i) \subseteq \Omega$, this axiom states that agent does not believe contradictory contexts,

A6 $B_i r \wedge \bigwedge_{\bar{r} \in \Re_{sel} \wedge P \in ant(\bar{r})} B_i P \wedge cp_i^{=n} \wedge \neg B_i cons(\bar{r}) \rightarrow EX(B_i cons(\bar{r}) \wedge cp_i^{=n})$, $i \in A_g$. This axiom describes that if a rule matches and is selected for execution, its consequent belongs to some successor state.

A7 $cp_i^{=m} \wedge \neg B_i \alpha \wedge B_j \alpha \rightarrow EX(B_i \alpha \wedge cp_i^{=m+1})$ where $\alpha$ is of the form $Ask(j, i, P)$ or $Tell(j, i, P)$, $i, j \in A_g$, $j \neq i$, $m < n_C(i)$. This axiom describes transitions made by *Copy* with communication counter increased.

A8 $EX(B_i \alpha \wedge B_i \beta) \rightarrow B_i \alpha \vee B_i \beta$, where $\alpha$ and $\beta$ are not of the form $Ask(j, i, P)$ and $Tell(j, i, P)$. This axiom says that at most one new belief is added in the next state.

A9 $B_i \alpha \rightarrow AX B_i \alpha$ for any $\alpha \in S_M(i) \cup \Re$. This axiom states that an agent $i \in A_g$ always believes formulas residing in its static memory and its rules.

A10 $EX(B_i \alpha \wedge cp_i^{=m}) \rightarrow B_i \alpha \vee ByRule_i(\alpha, m) \vee ByCopy_i(\alpha, m)$ for any $\alpha \in \cup \Omega$. This axiom says that a new belief can only be added by one of the valid reasoning actions.

A11a $start \rightarrow cp_i^{=0}$ for all $i \in A_g$. At the start state, the agent has not performed any *Copy* actions.

A11b $\neg EX\ start$. *start* holds only at the root of the tree.

A12 $B_i r$ where $r \in \Re$ and $i \in A_g$. This axiom tells agent $i$ believes its rules.

A13 $\neg B_i r$ where $r \notin \Re$ and $i \in A_g$. This axiom tells agent $i$ only believes its rules.

A14 $\varphi \rightarrow EX\varphi$, where $\varphi$ does not contain *start*. This axiom describes an *Idle* transition by all the agents.

A15 $\bigwedge_{i \in A_g} EX(\bigwedge_{\alpha \in \Gamma_i} B_i \alpha \wedge cp_i^{=m_i}) \rightarrow EX \bigwedge_{i \in A_g}(\bigwedge_{\alpha \in \Gamma_i} B_i \alpha \wedge cp_i^{=m_i})$ for any $\Gamma_i \subseteq \Omega$. This axiom describes that if each agent $i$ can separately reach a state where it believes formulas in $\Gamma_i$, then all agents together can reach a state where for each $i$, agent $i$ believes formulas in $\Gamma_i$.

Let us now define the logic obtained from the above axiomatisation system.

**Definition 6.** $\mathbb{L}(n_M, n_C)$ *is the logic defined by the axiomatisation* **A1** - **A15**.

**Theorem 1.** $\mathbb{L}(n_M, n_C)$ *is sound and complete with respect to* $\mathbb{M}(n_M, n_C)$.

*Sketch of Proof.* The proof of soundness is standard. The proofs for axioms and rules included in **A1** are given in [22]. Axiom **A2** assures that at a state, each agent can store maximally at most $n_M(i)$ formulas in its memory. Axioms **A3** and **A4** force the presence of a unique counter for each agent to record the number of copies it has performed so far. In particular, **A3** makes sure that at least a counter is available for any agent and **A4** guaranties that only one of them is present. Axiom **A5** assures that an agent does not believe contradictory contexts. In the following, we provide the proof for **A6** and **A7**. The proofs for other axioms are similar.

Let us consider **A6**. Let $\mathbb{M} = (S, T, V) \in \mathbb{M}(n_M, n_C)$, $\pi \in B(S, T)$ and $n \geq 0$. We assume that $\mathbb{M}, \pi, n \models B_i r \wedge \bigwedge_{\bar{r} \in \Re_{sel} \wedge P \in ant(\bar{r})} B_i P \wedge cp_i^{=m} \wedge \neg B_i cons(\bar{r})$, for some $r \in \Re$ such that $\bar{r} \in \Re_{sel}$, and $|V^M(s, i)| \leq n_M(i)$. Then $P \in V(\pi_n, i)$ for all $P \in ant(\bar{r})$, and $cons(\bar{r}) \notin V(\pi_n, i)$. This means that the action performed by $i$ is $Rule_{i,r,\beta}$. According to the definition of $\mathbb{M}(n_M, n_C)$, $\exists s' \in S \cdot \pi_n T s'$ and $V(s', i) = V(\pi_n, i) \setminus \{\beta\} \cup \{cons(\bar{r})\}$. Let $\pi'$ be a branch in $B(S, T)$ such that $\pi'_{\leq n} = \pi_{\leq n}$ and $\pi'_{n+1} = s'$. Then we have $\mathbb{M}, \pi', n + 1 \models B_i cons(\bar{r}) \wedge cp_i^{=m}$. Therefore, it is obvious that $\mathbb{M}, \pi, n \models EX(B_i cons(\bar{r}) \wedge cp_i^{=m})$.

Let us consider **A7**. Let $\mathbb{M} = (S, T, V) \in \mathbb{M}(n_M, n_C)$, $\pi \in B(S, T)$ and $n \geq 0$. We assume that $\mathbb{M}, \pi, n \models cp_i^{=m} \wedge \neg B_i \alpha \wedge B_j \alpha$, and $|V^M(s, i)| \leq n_M(i)$. Then $cp_i^{=m} \in V(\pi_n, i)$, $\alpha \notin V(\pi_n, i)$, and $\alpha \in V(\pi_n, j)$, for $i, j \in A_g$, $i \neq j$, and $m < n_C(i)$. This means that the action performed by $i$ is $Copy_{i,\alpha,\beta}$. According to the definition of $\mathbb{M}(n_M, n_C)$, $\exists s' \in S \cdot \pi_n T s'$ and $V(s', i) = V(\pi_n, i) \setminus \{\beta, cp_i^{=m}\} \cup \{\alpha, cp_i^{=m+1}\}$. Let $\pi'$ be a branch in $B(S, T)$ such that $\pi'_{\leq n} = \pi_{\leq n}$ and $\pi'_{n+1} = s'$. Then we have $\mathbb{M}, \pi', n + 1 \models B_i \alpha \wedge cp_i^{=m+1}$. Therefore, it is obvious that $\mathbb{M}, \pi, n \models EX(B_i \alpha \wedge cp_i^{=m+1})$.

Completeness can be shown by constructing a tree model for a consistent formula $\varphi$. This is constructed as in the completeness proof introduced in [22]. Then we use the axioms to show that this model is in $\mathbb{M}(n_M, n_C)$. Since the initial state of all agents does not restrict the set of formulas they may derive in the future, for simplicity we conjunctively add to $\varphi$ a tautology that contains all the potentially necessary formulas and message counters, in order to have enough sub-formulas for the construction. We construct a model $\mathbb{M} = (S, T, V)$ for

$$\varphi' = \varphi \wedge \bigwedge_{\alpha \in \Omega} (XB_i\alpha \vee \neg XB_i\alpha) \wedge \bigwedge_{n \in \{0...n_C(i)\}, i \in A_g} (Xcp_i^{=n} \vee \neg Xcp_i^{=n})$$

We then prove that $\mathbb{M}$ is in $\mathbb{M}(n_M, n_C)$ by showing that it satisfies all properties listed in Definition 5. Axioms **A3** and **A4** show that for any $i \in A_g$, there exists a unique $n \in \{0, \ldots, n_C\}$ such that at a state $s$ of $\mathbb{M}$, $cp_i^{=n} \in V(s, i)$. At the root $s_0$ of $(S, T)$, the construction of the model implies that there exists a maximally consistent set (MCS) $\Gamma_0$ such that $\Gamma_0 \supseteq V(s_0, i)$ and $start \in \Gamma_0$. Therefore, by axiom **A11**, it is trivial that $cp_i^{=0} \in V(s_0, i)$. We then need to prove that $\forall s \in S$, $act_i \in T_i(s)$, and $i \in A_g$, $\exists s' \in S \cdot sTs'$ and $V(s', i)$ is the result of $V(s, i)$ after $i$ has performed action $act_i$. Let us consider the case when $act_i$ is $Rule_{i,r,\beta} \in T_i(s)$ for some $r \in \Re$ such that $\bar{r} \in \Re_{sel}$. Since $Rule_{i,r,\beta}$ is applicable at $s$, $ant(\bar{r}) \subseteq V(s, i)$, $cons(\bar{r}) \notin V(s, i)$. Therefore there exists a MCS $\Gamma$ such that $\Gamma \supseteq V(s, i)$, and $\bigwedge_{\bar{r} \in \Re_{sel} \wedge P \in ant(\bar{r})} B_i P \wedge cp_i^{=m} \wedge \neg B_i cons(\bar{r}) \in \Gamma$, for some $m \in \{0, \ldots, n_C\}$ and $|V^M(s, i)| \leq n_M(i)$. By axiom **A6** and Modus Ponens (MP), $EX(B_i cons(\bar{r}) \wedge cp_i^{=m}) \in \Gamma$. Therefore, according to the construction, $\exists s' \in S \cdot sTs'$, $V(s', i) \subseteq \Gamma'$ for some $\Gamma'$, and $B_i cons(\bar{r}) \wedge cp_i^{=m} \in \Gamma'$. Therefore $V(s', i) = V(s, i) \setminus \{\beta\} \cup \{cons(\bar{r})\}$. For the $Copy_{i,\alpha,\beta} \in T_i(s)$ and $Idle_i \in T_i(s)$ actions, the proofs are similar by using MP and axioms **A7** and axiom **A14**. Then, using axiom **A15** we can show that, for any tuple of actions $\langle act_1, act_2, \ldots, act_{n_{A_g}} \rangle$, $act_i \in T_i(s)$ is applicable at $s \in S$ $\forall i \in A_g$, then $\exists s' \in S$ such that $V(s', i)$ is the result of $V(s, i)$ after performing $act_i$ at $s$ by agent $i$, $\forall i \in A_g$. Finally, we prove that $\forall s, s' \in S \cdot sTs'$, $\exists$ a tuple of actions $\langle act_1, act_2, \ldots, act_{n_{A_g}} \rangle$ and $V(s', i)$ is the result of $V(s, i)$ when agent $i$ performs $act_i$ for all $i \in A_g$. By axioms **A8** and **A2**, $V(s', i)$ is different from $V(s, i)$ by at most one formula added and possibly a formula is removed. If no formula is added or removed, we consider $act_i$ to be $Idle_i$. Let us now consider the case where a formula $\alpha$ is added. By axiom **A10**, if $cp_i^{=m} \in V(s, i)$ for some $m \in \{0, \ldots, n_C\}$ then either $cp_i^{=m}$ or $cp_i^{m+1} \in V(s', i)$. If $cp_i^{=m} \in V(s', i)$ then set $act_i$ to be $Rule_{i,r,\beta}$ for some $r \in V(s, i)$ such that $\bar{r} \in \Re_{sel}$, $\alpha = cons(\bar{r}) \notin V(s, i)$. If $cp_i^{=m+1} \in V(s', i)$ then set $act_i$ to be $Copy_{i,\alpha,\beta}$. Thus, we proved the existence of the tuple $\langle act_1, act_2, \ldots, act_{n_{A_g}} \rangle$ for $sTs'$. Therefore, $\mathbb{M}$ is in $\mathbb{M}(n_M, n_C)$. $\square$

## 4.1   An Illustrative Example

To illustrate the use of the proposed logical model, let us consider an example system consisting of four agents. A fragment of the context modelling ontology of the system is depicted in Fig. 1 (a). Fig. 1 (b) shows an individualised patient ontology and (c) depicts some SWRL rules. The set of translated rules and initial working memory facts that are distributed to the agents are shown in Table 1, and the goal is to infer the formula $B_4\ hasSituation('Mary,'\ Emergency)$ which states that agent 4 believes that the patient Mary has Emergency situation. The reasoning process includes resolving contradictory contextual information. One possible run of the system is shown in Table 2 and Table 3 (continuation). In the tables a newly inferred context at a particular step is shown in blue text. For example, antecedents of rule R11 of agent 1 match the contents of the memory configuration and infers new context $Patient('Mary)$ at step 1. A context which gets overwritten in the next state is shown in red text, and a context which is inferred in the current state and gets overwritten in the next state is shown in magenta text. In the memory configuration, for each agent, left side of the red vertical bar | represents $S_M(i)$ and its right side represents $D_M(i)$. It shows that the size of $D_M(1)$ is 3 units and the size of $D_M(i)$ is 1 unit for all $2 \leq i \leq 4$. We can observe that the resource requirements for the system to derive the goal

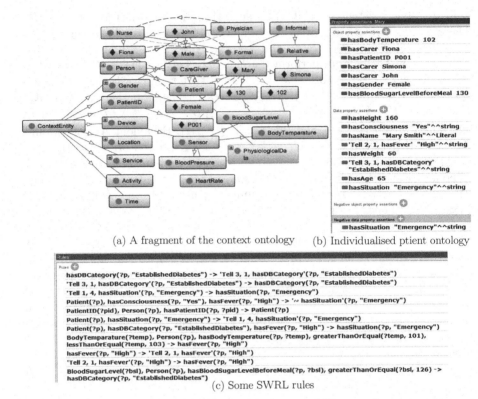

(a) A fragment of the context ontology     (b) Individualised ptient ontology

(c) Some SWRL rules

**Fig. 1.** A partial view of the context modelling ontology

formula $B_4$ $hasSituation('Mary,' Emergency)$ are 3 messages that need to be exchanged by agent 1 and 1 message that needs to be exchanged by each of the other three agents and 10 time steps. We can also observe that, if we reduce the dynamic memory size for agent 1 by 1, then the system will not be able to achieve the desired goal. We can prove that $X^{10}B_4$ $hasSituation('Mary,' Emergency)$ (i.e., from the start state, agent 4 believes $hasSituation('Mary,' Emergency)$ in 10 time steps), where $X^{10}$ is the concatenation of ten LTL next operators $X$. This is a very simple case; however, if we model a more realistic scenario and increase the problem size, the verification task would be hard to do by hand. Therefore it is more convenient to use an automatic method to verify them, for example using model checking techniques. Due to space constraints, we had to cut this discussion here, however, a $\mathcal{L_{DROCS}}$ model can be encoded using a standard model checker such as for example the Maude LTL model checker [11] and its interesting resource-bounded properties can be verified automatically.

## 5   Related Work

In general, rule-based systems have been studied for decades and traditionally rules have been used in theoretical computer science, databases, logic programming, and in particular, in Artificial Intelligence, to describe expert systems,

**Table 1.** Example rules for a homecare patients' monitoring context-aware system

| Agent 1: Patient care |
|---|
| Initial facts: Person('Mary),PatientID('P001), hasPatientID('Mary, 'P001), hasConsciousness('Mary, 'Yes) |
| R11: Person(?p), hasPatientID(?p, ?pid), PatientID(?pid) → Patient(?p) |
| R12: Tell(2,1, hasFever(?p, 'High)) → hasFever(?p, 'High) |
| R13: Tell(3,1, hasDBCategory(?p, 'EstablishedDiabetes)) → hasDBCategory(?p, 'EstablishedDiabetes) |
| R14: Patient(?p), hasFever(?p, 'High), hasConsciousness(?p, 'Yes)⇒ ∼ hasSituation(?p, 'Emergency) |
| R15: Patient(?p), hasFever(?p, 'High), hasDBCategory(?p, 'EstablishedDiabetes)⇒ hasSituation(?p, 'Emergency) |
| R16: Patient(?p), hasSituation(?p, 'Emergency) → Tell(1,4, hasSituation(?p, 'Emergency)) |
| Rule Priority: R15 ≻ R14 |
| Agent 2: Fever detector |
| Initial facts: Person('Mary),BodyTemperature('102), hasBodyTemperature('Mary,'102), greaterThanOrEqual('102, '101), lessThanOrEqual ('102, '103) |
| R21: Person(?p), BodyTemperature(?temp), hasBodyTemperature(?p,?temp), greaterThanOrEqual(?temp, '101), lessThanOrEqual (?temp, '103) → hasFever(?p, 'High) |
| R22: hasFever(?p, 'High)→ Tell(2,1, hasFever(?p, 'High)) |
| Agent 3: Diabetes tester |
| Initial facts: Person('Mary), BloodSugarLevel('130), hasBloodSugarLevelBeforeMeal('Mary,'130), greaterThan('130,'126) |
| R31: Person(?p), BloodSugarLevel(?bsl), hasBloodSugarLevelBeforeMeal(?p, ?bsl), greaterThan(?bsl,'126) → hasDBCategory(?p, 'EstablishedDiabetes) |
| R32: hasDBCategory(?p, 'EstablishedDiabetes) → Tell(3,1,hasDBCategory(?p,'EstablishedDiabetes)) |
| Agent 4: Emergency |
| Initial facts: |
| R41: Tell(1,4, hasSituation(?p, 'Emergency)) → hasSituation(?p, 'Emergency) |

robot behaviour, and behaviour of business. They have found significant application in practice and various researchers have proposed different approaches of defining a knowledge base as a pair of ontology and a set of rules including works by [16,18,23,9]. However, the approaches proposed by [14,13] have mostly influenced the work presented in this paper. In [14] Grosof et. al. have shown that the ontology based modelling techniques can be improved by using the concepts of logic programming. In their work they have noticed certain constraints while translating *DL* axioms into a set of rules. A similar approach proposed by [13] who show that a subset of *DL* languages can be effectively mapped into a set of strict and defeasible rules. Although we follow a similar approach proposed by [14,13] while constructing a set of strict and defeasible rules from an ontology, our purpose and application of those rules are quite different. We use those rules to build a context-aware system as a multi-agent non-monotonic rule-based agents and use a distributed problem solving approach to see whether agents can infer certain contexts while they are resource-bounded. In [21], it has been shown how context-aware systems can be modelled as resource-bounded rule-based systems using ontologies, however it is based on monotonic reasoning where beliefs of an agent cannot be revised based on some contradictory evidence. In [12], OWL ontologies are used to model context-aware systems, the authors exploited classes and properties from ontologies to write rules in Jess

**Table 2.** (a) One possible run (reasoning) of the system

| #Steps | Memory Config.1 | Action1 | #Msg1 | Memory Config.2 | Action2 | #Msg2 | Memory Config.3 | Action3 | #Msg3 | Memory Config.4 | Action4 | #Msg4 |
|---|---|---|---|---|---|---|---|---|---|---|---|---|
| | | Patient care | | | Fever detector | | | Diabetes tester | | | Emergency | |
| 0 | {Person('Mary), PatientID('P001), hasPatientID('Mary,' P001), hasConsciousness('Mary,'Yes) \|-, -, -\|} | - | 0 | {Person('Mary), BodyTemperature('102), hasBodyTemperature('Mary,'102), greaterThanOrEqual('102,'101), lessThanOrEqual('102,'103) \|-\|} | - | 0 | {Person('Mary), BloodSugarLevel('130), hasBloodSugarLevelBeforeMeal ('Mary,'130), greaterThan('130,'126) \|-\|} | - | 0 | {\|-\|} | - | 0 |
| 1 | {Person('Mary), PatientID('P001), hasPatientID('Mary,' P001), hasConsciousness('Mary,'Yes) \|Patient('Mary), -, -\|} | Rule (R11) | 0 | {Person('Mary), BodyTemperature('102), hasBodyTemperature('Mary,'102), greaterThanOrEqual('102,'101), lessThanOrEqual('102,'103) \|hasFever('Mary,' High)\|} | Rule (R21) | 0 | {Person('Mary), BloodSugarLevel('130), hasBloodSugarLevelBeforeMeal ('Mary,'130), greaterThan('130,'126) \|hasDBCategory('Mary,' EstablishedDiabetes)\|} | Rule (R31) | 0 | {\|-\|} | Idle | 0 |
| 2 | {Person('Mary), PatientID('P001), hasPatientID('Mary,' P001), hasConsciousness('Mary,'Yes) \|Patient('Mary), -, -\|} | Idle | 0 | {Person('Mary), BodyTemperature('102), hasBodyTemperature('Mary,'102), greaterThanOrEqual('102,'101), lessThanOrEqual('102,'103) \|Tell(2,1,hasFever('Mary,' High)\|} | Rule (R22) | 1 | {Person('Mary), BloodSugarLevel('130), hasBloodSugarLevelBeforeMeal ('Mary,'130), greaterThan('130,'126) \|Tell(3,1,hasDBCategory('Mary,' EstablishedDiabetes)\|} | Rule (R32) | 1 | {\|-\|} | Idle | 0 |
| 3 | {Person('Mary), PatientID('P001), hasPatientID('Mary,' P001), hasConsciousness('Mary,'Yes) \|Patient('Mary), Tell(2,1, hasFever('Mary, 'High),-\|} | Copy | 1 | {Person('Mary), BodyTemperature('102), hasBodyTemperature('Mary,'102), greaterThanOrEqual('102,'101), lessThanOrEqual('102,'103) \|Tell(2,1,hasFever('Mary,' High)\|} | Idle | 1 | {Person('Mary), BloodSugarLevel('130), hasBloodSugarLevelBeforeMeal ('Mary,'130), greaterThan('130,'126) \|Tell(3,1,hasDBCategory('Mary,' EstablishedDiabetes)\|} | Idle | 1 | {\|-\|} | Idle | 0 |
| 4 | {Person('Mary), PatientID('P001), hasPatientID('Mary,' P001), hasConsciousness('Mary,'Yes) \|Patient('Mary), Tell(2,1, hasFever('Mary, 'High), Tell(3,1, hasDBCategory('Mary,' EstablishedDiabetes)\|} | Copy | 2 | {Person('Mary), BodyTemperature('102), hasBodyTemperature('Mary,'102), greaterThanOrEqual('102,'101), lessThanOrEqual('102,'103) \|Tell(2,1,hasFever('Mary,' High)\|} | Idle | 1 | {Person('Mary), BloodSugarLevel('130), hasBloodSugarLevelBeforeMeal ('Mary,'130), greaterThan('130,'126) \|Tell(3,1,hasDBCategory('Mary,' EstablishedDiabetes)\|} | Idle | 1 | {\|-\|} | Idle | 0 |
| 5 | {Person('Mary), PatientID('P001), hasPatientID('Mary,' P001), hasConsciousness('Mary,'Yes) \|Patient('Mary), hasFever('Mary, 'High, Tell(3,1, hasDBCategory('Mary,' EstablishedDiabetes)\|} | Rule (R12) | 2 | {Person('Mary), BodyTemperature('102), hasBodyTemperature('Mary,'102), greaterThanOrEqual('102,'101), lessThanOrEqual('102,'103) \|Tell(2,1,hasFever('Mary,' High)\|} | Idle | 1 | {Person('Mary), BloodSugarLevel('130), hasBloodSugarLevelBeforeMeal ('Mary,'130), greaterThan('130,'126) \|Tell(3,1,hasDBCategory('Mary,' EstablishedDiabetes)\|} | Idle | 1 | {\|-\|} | Idle | 0 |

**Table 3.** (b) One possible run (reasoning) of the system

| | | Patient care | | | Fever detector | | | Diabetes tester | | | Emergency | |
|---|---|---|---|---|---|---|---|---|---|---|---|---|
| #Steps | Memory Config.1 | Action1 | #Msg1 | Memory Config.2 | Action2 | #Msg2 | Memory Config.3 | Action3 | #Msg3 | Memory Config.4 | Action4 | #Msg4 |
| 6 | {Person('Mary),<br>PatientID('P001),<br>hasPatientID('Mary,'P001),<br>hasConsciousness('Mary,'Yes)<br>Patient('Mary),<br>hasFever('Mary,'High),<br>hasDBCategory('Mary,'EstablishedDiabetes)}} | Rule (R13) | 2 | {Person('Mary),<br>BodyTemperature('102),<br>hasBodyTemperature('Mary,'102),<br>greaterThanOrEqual('102,'101),<br>lessThanOrEqual('102,'103)<br>Tell(2,1,hasFever('Mary,'High))}} | Idle | 1 | {Person('Mary),<br>BloodSugarLevel('130),<br>hasBloodSugarLevelBeforeMeal<br>('Mary,'130),<br>greaterThan('130,'126)<br>Tell(3,1,hasDBCategory(<br>'Mary,'EstablishedDiabetes))}} | Idle | 1 | {[−]} | Idle | 0 |
| 7 | {Person('Mary),<br>PatientID('P001),<br>hasPatientID('Mary,'P001),<br>hasConsciousness('Mary,'Yes)<br>Patient('Mary),<br>hasSituation('Mary,'Emergency),<br>hasDBCategory('Mary,'EstablishedDiabetes)}} | Rule (R15~R14 Resolving conflicting context) | 2 | {Person('Mary),<br>BodyTemperature('102),<br>hasBodyTemperature('Mary,'102),<br>greaterThanOrEqual('102,'101),<br>lessThanOrEqual('102,'103)<br>Tell(2,1,hasFever('Mary,'High))}} | Idle | 1 | {Person('Mary),<br>BloodSugarLevel('130),<br>hasBloodSugarLevelBeforeMeal<br>('Mary,'130),<br>greaterThan('130,'126)<br>Tell(3,1,hasDBCategory(<br>'Mary,'EstablishedDiabetes))}} | Idle | 1 | {[−]} | Idle | 0 |
| 8 | {Person('Mary),<br>PatientID('P001),<br>hasPatientID('Mary,'P001),<br>hasConsciousness('Mary,'Yes)<br>Patient('Mary),<br>hasSituation('Mary,'Emergency),<br>Tell(1,4,hasSituation('Mary,'Emergency))}} | Rule (R16) | 3 | {Person('Mary),<br>BodyTemperature('102),<br>hasBodyTemperature('Mary,'102),<br>greaterThanOrEqual('102,'101),<br>lessThanOrEqual('102,'103)<br>Tell(2,1,hasFever('Mary,'High))}} | Idle | 1 | {Person('Mary),<br>BloodSugarLevel('130),<br>hasBloodSugarLevelBeforeMeal<br>('Mary,'130),<br>greaterThan('130,'126)<br>Tell(3,1,hasDBCategory(<br>'Mary,'EstablishedDiabetes))}} | Idle | 1 | {[−]} | Idle | 0 |
| 9 | {Person('Mary),<br>PatientID('P001),<br>hasPatientID('Mary,'P001),<br>hasConsciousness('Mary,'Yes)<br>Patient('Mary),<br>hasSituation('Mary,'Emergency),<br>Tell(1,4,hasSituation('Mary,'Emergency))}} | Idle | 3 | {Person('Mary),<br>BodyTemperature('102),<br>hasBodyTemperature('Mary,'102),<br>greaterThanOrEqual('102,'101),<br>lessThanOrEqual('102,'103)<br>Tell(2,1,hasFever('Mary,'High))}} | Idle | 1 | {Person('Mary),<br>BloodSugarLevel('130),<br>hasBloodSugarLevelBeforeMeal<br>('Mary,'130),<br>greaterThan('130,'126)<br>Tell(3,1,hasDBCategory(<br>'Mary,'EstablishedDiabetes))}} | Idle | 1 | {{Tell(1,4,hasSituation('Copy<br>'Mary,'Emergency))}} | Idle | 1 |
| 10 | {Person('Mary),<br>PatientID('P001),<br>hasPatientID('Mary,'P001),<br>hasConsciousness('Mary,'Yes)<br>Patient('Mary),<br>hasSituation('Mary,'Emergency),<br>Tell(1,4,hasSituation('Mary,'Emergency))}} | Idle | 3 | {Person('Mary),<br>BodyTemperature('102),<br>hasBodyTemperature('Mary,'102),<br>greaterThanOrEqual('102,'101),<br>lessThanOrEqual('102,'103)<br>Tell(2,1,hasFever('Mary,'High))}} | Idle | 1 | {Person('Mary),<br>BloodSugarLevel('130),<br>hasBloodSugarLevelBeforeMeal<br>('Mary,'130),<br>greaterThan('130,'126)<br>Tell(3,1,hasDBCategory(<br>'Mary,'EstablishedDiabetes))}} | Idle | 1 | {hasSituation(<br>'Mary,'Emergency)} | Infer (R41) | 1 |

to derive multi-agent rules based system. Thus their modelling part of the system only reflects the static behaviour. In contrast, our ontology-based modelling captures both static and dynamic behaviour of the system using OWL 2 RL and SWRL. A prototype of context management model is presented in [10] that supports collaborative reasoning in a multi-domain pervasive context-aware application. The model facilitates the context reasoning by providing structure for contexts, rules and their semantics. In [5], authors have proposed a distributed algorithm for query evaluation in a Multi-Context Systems framework based on defeasible logic. In their work, contexts are built using defeasible rules, and the proposed algorithm can determine for a given literal $P$ whether $P$ is (not) a logical conclusion of the Multi-Context Systems, or whether it cannot be proved that $P$ is a logical conclusion. However, none of these approaches studies formal specification of context-aware systems considering their resource-boundedness features.

## 6    Conclusions and Future Work

In this paper, we propose a logical framework for modelling context-aware systems as multi-agent non-monotonic rule-based agents, and the resulting logic $\mathcal{L}_{\mathcal{DROCS}}$ allows us to describe a set of ontology-driven rule-based non-monotonic reasoning agents with bounds on time, memory, and communication. Agents use defeasible reasoning technique to reason with inconsistent information. In future work, we will show how we can encode a $\mathcal{L}_{\mathcal{DROCS}}$ model considering a more realistic system and verify its interesting resource-bounded properties automatically.

## References

1. Alechina, N., Logan, B., Nga, N.H., Rakib, A.: Verifying time and communication costs of rule-based reasoners. In: Peled, D.A., Wooldridge, M.J. (eds.) MoChArt 2008. LNCS, vol. 5348, pp. 1–14. Springer, Heidelberg (2009)
2. Antoniou, G., Billington, D., Governatori, G., Maher, M.J.: Representation results for defeasible logic. ACM Transactions on Computational Logic 2(2), 255–287 (2001)
3. Baader, F., McGuinness, D.L., Nardi, D. (eds.): P.F.P.S.: The Description Logic Handbook: Theory, Implementation, and Applications. Cambridge University Press (2003)
4. Baldauf, M., Dustdar, S., Rosenberg, F.: A survey on context-aware systems. International Journal of Ad Hoc and Ubiquitous Computing 2(4), 263–277 (2007)
5. Bikakis, A., Antoniou, G., Hasapis, P.: Strategies for contextual reasoning with conflicts in ambient intelligence. Knowledge and Information Systems 27(1), 45–84 (2011)
6. Byun, H.E., Chevers, K.: Utilizing context history to provide dynamic adaptations. Applied Artificial Intelligence 18(6), 533–548 (2004)
7. Daniele, L., Costa, P.D., Pires, L.F.: Towards a rule-based approach for context-aware applications. In: Pras, A., van Sinderen, M. (eds.) EUNICE 2007. LNCS, vol. 4606, pp. 33–43. Springer, Heidelberg (2007)
8. Dey, A., Abwowd, G.: Towards a better understanding of context and context-awareness. Technical Report GIT-GVU-99-22, Georgia Institute of Technology

9. Eiter, T., Ianni, G., Lukasiewicz, T., Schindlauer, R.: Well-founded semantics for description logic programs in the semantic web. ACM Trans. Comput. Logic 12(2), 1–11 (2011)

10. Ejigu, D., Scuturici, M., Brunie, L.: An ontology-based approach to context modeling and reasoning in pervasive computing. In: PerCom Workshops 2007, pp. 14–19 (2007)

11. Eker, S., Meseguer, J., Sridharanarayanan, A.: The maude LTL model checker and its implementation. In: Ball, T., Rajamani, S.K. (eds.) SPIN 2003. LNCS, vol. 2648, pp. 230–234. Springer, Heidelberg (2003)

12. Esposito, A., Tarricone, L., Zappatore, M., Catarinucci, L., Colella, R., DiBari, A.: A framework for context-aware home-health monitoring. In: Sandnes, F.E., Zhang, Y., Rong, C., Yang, L.T., Ma, J. (eds.) UIC 2008. LNCS, vol. 5061, pp. 119–130. Springer, Heidelberg (2008)

13. Gómez, S.A., Chesñevar, C.I., Simari, G.R.: Inconsistent ontology handling by translating description logics into defeasible logic programming. Inteligencia Artificial, Revista Iberoamericana de Inteligencia Artificial 11(35), 11–22 (2007)

14. Grosof, B.N., Horrocks, I., Volz, R., Decker, S.: Description logic programs: Combining logic programs with description logic. In: WWW 2003, pp. 48–57. ACM Press (2003)

15. Horridge, M., Bechhofer, S.: The OWL API: A java API for working with OWL 2 Ontologies. In: 6th OWL Experienced and Directions Workshop (OWLED) (October 2009)

16. Levy, A.Y., Rousset, M.C.: Combining horn rules and description logics in CARIN. Artif. Intell. 104(1-2), 165–209 (1998)

17. Motik, B., Grau, B., Horrocks, I., Wu, Z., Fokoue, A., Lutz, C.: OWL 2 Web Ontology Language: Profiles, W3C Recommendation. (October 2009), http://www.w3.org/TR/owl2-profiles/

18. Motik, B., Sattler, U., Studer, R.: Query answering for OWL-DL with rules. Journal of Web Semantics: Science, Services and Agents on the World Wide Web 3, 41–60 (2005)

19. Pollock, J.L.: Defeasible reasoning. Cognitive Science 11(4), 481–518 (1987)

20. Protégé: The Protégé ontology editor and knowledge-base framework (Version 4.1) (July 2011), http://protege.stanford.edu/

21. Rakib, A., Haque, H.M.U., Faruqui, R.U.: A temporal description logic for resource-bounded rule-based context-aware agents. In: Vinh, P.C., Alagar, V., Vassev, E., Khare, A. (eds.) ICCASA 2013. LNICST, vol. 128, pp. 3–14. Springer, Heidelberg (2014)

22. Reynolds, M.: An axiomatization of full computation tree logic. J. Symb. Log. 66(3), 1011–1057 (2001)

23. Rosati, R.: DL+log: Tight integration of description logics and disjunctive datalog. In: Proceedings of the Tenth International Conference on Principles of Knowledge Representation and Reasoning, pp. 68–78. AAAI Press (2006)

24. Schilit, B., Adams, N., Want, R.: Context-aware computing applications. In: Proceedings of the First Workshop on Mobile Computing Systems and Applications, pp. 85–90. IEEE Computer Society, Washington, DC (1994)

25. Schmidt, A., Beigl, M., Gellersen, H.W.: There is more to context than location. Computers and Graphics 23, 893–901 (1998)

26. Viterbo, F.J., da G. Malcher, M., Endler, M.: Supporting the development of context-aware agent-based systems for mobile networks. In: Proceedings of the 2008 ACM Symposium on Applied Computing, pp. 1872–1873. ACM (2008)

# MAS-td: An Approach to Termination Detection of Multi-agent Systems

Ammar Lahlouhi[*]

Department of Computer Science, University of Batna, 05000 Batna, Algeria
ammar.lahlouhi@gmail.com

**Abstract.** Current multi-agent systems (MASs) don't include the detection of their termination. Without such detection, the MAS will be either incomplete or incoherent. It is incomplete if it is a MAS lacking the detection of its termination. It is incoherent if it is other kind of systems than a MAS even if it terminates correctly. The problem of termination detection is borrowed from distributed systems where several solutions are proposed and/or improved. However, few works deal with this problem in the MAS context. In such context, the proposed solutions don't meet MASs requirements. This paper proposes MAS-td approach to the problem of termination detection in the MAS context. MAS-td improves the probe algorithm and meets the MASs requirements.

**Keywords:** Distributed Systems, Distributed Termination Detection, Multi-Agent Systems.

## 1 Introduction

Multi-agent systems must consider the detection of their termination. Without such detection, a multi-agent system will be either incomplete or incoherent. It is incomplete if it is effectively a multi-agent system (MAS) which lacks termination detection, since such detection is needed. It is incoherent if it is other kind of systems (such as procedural system) than a MAS, even if such system terminates correctly. The rest of this introduction explains the necessity of endowing MASs with termination detection and describes the organization of the paper.

An agent is an autonomous entity that integrates aspects allowing it to react to an environment's evolution to carry out its mission. Since the agents are autonomous, the agent's termination detection will be independent from other agents. Any agent can know neither the details of another agent's mission nor the progress of its activities. However, MASs are complex systems composed of agents. There are interactions between such agents. An agent can be influenced by other agents by receiving messages or through the modification of the common environment. Consequently, any agent cannot know if it will be influenced by other agents. In addition, when an agent terminates a task, it is not sure that it terminates its mission entirely in the MAS since it can be influenced. The

---

[*] Corresponding author.

A. Gelbukh et al. (Eds.): MICAI 2014, Part I, LNAI 8856, pp. 472–482, 2014.
© Springer International Publishing Switzerland 2014

termination of an agent cannot be decided basing only on local decisions of one agent. It depends on the termination of the entire MAS which must be determined collectively, i.e., all the agents of the MAS must cooperate to reach such objective.

The termination detection problem is independent from the problem domain that addresses a particular MAS. The aspects of an adapted solution of this termination must be added methodically to the MASs so they can detect their termination. Otherwise the MAS remains infinitely busy or terminates incorrectly. It is important then to treat the termination detection problem at the methodological level and don't leave it at a development level.

The problem of termination detection is a well-known problem in distributed systems where several solutions are proposed or improved, such as [1–7], [8, 9], [11–13]. However, few works deal with this problem in MAS context, such as [10], [14]. The proposed solutions in such a context are borrowed from termination detection in the distributed systems context. This paper describes the MAS-td approach to equip the MAS agents with their termination detection. MAS-td is an improvement of the probe algorithm, described by Dijkstra, Feijen & Van Gasteren in [4], which is developed in the context of distributed systems.

The rest of the paper is organized in three sections. Section 2 explains the problem of termination detection in the context of distributed systems. It includes the description of tracing algorithms and details the probe one, on which MAS-td is based. Section 3 presents MAS-td approach to equip the agents of the MASs with their termination detection. Finally, section 4 concludes the paper.

## 2   Termination Detection of Distributed Systems

The problem of termination detection of distributed systems is sufficiently easy to define but yet nontrivial to solve [11]. It is well-studied in the context of distributed systems. Several solutions are proposed or improved such as [1–7], [8, 9], [11–13]. This section presents the main ideas proposed for the termination detection in the context of distributed systems.

The termination detection can be described as follows. A distributed system is a set of processes communicating by message passing only. There are neither shared variables nor a common clock. A process is either passive or active. Active processes may send messages, but passive processes cannot. An active process may spontaneously become passive, but a passive process may become active by receiving a message only. The termination is detected if the following condition is verified: no process is active and, then, if the communication is asynchronous, no messages are in transit. Massages in transit are messages sent by source processes but not yet received by destination processes.

The evaluation of such condition in the context of distributed systems is difficult because each process has only partial information on the global system. A process knows its state (active or idle) but, it cannot know the state of other processes nor the messages in transit. It cannot detect then the termination of the task of the entire distributed system. The termination detection necessitates

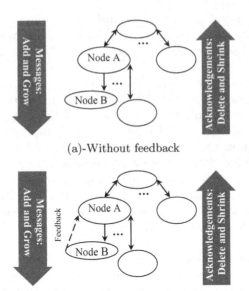

(a)-Without feedback

(b)-With a feedback (the feedback is presented by a dotted arrow)

**Fig. 1.** Spanning tree with and without feedbacks

then a distributed solution. Such solution has received considerable attention. These works roughly fall into two categories [12]: Tracing algorithms and probe algorithms.

## 2.1  Tracing Algorithms

Tracing algorithms follow the computation flow by tracing active nodes along with the message chains and call termination when all traced activity has ceased. The best known example in this class is the algorithm by Dijkstra & Scholten [5]. In this algorithm, the underlying computation is augmented with the construction and the maintenance of a spanning tree (Fig. 1 part a). Such tree is rooted at a source node representing the process with the initial input. The tree construction allows such tree to grow and shrink repeatedly. When a non-source process receives the first computation message, it sets the sender as parent and no acknowledgment is sent. Subsequent messages are acknowledged and the source acknowledges all messages. When a process is in a quiescent state and all its messages have been acknowledged, it sends an acknowledgment to its parent and deletes itself from the tree. If the deleting node is the source process, the termination is announced.

## 2.2  Probe Algorithm

Probe algorithms repeatedly scan the entire network for active processes and computation messages. They are based on the principle laid out by Dijkstra,

Feijen & Van Gasteren [4]. In the following, we describe such algorithm in more details.

For simplicity of explanation, we assume the existence of a special process (called controller) that coordinates the termination detection. Such a controller exchanges status reports with all processes. Instead of having an additional controller, it is possible that one of the processes of the computation performs the task of the controller in addition to its computation task. In this way, it is not necessary to add either processes or communication channels solely for the purpose of termination detection. In order to establish the absence of computation messages in transit, each process maintains a message deficit, which is computed as follows:

$$Deficit = (NumberOfSentMessages) - (NumberOfReceivedMessages).$$
$$(1)$$

At any time, the number of messages in transit equals the sum of all processes deficits; hence empty channels mean zero deficit sum. In a reply to a request from the controller, each process sends, immediately before it becomes passive, a status report.

It is not correct to believe that, because the processes were passive when sending the reports, the controller can detect termination if it receives status reports from all the processes and the sum of the deficits equal zero. Incoherent results from the status reports being produced at different times. Taking the status reports can be coordinated so as to prevent any message from crossing the probe backwards, which would render the algorithm safe; the status reports would then form a consistent snapshot. To detect the possibility of compensated behind-the-back activation, each process also includes in its status report, whether any message was received since sending the previous report. If this is the case, termination is not concluded; thus the receipt of a compensating backward message prevents detection. The status report must then include the process's state, the deficit number and an indication "if whether any message was received since sending the previous report".

In the probe algorithm (see the algorithms anyProcess and controllerProcess), the controller starts a wave (sends messages to the processes and then recovers their reports). The termination is detected when the deficits sum is nil and all processes are remained passive since the last wave. If the termination is detected, the controller ends the system otherwise it starts another wave. The termination detection requires two waves only. The first allows detecting the passivity of all the processes. The second allows confirming that all the processes remained passive since the last wave. The other waves are added to make up-to-date the information about the processes states. These additional waves use several communications which are time consuming. Any reduction of the number of these waves or the number of the communications in the waves will be then valuable.

*Probe algorithm (Algorithms of anyProcess and controllerProcess)*

Algorithm anyProcess (Adapted from [12])

```
Initialization:
  Deficit := 0; RemainedActive := false;
At any moment:
 // Pi's state is active: on sending a message
    send a message to some process;
    Deficit := Deficit + 1;
 //Pi's state is active: on terminating the processing
    State := Passive;
 //Pi's state is passive: on receiving a message from a process
    Receive the message from a process;  State := Active;
    RemainedActive := True; Deficit := Deficit - 1;
 // Pi's state = passive:
 //          on receiving a request from the controller
    send(State, Deficit, RemainedActive) to controllerProcess;
    RemainedActive := False;
```

Algorithm controllerProcess (Adapted from [12])

```
Repeat
  Confirmed:=true;      sumDeficit:=0;
  For i:=1 to nbProcesses do send (req) to Pi;
  For i:=1 to nbProcesses do
     receive (State, Deficit, remainedPassive) from Pi;
     Confirmed := (Confirmed and remainedPassive);
     sumDeficit := sumDeficit + Deficit;
  End For;
Until (Confirmed and (sumDeficit=0));
```

# 3   Termination Detection of Multi-agent Systems

It is interesting that the solutions for the termination detection in the context of MAS beneficiate from the solutions developed in the context of distributed systems as it is made in [14]. However, such solutions must meet MASs requirements so that they will be accepted, such as:

1. Meet the main notions of MASs,
2. Since the processing of termination detection is not directly devoted to the problem domain, they must be reduced and made out of the processing related to the solutions of the problem domain.

In addition, it is preferable that such solutions:

1. Use MAS mechanisms only (such as communication, coordination, cooperation ... ). This allows avoiding the modification of agents' controls to make them comply with the special termination detection tasks,
2. Benefit from the multi-agent advances such as the agents' proactivity and their cooperation.

This section describes MAS-td approach to termination detection of MAS. MAS-td is based on an improved probe algorithm. The rest of this section describes the probe algorithm and its improvement, in subsection 3.1, and shows how it can be applied in the context of MAS, in subsection 3.2.

## 3.1   Termination Detection in Multi-agent Systems Context

Some fundamental properties of the agents prevent the application of the methods developed for processes in the context of distributed systems to the MASs without substantial modification. In the following subsections, we explain the fundamental differences between processes in the context of distributed systems and the agents, and, then, we describe some works on the termination detection in the MASs context.

**Main Differences between Processes and Agents.** Firstly, distributed systems termination algorithms suppose that initially only some processes are active. The passive processes will be activated by sending them messages from active processes. This allows active processes to govern the termination detection of passive ones. This is not the case of the agents which are active at MAS starting and remain active until the MAS's termination.

Secondly, before an agent becomes passive, it must terminate its mission. However, when the environment doesn't comply with some conditions required by its behavior, the agent waits where it doesn't make any thing in relation to the MAS's task while it remains active. We prefer then to qualify an agent of "idle" instead of passive and "busy" instead of active. For example, a passive process cannot respond to the requests of the controller of the termination detection. Such response is delayed until the process becomes active. But an idle agent can respond since it remains active.

Thirdly, while a passive process may become active on its reception of an activation message only; an idle agent may also become busy on environment's evolution since it is proactive. The transition from busy state to idle state is not subject to message passing only but also it may be subject of the environment's evolution. In the case of the processes, it is sufficient to determine if there are messages in transit which can activate passive processes. In the case of the agents, however, it is necessary to be sure that the environment is not evolved; otherwise, there can be idle agents that can be influenced to become busy. However, an agent isnt influenced by the environment evolutions randomly but rather it knows if it waits for an environment's evolution to complete its mission. If its mission finishes temporarily, the environment's evolution doesn't influence it. Since an agent is autonomous, other agents do not know the achieved part of its mission. Only the agent itself knows if, at a given moment, the environment can influence it; the agent's state cannot be known by another agent.

Fourthly, MASs are complex systems of interacting agents. Such interactions prevent the use of tracing techniques such as that by Dijkstra & Scholten in [5] to detect termination since the spanning tree becomes cyclic (see Fig. 1 part b). The use of such techniques can brought either to use the method incorrectly or to not meet the main notions of multi-agent systems.

**Related Works.** Few works deal with the problem of termination detection of MAS. The work described in [14] is the first which explained the problem of MAS termination detection. It uses the tracing algorithm (per se) of Dijkstra & Scholten [5] developed for the distributed systems in order to detect the quiescence of the agents. As explained previously (see the previous subsection "main differences between processes and agents"), the direct use of such algorithms in the context of MAS is incoherent. The algorithm of Dijkstra & Scholten is based on the construction of a spanning tree (Fig. 1). However, as showed in Fig. 1 part b, such algorithm cannot terminate correctly with the presence of interactions between agents (since it introduces a cycle in the spanning tree).

The work described in [10] addresses the larger problem of deriving a global view of systems of interacting agents given individual agent partial local views. In the setup, the agents must communicate information about protocols and their execution when queried by a monitor. The monitor can deduce termination based on information provided by individual agents. The proposed solution becomes more difficult than the problem of termination detection that MAS requires. This is showed particularly in the assumption described as follows [10] "Agents have incentives to communicate information regarding their protocol". This assumption is not required by the termination detection, cumbersome the system and can be problematic in some systems preventing the communication of such information. In addition, MAS are complex systems where the global view emerges and its derivation is not always viable.

*MAS-td algorithm: anyAgent and controllerAgent algorithms*

anyAgent algorithm

```
Initialization:  // Initially, any agent is busy
    Busy := -1; Idle := 1; // Constants initialization
    Deficit := 0;
At any moment:
  // Agent initiates a task
    State := Busy; remainedBusy := True;
    send(State, Deficit, remainedBusy) to controllerAgent;
  // Agent terminates the task at hand
    State := Idle;
```

```
      send(State, Deficit, remainedBusy) to controllerAgent;
      remainedBusy := False;
   // Agent sends a message to an agent Ai
      send(message) to Ai; Deficit := Deficit + 1;
   // Agent receives a message from an agent Aj
      Receive(message) from Aj; Deficit := Deficit - 1;
   // Agent receives "confirm idleness" from controllerAgent
      Receive("confirm idleness") from controllerAgent;
      send(State, Deficit, remainedBusy) to controllerAgent;
   // Agent receives "termination reached" from controllerAgent
      Receive ("termination reached") from controllerAgent;
      Stop agent's execution;

controllerAgent algorithm

Initialization:
   //We start by gathering information on the agents' idleness
   idleInf := True; nbIdle := 0;
At any moment:
   // On receiving a message from an agent Ai
   receive(State, Deficit, remainedIdle) from Ai;
 If idleInf Then // We are in Gathering information phase
 |  // State will be: (-1) if Ai is busy and (+1) if Ai is idle
 |  nbIdle := nbIdle + State;
 |  if (nbIdle = nbAgents) Then
 |  |  // Gathering information phase is completed
 |  |  idleInf := False;
 |  |  // and then we enter the confirmation phase
 |  |  nbConfirmations:= 0; notConfirmed:= false; sumDeficit:= 0;
 |  |  For i := 1 to nbAgents Do
 |  |     send ("confirm idleness") message to Ai;
 |
 else // We are in Confirmation phase
 | If not remainedIdle Then  notConfirmed := true;
 | sumDeficit := sumDeficit + Deficit;
 | nbConfirmations := nbConfirmations + 1;
 | If (nbConfirmations = nbAgents) Then
      If ((notConfirmed) or (sumDeficit <> 0)) Then
      |  // Returning to gathering information phase
      |  idleInf := True; nbIdle := 0;
      else
      |  For i := 1 to nbAgents Do // Termination reached
      |     send ("Termination reached") message to Ai;
```

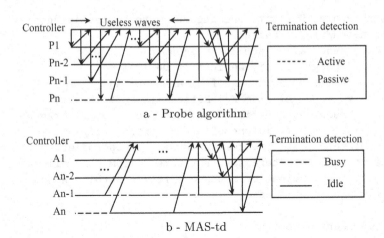

a - Probe algorithm

b - MAS-td

**Fig. 2.** MAS-td vs Probe algorithm: Decreasing the number of waves (P for process and A for agent)

## 3.2  MAS-td Approach for Termination Detection of Multi-agent Systems

In the probe algorithm (see subsection 2.2), the controller requests the processes to provide it with reports on their status. Assume the following situation (Fig. 2):

1. The system contains n processes p1...pn,
2. At the moment t, (n-2) processes p1...pn-2 become and remain passive,
3. The two remaining processes (pn and pn-1) become alternatively passive and active.

In such situation, assume also that the process Pn-1 becomes passive (n-1 processes are now passive) and only Pn is active. When Pn-1 becomes active and Pn become passive, the controller starts a wave. The n-1 passive processes (including Pn-1) will respond by "remained passive" while Pn delays its response until it becomes passive. After the response of Pn, the controller initiates another wave (since there is an active process Pn) by requesting all the processes, a second time.

Each time a process (Pn-1 or Pn) becomes active and the other becomes passive, the controller starts a new wave until these two processes become and remain passive; where the controller detects the system's termination. Several situations similar to that described here can be identified.

When i processes alternate between passivity and activity and j processes remain passive, in a time interval, the processes remained passive will be solicited by the controller uselessly. Such situations are the consequence of the fact that the controller doesn't know the existence of active processes since this information is not provided by the probe algorithm. The system makes then several waves uselessly (see useless waves in Fig. 2 part a). A wave requires the communication of the request from the controller to all the processes and the responses from such processes.

To decrease the number of the waves, MAS-td approach allows the agent to be more precise by notifying the controller of its activities without that the controller initiates a wave. The communication of the information, indicating that an agent is busy, needs communications from the agents only; it doesn't need communications from the controller. Before an idle agent becomes busy, it informs the controller and, before a busy agent becomes idle, it informs the controller also. The controller doesn't initiate any wave until it has information indicating that all agents are idles. In Fig. 2 part b, the only information to communicate concerns the status of the agents Pn and Pn-1. The agents remained idle will not be concerned with the communication of such information. However, since this information is not up-to-date, a wave must be launched to confirm that all agents remained idle (see algorithms anyAgent and controllerAgent).

The necessary actions of the termination detection must be integrated in the agents' behaviors in order to that they can carry them out during their functioning. For an organizational development of MASs, these actions will be designed as roles. We have then several roles anyAgent and one role controllerAgent. The anyAgent role will be assumed by all the agents while the controllerAgent role will be assumed by only one agent. The controllerAgent can be not a special agent but one of the agents of the problem domain of MAS.

# 4 Discussion and Conclusion

In this paper, we described MAS-td, an approach to the termination detection of MASs. MAS-td meets the main notions of MASs. In addition, it improves an existing approach, the probe algorithm, in two aspects.

Firstly, in the probe algorithm, the controller must initiate a wave so the processes will send reports to it. If all the reports indicate that all the processes are passive, the controller must also send another wave so the processes confirm their passivity. It requires then four times the number of the processes communication. MAS-td doesn't need the first wave. It needs only three times the number of the agents' communication. Consequently, MAS-td removes, at least, the initial communications.

Secondly, in the probe algorithm, a process which remained passive will be solicited by the controller several times so it sends its report (at each time, it confirms its passivity only). With MAS-td, this is not needed since the agents send information about their states to the controller which knows then their states. However, since this information is not up-to-date, the controller must confirm this information, as in probe algorithm, when the agents' reports that they are all idles, before deciding on the termination of the MAS. MAS-td avoids then several solicitations of idle agents.

Finally, MAS-td uses MAS mechanisms only and it doesn't introduce any other special mechanism, such that of [10], which is made on a special specification of interaction protocols, or that of [14], which introduces intermediate agents.

# References

1. Apt, K.R.: Correctness proofs of distributed termination algorithms. ACM Transactions on Programming Languages and Systems (TOPLAS) 8(3), 388–405 (1986)
2. Apt, K.R., Francez, N.: Modeling the distributed termination convention of csp. ACM Transactions on Programming Languages and Systems (TOPLAS) 6(3), 370–379 (1984)
3. Chandrasekaran, S., Venkatesan, S.: A message-optimal algorithm for distributed termination detection. Journal of Parallel and Distributed Computing 8(3), 245–252 (1990)
4. Dijkstra, E.W., Feijen, W., Van Gasteren, A.J.M.: Derivation of a termination detection algorithm for distributed computations. Information Processing Letters 16(5), 217–219 (1983)
5. Dijkstra, E.W., Scholten, C.S.: Termination detection for diffusing computations. Information Processing Letters 11(1), 1–4 (1980)
6. Francez, N.: Distributed termination. ACM Transactions on Programming Languages and Systems (TOPLAS) 2(1), 42–55 (1980)
7. Francez, N., Rodeh, M.: Achieving distributed termination without freezing. IEEE Transactions on Software Engineering 8(3), 287–292 (1982)
8. Mattern, F.: Algorithms for distributed termination detection. Distributed Computing 2(3), 161–175 (1987)
9. Mattern, F.: Global quiescence detection based on credit distribution and recovery. Information Processing Letters 30(4), 195–200 (1989)
10. Motshegwa, T., Schroeder, M.: Interaction monitoring and termination detection for agent societies: Preliminary results. In: Omicini, A., Petta, P., Pitt, J. (eds.) ESAW 2003. LNCS (LNAI), vol. 3071, pp. 136–154. Springer, Heidelberg (2004)
11. Tel, G., Mattern, F.: The derivation of distributed termination detection algorithms from garbage collection schemes. ACM Transactions on Programming Languages and Systems (TOPLAS) 15(1), 1–35 (1993)
12. Tel, G.: Distributed control algorithms for AI. In: Multiagent Systems, pp. 539–580. MIT Press (1999)
13. Topor, R.W.: Termination detection for distributed computations. Information Processing Letters 18(1), 33–36 (1984)
14. Wellman, P.P., Walsh, W.E.: Distributed quiescence detection in multiagent negotiation. In: Proceedings of the Fourth International Conference on MultiAgent Systems, pp. 317–324. IEEE (2000)

# Intelligent Tutoring System with Affective Learning for Mathematics

Ramón Zataraín Cabada, María Lucía Barrón Estrada,
Francisco González Hernández, and Raúl Oramas Bustillos

Instituto Tecnológico de Culiacán, Juan de Dios Bátiz s/n,
Col. Guadalupe, Culiacán Sinaloa, 80220, México
{rzatarain,lbarron}@itculiacan.edu.mx

**Abstract.** In this paper we present an intelligent tutoring system with affective learning, which is integrated into a social network for learning mathematics. The system is designed to help students of the second grade of primary education to improve the teaching-learning process. The system evaluates cognitive and affective aspects of the student by using a neural network and a fuzzy expert system to decide the following exercise to be resolved by the student, enabling personalized learning. We evaluate and compare our tutoring system against other well-known tutoring systems.

**Keywords:** Intelligent Tutoring System, Social Networks, Neural Network, Expert System, Recognition of Emotions.

## 1   Introduction

Reports published by the OCDE [1] and SEP [2] in 2010 showed that a high percentage of Mexican students failed in the mathematic subject. Other studies noted a general lack of mathematical knowledge, cognitive skills, and motivation [3].

Traditionally, Intelligent Tutoring Systems (ITS) only considered student cognitive states. But, in recent years ITS also consider the identification and response of emotions to improve performance, usability and more generally, the quality of human-computer interaction with the students [4] [5] [6].

This paper presents the implementation of an Intelligent and Affective Tutoring System for learning second-grade mathematics that is integrated into a learning social network. The system uses a feed-forward neural network to recognize the affective state of the student and a fuzzy expert system which integrates cognitive student data (such as mistakes, time and number of aids to solve a problem) with affective data as the student emotional state. This allows the system to calculate the complexity of the following exercise that will solve the student.

This paper is organized as follows: in section 2, we describe the design and implementation of the system with its layered architecture, components and algorithms. Results and software evaluation are presented in Section 3 and conclusions and future work are discussed in section 4.

A. Gelbukh et al. (Eds.): MICAI 2014, Part I, LNAI 8856, pp. 483–493, 2014.

# 2    System Design and Implementation

## 2.1    System Architecture

The structure of the ITS follows the traditional model for such systems [7] which include a domain model, a student model, a tutoring model, and a user interface. In our tutoring system the user interface is represented by a social network, from where the communication with the students and the other three components is established.

The architectural design of the system is organized into a model containing five layers: presentation, server, logic, management of models, and data access. The system architecture is shown in Figure 1.

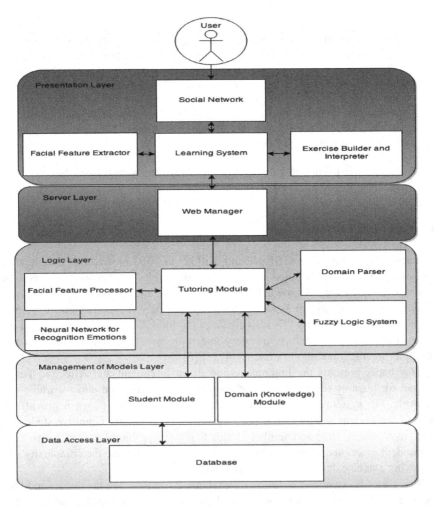

**Fig. 1.** Architecture of the Intelligent and Affective Tutoring System

In a typical scenario of the system, the student has access through the social network and interacts with its own interface that is responsible for displaying the items with a block of exercises; for different time intervals the user's face is captured to recognize their affective state. The student solves a math problem and depending on the time taken to solve the problem, the number of requested aid, the mistakes, and the emotional state of the student, the fuzzy system of the ITS calculates the complexity of the following problem.

## 2.2  The Presentation Layer

The Presentation Layer is the graphical interface of the system; its task is to interact with the user (a student) through a web interface that is displayed on a desktop or mobile device. Math exercises that the student must solve are presented in the web interface. For each student response, cognitive and affective data are processed, allowing building the next exercise. This layer contains three components:

- **Facial Feature Extractor:** It obtains an image of the student's face at predefined time intervals and sends it to the Learning System component in JPEG format. To capture the image we use the HTML 5 API to manage the webcam of a PC computer or a smartphone.
- **Learning System:** It is responsible for presenting the web interface with mathematical exercises that the student must solve. It contains different kind of aid and information of the target (goal) that the student must achieve. The component uses the cognitive and affective data obtained from component *Facial Feature Extractor*. This data is sent to *Web Manager*, which forwards it to *Tutoring Module*. This component processes the information and returns it to *Web Manager*, who returns it to *Learning System*. These cognitive and affective data are processed it by the Learning System and the Exercise Builder and Interpreter components to generate new math exercises that the student must solve. The web interface uses jQuery Mobile (for smartphones), HTML 5, CSS 3 and JavaScript.
- **Exercise Builder and Interpreter:** It has the task of interpreting the information it receives from the Tutoring Module. It also generates and supports the user goals to be achieved. It helps the Learning System component as each mathematics exercise is interpreted and constructed according to the student interaction.

## 2.3  The Server Layer

The server layer is an intermediary between the Presentation Layer and Logic Layer. This layer contains only one component:

- **Web Manager:** It receives the data sent from the Presentation Layer and builds objects which are processed by *Tutoring Module*. The Tutoring Module component returns the processed information which is to be sent to clients (students) who are in the Presentation Layer.

## 2.4 Logic Layer

This layer interacts with the server layer. It provides the intelligent part (neural network and fuzzy-logic system) to our system. It receives and process cognitive and affective user data and later generates the following math exercises with the appropriate level of difficulty for the students. This layer contains five components that are described below.

- **Tutoring Module:** It is the main component of the system. It contains the algorithm for constructing mathematical exercises (see Figure 2). The component uses the cognitive and affective student data obtained from Facial Feature Extractor, Domain Analyzer/Parser, and Fuzzy-Logic System components.
- **Facial Feature Processor:** It analyzes a JPEG image and extracts certain features of the face. These features create a set of 10 coordinates that are sent to the neural network to recognize emotions and return the student's affective state.
- **Neural Network for Recognizing Emotions:** it uses a back propagation (Feed-Forward) neural network previously trained with a corpus of facial emotions to determine the affective state of the student. This component receives a set of 10 coordinates and determines the emotional state of the student.
- **Domain Analyzer/Parser:** It is responsible for analyzing a domain pattern sent by the Tutoring Module. The component has the knowledge of how to process different tasks of different domains that are in different formats. For example, the domain or knowledge for second-grade Math is encoded in XML format. To analyze and process this file we use the xPath language.
- **Fuzzy Logic System:** It receives data (fuzzy variables *time, aid, error*, and *emotion*) sent by *Tutoring Module* which are evaluated by using a set of pre-defined fuzzy logic rules. The component uses the API jFuzzyLogic [8] for evaluation of cognitive data. The definition of input and output variables, fuzzy logic rules and defuzzification method is in a text file using API jFuzzyLogic.

**Description of the Algorithm**
Figure 2 presents the algorithm that uses the Tutoring Module to build the math exercises.

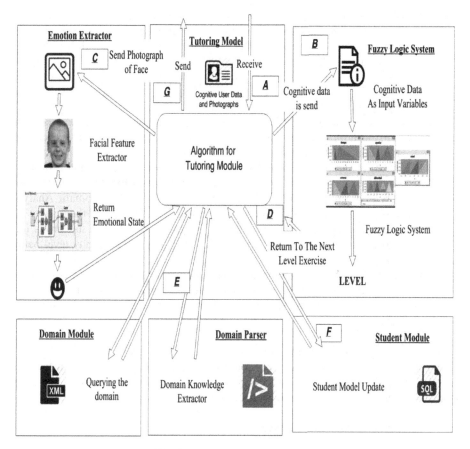

**Fig. 2.** Algorithm for Tutor Model

The algorithm works as follows:

A. The Tutoring Module receives an object that contains the student cognitive data, its facial image, and information about the problem (exercise) that the student has solved.

B. Then, it sends cognitive and affective data to the Fuzzy Logic System which outputs the result to the Tutoring Module. This output represents the recommended level for the next exercise.

C. Next, it sends the student facial image to the Emotion Extractor component. A Haar-like features Cascades method [9] is applied, for face detection of student. The detection created by this method allows the creation of boundary areas in the image. These areas are well-known as regions of interest (ROI). The Haar-like features Cascades method is again applied to the ROI created in the previous step to detect the person's mouth. A rectangle is drawn around the new ROI and it is transformed to gray scale. Then, histogram equalization is applied to the gray scale image enclosed in the ROI and a threshold is also applied to reduce the light and the colors (only black and white).The image result is stored in an array of pixels. Again, the Haar-like features Cascades method is applied to detect the right and left eye of the student. Some lines are drawn among coordinates. These lines represent "distances" which are used to detect the emotion of the person. For each distance, the Pythagorean Theorem is applied between the two coordinates of each distance and the result of the hypotenuse of the triangle is obtained.

D. The Tutoring Module begins to take decisions on the next exercise that will be built, considering the values of emotion and cognitive data obtained in steps B and C.

E. Next, it requests a particular domain or topic from the Domain Module. Then, it sends the topic to *Domain Analyzer/Parser* together with parameters of what you need to do or get. Subsequently, the Domain Analyzer/Parser component executes those instructions and returns the results.

F. Then, it sends information to the Student Model to establish its current improvement over the domain, their emotional state and difficulty level being managed.

G. Last, the Tutoring Module completes the building of the next exercise and transforms it into a format that the interpreter understands. This exercise or problem is sent to the Server Layer that handles it to the student (presentation layer).

In step B the system needs to load a FCL file (Fuzzy Control Language) [10] containing all information about the fuzzy logic system. This is a configuration file that contains 4 input variables, 1 output variable and 74 fuzzy rules. The defuzzification method is *center of gravity* and rule evaluation is restricted to *AND type*.

### 2.5    Management of Model Layer

This layer contains the Domain Module and the Student Module components. Each component manages their respective models and responds to requests from the Tutoring Module.

- **Domain Model (Knowledge):** the domain represented in this system of math learning is elementary second grade. The domain models are quantitative representations of expert knowledge in a specific domain [7]; therefore we try to define a knowledge representation that matches the structure shown in second grade books for the official program in Mexico (see Figure 3). To represent the domain, we applied the theory of knowledge spaces [11]. This theory uses concepts of combinatory and probability theory to model and empirically describe particular areas of knowledge. In formal terms, the theory tells us that a knowledge structure is a pair (Q, K) in which Q is a nonempty set, and K is a family of subsets of Q, which contains at least one Q and one empty set $\emptyset$. The set Q is called the domain of knowledge structure. Its elements are called questions or items and the subsets in the K family are labeled (knowledge) as states. Occasionally it may be said that K is a knowledge structure on a Q set in the sense that (Q, K) is a knowledge structure. The specification of the domain can be omitted without ambiguity since we have $\cup K = Q$. For example, we can represent the model of knowledge as:

*Knowledge = {Ø, {Block 1, Lesson 1.1, Lesson 1.2}, {Block 2, Lesson 2.1}}.*

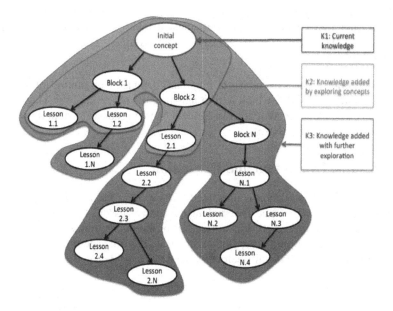

**Fig. 3.** Knowledge representation for second grade math

- **Student Model:** It is the representation of knowledge that the student has with respect to the domain model. However as our system is an ITS handling emotions, a representation that includes more than just knowledge is required. For this purpose a semantic network was selected to represent the student knowledge (see Figure 4). This representation has been used in ITS such as ActiveMath, Wayang Outpost, and Guru Tutor [7]. We may expand it by adding the affective part of the student. The category used was a Red IS-A [12].

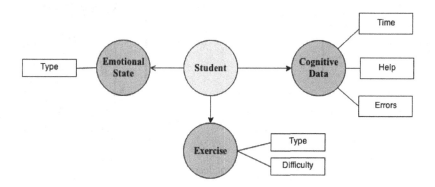

**Fig. 4.** Representation of student knowledge in a semantic network

## 2.6    The Data Access Layer

It contains components that manage access to external data sources such as text files with XML and JSON formats, and a relational database. The component goal is to bring a bridge of technology with the various data sources. This layer contains only one component:

- **Database:** The system has a relational database containing information of the Student Model, which in turn manages the requests of the Tutoring Module. The Database will convert Student Model requests to running requests in the relational database.

# 3    Results, Evaluation and Discussion

In Figure 5 a small test session is presented. The student has to select a block which in turn contains lessons. Once the student chooses a lesson, the system presents a series of exercises to be solved. It is in this part of the interaction with the student that the tutoring system recognizes the student emotion, the time spent in the exercise, the number of requested petitions for help, and the number of detected errors.

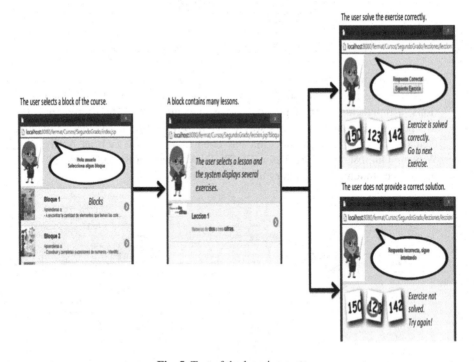

**Fig. 5.** Test of the learning system

For the evaluation of our system we took as reference the seven features that distinguish a modern ITS from traditional instructional systems Woolf [7]. Table 1 shows the evaluation results.

**Table 1.** Distinguishing Features desired in an ITS

| Characteristics of ITS | Description | Implementation in the ITS |
|---|---|---|
| Generality | The ability to generate appropriate problems and personal advice. | The system evaluates the user's cognitive and affective data. The system selects the complexity of next exercise that the user must solve based on these data. |
| Student Model | The ability to represent and reason about knowledge of the student and their learning needs. | The system works and updates a Student Model from solving exercises. |
| Expert Model | Represents the expert's knowledge and their reasoning. | The system has the ability to modify the Domain Model. |
| Mixed Initiative | The ability to interact with the student individually. | In this version of the system this feature is not implemented. |
| Interactive Learning | Activities that require a commitment to learning by the student. | This feature is achieved by identifying the affective state of the student. The system uses a neural network and a fuzzy expert system. |
| Instructional Model | The ability to change the mode of teaching based on inferences depending on student learning. | The system uses the problem solving model. |
| Self-improvement | The system's ability to learn from their own experience. | In this version of the system, we do not considered this feature. |

Table 2 shows the system evaluation with a metric with values 0, 1 and 3. 0 represents the features that will be added in future versions or are not covered. 1 represents an incomplete feature and 3 is a complete feature. The system was compared against ITSs *ActiveMath, Wayang Outpost* and *Animal Watch* [7].

**Table 2.** Comparison against other ITS system

| Characteristic | Intelligent and Affective Tutoring Sys. | ActiveMath | Wayang Outpost | Animal Watch |
|---|---|---|---|---|
| Generality | 3 | 3 | 0 | 0 |
| Student Model | 3 | 3 | 3 | 3 |
| Expert Model | 3 | 3 | 3 | 3 |
| Mixed Initiative | 1 | 1 | 0 | 0 |
| Interactive Learning | 1 | 3 | 3 | 3 |
| Instructional Model | 1 | 1 | 3 | 1 |
| Self-improvement | 0 | 1 | 0 | 1 |
| **Total assessment** | **12** | **15** | **12** | **11** |

According to the total assessment, the intelligent and affective tutoring system achieves a score of 12 points, which leaves him with the same score as Wayang Outpost and a greater score than Animal Watch. ActiveMath achieved a score of 15 points. We still are working to include Mixed Initiative and Self-improvement features.

## 4    Conclusions and Future Work

Emotions play an important role in the teaching-learning process of a person. In recent years, intelligent tutoring systems already integrate automatic recognition of emotions. This functionality improves the teaching-learning process through interactions tailored to each student for their cognitive and affective states.

In the process of developing this system we noticed the complexity associated with these systems and the diversity of specialists needed to run a large-scale project. For this reason it was necessary to use various (open) source software such as: HTML 5 for web content; CSS3 for visual representation of the content; Java Technology for the ITS program in the server side; JavaScript language and frameworks jQuery, jQuery Mobile, to set the client-side interface; MySQL relational database to store student information. We also used other tools such as JavaScript Object Notation (JSON), eXtensible Markup Language (XML) and XML Path Language (XPath). Besides that, we used OpenCV, JavaCV, and Weka for building the Facial Feature Extractor and the Neural Network.

In the future it is planned to include a pedagogical agent with the ability to interact with the student in natural language. In relation to the instructional model we plan to include a module to manage learning styles. For the interactive learning, it is thought to include more activities that involve interaction among students using the social network functionalities.

## References

1. PISA Country Profiles, http://pisacountry.acer.edu.au/
2. Secretaría de Educación Pública (2013),
   http://enlace.sep.gob.mx/content/gr/docs/2013/historico/
   00_EB_2013.pdf
3. Díaz Velarde, M.E., Villegas, Q.C.: Las matemáticas y el dominio afectivo. Revista Multidisciplinar, Matemáticas e Ingeniería 16, 139–164 (2013)
4. Arroyo, I., Cooper, D.G., Burleson, W., Woolf, B.P., Muldner, K., Christopherson, R.: Emotions sensors go to school. In: Proceedings of the 14th International Conference on Artificial Intelligence in Education, pp. 17–24 (2009)
5. D'Mello, S.K., Picard, R.W., Graesser, A.C.: Towards an affective-sensitive AutoTutor. Special Issue on Intelligent Educational Systems IEEE Intelligent Systems 22(4), 53–61 (2007)
6. Conati, C.Y., Maclaren, H.: Empirically building and evaluating a probabilistic model of user affect. User Modeling and User Adapted Interaction 19(3), 267–303 (2009)

7. Woolf, B.P.: Building intelligent interactive tutors: Student-centered strategies for revolutionizing e-learning. Morgan Kauffman Publishers/Elsevier, USA (2009)

8. jFuzzyLogic, http://jfuzzylogic.sourceforge.net/html/index.html

9. Bradski, G., Kaehler, A.: Learning computer Vision with OpenCV library. Oreally (2008)

10. Cingolani, P., Alcalá-Fdez, J.: jFuzzyLogic: a Java Library to Design Fuzzy Logic Controllers According to the Standard for Fuzzy Control Programming. International Journal of Computational Intelligence Systems 6(suppl. 1), 61–75 (2013)

11. Doignon, J.-P., Falmagne, J.C.: Knowledge Spaces. Springer (1999)

12. Brachman, R.J.: What IS-A Is and Isn't: An analysis of Taxonomic Links in Semantic Networks. IEEE Computer 16(10), 30–36 (1983)

# Emotion Recognition in Intelligent Tutoring Systems for Android-Based Mobile Devices

Ramón Zataraín Cabada[1], María Lucía Barrón-Estrada[1], Giner Alor-Hernández[2], and Carlos Alberto Reyes-García[3]

[1] Instituto Tecnológico de Culiacán, Juan de Dios Bátiz s/n,
Col. Guadalupe, Culiacán Sinaloa, 80220, México
[2] Instituto Tecnológico de Orizaba, Avenida Oriente 9 No. 852,
Col. Emiliano Zapata, C.P. 94320, Orizaba, Veracruz, México
[3] Instituto Nacional de Astrofísica, Óptica y Electrónica (INAOE)
Luis Enrique Erro No. 1, Sta. Ma. Tonanzintla, Puebla, 72840, México
{rzatarain,lbarron}@itculiacan.edu.mx,
galor@itorizaba.edu.mx, kargaxxi@inaoep.mx

**Abstract.** In this paper, we present a Web-based system aimed at learning basic mathematics. The Web-based system includes different components like a social network for learning, an intelligent tutoring system and an emotion recognizer. We have developed the system with the goal of being accessed from any kind of computer platform and Android-based mobile device. We have also built a neural-fuzzy system for the identification of student emotions and a fuzzy system for tracking student´s pedagogical states. We carried out different experiments with the emotion recognizer where we obtained a success rate of 96%. Furthermore, the system (including the social network and the intelligent tutoring system) was tested with real students and the obtained results were very satisfying.

**Keywords:** Intelligent Tutoring Systems, Affective Computing, Social Intelligence, Artificial Neural Networks, Mobile learning.

## 1 Introduction

The use of new technologies such as social networking in education – specifically in intelligent tutoring systems, affective computing applied to learning systems, and mobile computing – is creating a point of inflection in the ways of learning. An inflection point is a new paradigm change used to carry out a process, such as in the case of education, where traditional methods used to learn certain activities, particularly academics, are fully renovated.

In recent years, the Web has evolved from being a static platform with content information to an entity that is constantly producing, renewing, and sharing not only information but also knowledge. This way of operating, where users not only consume information and knowledge but also produce it, has been called "Web 2.0" [1] or harnessing collective intelligence [2]. Moreover, the concept of social software has emerged as part of the Web 2.0, which is a medium that allows people to not only

A. Gelbukh et al. (Eds.): MICAI 2014, Part I, LNAI 8856, pp. 494–504, 2014.

connect to repositories containing information and knowledge (e.g. learning objects), but also connect to other people. Blogs, wikis and social networks are examples of communities of knowledge or social software, where the case of the latter is the most significant because of its explosive growth in our society. For example, social networks such as Facebook© has over 1.11 billion users and Twitter© over 645 million. A social network is an online communication tool that allows users to create public or private profiles, create and display their own as well as other users' online social networks and interact with people in their networks [3].

Affective computing [4] is a field of research that integrates different scientific disciplines, seeking to enable computers in order to behave intelligently, interacting naturally with users through the ability to recognize, understand and express emotions. Knowing the emotional state of a person provides relevant information about his/her psychological state and offers the possibility to decide on how to respond to it. Research in this field aims to develop software systems that identify and respond to the emotions of a user (e.g. a student). Emotions are detected by different devices (PC camera, PC microphone, special mouse, neuro-headset, among others) that can be placed on a computer or person [5]. These devices are responsible for picking up the users' signals (facial image, voice, mouse applied pressure, heart rate, stress level, to mention but a few) and sending them to the computer to be processed. Then, the resulting emotional state is obtained in real time. In the field of education, an affective system seeks to change a user's negative emotional state (e.g. confused) into a positive emotional state (e.g. committed), in order to facilitate an appropriate emotional state for learning. The latest related works on emotion recognition in intelligent tutoring systems (ITS) incorporates different hardware and software-based methods to recognize student emotions [5, 6, 7, 8].

In the last several years, many studies have proved the benefits of web-based learning and mobile learning [9, 10, 11]. Different learning methodologies such as hybrid learning, blended learning, and mobile learning have been proposed for increasing the efficacy of web-based learning. We decided to implement our social software system as a Web-based and mobile application instead of a desktop application, due to the advantages posed by the former (platform independence, access from anywhere-anytime-anyplace, no software installation, among others).

In this work, we present a software system that incorporates emotion recognition and support to an ITS for mathematics, which are part of a learning social network. Our main contribution is the integration of different components like a social network for learning, an intelligent tutoring system and an emotion recognizer. The emotion is recognized by capturing the students' facial expressions. Another contribution is the integration of an ITS inside a social network. This allows students to collaboratively work in a natural way.

The output of the affective recognizer (the actual student emotion) is merged with the pedagogical or cognitive results in the math exercises, forming the input for a fuzzy system that decides what kind of exercise to present to the student. To implement this process we built a neural network for emotion recognition and a fuzzy system for tracking student's pedagogical states.

## 2     Explicit Invocation Architecture

We developed an application for web browsers and Android-based mobile devices, allowing the Intelligent Tutoring System (ITS) to be accessed from both PC and mobile devices (e.g. smartphones and tablets). The ITS requests the execution of an application in order to extract the facial features. This task is done via web browser by executing an invocation to the program installed on the PC or mobile device. This program takes a picture of the student's face to obtain features of the eyes and mouth, which are submitted to the ITS. The information obtained is sent to a Web server with a neural network in order to determine the corresponding emotion, providing such information to the ITS. Once the emotion is obtained, the ITS uses it as an input with other related values from results of the student's exercises. Figure 1 shows the Explicit Invocation Architecture where some of the components are briefly explained.

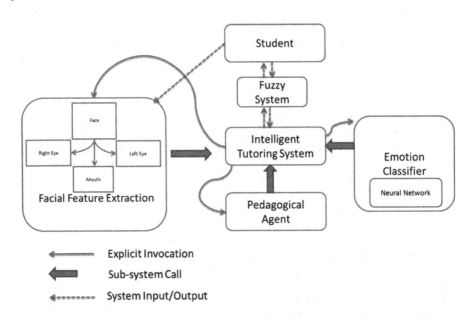

**Fig. 1.** Explicit Invocation Architecture

**Facial Feature Extraction**
**Face.** This component is responsible for finding the human face in the picture by using a Haar-like features Cascades method, implemented with the *OpenCV* library.

**Mouth, Right and Left Eye.** Once the student's face is detected, the components are invoked in order to find the mouth, right eye and left eye. For optimal image processing, a ROI (Region of Interest) method was used delimiting the search space and discarding the rest of the image. Once the objects in the image are found, a series of transformations are performed, facilitating the search for edges on objects and calculating their opening distances. These data feed the input to the neural network for emotion classification.

Next, the eight steps of the algorithm for Facial Feature Extraction process are described.

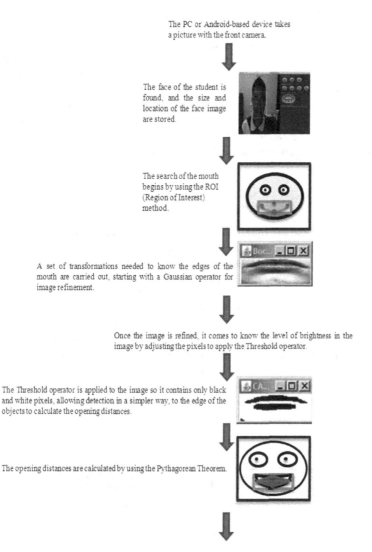

The PC or Android-based device takes a picture with the front camera.

The face of the student is found, and the size and location of the face image are stored.

The search of the mouth begins by using the ROI (Region of Interest) method.

A set of transformations needed to know the edges of the mouth are carried out, starting with a Gaussian operator for image refinement.

Once the image is refined, it comes to know the level of brightness in the image by adjusting the pixels to apply the Threshold operator.

The Threshold operator is applied to the image so it contains only black and white pixels, allowing detection in a simpler way, to the edge of the objects to calculate the opening distances.

The opening distances are calculated by using the Pythagorean Theorem.

Steps III to VII are performed for the left and right eyes

To calculate the opening distance (points) of the mouth, left and right eye, different transformations were performed in regions of interest where the objects are found in the image. These modifications allow the application to perform feature extraction, with optimal performance in image size, besides image noise cleaning and handling of certain pixels to identify objects in regions of interest.

The Gaussian average operator was considered to allow cleaning the image obtained by the application. Initially, Gaussian g was used where the coordinates x, y are controlled by the difference σ2 according to equation 1 [12]:

$$g(x, y, \sigma) = \frac{1}{2\pi\sigma} \, e^{\cdot \left( -\frac{x^2 + y^2}{2\sigma^2} \right)} \tag{1}$$

The results obtained using the Gaussian average operator were smoother images, removing details of the photo, allowing a greater focus on long structures.

Another influential factor in the images is the brightness, which may hinder the transformation process because it does not allow the definition of some edges and structures. So we applied the histogram equalization process where the image obtained passes through a non-linear process, which tends to emphasize the brightness in a particular way to make it more suitable for recognition. With this application, the process makes changes producing an image with a flat histogram, where all levels are very similar. Then, for a range of $M$ levels the histogram draws the points. For the input (old) and output (new) image, the number of points per level is denoted as $O$ ($l$) and $N$ ($l$) (for $O \leq l \leq N$) respectively (Equation 2).

$$\sum_{l=0}^{M} O(l) = \sum_{l=0}^{M} N(l) \tag{2}$$

Since the output of the histogram is uniformly smooth, the cumulative histogram to the p level (for an arbitrarily chosen level p) should be a fraction of the total sum. Then the number of points in the output image is the ratio of the number of points in the range of levels of the output image (Equation 3).

$$N(l) = \frac{N^2}{N_{max} - N_{min}} \tag{3}$$

The last transformation is a thresholding that allows distinguishing the starting point for calculating opening distances in order to determine the border points of the mouth, right eye, and left eye. Specifying a certain level, the pixels are only set in two colors, white for high-level and black for low-level (figure 2). To represent the probability of distribution of the intensity levels, the following equation (equation 4) is used.

$$P(l) = \frac{N(l)}{N^2} \tag{4}$$

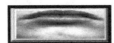 

**Fig. 2.** Aplication of Thresholding operator

## 3    Intelligent Tutoring System (ITS)

Figure 3 shows the architecture of the ITS, which is similar to traditional tutoring systems. This architecture has three main modules: The **Domain Module** represents the knowledge of the expert and handles different concepts related to Knowledge Space Theory [13]. This theory provides a sound foundation for structuring and representing the domain module for personalized or adapted learning. It applies concepts from combinatory theory and we use it to model particular or personalized courses. The knowledge base of this module is stored by using a particular kind of XML-based format. The **Student Module** provides the information about student competencies and learning capabilities through a diagnostic test. The **Student Module** can be seen as a sub-tree of all knowledge stored in the domain. For every student there is a static profile, which stores particular and academic information, and a dynamic profile, which stores information obtained from the navigation on the tutor and from the emotion recognition process. The **Tutoring Module** presents the exercises to the students according to the level in the problem. We implemented production rules (procedural memory) and facts (declarative memory) via a set of XML-based rules. Furthermore, we developed a new knowledge tracing algorithm based on fuzzy logic, which is used to track student's cognitive states, applying the set of rules (XML-based and Fuzzy rules) to the set of facts.

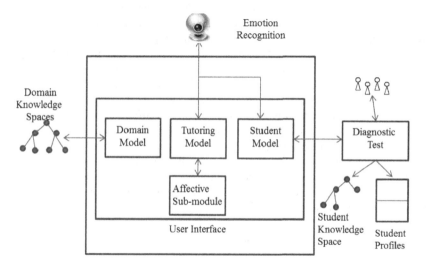

**Fig. 3.** ITS Architecture

As it was mentioned, the emotion recognition is done by using a face feature extraction process that follows the Ekman's theory [14]. We considered five types of emotional states: anger, happiness, sadness, surprise, and neutral. The ITS also has, as part of the affective sub-module, an affective/pedagogical agent. The agent shows up when the student makes a mistake or error (pay attention, explain, suggest, or think actions) during the exercise, when the student correctly completes the problem (acknowledge or congratulate actions), or when the student asks for help (announce or confuse actions). Figure 4 shows an interface of the ITS developed in Spanish language, where "Genie" is delivering a congratulatory message and a reminder to ask for help if needed.

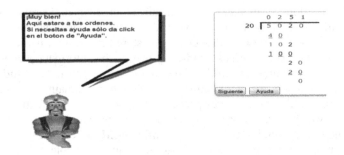

**Fig. 4.** Genie: An Affective Agent (the message in Spanish language)

## 3.1    The Neural Network for Recognizing Emotional States

The emotion recognition system was built in three steps: the first one was an implementation to extract features from face images (algorithm explained before) in a corpus used to train the neural network. The second step was the implementation of the neural network. We used the Java-based algorithms implemented in Weka [15] to implement classification by using neural network (feed-forward method). The third step integrated extraction and recognition into a fuzzy system, which is part of the ITS. For training and testing the neural network, we used the corpus RAFD (Radboud Faces Database) [16], which is a database with 8040 different facial expressions that contains a set of 67 models including men and women. Once the emotional state is extracted from the student, the emotional state is sent to the fuzzy system. The fuzzy system takes the emotion value together with other parameters such as time, number of errors, and requests for help from the student exercise, and produces a math exercise (see figure 5). The difficulty of the math exercise depends on the parameters entering the fuzzy system.

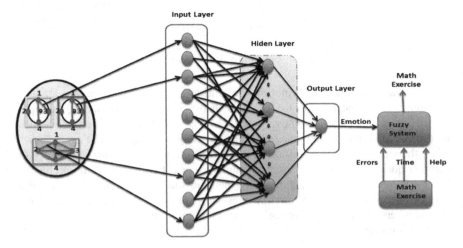

**Fig. 5.** Feature Extraction and Emotion Classification

## 3.2    The Fuzzy Expert System

In the ITS, a fuzzy expert system was implemented with a new knowledge tracing algorithm, which is used to track student's pedagogical states, applying a set of rules. The benefit of using fuzzy rules is that they allow inferences even when the conditions are only partially satisfied. As it was established, the fuzzy system uses four input linguistic variables: *error, help, time*, and *emotion*. These variables are loaded when the student solves an exercise. The output variable of the fuzzy system is the difficulty and type of the next exercise.

# 4    Results

Figure 6 illustrates the interfaces of the software in two different versions: Android-based version (upper of figure) and Web-based version (bottom of figure). The Android-based version shows the emotion recognition of a user, part of an exercise and a message (left). The Web-based version interface shows the social network, a Math exercise (an integer division), and the pedagogical or affective agent. The social network contains all the functionalities common in this type of Web 2.0 applications (creating a user profile, a community, making friends, accessing a course (ITS), ), among others).

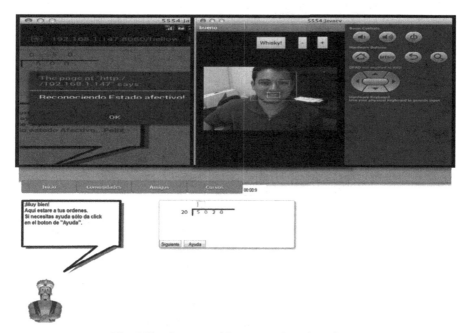

**Fig. 6.** Emotion recognition process into the software

In our evaluation design method (Pretest –intervention- posttest) [17], we tested the classification precision of the neural network with two different tools: Weka and Matlab, and the intelligent tutoring system (Web-based version) with students of two schools (public and private) in Mexico.

The results of the neural networks (left corner of Figure 7) trained with Matlab can be observed. We created a two-layer feed-forward network with sigmoid hidden neurons and linear output neurons. The network was trained with the Levenberg-Marquardt back-propagation algorithm. Regression Values that measure the correlation between outputs and targets had values very close to 1, meaning an almost perfect lineal association between target and actual output values (independent and dependent variables). In other words, predicted values Y (actual output), from X (target values) according to the regression model coincide almost exactly with the values observed in Y, and very few prediction errors will occur. The right part of Figure 7 shows the results with the Weka tool. We can observe the error levels when applying the classifier to corpus RAFD. We obtained excellent results with a success rate of 96.9466 % in the emotion recognition process. Small prediction errors shown with Matlab are equivalent to errors detected in Weka instances classified as incorrect (3.0534 %).

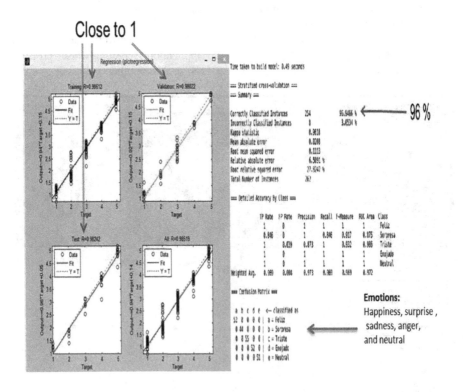

**Fig. 7.** Training and testing the neural network with Matlab and Weka

Figure 8 shows the evaluation results considering multiplication and division operations applied to 33 students (9 from public schools and 24 from private schools; all of them in Culiacán, Mexico). We can observe the progress of 27 students (six of them did not change their rating).

Based on the results obtained with Weka and because this tool is open source, we decided to integrate this classifier with the feature extractor and the intelligent tutoring system (as it was mentioned). Another reason for implementing the tutoring system by using Weka tool is that the source code used was Java, which is the programming language to develop Android-based applications. The intelligent tutoring system and the fuzzy expert system were implemented with CCS3, HTML 5, Java, and JSP. We tested the Web applications with real students and soon we are starting to test the Android-based version.

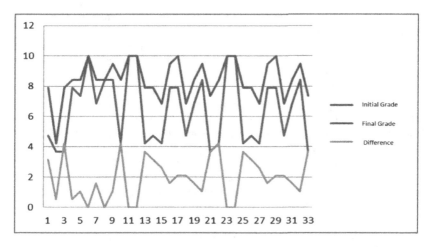

**Fig. 8.** Results of using the ITS with 33 students

# 5     Conclusions and Future Work

The implementation of this work has been a very complex job because we integrate different technologies like a social network implemented with web programming languages (HTML, JavaScript, and Java Servlets, and MySQL database), emotion recognition (Java programming, OpenCV and JavaCV libraries), Feed-Forward Neural networks (taken and adapted to our system from Weka software), a fuzzy system implemented also in Java language, and the software for the Android-based mobile device (Java for Android).

As future work, we are considering creating our own corpus of emotions oriented to the teaching-learning process, covering more math material in the ITS, and making more experiments with more students

**Funding**
The work described in this paper is fully supported by a grant from the DGEST (Dirección General de Educación Superior Tecnológica) in Mexico under the program "Projects of Scientific Research and Technological Innovation". Additionally, this work was sponsored by the National Council of Science and Technology (CONACYT) and the Public Education Secretary (SEP) through PROMEP.

# References

1. O'Reilly, T. What is Web 2.0 (2005), http://www.oreillynet.com
2. Hage, H., Aïmeur, E.: Harnessing Learner's Collective Intelligence: A Web2.0 Approach to E-Learning. In: Woolf, B.P., Aïmeur, E., Nkambou, R., Lajoie, S. (eds.) ITS 2008. LNCS, vol. 5091, pp. 438–447. Springer, Heidelberg (2008)
3. Boyd, D., Ellison, N.B.: Social network sites: Definition, history and scholarship. Journal of Computer-Mediated Communication 13(1), article 11 (2007), http://jcmc.indiana.edu/vol13/issue1/boyd.ellison.html
4. Picard, R.W.: Affective Computing. M.I.T Media Laboratory Perceptual Computing Section Technical Report No. 321 (1995)
5. Arroyo, I., Woolf, B., Cooper, D., Burleson, W., Muldner, K., Christopherson, R.: Emotions sensors go to school. In: Proceedings of the 14th International Conference on Artificial Intelligence in Education, pp. 17–24. IOS Press, Amsterdam (2009)
6. Calvo, R.A., D'Mello, S.: Affect Detection: An interdisciplinary review of models, methods, and their applications. IEEE Transactions on Affect Computing 1, 18–37 (2010)
7. Baker, R.S.J.D., D'Mello, S.K., Rodrigo, M.M.T., Graesser, A.C.: Better to be Frustrated than Bored: The Incidence, Persistence, and Impact of learners' Cognitive-affective States During Interactions with three Different Computer-Based Learning Environments. International Journal of Human-Computer Studies 68(4), 223–241 (2010)
8. Sabourin, J., Rowe, J.P., Mott, B.W., Lester, J.C.: When Off-Task is On-Task: The Affective Role of Off-Task Behavior in Narrative-Centered Learning Environments. In: Biswas, G., Bull, S., Kay, J., Mitrovic, A. (eds.) AIED 2011. LNCS, vol. 6738, pp. 534–536. Springer, Heidelberg (2011)
9. Gardner, L., Sheridan, D., White, D.: A Web-based learning and assessment system to support flexible education. Journal of Computer Assisted Learning 18, 125–136 (2002)
10. Costa, D.S.J., Mullan, B.A., Kothe, E.J., Butow, P.: A web-based formative assessment tool for Masters students: a pilot study. Computers & Education 54(4), 1248–1253 (2010)
11. Chen, G.D., Chang, C.K., Wang, C.Y.: Ubiquitous learning website: scaffold learners by mobile devices with information-aware techniques. Computers & Education 50, 77–90 (2008)
12. Nixon, M., Aguado, A.: Feature Extraction & Image Processing, 2nd edn. Academic Press (2008)
13. Doignon, J.-P., Falmagne, J.C.: Knowledge Spaces. Springer (1999)
14. Ekman, P., Oster, H.: Facial expressions of emotion. Annual Review of Psychology 30, 527–554 (1979)
15. Weka Oficial Homepage. University of Waikato, New Zealand, http://www.cs.waikato.ac.nz/ml/weka/
16. Langner, O., Dotsch, R., Bijlstra, G., Wigboldus, D., Hawk, S., van Knippenberg, A.: Presentation and validation of the Radboud Faces Database. Cognition & Emotion 24(8), 1377–1388 (2010), doi:10.1080/02699930903485076
17. Ainsworth, S.: Evaluation methods for learning environments (2005), Tutorial at AIED 2005 available at http://www.psychology.nottingham.ac.uk/staff/ Shaaron.Ainsworth/aied_tutorialslides2005.pdf

# Author Index